te of Ca

ANTIFOLATE DRUGS IN CANCER THERAPY

CANCER DRUG DISCOVERY AND DEVELOPMENT

Apoptosis and Cancer Chemotherapy, edited by *John A. Hickman and Caroline Dive,* 1999
Signal Transduction and Cell Cycle Inhibitors in Cancer Therapy, edited by *J. Silvio Gutkind,* 1999
Antifolate Drugs in Cancer Therapy, edited by *Ann L. Jackman,* 1999
Antiangiogenic Agents in Cancer Therapy, edited by *Beverly A. Teicher,* 1999
Anticancer Drug Development Guide: *Preclinical Screening, Clinical Trials, and Approval,* edited by *Beverly A. Teicher,* 1997
Cancer Therapeutics: *Experimental and Clinical Agents,* edited by *Beverly A. Teicher,* 1997

ANTIFOLATE DRUGS IN CANCER THERAPY

Edited by

ANN L. JACKMAN

*The Cancer Research Campaign Centre
for Cancer Therapeutics,
The Institute of Cancer Research,
Sutton, Surrey, UK*

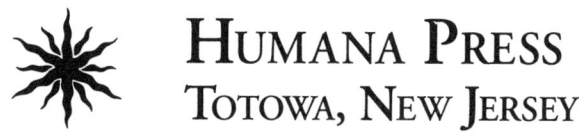

HUMANA PRESS
TOTOWA, NEW JERSEY

© 1999 Humana Press Inc.
999 Riverview Drive, Suite 208
Totowa, New Jersey 07512

All rights reserved.

No part of this book may be reproduced, stored in a retrieval system, or transmitted in any form or by any means, electronic, mechanical, photocopying, microfilming, recording, or otherwise without written permission from the Publisher.

All authored papers, comments, opinions, conclusions, or recommendations are those of the author(s), and do not necessarily reflect the views of the publisher.

For additional copies, pricing for bulk purchases, and/or information about other Humana titles, contact Humana at the above address or at any of the following numbers: Tel.: 973-256-1699; Fax: 973-256-8341; E-mail: humana@humanapr.com

This publication is printed on acid-free paper. ∞
ANSI Z39.48-1984 (American Standards Institute) Permanence of Paper for Printed Library Materials.

Cover illustration:

Cover design by Patricia F. Cleary.

Photocopy Authorization Policy:
Authorization to photocopy items for internal or personal use, or the internal or personal use of specific clients, is granted by Humana Press Inc., provided that the base fee of US $5.00 per copy, plus US $00.25 per page, is paid directly to the Copyright Clearance Center at 222 Rosewood Drive, Danvers, MA 01923. For those organizations that have been granted a photocopy license from the CCC, a separate system of payment has been arranged and is acceptable to Humana Press Inc. The fee code for users of the Transactional Reporting Service is: [0-89603-460-7/97 $5.00 + $00.25].

Printed in the United States of America.   10 9 8 7 6 5 4 3 2 1

PREFACE

Antifolates are an important class of anticancer drugs originally developed as antileukemic agents, but now used, usually in combination with other drugs, for the treatment of a wide range of tumors, notably carcinomas of the head and neck, breast, germ cell tumors, non-Hodgkin's lymphoma, acute lymphoblastic leukemia, and osteogenic sarcomas. 5-Fluorouracil and its prodrugs also target, in part, the folate-dependent enzyme, thymidylate synthase. Furthermore, folate supplementation in the form of leucovorin, modulates 5-fluororuacil activity. 5-Fluorouracil is widely used in the treatment of colorectal and gastric cancer and in combination for other solid tumors such as breast and head and neck cancers. Ongoing clinical trials with the newer antifolates suggest that the range of solid tumors where these agents will be of use may broaden further.

Half a century ago, interesting scientific and clinical discoveries suggested that folic acid was a vitamin involved in vital cellular metabolic processes. The folate analogs, aminopterin and methotrexate, were synthesized by the American Cyanamid Company in an attempt to interfere with these processes and were shown to have anticancer activity by Farber and his colleagues. Hence, the principle of antimetabolite therapy for the treatment of cancer was established. Biomedical research over the following years led to a deeper understanding of the complex biochemical pharmacology of folates and antifolates. Selective antimicrobial agents were discovered, but more tumor-selective anticancer agents did not immediately emerge. However, advances in drug development practice in recent years has led to the discovery of novel antifolates with encouraging clinical anticancer activity. As the new millenium approaches, it is timely to assess progress so that future research will expand on these promising foundations. Importantly, it is necessary to embrace and exploit exciting new technologies and knowledge relating to the oncological process and selective approaches to therapy.

The contributors to *Antifolate Drugs in Cancer Therapy* are largely drawn from researchers highly regarded in the field of folate biochemistry and antifolate drug development. However, there is the deliberate inclusion of some laboratory and clinical scientists whose work has only recently encompassed the antifolate area or is peripheral to their main research areas. I believe this has led to a book that provides a contextual review and exciting new avenues for future research.

Antifolate Drugs in Cancer Therapy is divided broadly into five areas. First, an historical and future perspective, along with an overview of folate biochemistry, are given. This is followed by the preclinical and clinical pharmacology of methotrexate, other dihydrofolate reductase inhibitors, and 5-fluorouracil. Eight chapters review the preclinical development and clinical activity of the new generation of antifolates, the thymidylate synthase and glycinamide ribonucleotide formyltransferase inhibitors. The fourth area draws together experience from all of the above and reviews in depth subjects such as folate and antifolate transport mechanisms, modulation of antifolate drugs, polyglutamation, resistance, and drug combinations. Finally, the rapidly expanding topics of pharmacogenomics, pharmacodynamics, regulation of gene expression, and mechanisms of cell death bring this volume to a close. The wide and progressive scope of *Antifolate Drugs in Cancer Therapy* makes it an important point of reference for basic scientists and clinicians and provides a platform on which to build further reading in areas of interest. Editing this volume has been an exciting project, and I am very grateful to all the contributors for their participation.

Ann L. Jackman

CONTENTS

Preface v

Contributors ix

1 Antifolate Drugs: *Past and Future Perspectives* 1
  Robert C. Jackson

2 Folate Biochemistry in Relation to Antifolate Selectivity 13
  Roy L. Kisliuk

3 Clinical Pharmacology and Resistance to Dihydrofolate
  Reductase Inhibitors 37
  Richard Gorlick and Joseph R. Bertino

4 Development of Nonpolyglutamatable DHFR Inhibitors 59
  Andre Rosowsky

5 Fluoropyrimidines as Antifolate Drugs 101
  G. J. Peters and C. H. Köhne

6 Raltitrexed (Tomudex™), a Highly Polyglutamatable
  Antifolate Thymidylate Synthase Inhibitor:
  Design and Preclinical Activity 147
  Leslie R. Hughes, Trevor C. Stephens, F. Thomas Boyle,
  and Ann L. Jackman

7 Tomudex: *Clinical Development* 167
  Philip Beale and Stephen Clarke

8 Preclinical Pharmacology Studies and the Clinical
  Development of a Novel Multitargeted Antifolate,
  MTA (LY231514) 183
  Chuan Shih and Donald E. Thornton

9 GW1843: *A Potent, Noncompetitive Thymidylate Synthase
  Inhibitor—Preclinical and Preliminary Clinical Studies* 203
  Gary K. Smith, Joseph W. Bigley, Inderjit K. Dev,
  David S. Duch, Robert Ferone, and William Pendergast

10 Preclinical and Clinical Studies with the Novel Thymidylate
   Synthase Inhibitor Nolatrexed Dihydrochloride
   (Thymitaq™, AG337) 229
   Andy Hughes and A. Hilary Calvert

11 ZD9331: *Preclinical and Clinical Studies* 243
   F. Thomas Boyle, Trevor C. Stephens, S. D. Averbuch,
   and Ann L. Jackman

12	Preclinical and Clinical Evaluation of the Glycinamide Ribonucleotide Formyltransferase Inhibitors Lometrexol and LY309887 .... *261*	
	Laurane G. Mendelsohn, John F. Worzalla, and Jackie M. Walling	
13	AG2034: *A GARFT Inhibitor with Selective Cytotoxicity to Cells that Lack a G1 Checkpoint* *281*	
	Theodore J. Boritzki, Cathy Zhang, Charlotte A. Bartlett, and Robert C. Jackson	
14	Receptor- and Carrier-Mediated Transport Systems for Folates and Antifolates: *Exploitation for Folate-Based Chemotherapy and Immunotherapy* *293*	
	G. Jansen	
15	Folates as Chemotherapeutic Modulators *323*	
	Julio Barredo, Marlene A. Bunni, Raghunathan Kamasamudram, and David G. Priest	
16	Antifolate Polyglutamylation in Preclinical and Clinical Antifolate Resistance *339*	
	John J. McGuire	
17	Antifolates in Combination Therapy *365*	
	Stephen P. Ackland and Rosemary Kimbell	
18	Pharmacodynamic Measurements and Predictors of Response to Thymidylate Synthase Inhibitors *383*	
	David Farrugia and Patrick G. Johnston	
19	Molecular Regulation of Expression of Thymidylate Synthase *397*	
	Edward Chu, Jingfang Ju, and John C. Schmitz	
20	The Role of Uracil Misincorporation in Thymineless Death *409*	
	G. Wynne Aherne and Sherael Brown	
21	Thymineless Death *423*	
	Peter J. Houghton	
22	Genetic Determinants of Cell Death and Toxicity *437*	
	D. Mark Pritchard and John A. Hickman	
Index *453*		

CONTRIBUTORS

STEPHEN P. ACKLAND • *Department of Medical Oncology, Newcastle Mater Misericordiae Hospital, Hunter Region Mail Center, New South Wales, Australia*

G. WYNNE AHERNE • *CRC Centre for Cancer Therapeutics, The Institute of Cancer Research, Sutton, Surrey, UK*

S. D. AVERBUCH • *Zeneca Pharmaceuticals, Wilmington, DE*

JULIO BARREDO • *Department of Biochemistry and Molecular Biology, Medical University of South Carolina, Charleston, SC*

CHARLOTTE A. BARTLETT • *Agouron Pharmaceuticals, San Diego, CA*

PHILIP BEALE • *CRC Centre for Cancer Therapeutics, The Institute of Cancer Research, Sutton, Surrey, UK*

JOSEPH R. BERTINO • *American Cancer Society Professor of Medicine & Pharmacology, Memorial Sloan-Kettering Cancer Center, New York, NY*

JOSEPH W. BIGLEY • *Oncology Clinical Research, Glaxo Wellcome, Research Triangle Park, NC*

THEODORE J. BORITZKI • *Agouron Pharmaceuticals, San Diego, CA*

F. THOMAS BOYLE • *Zeneca Pharmaceuticals, Chesire, UK*

SHERAEL BROWN • *CRC Centre for Cancer Therapeutics, The Institute of Cancer Research, Sutton, Surrey, UK*

MARLENE A. BUNNI • *Department of Biochemistry and Molecular Biology, Medical University of South Carolina, Charleston, SC*

A. HILARY CALVERT • *Department of Oncology, Newcastle General Hospital, Newcastle upon Tyne, UK*

EDWARD CHU • *Yale Cancer Center, Yale University School of Medicine, and VA Connecticut Healthcare System, New Haven, CT*

STEPHEN CLARKE • *Department of Medical Oncology, Concord Repatriation General Hospital, Concord, Australia*

INDERJIT K. DEV • *Department of Cancer Biology, Glaxo Wellcome, Research Triangle Park, NC*

DAVID S. DUCH • *Cato Research, Durham, NC*

ROBERT FERONE • *Cary, NC*

DAVID FARRUGIA • *CRC Center for Cancer Thera[eutics, The Institute of Cancer Research, Sutton, Surrey, UK*

RICHARD GORLICK • *Memorial Sloan-Kettering Cancer, New York, NY*

JOHN A. HICKMAN • *School of Biological Sciences, Manchester, UK*

PETER J. HOUGHTON • *Department of Molecular Pharmacology, St. Jude Children's Research Hospital, Memphis, TN*

ANDY HUGHES • *Department of Oncology, Newcastle General Hospital, Newcastle upon Tyne, UK*

LESLIE R. HUGHES • *Zeneca Pharmaceuticals, Chesire, UK*

ANN L. JACKMAN • *The Cancer Research Campaign Centre for Cancer Therapeutics, The Institute of Cancer Research, Surrey, UK*

ROBERT C. JACKSON • *Chiroscience Ltd., Cambridge, UK*
G. JANSEN • *Department of Oncology, Queens University of Belfast, City Hospital, Belfast, Northern Ireland*
PATRICK G. JOHNSTON • *Department of Oncology, The Queen's University of Belfast, Belfaast, Northern Ireland*
JINGFANG JU • *Yale Cancer Center, Yale University School of Medicine, and VA Connecticut Healthcare System, New Haven, CT*
RAGHUNATHAN KAMASAMUDRAM • *Department of Biochemistry and Molecular Biology, Medical University of South Carolina, Charleston, SC*
ROSEMARY KIMBELL • *CRC Centre for Cancer Therapeutics, Institute for Cancer Research, Royal Marsden Hospital, UK*
ROY L. KISLIUK • *Department of Biochemistry, Tufts University, Boston, MA*
C. H. KÖHNE • *Department of Hematology/Oncology and Tumor Immunology, Rober Rössle Klinik, Charite Campius Berlin–Buch, Berlin, Germany*
LAURANE G. MENDELSOHN • *Cancer Research Division, Lilly Research Laboratories, Eli Lilly & Co., Indianapolis, IN*
JOHN J. MCGUIRE • *Department of Experimental Therapeutics, Grace Cancer Drug Center, Roswell Park Cancer Institute, Buffalo, NY*
WILLIAM PENDERGAST • *Inspire Pharmaceuticals, Durham, NC*
G. J. PETERS • *Department of Medical Oncology, Academic Hospital, Vrije Universiteit, Amsterdam, The Netherlands*
DAVID G. PRIEST • *Department of Biochemistry and Molecular Biology, Medical University of South Carolina, Charleston, SC*
D. MARK PRITCHARD • *School of Biological Sciences, Manchester, UK*
ANDRE ROSOWSKY • *Department of Adult Oncology, Dana-Faber Cancer Institute, Boston, MA*
JOHN C. SCHMITZ • *Yale Cancer Center, Yale University School of Medicine, and VA Connecticut Healthcare System, New Haven, CT*
CHUAN SHIH • *Lilly Research Laboratories, Eli Lilly & Co., Indianapolis, IN*
GARY K. SMITH • *Department of Molecular Biochemistry, Glaxo Wellcome, Research Triangle Park, NC*
TREVOR C. STEPHENS • *Zeneca Pharmaceuticals, Cheshire, UK*
DONALD E. THORNTON • *Division of Oncology, Lilly Corporate Center, Eli Lilly & Co., Indianapolis, IN*
JACKIE M. WALLING • *Cancer Research Division, Lilly Research Laboratories, Eli Lilly & Co., Indianapolis, IN*
JOHN F. WORZALLA • *Cancer Research Division, Lilly Research Laboratories, Eli Lilly & Co., Indianapolis, IN*
CATHY ZHANG • *Agouron Pharmaceuticals, San Diego, CA*

1 Antifolate Drugs
Past and Future Perspectives

Robert C. Jackson

CONTENTS

INTRODUCTION
DHFR INHIBITORS AND THE CONCEPT OF THYMINELESS DEATH
MTX AND TIGHT-BINDING INHIBITION
TRANSPORT AS A DETERMINANT OF SELECTIVITY AND RESISTANCE
HOMOGENEOUSLY STAINING REGIONS, DOUBLE MINUTES, AND
    GENE AMPLIFICATION
ANTITHYMIDYLATE AND ANTIPURINE EFFECTS OF MTX
POLYGLUTAMYLATION IN RELATION TO SELECTIVITY AND
    RESISTANCE
LIPOPHILIC ANTIFOLATES
INHIBITORS OF GLYCINAMIDE RIBONUCLEOTIDE
    FORMYLTRANSFERASE
ANTIFOLATES IN COMBINATION CHEMOTHERAPY
DNA STRAND BREAKS, APOPTOSIS, CHECKPOINTS, AND
    ANTIFOLATE SELECTIVITY
CONCLUSIONS: WHERE NEXT WITH ANTIFOLATES?
REFERENCES

1. INTRODUCTION

The antifolates remain a topic of continuing fascination to pharmacologists. This interest is not entirely theoretical. Recent years have seen two new antifolate drugs approved for marketing: trimetrexate (Neutrexin), a lipophilic inhibitor of dihydrofolate reductase (DHFR) for treatment of the life-threatening fungal infection, *Pneumocystis carinii* pneumonia; and the thymidylate synthase (TS) inhibitor, raltitrexed (Tomudex), for colorectal cancer. In addition to their importance as drugs, however, the antifolates have taught us some important lessons about general principles of pharmacology—how to use drugs optimally, how to design improved selectivity into next-generation compounds, how cells become drug resistant and how to use biochemical modulation ap-

From: *Anticancer Drug Development Guide: Antifolate Drugs in Cancer Therapy*
Edited by: A.L. Jackman © Humana Press Inc., Totowa, NJ

proaches. They have also been valuable probes for exploring basic biology. These points will be made using 10 examples of topics in antifolate pharmacology that have sparked major debates over the years. Several of these areas will be dealt with very briefly, because they are covered in more detail in subsequent chapters. The final section touches on some unanswered questions, which are areas of current debate, and which are likely to be the focus of ongoing research.

Much of the work discussed in this volume had its origins in programs of analog development, often considered to be uncreative "fine tuning," rather than innovative research, and thus an area in which it is difficult to obtain funding, both from government agencies and from pharmaceutical companies. In fact, as this book demonstrates, the antifolate field continues to be a productive source not only of new drugs, but of new therapeutic strategies, and important findings in basic biology.

2. DHFR INHIBITORS AND THE CONCEPT OF THYMINELESS DEATH

The antimetabolite drugs arose from two distinct lines of research. The first of these approaches, which used inhibitors of enzymes involved in essential biosynthetic processes, emerged from the studies of D. D. Woods (1) on the mechanism of action of the sulfa group of antibacterial drugs. Sulfa drugs are structural analogs of *p*-aminobenzoate in which the carboxylate group has been replaced by a sulfonamide function. These agents act as potent competitive inhibitors of the dihydrofolate synthetase reaction (which occurs in many bacteria but not in eukaryotic cells) in which *p*-aminobenzoate is condensed with a pteroate to form dihydrofolate. It is characteristic of this kind of antimetabolites that they are structural analogs of normal metabolites, that they are potent inhibitors of biosynthetic reactions, that they are competitively antagonized by the corresponding normal substrate (which generally accumulates behind the block), and that the product of the inhibited reaction will give a noncompetitive reversal of the antimetabolite effect. There is another kind of antimetabolite (exemplified by 6-thioguanine) that is a substrate analog that is incorporated into macromolecules, producing, in this case, defective or misfunctional RNA and DNA molecules, a process known as "lethal synthesis." Whereas many analogs of purines and pyrimidines exert both types of effect, antifolates are not incorporated into macromolecules, and their effects must therefore be understood in terms of depletion of purine and pyrimidine precursors. It was originally suggested that antimetabolites of the first class must be cytostatic, rather than cytotoxic, since they were believed to act by starving cells of synthetic precursors. Although antifolates are sometimes cytostatic, in other cases they are clearly cytotoxic. The question thus arose: Why should precursor depletion be lethal? Seymour Cohen, working with bacteria, formulated the concept of unbalanced growth, that if cells could not synthesize DNA, but could still synthesize RNA and protein, then giant cells would result (as he observed experimentally) which would be nonviable. He proposed that thymineless death represented a form of unbalanced growth. Cohen showed that, though selective thymine starvation was often lethal to bacteria, simultaneous depletion of thymine and purines was simply cytostatic, which, he claimed, was because unbalanced growth could not occur in the absence of purines (2). The development of the early DHFR inhibitors, e.g., aminopterin, methotrexate (MTX), pyrimethamine, and trimethoprim, indicated that their cellular effects on bacteria were similar to those of sulfa drugs, and, in the case of aminopterin and methotrexate, that similar effects were seen in mammalian cells. The unbalanced growth hypothesis prompted much fruitful thought and experiment, but although it explained many of the experimental data, it did not give any insight into drug selectivity. The antibacterial selectivity of sulfa drugs is explained by the fact that mammalian cells do not possess dihydrofolate synthetase, obtaining their folates from the diet. The antitumor selectivity of methotrexate, although quantitatively much less than the selectivity of sulfa drugs, nevertheless exists, and could not be easily explained, since the DHFR enzymes of normal and transformed cells were identical, and were inhibited by MTX to a similar extent. Current explanations of thymineless death are discussed in Chapter 21.

3. MTX AND TIGHT-BINDING INHIBITION

Straus and Goldstein (3) pointed out that inhibitors whose binding constants for their target enzyme were of the same order of magnitude as the molar concentration of enzyme in the system, or lower, could not be assumed to follow Michaelis-Menten kinetics. Puzzling early observations reported that aminopterin and methotrexate, despite being close structural analogs of folic acid, appeared to be noncompetitive inhibitors of DHFR. This conclusion was a consequence of inappropriate kinetic analysis; when methods appropriate for tight-binding inhibitors were used, the inhibition was shown to be competitive. Most new inhibitors of TS and of glycinamide ribonucleotide formyltransferase (GARFT) are sufficiently potent that tight-binding kinetic analysis is also appropriate in these cases. However, many investigators continue to report inhibition constants obtained with conventional kinetic analysis. These reported K_i values are not in fact constants, but will depend upon the concentration of enzyme used in the assay system, since for a tight-binding inhibitor the apparent K_i will approximate [E]/2.

Having grasped the tight-binding nature of inhibition of DHFR by methotrexate, some investigators then made the opposite error and assumed that it was virtually irreversible. In fact, MTX has an off rate constant from human DHFR that corresponds to a half-life for the complex of approx 15 min. In a cell-free system in which the concentration of the competing substrate, dihydrofolate (actually as polyglutamates), may be very low, a newly dissociated molecule of MTX may rapidly rebind to DHFR, so that it may appear that the inhibition is functionally irreversible. However, in the cell the system shows more complex behavior: DHFR activity is often in 10- to 50-fold excess over that of TS, which is the ratelimiting enzyme in the cycle of dihydrofolate oxido-reduction (DHFR, serine hydroxymethyltransferase, TS). Thus the steady-state concentration of dihydrofolate is very low, typically below 0.1 μM. When DHFR is inhibited, dihydrofolate is now being produced faster than it is re-reduced, so that dihydrofolate accumulates until the flux through the three enzymes of the cycle again becomes equal. In this way, the dihydrofolate concentration may increase by as much as three logs, at which point it represents a significant fraction of total cellular folate cofactors. At some point, the system can no longer generate enough additional dihydrofolate to overcome the DHFR inhibition, DHFR then becomes rate limiting for the cycle, and the flux through the cycle will fall. The pool size of methylenetetrahydrofolate polyglutamates will now be depleted, and biosynthesis of thymidylate and of purine ribonucleotides will decrease. The kinetics of the system are such that by the time this point is reached, there will be free MTX (i.e., MTX that is not bound to DHFR) in the cell. In early studies it was sometimes concluded that the need for free MTX to be measurable in the cell before a growth-inhibitory effect was observed indicated that there must be a second site of action of MTX, other than DHFR, that was required for its pharmacological effect. Computer simulation of the biochemical pathways showed that the observed kinetics were consistent with inhibition of DHFR being the primary site of action of MTX, and that the necessity for free MTX was an inherent consequence of the kinetics of this cyclic multienzyme system.

4. TRANSPORT AS A DETERMINANT OF SELECTIVITY AND RESISTANCE

The early antifolates that were developed as anti-infective drugs (e.g. pyrimethamine, trimethoprin) were lipophilic compounds that entered cells by passive diffusion. This is an advantageous property since some microorganisms are unable to transport folic acid and its analogs. However, the early anticancer folate analogs, such as MTX are polyanions, and thus require facilitated or active transport to get across cell membranes. It was observed that some transformed cells (and embryonic cells in general) tended to have relatively high rates of folate and antifolate transport, and it was thus suggested that transport was a determinant of antifolate selectivity. Studies with mouse tumors indicated that experimental mouse leukemias often had high levels of MTX transport, and were MTX-sensitive, whereas mouse carcinomas frequently were relatively inefficient at transporting MTX, and tended to be MTX-insensitive. It was thus widely believed for a time that antifolates should be regarded as antileukemic drugs, without much potential against solid tumors. One line of approach to developing more active DHFR inhibitors was to optimize transport parameters (to increase V_{max} and decrease K_m) for the reduced folate carrier, and this was one of the principles that guided development of 10-ethyl-10-deazaaminopterin, which did indeed possess better activity than MTX against murine carcinomas (4). A second line of evidence that transport was a major determinant of the antifolate response of tumors was the observation that acquired resistance of tumor cells to MTX was frequently associated with decreased MTX transport. The current view is that, although the selectivity of antifolates and cellular resistance to them are multifactorial, transport is an important determinant of therapeutic effect and toxicity. This subject is discussed in detail in Chapter 14. Another view is that transport is not necessary for antitumor selectivity, since lipophilic antifolates such as trimetrexate and Thymitaq have shown clinical anticancer activity, but that being a good substrate for the carrier confers potency upon a drug.

This topic was made more interesting, and more complex, by the discovery that in addition to the high capacity, low-affinity carrier that transports MTX, leucovorin, and 5-methyltetrahydrofolate (the reduced folate carrier, or RFC) some tissues possessed a high-affinity, low-capacity membrane folate-binding protein (mFBP) whose physiological function appeared to be binding and uptake of folic acid. When lometrexol was developed, it was found to be an excellent ligand for mFBP, and a subject of ongoing research is whether this contributes to lometrexol's broad antitumor spectrum, whether it contributes to lometrexol's severe delayed toxicity, and whether mFBP binding is a desirable attribute for an antitumor drug or not. The discovery (discussed in Chapter 13) of closely related compounds with very different affinity for mFBP will help to resolve these questions.

5. HOMOGENEOUSLY STAINING REGIONS, DOUBLE MINUTES, AND GENE AMPLIFICATION

Early studies on resistance of tumor cells to methotrexate elicited two frequent mechanisms: transport defects as discussed above, and overproduction of the target enzyme, DHFR. Whereas in principle enzyme overproduction might be achieved by increasing the expression level of the DHFR gene, it was found that MTX-resistant cells often had multiple copies of the DHFR gene. Gene amplification is an aspect of the genetic instability of transformed cells, and has been reported for several other enzymes, including TS. The additional genetic material may either occur as pairs of small additional chromosomes (double minutes) or as a large piece of extra DNA in one of the normal set of chromosomes, referred to as a homogeneously staining region (HSR). In cells that have extra DHFR gene copies, the expression level of active enzyme roughly parallels the gene copy number, and the amount of tight-binding inhibitor required to inhibit the enzyme is somewhat more than proportionately greater, so that a cell with a 10-fold gene amplification will have an IC_{50} that is increased by more than 10-fold relative to the wild-type. Kinetic analysis indicates that, regardless of whether an enzyme is normally rate limiting in its pathway or not, and regardless of whether the inhibitor exhibits conventional or tight-binding kinetics, increased expression of target enzyme will always tend to confer increased resistance to the inhibitor. Recent clinical studies that relate response rates to expression levels of target enzyme are discussed in Chapter 18 which reports that tumors with high levels of TS were less likely to respond to 5-FU than the subgroup with lower TS expression.

6. ANTITHYMIDYLATE AND ANTIPURINE EFFECTS OF MTX

An early debate concerned the issue of whether the antithymidylate effect or the antipurine effect of MTX was the primary cause of its antitumor effect. The work of Cohen *(2)* in bacteria, and of Borsa and Whitmore *(5)* with murine cells appeared to implicate thymidylate depletion as the primary cause of cytotoxicity, since addition of a purine to methotrexate-treated cultures decreased the amount of cytotoxicity. Opposing this viewpoint was the work of Hryniuk *(6)*, who studied the L5178Y leukaemia in mice, and found that the primary lesion caused by MTX in this system was purine depletion. A possible explanation of this discrepancy was suggested by Jackman and colleagues *(7)*, who found that mice have relatively high concentrations of circulating thymidine, whereas the plasma thymidine concentration is much lower in humans. As a result, mice tend to underpredict for the activity of TS inhibitors in humans; with DHFR inhibitors responses are seen in certain murine tumor systems, but it is likely that the effect in mice is primarily a consequence of purine depletion (as suggested by Hryniuk) rather than of thymidylate depletion as may be the case in humans.

The suggestion that the antitumor activity of DHFR inhibitors, at least in humans, is primarily an antithymidylate effect, and that the antipurine effect actually limits the degree of cytotoxicity, suggests that a pure TS inhibitor should be a more effective drug than a DHFR inhibitor. It is still not clear whether this is, in fact, the case and since this subject cannot be studied in mice it is difficult to design definitive in vivo experiments to address this question. What is clear is that antifolate drugs that have a pure antithymidylate effect (the TS inhibitors) or a pure antipurine effect (the GARFT inhibitors) have clinical anticancer activity, despite having different cell cycle effects. The present indications are that the effect of DHFR inhibitors in humans is primarily a consequence of thymidylate depletion.

7. POLYGLUTAMYLATION IN RELATION TO SELECTIVITY AND RESISTANCE

It has been known from the early days of folate biochemistry that cellular folate cofactors existed primarily as poly-gamma-glutamates, and that enzymes—initially termed conjugases, now more formally termed folylpolyglutamate hydrolases (FPGH)—existed in plasma and intestine that could hydrolyze these polyglutamates to the corresponding monoglutamates. It was subsequently shown that FPGH existed within most cells, as did the enzyme folylpolyglutamate synthetase (FPGS) that formed polyglutamates from folate cofactors, glutamate, and ATP. It then became clear that classical antifolates, as well as natural cofactors, existed as polyglutamates, and that MTX, for example, exerted most of its pharmacological effect as a polyglutamate. Antifolate polyglutamates are pharmacologically important for two reasons: In some cases the long-chain polyglutamates (e.g., heptaglutamate) may be hundreds of times more potent as enzyme inhibitors than the parent monoglutamate (though this is not generally the case with DHFR inhibitors), and secondly, since polyglutamates above diglutamate cannot readily efflux from cells, they represent a long-acting cellular repository of drug, and have a profound effect on the cellular pharmacokinetics of the antifolate drug. Thus all classical antifolates (i.e., drugs that are close structural analogs of natural folates, and that have a glutamate function) must be regarded as prodrugs, requiring cellular activation by FPGS to exert their full effect. It follows from this that if the FPGS activity of a tumor cell is decreased, or if its active site is mutated in a way that decreases the substrate affinity of the antifolate, some degree of drug resistance will result. This subject is treated in detail in Chapter 16. It also follows that the FPGS activity of a tissue will be a major determinant of drug selectivity for a classical antifolate drug. Cancer cells, and embryonic tissues, tend to have high activity of FPGS, and this probably contributes to the antitumor selectivity and teratogenic activity of classical antifolates. Another consequence of polyglutamylation of classical antifolates is to increase their potency, since the trapping effect within the cell of polyglutamylation greatly increases the area under the curve (AUC, the concentration × time integral) of the drug.

It was mentioned above that some enzymes are more sensitive than others to the degree of polyglutamylation of their reduced folate cofactors, or to that of antifolate inhibitors. DHFR appears to be almost indifferent to polyglutamate chain length, and TS is also relatively insensitive to chain length. GARFT appears to have a marked preference for longer chain length, with cofactors or inhibitors increasing in binding affinity up to a chain length of seven glutamates. 5-Aminoimidazole-4-carboxamide ribonucleotide formyltransferase (AICARFT) is even more affected by chain length. These differences have given rise to speculation that folate cofactors may be functionally compartmented within the cell according to their number of glutamate residues. There does not appear to be any strong evidence for this; however, in the case of an antifolate that inhibits, for example, both GARFT and AICARFT, it is probable that the latter effect may become relatively more important as the polyglutamate chain length increases, so that the partitioning of the inhibitor between its two targets may change with increasing chain length.

From the drug-design perspective, susceptibility to polyglutamylation by FPGS has generally been considered a positive attribute, endowing a molecule with some degree of antitumor selectivity, with long-acting cellular pharmacokinetics, and with high dose potency. However, it confers vulnerability to an additional mechanism of drug resistance. A few counter-examples are emerging that suggest we may sometimes have too much of a good thing: The long-chain polyglutamates of lometrexol appear to turn over so slowly (if at all) that the drug is effectively permanently trapped within the cell. It is possible that the severe, delayed thrombocytopoenia caused by lometrexol may be related to too-effective retention of its polyglutamates within megakaryocytes. Perhaps analogs of lometrexol whose polyglutamates are better substrates for FPGH may be safer drugs.

8. LIPOPHILIC ANTIFOLATES

Having made the case that transport and polyglutamylation of classical antifolates contribute to their antitumor selectivity, one must question whether the effort to develop nonclassical, lipophilic antifolates has been fundamentally misdirected. In the anti-infective arena, the rationale is clear: Many microorganisms cannot transport folate-like molecules, so that the lipophilic nature of the antimalarial, pyrimethamine, or the antibacterial, trimethoprim, was a desirable, even essential, attribute. But what is the justification for the development of the lipophilic anticancer DHFR inhibitor, trimetrexate, or the lipophilic anticancer TS inhibitor, Thymitaq? The development of trimetrexate was certainly influenced by the observation that mouse carcinomas tend to transport folates poorly, and tend to be relatively insensitive to MTX. Broome et al. *(8)* showed that the M5076 murine sarcoma, and several murine colon carcinomas, were responsive to trimetrexate but not to MTX. Thus, for murine solid tumors, avoiding the necessity for facilitated transport seems to confer a broader antitumor spectrum to a drug. It is not at all clear whether this argument can be directly extrapolated to human solid tumors, since some of these are undoubtedly responsive to MTX and to other classical antifolate drugs. However, it seems likely that there is a subset of human solid tumors with relatively low activity of the RFC, and against such cancer cells a lipophilic antifolate should be a better drug. In theory, lipophilic antifolates should have a broader spectrum than classical antifolates; against mouse tumours, there is considerable evidence that this is the case. Clinically, there are suggestions that lipophilic inhibitors of DHFR or TS may have a different antitumour spectrum than their classical counterparts. A price is paid for this putative increase in spectrum, in two ways: Since transport and polyglutamylation contribute partially to antitumor selectivity, removing these two factors could make lipophilic antifolates less selective, i.e., more toxic. This is an example of the drug designers' maxim that broader spectrum is usually bought at the price of greater toxicity. Second, comparing trimetrexate with MTX, or Thymitaq with Tomudex, it is clear that removing the capacity for polyglutamylation results in a marked loss of dose potency.

One special case in which lipophilic drugs will clearly have an advantage as antitumor agents is when a tumor has acquired resistance to a classical antifolate though a deletion either of transport or of FPGS, both established mechanisms of resistance of human cancer cells to classical antifolates. On the down side, lipophilic antifolates are themselves vulnerable to some resistance mechanisms that do not affect response to classical antifolates, notably the p170 glycoprotein-mediated form of multidrug resistance. The fact is that the target mechanism of action of a drug is only one of its determinants of activity, and cellular pharmacokinetic factors—routes of cellular uptake and cellular activation and retention, are at least as important as the nature of the molecular target in determining a drug's properties. The lipophilic antifolates are very different drugs from their classical counterparts, with differences in spectrum, toxicity profiles, and susceptibility to resistance. So far as antitumor selectivity is concerned, the nonclassical antifolates undoubtedly sacrifice the contributions to selectivity that could be made by exploiting a tumor cell's generally high activity of RFC and FPGS. However, the major determinant of the antifolate drugs' anticancer selectivity is probably the changes in cell-cycle control in transformed cells that make a cancer cell more likely to respond to depletion of thymidylate or purine by triggering apoptosis; a glutamate sidechain is not required to take advantage of this.

Finally the work of Allegra and his colleagues *(9)* in developing trimetrexate as an agent for treatment of *Pneumocystis carinii* pneumonia deserves mention as an elegant example of biochemical modulation. The fungus that causes this infection does not transport reduced folates, but the lipophilic molecule trimetrexate is able to enter cells of both the fungus and the host. The trimetrexate treatment is then followed by leucovorin, which rescues the host cells, but not those of the fungus, which it is unable to penetrate.

9. INHIBITORS OF GLYCINAMIDE RIBONUCLEOTIDE FORMYLTRANSFERASE

There are numerous antimetabolites that inhibit purine biosynthesis, and some of them have anticancer activity. Until recently these drugs fell into two classes: Several were analogs of purine bases or nucleosides (e.g. 6-mercaptopurine, methylmercaptopurine riboside, MMPR). Although these compounds (or their nucleotide derivatives) are often inhibitors of *de novo* purine biosynthesis (the 5'-phosphate of MMPR, for example, is a potent inhibitor of PRPP amidotransferase), their pharmacological effects are complicated by their incorporation into RNA or DNA or both, so that it is impossible to determine whether their therapeutic and toxic effects are a direct consequence of purine depletion. The second class of antipurines is the glutamine antagonists, such as azaserine, diazooxonorleucine, and acivicin; since two enzymes of the purine *de novo* pathway are glutamine-dependent amidotransferases, these compounds are certainly antipurine agents. However, in this case the interpretation of their effects is complicated by the fact that these glutamine analogs inhibit numerous other glutamine-requiring enzymes. The development of lometrexol (5,10-dideazatetrahydrofolate), which was shown to act on GARFT was thus of great interest as the first antimetabolite that unequivocally acted through depletion of purine ribonucleotide formation. Lometrexol and other GARFT inhibitors clearly had experimental antitumor activity in mice, and were active against tumors that were unresponsive to MTX. However, there was a debate as to whether GARFT inhibitors were cytotoxic or cytostatic. More recent work *(10,11)* indicates that GARFT inhibitors are indeed cytotoxic to certain cell lines, but take much longer to kill cells (72 or more) than do inhibitors of TS. Moreover, the GARFT inhibitor AG2034 was only cytotoxic at low concentrations of folic acid; in standard tissue-culture medium, containing 2.2 μM folate, it was cytostatic. Also, AG2034 was much more cytotoxic to cells that lacked a functional G1 checkpoint; in cells that had a functional checkpoint, purine starvation appeared to induce a G1 cell-cycle block in which cells could remain arrested for many days without losing viability.

Despite showing promising preliminary clinical anticancer activity, lometrexol's usefulness was compromised by severe delayed thrombocytopoenia; for a discussion of this, and of the use of folic acid supplementation to prevent it, *see* Chapter 12). The biochemical basis for the thrombocytopoenia is still under investigation. Since platelets have a higher requirement for ATP than any other cell of the body, it seems likely that it is an antipurine effect. It is delayed because of the long maturation time of megakaryocytes (which is probably further extended under conditions of purine shortage), and it may be irreversible because the polyglutamate forms of lometrexol turn over so slowly that, once formed, they are effectively impossible to eliminate.

Whether these disadvantages of lometrexol can be designed out may be clarified by studies with two newer GARFT inhibitors; these compounds are reviewed in Chapters 12 and 13. It seems clear, however that GARFT inhibitors have clearly distinct properties from those of TS inhibitors, and as a class they have therapeutic potential, and perhaps the unusual property of selectivity against p53-defective cells.

10. ANTIFOLATES IN COMBINATION CHEMOTHERAPY

The most useful applications of antifolates as anticancer treatments involve using the antifolate as part of a combination chemotherapy regimen; a well-known example is the combination of methotrexate with cytoxan and 5-fluorouracil (CMF) for treatment of breast cancer. This topic is discussed in Chapter 17, and the present chapter will be confined to a couple of general observations on the design of antifolate-containing combinations.

Several investigators have explored the combination of DHFR inhibitors with inhibitors of TS, sometimes under the impression that inhibition of sequential sites in a cyclic pathway results in an inherently synergistic combination. In fact, this combination when studied (e.g. with Thymitaq and methotrexate) in cell culture generally results in additivity. Theoretically, such combinations may give interactions that are synergistic, additive, or antagonistic *(12,13)*. If the TS inhibitor is 5-fluorouracil (5-FU), the situation is complicated by the fact (first shown by Bertino, ref. *14*) that DHFR inhibitors cause accumulation of PRPP within cells, which results in more efficient conversion of 5-FU to its active TS-inhibiting metabolite, 5-FdUMP, so that MTX and other DHFR inhibitors generally do make 5-FU (but not antifolate TS inhibitors) more effective.

One kind of antifolate combination that gives a very marked synergistic interaction is the use of a lipophilic DHFR inhibitor (e.g., trimetrexate) in combination with a classical antifolate that inhibits TS, GARFT, or AICARFT. The very pronounced synergism observed with this kind of combination is referred to as the "Kisliuk effect," after the investigator who first demonstrated the phenomenon in bacteria. The mechanism of the effect has been elucidated by Galivan, Greco, and others *(15,16)*. Briefly, trimetrexate depletes cellular levels of tetrahydrofolate polyglutamates, and results in formation of much higher levels of polyglutamates of the classical antifolate drug than would otherwise be the case. This postulated mechanism is supported by the fact that the Kisliuk effect is not seen in mutant cells that lack FPGS, and also that trimetrexate does not potentiate the effect of nonclassical inhibitors of TS or GARFT. So far, most studies of the Kisliuk effect have been in vitro, but trimetrexate has been shown to be synergistic with the classical GARFT inhibitor, AG2034, against a number of in vivo tumor models, and there is great interest in exploring the therapeutic utility of this class of antifolate combinations.

Another kind of combination regimen that frequently gives therapeutic synergism is the use of an antifolate with a DNA-damaging drug. The CMF combination is an example of this kind. In this case, it does not seem to matter whether the antifolate component of the combination is classical or lipophilic, and synergism is obtained with several kinds of DNA strand-breaking drugs. Two possible explanations have been advanced for this synergistic interaction. Since antifolates deplete cellular pools of deoxyribonucleoside 5'-triphosphates (dNTP), it has been proposed that this inhibits repair of the DNA damage. However, in some cases the synergism seems to be greatest when the antifolate precedes the DNA-damaging agent, which seems inconsistent with potentiation of DNA damage by repair inhibition. In this case it has been proposed that antifolates may have a cell-synchronizing effect that maximizes the number of tumor cells in the part of the cell cycle where they are most sensitive to DNA damage. The study of cell-cycle changes induced by TS inhibitors has been facilitated by the availability of Thymitaq, which can be rapidly washed out of cells, so that the timing of cell-cycle perturbations can be precisely correlated with drug effects. It is possible that combinations of antifolates with DNA strand-breaking drugs draw their efficacy from a combination of these two mechanisms. In any event, further mechanistic studies of these effects should make possible the design of optimal clinical combinations of this type.

11. DNA STRAND BREAKS, APOPTOSIS, CHECKPOINTS, AND ANTIFOLATE SELECTIVITY

Antifolates deplete cellular pools of thymidylate or purines or both, they cause cell-cycle arrest, which may or may not be followed by programmed cell death (apoptosis); and in the case of inhibitors of DHFR and of TS, but not GARFT, they cause DNA strand breaks. The relationship of these various effects to drug efficacy and selectivity, and the extent to which antifolate selectivity is mediated by altered cell-cycle checkpoint function in cancer cells, is one of the hottest topics in the current investigation of antifolate drugs. In certain cell lines, inhibitors of DHFR and of TS cause an imbalance in the ratio of dTTP to dUTP (largely mediated by release of dCMP deaminase from feedback inhibition by dTTP) that results in misincorporation of uracil into DNA. Uracil bases are excised, resulting in apyrimidinic sites, and a futile cycle of misincorporation and misrepair results that can lead to DNA strand breaks and irreparable DNA damage. The extent to which this process is a primary cause of cell death in antifolate-treated cells is discussed in Chapter 20. Do these DNA strand breaks result in a cell-cycle block by the p53-associated checkpoint mechanism? In the case of inhibitors of DHFR and TS, this seems possible, and there is evidence that cells that lack a functional p53 checkpoint are less sensitive to these antifolates than cells that have such a checkpoint. However, some flow-cytometric studies seem to indicate that TS inhibitors cause arrest in very early S-phase, rather than at the G1:S boundary, as seen with DNA-damaging agents. This is what would be expected if the cells are arrested because of lack of dTTP for DNA synthesis, rather than because unrepaired DNA damage has triggered the G1 checkpoint. After this cell-cycle arrest has been sustained for a certain period of time (often approx 12h), the arrested cells move into apoptosis. Some cells are more apt to do this than others, so that, for example, bcl-2 overexpression makes cells less subject to antifolate-induced apoptosis (*see* Chapter 22). The expression or not of those genes that make cells sensitive to programmed cell death are thus important discriminants of response to antifolates.

GARFT inhibitors kill cells much more slowly than do inhibitors of TS or of DHFR *(10)*. Unlike TS and DHFR inhibitors, GARFT inhibitors do not cause DNA strand breaks within 24h of drug treatment (though DNA breaks appear much later when the purine-starved cells undergo apoptosis). Unlike inhibitors of TS and DHFR, which seem to block cell-cycle progression in early S-phase, GARFT inhibitors block in late G1, or at the G1:S transition. This is consistent with the metabolite depletion hypothesis of Wahl and his collaborators, who claim that depletion of cellular ribonucleotide pools can trigger the p53-dependent G1 checkpoint in the absence of DNA strand breaks *(17)*. The cells that are arrested in this way by the GARFT inhibitor AG2034 do not die, at least for several days, but remain arrested, and can move back into the cell cycle if a purine source is added to the medium. However, this nonlethal arrest state appears to require a functional G1 checkpoint: Cells that lack such a checkpoint, when treated with AG2034, progress slowly through S-phase, and die, either in S-phase or in G2 (*see* Chapter 13). Thus p53-competent cells are less sensitive to GARFT inhibitors than p53-defective cells; this pattern of selectivity is the reverse of the situation for inhibitors of TS and DHFR.

12. CONCLUSIONS: WHERE NEXT WITH ANTIFOLATES?

The antifolate field remains a rich source of new drugs, new mechanistic approaches, and new therapeutic ideas. Investigators in this field have a wide choice of compounds to study, including potent, selective inhibitors of DHFR, TS, GARFT, and AICARFT, as well as compounds that inhibit more than one of these targets to varying degrees. We can choose between classical antifolates that are subject to facilitated transport and to polyglutamylation, lipophilic compounds that are neither transported nor polyglutamylated, or compounds that require transport but are not polyglutamylated (as well as some intermediate situations such as that of GW1843, which is converted to a diglutamate, but no further; *see* Chapter 9).

Many questions remain, some of which can only be answered by extensive clinical trials. Are selective TS inhibitors, such as Tomudex, in fact better drugs than 5-FU? Can novel GARFT inhibitors reproduce the clinical activity of lometrexol without its serious delayed toxicity? Will selective AICARFT inhibitors show antiarthritic activity; as may be the case if the hypothesis of Cronstein *(18)* is correct, that this enzyme is the target for the anti-inflammatory activity of methotrexate?

Studies to date have clearly established the major influence of cellular pharmacokinetics on drug efficacy, selectivity, and potency, but many interesting questions remain unanswered: would a classical antifolate that was transported exclusively by the mFBP have a radically different spectrum from an otherwise similar compound that was transported exclusively by the RFC? Would drug polyglutamates that are good substrates for FPGH be less toxic without compromising potency and selectivity? Are there circumstances in which the rapid loss of a lipophilic antifolate from the cell could be turned to therapeutic advantage, e.g., by giving a tightly synchronized target cell population whose response to a second agent acting later in the cell cycle would thus be optimized? The availability of a group of inhibitors designed against a set of related target molecules, and with a wide range of physicochemical and pharmacokinetic properties, provides us with the opportunity to tailor chemotherapy rationally against tumors with particular biochemical profiles. Antifolates are thus a class of drugs in which the prospects for designing more efficacious and more selective chemotherapy remain unusually promising.

REFERENCES

1. Woods DD. Relation of p-aminobenzoic acid to mechanism of action of sulphanilamide. *Br J Exp Pathol* 1940;21:74–90.
2. Cohen SS. On the nature of thymineless death. *Ann NY Acad Sci* 1971;186:292–301.
3. Straus OH, Goldstein A. Zone behavior of enzymes. *J Gen Physiol* 1943;26:559–585.
4. Sirotnak FM. Biochemical pharmacologic and antitumor properties of 10-ethyl-10-deazaaminopterin. 1987; NCI Monograph 5:127–131.
5. Borsa J, Whitmore GF. Studies relating to the mode of action of methotrexate II. Studies on sites of action on L-cells in vitro. *Molec Pharmacol* 1969;5:303–317.
6. Hryniuk WM. Purineless death as a link between growth rate and cytotoxicity by methotrexate. *Cancer Res* 1972;32:1506–1511.
7. Jackman AL, Taylor GA, Calvert AH, Harrap KR. Modulation of antimetabolite effects. Effects of thymidine on the efficacy of the quinazoline-based thymidylate synthase inhibitor, CB3717. *Biochem Pharmacol* 1984;33:3269–3275.
8. Broome MG, Johnson RK, Evans SF, Wodinsky I. Leucovorin reversal studies with TMQ and a triazine antifol in comparison with methotrexate. *Proc Am Assoc Cancer Res* 1982;23:178.
9. Walzer PD, Foy J, Steele P, Kim CK, White M, Klein RS, Otten BA, Allegra C. Activities of antifolate, antiviral and other drugs in an immunosuppressed rat model of Pneumocystis carinii pneumonia. *Antimicrob Agents Chemother* 1992;36:1935–1942.
10. Smith SG, Lehman NL, Moran RG. Cytotoxicity of antifolate inhibitors of thymidylate and purine synthesis to WiDr colonic carcinoma cells. *Cancer Res* 1993;53:5697–5706.
11. Zhang CC, Boritzki TJ, Jackson RC. An Inhibitor of glycinamide ribonucleotide formyltransferase is selectively cytotoxic to cells that lack a functional G1 checkpoint. *Cancer Chemother Pharmacol*, 1998;41:223–228.
12. Harvey RJ. Interaction of two inhibitors which act on different enzymes of a metabolic pathway. *J Theoret Biol* 1978;74:411–437.
13. Jackson RC. Amphibolic drug combinations: the design of selective antimetabolite protocols based upon the kinetic properties of multienzyme systems. *Cancer Res* 1993;53:3998–4003.
14. Bertino JR, Sawicki WL, Lindquist CA, Gupta VS. Schedule-dependent antitumor effects of methotrexate and 5-fluorouracil. *Cancer Res* 1977;37:327–328.
15. Galivan J, Rhee MS, Johnson TB, Dilwith R, Nair MG, Bunni M, Priest DG. The role of cellular folates in the enhancement of activity of the thymidylate synthase inhibitor 10-propargyl-5,8-dideazafolate against hepatoma cells in vitro by inhibitors of dihydrofolate reductase. *J Biol Chem* 1989;264:10,685–10,692.
16. Gaumont Y, Kisliuk RL, Parsons JC, Greco WR. Quantitation of folic acid enhancement of antifolate synergism. *Cancer Res* 1992;52:2228–2235.
17. Yin Y, Tainsky MA, Bischoff FZ, Strong LC, Wahl GM. Wild-type p53 restores cell cycle control and inhibits gene amplification in cells with mutant p53 alleles. *Cell* 1992;70:937–948.
18. Cronstein BN. Molecular therapeutics: methotrexate and its mechanism of action. *Arthritis Rheum* 1996;39:1951–1960.

2 Folate Biochemistry in Relation to Antifolate Selectivity

Roy L. Kisliuk

CONTENTS

INTRODUCTION
METHIONINE
THYMIDYLATE CYCLE
C1-THF-SYNTHASE
5,10-METHENYLTETRAHYDROFOLATE SYNTHETASE
GLYCINAMIDE RIBONUCLEOTIDE FORMYLTRANSFERASE (GARFT)
AMINOIMIDAZOLECARBOXAMIDE RIBONUCLEOTIDE
    FORMYLTRANSFERASE (AICARFT)
METHIONYL tRNA$_f^{met}$ FORMYLTRANSFERASE
FORMIMINOTRANSFERASE-CYCLODEAMINASE
GLYCINE CLEAVAGE SYSTEM
DIMETHYLGLYCINE DEHYDROGENASE AND SARCOSINE
    DEHYDROGENASE
FOLYLPOLY-γ-GLUTAMATE SYNTHETASE
GLUTAMYL HYDROLASE
CONCLUSIONS
ACKNOWLEDGMENTS
REFERENCES

1. INTRODUCTION

This review will deal with advances in folate biochemistry related to antifolate toxicity and selectivity. Because of the interrelatedness of reactions of folate metabolism, alterations in the activity of any folate enzyme, cellular transport system, as well as the concentration of any folate metabolite may be relevant to antifolate cytotoxicity and selectivity. Therefore, it is difficult to predict the results of inhibiting a given folate enzyme on antifolate selectivity. For example, in many experimental systems, the *cytotoxicity* of methotrexate is caused by its ability to inhibit dihydrofolate reductase, resulting

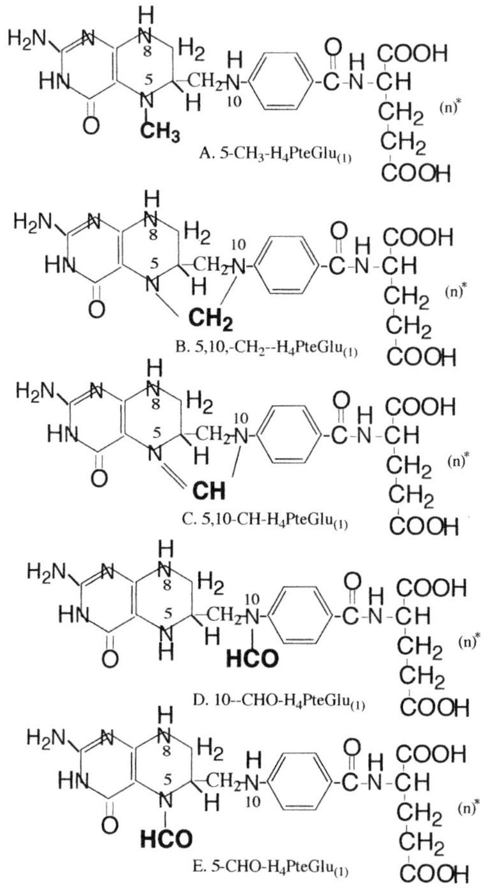

Fig. 1. Structures of tetrahydrofolic acid (THF) derivatives: **(A)** 5-methylTHF; **(B)** 5,10-methyleneTHF; **(C)** 5,10-methenylTHF; **(D)** 10-formylTHF; **(E)** 5-formylTHF (also called folinic acid, leucovorin or citrovorum factor). Pte stands for pteroic acid (p-[(2-amino-4-oxy-6-pteridyl-methyl)amino]benzoic acid).*n refers to the total number of glutamate residues attached to pteroic acid. All additional Glu residues are joined by amide bonds to the γ-carboxyl group of Glu(1).

in lowered thymidylate formation, leading to lethal defects in DNA. However, its *selectivity* is often dependent on differential cellular uptake and polyglutamylation. Favorable clinical results with aminopterin, the forerunner of methotrexate, in acute leukemia in children were reported by Farber et al. *(1)* in 1948. This work depended on knowledge generated at the American Cyanamid Company, Pearl River, NY, on the structure of folic acid and the chemical synthesis of analogs in addition to the insightful clinical observations of the Farber group *(1)*. This work was done before the role of tetrahydrofolates in the metabolism of single carbon units was known. The present discussion of the current literature on folates is offered in the hope that, given the powerful analytical, structural, molecular genetic, and synthetic methods now available, new approaches to selective toxicity can be generated.

We focus on the metabolic interconversions and enzymology of three areas of folate metabolism, areas related to the essential metabolites methionine, thymidylate, and purine

Table 1
Folate Enzymes in Mammalian Cells

Enzyme	Abbreviation	Cellular Location	Review Section
1. methylenetetrahydrofolate reductase (Fig. 2)	MTHFR	cytoplasm	(2.2.)
2. methionine synthase (Fig. 2)	MS	cytoplasm	(2.2.)
3. serine hydroxymethyltransferase (Figs. 5,6)	SHMT	cytoplasm, mitochondria	(3.2.)
4. thymidylate synthase (Fig. 5)	TS	cytoplasm, nucleus	(3.3.)
5. dihydrofolate reductase (Fig. 5)	DHFR	cytoplasm	(3.4.)
[a]C_1THF synthase: [c](Fig. 6)			(4.)
6. *methylenetetrahydrofolate dehydrogenase*	D	cytoplasm, mitochondria	
7. *methenyltetrahydrofolate cyclohydrolase*	C	cytoplasm, mitochondria	
8. *10-formyltetrahydrofolate synthetase*	S	cytoplasm	
9. 10-formyltetrahydrofolate dehydrogenase (Fig. 6)	FDH	cytoplasm	(5.)
10. 5,10-methenyltetrahydrofolate synthetase (Fig. 6)	MTHFS	cytoplasm, mitochondria	(6.)
11. *glycinamide ribonucleotide formyltransferase*[c] (Fig. 7)	GARFT	cytoplasm	(7.)
12. *aminoimidazolecarboxamide ribonucleotide formyltransferase*[b] (Fig. 7)	AICARFT	cytoplasm	(8.)
13. methionyl tRNA$_f^{met}$ formyltransferase	FMT	mitochondria	(9.)
14. *formiminotransferase*[b]	FTCD	cytoplasm	(10.)
15. *formiminocyclodeaminase*[b]	FTCD	cytoplasm	(10.)
16. glycine cleavage system[d]		mitochondria	(11.)
17. dimethylglycine dehydrogenase		mitochondria	(12.)
18. sarcosine dehydrogenase (Fig.3)		mitochondria	(12.)
19. folylpolyglutamate synthetase	FPGS	cytoplasm, mitochondria	(13.)
20. folylpolyglutamate hydrolase	GH	lysosomes, excreted	(14.)

[a] Italics indicate that the enzymes are part of a bifunctional[b], trifunctional[c], or tetrafunctional[d] protein complex.

nucleotides. In this order we proceed from the most reduced form of the single carbon unit encountered in mammalian metabolism to the more oxidized forms, that is, from methyl (methanol level) through methylene (formaldehyde level) to methenyl and formyl (formate level) (Fig. 1). We then consider the enzymes of folylpolyglutamate formation and hydrolysis. The enzymes discussed are listed in Table 1 with abbreviations, cellular location, and

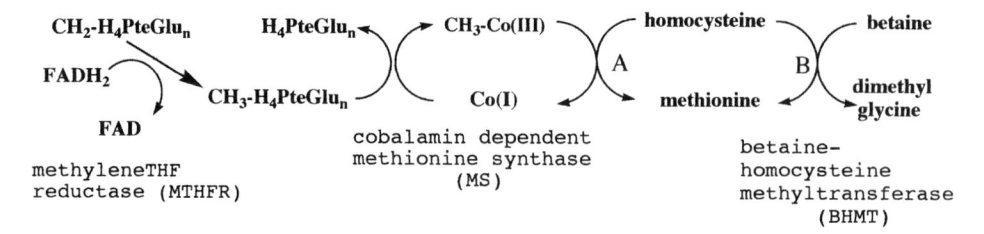

Fig. 2. Methylation of homocysteine to form methionine: (**A**) from 5-CH$_3$-H$_4$PteGlu$_n$ via methylcobalamin (CH$_3$-Co[III]), (**B**) from betaine.

location in the text. Human systems are emphasized. In order to keep the number of citations within bounds, key references serve as the source of additional current literature. Earlier folate studies are summarized in the treatise edited by Blakley and Benkovic *(2)* as well as in reviews by Kisliuk *(3)*, Shane *(4)*, and Wagner *(5)*.

2. METHIONINE

2.1 Introduction

In addition to its essential role as a constituent of proteins, methionine is a major metabolite, being at the confluence of the metabolism of folate, cobalamin, methyl groups, and polyamines. Our discussion will be divided into three sections: methionine methyl formation (Fig. 2), methionine methyl donation (Fig. 3), and propylamine donation (Fig. 4).

2.2 Methionine Methyl Formation

Methionine is required in the diet for normal growth but it is only the homocysteine portion that animals are unable to synthesize. Given adequate dietary folate and cobalamin, methyl groups are readily formed from CH$_2$-H$_4$PteGlu$_n$ by sequential reactions catalyzed by CH$_2$-H$_4$PteGlu reductase (MTHFR) and cobalamin-dependent methionine synthase (MS) (Fig. 2), which result in the methylation of homocysteine to form methionine. Interest in these enzymes is intense because low activity of either one leads to elevated blood levels of homocysteine, an important correlate in coronary disease *(6)*. Homocysteine has been implicated as a toxin of the endothelium of blood vessels *(7)* and has been shown to inhibit growth and p21ras methylation in cultured vascular endothelial cells *(8)*. The incidence of both coronary disease *(6)* and neural tube defects *(9)* is diminished by supplemental dietary folate.

Another enzyme catalyzing the methylation of homocysteine to methionine is betaine-homocysteine methyltransferase (Fig. 2). This enzyme has so far only been found in liver and kidney and its activity does not suffice to alleviate homocysteinemia *(7,10)*.

MTHFR catalyzes the reduction of CH$_2$-H$_4$PteGlu$_n$ to CH$_3$-H$_4$PteGlu$_n$ (Fig. 2). The hydrogen donor bound to the pig liver enzyme is FAD, which is itself reduced by NADPH. The K_m for CH$_2$-H$_4$PteGlu$_6$ is 0.1 μM as compared with 7 μM for CH$_2$-H$_4$PteGlu$_1$ *(11)*. MTHFR can catalyze the reverse reaction, the formation of CH$_2$-H$_4$PteGlu$_n$ from CH$_3$-H$_4$PteGlu$_n$, in the presence of the artificial electron acceptor menadione *(12)*, but this reaction is insignificant under physiological conditions in vitro *(7)* and in vivo *(13)*.

Sequencing of the cDNA for human MTHFR led to the discovery of an important variant (Ala222Val) which, in the homozygous state, leads to decreased MTHFR activ-

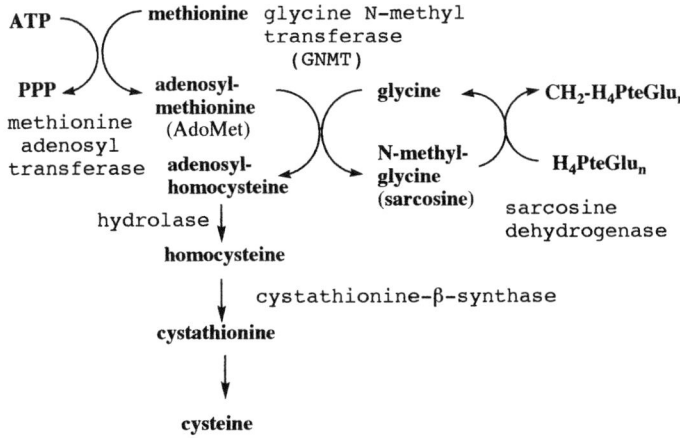

Fig. 3. Methionine as methyl donor; formation of homocysteine.

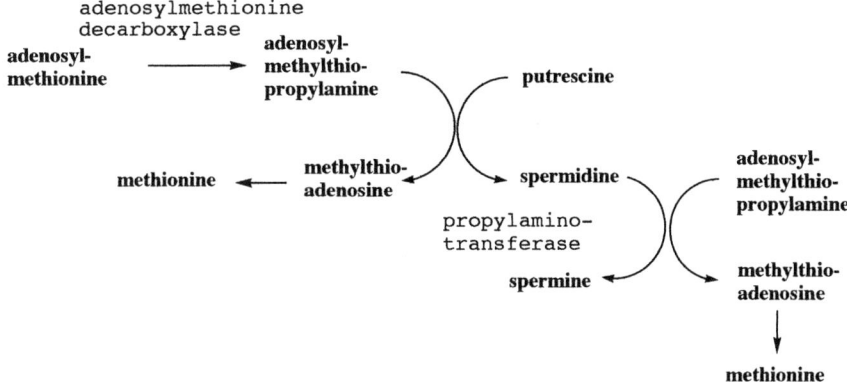

Fig. 4. Methionine as propylamine donor; formation of polyamines; putrescine, spermidine, and spermine.

ity which can lead to homocysteinemia *(14)*. Studies with an analogous mutation in *E. coli* MTHFR showed that FAD is more loosely bound to the mutant enzyme, leading to lower activity *(15)*. Addition of CH_3-$H_4PteGlu_1$ greatly slowed FAD dissociation. These results provide a reasonable explanation for the ability of high folate diets to lower blood levels of homocysteine in that MTHFR activity would be maintained even in the presence of the variant enzyme provided that, as is likely, CH_2-$H_4PteGlu_n$ in vivo also slows FAD dissociation and stabilizes MTHFR.

MTHFR is inhibited by adenosylmethionine (AdoMet) providing a system for decreasing methionine methyl group synthesis when dietary methionine is provided *(11)*.

Methionine synthase (Fig. 2) catalyzes the transfer of the methyl group of CH_3-$H_4PteGlu_n$ to homocysteine to form methionine. The human enzyme has been cloned in three laboratories *(16–18)* and consists of 1265 amino acids with a kDa of 140. Based on studies with the *E. coli* enzyme, which is highly homologous to the human enzyme, the cobalamin prosthetic group in the central portion of the protein interacts with homocysteine, CH_3-$H_4PteGlu_n$ and AdoMet, each of which is activated by a specific region of the protein *(19)*. The C-terminal AdoMet binding region is required because MS is occasionally inactivated by oxidation of the cob(I)alamin cofactor to an inactive cob(II)alamin form. Reactivation requires reductive methylation of cob(II)alamin to methylcob(I)alamin. The methyl group is provided by AdoMet. The reducing system is provided by a flavodoxin system in *E. coli*. In animals the auxiliary redox proteins have not been characterized, but defects in these proteins lead to functional MS deficiency *(20)*. The AdoMet requirement for the maintenance of MS activity is important in view of the essential role of MS in the incorporation of CH_3-$H_4PteGlu_1$ into cellular metabolism.

MS provides the only pathway by which the methyl group of CH_3-$H_4PteGlu_n$ can be removed in vivo, which makes MS activity essential for providing $H_4PteGlu_n$ from CH_3-$H_4PteGlu_n$. When MS activity is low because of either defective enzyme(s), cobalamin deficiency, or nitrous oxide inhibition, CH_3-$H_4PteGlu_n$ accumulates. The major source of cellular folates is usually blood CH_3-$H_4PteGlu_1$ which must be demethylated and then polyglutamylated before functioning as a coenzyme in thymidylate and purine nucleotide formation. Thus MS deficiency causes folate deficiency by trapping methyl groups in the form of CH_3-$H_4PteGlu_1$. CH_3-$H_4PteGlu_1$ is not retained in cells because it is a poor substrate for folylpolyglutamate synthetase and the monoglutamate form is not as tightly bound to folate enzymes or other folate binding proteins in cells as are the polyglutamate forms. Polyglutamate forms of CH_3-$H_4PteGlu$ are reported to have lower K_m values than the monoglutamate form for *E. coli* and bovine brain MS, but studies on the effect of polyglutamate chain length on substrate activity for human MS have not been reported. However, the fact that cultured cells can grow when supplied with CH_3-$H_4PteGlu_1$ indicates that it is demethylated to some extent by the action of MS.

Two interrelated aspects of methionine metabolism that have received attention in relation to chemotherapy are: the inhibition of MS by nitrous oxide *(21)* and the inability of many tumor cell lines to synthesize the methionine methyl group *(22)*. These cell lines are unable to grow when supplied with homocysteine and must be provided with methionine in the medium. In one such instance, a glioma cell line requires methionine because of lowered levels of cobalamin on MS *(23)*. MS-deficient cells should be especially sensitive to inhibition of methionine adenosyl transferase, which would deprive cells of AdoMet rendering them incapable of utilizing exogenous methionine as a source of methyl groups or polyamines.

Nitrous oxide specifically inactivates MS by reacting with cob(I)alamin and exposure to nitrous oxide leads to megaloblastic anemia *(24)*. Short-term remissions were observed in cases of chronic myeloid leukemia and childhood acute myeloid leukemia after treatment with nitrous oxide *(21)*. Methotrexate enhances nitrous oxide toxicity *(23)*. Methotrexate decreases MS activity by depleting cells of CH_3-$H_4PteGlu_n$ and of methylcobalamin. It is proposed that this leads to lower AdoMet levels and decreased methylation reactions that contribute to the cytotoxic action of methotrexate *(23)*. A reasonable explanation for methotrexate enhancement of nitrous oxide toxicity would be that both agents reduce MS activity, methotrexate by lowering cofactor levels, and nitrous oxide by inactivating cobalamin remaining on MS.

Recently cobalamin analogs were shown to inhibit the growth of BW5147 mouse lymphoma cells in culture *(25)*.

2.3 Methionine Methyl Donation

Methionine is converted to the active methyl donor, AdoMet, through the action of methionine adenosyl transferase (Fig. 3). Acceptors of the methyl group include glycine, DNA, RNA, norepinephrine, and at least 100 additional compounds *(5)* including arsenic compounds *(26)*. We limit our discussion to methylation of glycine and DNA. Glycine methylation serves as a route to recycle uneeded methionine methyl groups and is regulated by CH_3-$H_4PteGlu_n$ *(5)*. DNA methylation regulates gene expression *(27)*.

Glycine *N*-methyltransferase (GNMT) makes up 1–3% of the soluble protein in rat liver cytosol and is a major folate-binding protein even though it does not require a folate coenzyme for its activity *(5)*. It is a tetramer containing identical 292-amino acid residue 34-kDa subunits. When dietary methionine intake is high, glycine is methylated to sarcosine which is metabolized to CH_2-$H_4PteGlu_n$ and glycine in mitochondria. When dietary methionine is low, synthesis of CH_3-$H_4PteGlu_n$ is elevated because the inhibition of MTHFR by AdoMet is released. CH_3-$H_4PteGlu_n$ is an allosteric inhibitor of GNMT under conditions in which conserving methionine is advantageous. Thus AdoMet and CH_3-$H_4PteGlu_n$ regulate methionine methyl synthesis and disposal, respectively.

GNMT is also present at high levels in the exocrine pancreas in which methylation plays a role in exocrine secretion *(28)*.

Rat liver GNMT appears to be identical to the cytosolic receptor for benzo[a]pyrene which induces cytochrome P450 1A1 gene expression. Consistent with this proposed role for GNMT, its subunits are transported into the nucleus *(29)*.

The methylation of specific CpG sites in the DNA of the tumor suppressor gene p53 decreases when rats are maintained on a diet deficient in folate and methyl donors. The amount of p53 protein increases in response to many signals including DNA damage and nucleotide depletion *(30)*. p53 function is lost in about half of all human cancers. Alteration of the pattern of DNA methylation is postulated to be a factor in the increase in spontaneous liver cancer and in susceptibility to dimethylhydrazine-induced colon tumors *(31)*.

The adenosylhomocysteine arising from the action of AdoMet-dependent methyltransferases is hydrolyzed to homocysteine and adenosine (Fig. 3), an important reaction because adenosylhomocysteine is a potent inhibitor of AdoMet-dependent methylation reactions. Homocysteine may either be remethylated or metabolized to cysteine through the transsulfuration pathway that requires the action of cystathionine-β-synthase (Fig. 3) *(7)*. In mammalian liver, about half of the homocysteine is remethylated and half proceeds through the transsulfuration pathway. Many tissues however, lack cystathionine-β-synthase and are incapable of transsulfuration *(7)*. Genetic polymorphisms can result in decreased cystathionine-β-synthase activity which leads to homocysteinemia. One type of cystathionine-β-synthase deficiency responds to an increased supply of vitamin B_6 because the variant enzyme in this instance has a lowered affinity for its coenzyme, pyridoxal phosphate *(7)*.

2.4 Propylamine Donation

The polyamines putrescine, spermidine, and spermine are necessary for the growth of all cells *(32)*. Putrescine arises from the decarboxylation of ornithine. Spermidine and spermine are formed by sequential addition of propylamine residues to putrescine (Fig. 4). Adenosylmethylthiopropylamine arising from the decarboxylation of AdoMet is the donor of propylamine. Thus ornithine decarboxylase and AdoMet decarboxylase are key enzymes involved in polyamine synthesis and the level of these enzymes is regulated by hormones, tumor promoters, and by polyamine levels *(32)*. A polyamine-responsive element has been identified in the 5'-leader sequence of the mRNA for AdoMet decarboxylase. This element codes for the peptide MAGDIS which plays a role in polyamine regulation of polyamine biosynthesis.

Spermine stimulates the activity of partially purified rat liver MS *(33)*. Since methionine provides propylamine for spermine synthesis (Fig. 4), stimulation of methionine synthesis by spermine could be part of a positive feedback loop related to the association of polyamine formation and growth. Polyamine analogs can cause cell-cycle arrest and apoptosis in human melanoma cells. One such analog is currently in Phase I clinical trial against solid tumors *(34)*.

3. THYMIDYLATE CYCLE

3.1 Introduction

Growing cells undergo apoptosis if *de novo* thymidylate synthesis is blocked. In colon carcinoma cells, thymineless apoptosis is mediated via Fas signaling *(35)*. Although cell death can be prevented if thymidine is supplied, under the usual in vivo conditions, plasma thymidine levels are too low for protection *(36)*. The three enzymes of the thymidylate synthesis cycle (Fig. 5) are serine hydroxymethytransferase (SHMT) *(37)*, thymidylate synthase (TS) *(38)*, and dihydrofolate reductase (DHFR) *(39)*. SHMT catalyzes the formation of CH_2-$H_4PteGlu_n$ from serine and $H_4PteGlu_n$. CH_2-$H_4PteGlu_n$ is then the substrate for the reductive methylation of dUMP to dTMP. Reducing equivalents are supplied by the conversion of $H_4PteGlu_n$ to $H_2PteGlu_n$, which makes it necessary to regenerate a molecule of $H_4PteGlu_n$ for every molecule of dTMP formed. DHFR enables completion of the cycle by catalyzing the reduction of $H_2PteGlu_n$ to $H_4PteGlu_n$, utilizing NADPH as the reductant.

3.2 Serine Hydroxymethyltransferase

Serine and glycine both provide CH_2-$H_4PteGlu_n$ which, in turn, is the major source of single carbon units for methionine, thymidylate and purine nucleotide synthesis. SHMT catalyzes the conversion of serine to glycine and CH_2-$H_4PteGlu_n$, whereas glycine is metabolized to CH_2-$H_4PteGlu_n$, CO_2, and NH_3^+ in mitochondria via the glycine cleavage system *(40)*. SHMT is found both in mitochondria (mSHMT) and in the cytosol (cSHMT). Chinese hamster ovary cells become auxotrophic for glycine when mSHMT is absent, which shows that the presence of cSHMT is insufficient to provide the cells need for glycine *(4)*. cSHMT may serve in gluconeogenesis by catalyzing the conversion of dietary glycine to serine, which then gives rise to pyruvate.

Human cDNAs that encode the two isozymes of SHMT have been cloned and sequenced *(41,42)*. Human mSHMT and cSHMT monomers (approx 55 kDa) contain 474 and 483 amino acid residues, respectively, and the deduced amino acid sequences show 63% identity. SHMT is a highly conserved enzyme, the human isozymes having approx 43% sequence identity with *E. coli* SHMT. All of the purified enzymes have four identical subunits that are yellow because of the presence of one molecule of pyridoxal phosphate on each subunit. Experiments with pig liver SHMT show that folylpolyglutamate

Chapter 2 / Folate Biochemistry

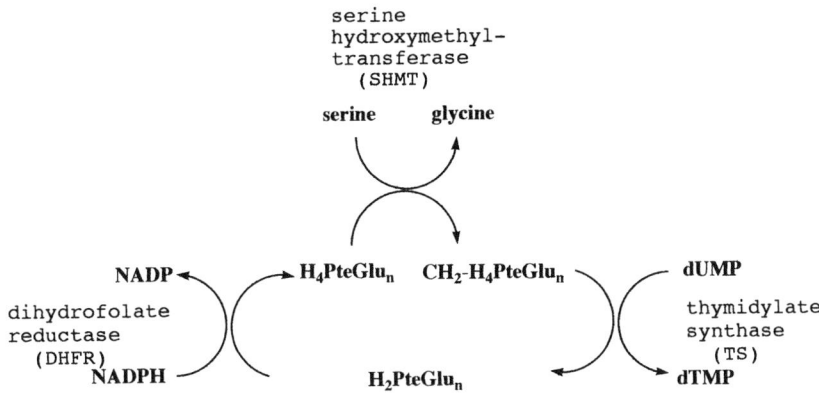

Fig. 5. The thymidylate cycle.

substrates and inhibitors bind more tightly to the enzyme than the monoglutamate forms *(43)*. Similar results were obtained with rabbit liver SHMT where it was shown, in addition, that cytosolic and mitochondrial SHMT have similar affinities for polyglutamate forms *(44)*.

An additional reaction catalyzed by both mSHMT and cSHMT is the hydrolysis of 5,10-CH-H_4PteGlu$_n$ to form 5-CHO-H_4PteGlu$_n$ (Fig. 6) *(45)*. A hydrated form of 5,10-CH-H_4PteGlu$_n$, (6R,11R)-5,10-hydroxymethylene-H_4PteGlu$_n$ is a likely intermediate in this reaction *(46)*. 5-CHO-H_4PteGlu$_{(n)}$ inhibits SHMT *(47)*, TS *(48)*, and AICARFT *(49)* and could therefore be an important compound in regulating one-carbon metabolism in that it could diminish both the formation and utilization of single-carbon units *(50)*. 5-CH_3-H_4PteGlu$_n$ also inhibits SHMT and thus could also act to diminish formation of single-carbon units along with 10-CHO-H_4PteGlu$_n$ which inhibits L1210 dihydrofolate reductase *(48)*. 5-CHO-H_4PteGlu$_n$, 10-CHO-H_4PteGlu$_n$ and 5-CH_3-H_4PteGlu$_n$ could all be feedback-signaling agents responding to increased levels of single-carbon folate metabolites at the formyl, hydroxymethyl, and methyl levels of oxidation. Consistent with this view, depletion of 5-CHO-H_4PteGlu$_n$ in neuroblastoma cells by overexpressing the cDNA for methenyltetrahydrofolate synthetase enhanced serine levels but lowered methionine levels, leading to the suggestion that serine synthesis and homocysteine remethylation compete for one-carbon units in the cytoplasm *(51)*.

Although SHMT as provider of the methylene group for the methyl group of thymidylate has been considered as a target for chemotherapeutic agents, specific antifolate inhibitors of SHMT have not been described. Perhaps an analog that bridges the folate site with the pyridoxal phosphate site would be effective. The serine analogs, D-fluoroalanine *(52)* and 4-chlorothreonine *(53)* are mechanism-based inhibitors of SHMT at millimolar levels.

3.3 Thymidylate Synthase

Thymidylate synthase catalyzes the reductive methylation of dUMP to dTMP. It is a dimeric enzyme (70 kD) with two catalytic sites per dimer, whose amino acid sequences are highly conserved *(54)*. Each monomer contributes amino acids to the catalytic site *(54)*. X-ray crystal structures of the *Lactobacillus casei* and *E. coli* enzymes show the folate cofactor bound above and trapping dUMP. Polyglutamate forms of the folate cofactor may tether it to the enzyme and allow access of the site to nucleotide substrate and release of product. The bifunctional DHFR-TS from *Leishmania major* has an unusual charge distribution that could account for channelling of folate cofactors between active sites *(55)*. Human TS has been cloned, sequenced, expressed *(56,57)*, and crystallized *(58)*. The crystal structure suggests a mechanism for docking of substrates involving the pivoting of an active site loop.

Purified cellular human and rat thymidylate synthases are acetylated at their N-terminal amino acids and have a lower specific activity than the corresponding recombinant enzymes *(57)*. In H35 rat hepatoma cells, TS has been localized to the nucleolar region but appears in the cytoplasm when overexpressed *(59)*. TS was also present in the mitochondria of H35 cells and a small amount of phosphorylated TS was identified. TS binds to its own mRNA as a negative regulator *(60)*. This binding requires that TS be blocked at its N-terminal position. Elements in the promoter region of the human TS gene have been identified and the nuclear factor Sp1 is a major contributor to promoter activity, but other positive and negative regulators have been identified *(61)*. Further studies of these modifications and interactions should elucidate the relationship of thymidylate synthase to the cell division cycle.

Accumulation of dUTP and its misincorporation into DNA is a major factor in the cytotoxicity resulting from the inhibition of TS. dUTPase catalyzes the conversion of dUTP to dUMP and therefore acts to counteract the toxic action of dUTP *(62)*. Conversely, inhibitors of dUTPase should enhance the toxicity of TS inhibitors. X-ray crystallographic studies show that the active site of human dUTPase, a trimeric enzyme, consists of residues from all three subunits *(63)*. The human dUTPase gene codes for both nuclear and mitochondrial isoforms of the enzyme *(62)*.

3.4 Dihydrofolate Reductase

In contrast with SHMT (a tetramer) and TS (a dimer), human DHFR is monomeric (22 kDa). It catalyzes the reduction of $7,8\text{-}H_2PteGlu_n$ to $5,6,7,8\text{-}H_4PteGlu_n$ *(64)*. The human enzyme has been cloned, expressed, and crystallized *(65)* and the 1H and 15N nuclear magnetic resonance assignments obtained *(66)*. Again in contrast with SHMT and TS, the primary structures of eukaryotic DHFRs are not highly homologous, only 20% of the residues of human DHFR are identical to those found in eight other eukaryotic DHFRs *(64)*.

Site-directed mutagenesis studies have led to the production of variants of human DHFR resistant to methotrexate *(67,68)*. Current studies in mice are testing the concept that cDNA coding for methotrexate-resistant DHFR transduced into bone marrow progenitor cells will lead to improved curability of mice bearing a methotrexate-sensitive tumor *(67,68)*.

Folate polyglutamates and antifolate polyglutamates often have a modest two- to 10-fold enhanced affinity for human DHFR as compared with monoglutamate forms *(64,69)*. An interesting exception is 2-desamino-2-methylaminopterin, which has an IC_{50} value greater than 50 μM but the addition of four γ-linked glutamyl residues lowers the IC_{50} >200-fold to 0.25 μM *(70)*.

The cellular synthesis of human DHFR is negatively regulated by the binding of the enzyme to its cognate mRNA *(71,72)*. Methotrexate binding to DHFR prevents this interaction and promotes DHFR production.

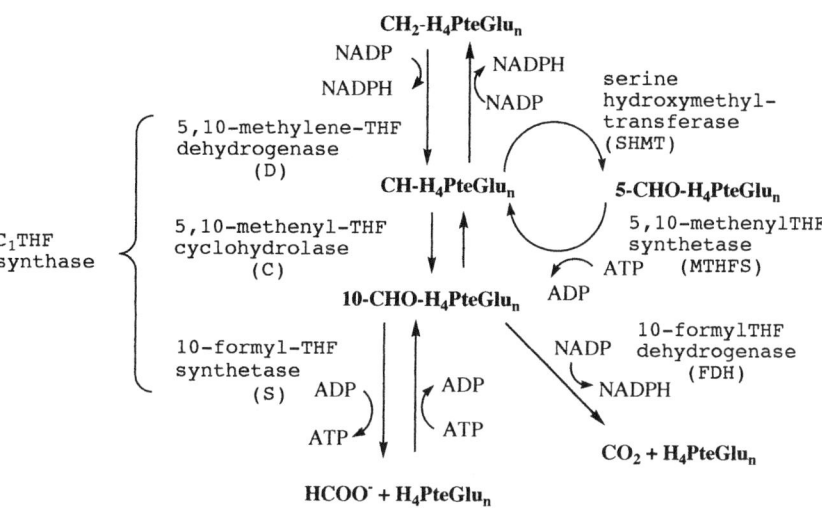

Fig. 6. Interconversion of methylene and formyl tetrahydrofolate derivatives.

The activity of the murine DHFR gene promoter increases at the G1-S-phase boundary of the cell cycle, mediated by a member of the E2F family of transcription factors *(73)*.

4. C1-THF-SYNTHASE

C1-THF-synthase is a homodimeric enzyme complex that occurs in two forms in mammalian cells *(74)*. One form is a trifunctional, cytoplasmic, 100 kDa, $NADP^+$-dependent 5,10-CH_2-$H_4PteGlu_n$ dehydrogenase-5,10-CH-$H_4PteGlu_n$ cyclohydrolase-10-CHO-$H_4PteGlu_n$ synthetase (Fig. 6). The three enzyme activities are abbreviated D, C, and S for dehydrogenase, cyclohydrolase, and synthetase, respectively. The human trifunctional enzyme has been cloned, sequenced, and expressed *(75)*. The amino-terminal 34-kDa DC portion of the trifunctional enzyme has been expressed separately and is convenient for kinetic studies. The trifunctional cytoplasmic DCS complex is most likely necessary to catalyze the incorporation of formate, arising from serine, glycine, and methyl groups in mitochondria, into 10-CHO-$H_4PteGlu_n$ for use in purine nucleotide synthesis and into 5,10-CH_2-$H_4PteGlu_n$ for use in dTMP and methionine synthesis *(76–78)*. This role for the trifunctional enzyme is supported by kinetic and metabolic studies.

The second form is bifunctional NAD^+-dependent DC, which is a nuclear-encoded 34-kDa mitochondrial enzyme. The human and murine bifunctional mitochondrial enzymes have been cloned, sequenced, and expressed *(79)*. This system has been suggested to serve as the source of formyl groups for the synthesis of formylmethionyl tRNA required for protein synthesis in mitochondria. Its location in mitochondria is consistent with its resemblence to DC enzyme complex found in bacteria *(79)*. In contrast to the DC portion of the cytosolic trifunctional enzyme complex, it has an absolute requirement for Mg^{2+} and P_i *(80)*. It is proposed that Mg^{2+} and P_i substitute for the 2′ phosphate on the adenosine portion of NADPH because it has a 44% amino acid sequence identity with the DC domain of yeast mitochondrial NADP-dependent trifunctional enzyme, the human NAD-dependent enzyme has a low, Mg^{2+}-dependent turnover with NADP, and P_i competes for NADP binding.

Kinetic studies provide an explanation of the mechanism by which the mitochondrial NAD-dependent DC enzyme functions to convert 5,10-CH_2-$H_4PteGlu_n$ to 10-CHO-$H_4PteGlu_n$, whereas the cytosolic NADP-dependent enzyme functions in the reverse direction (78). In the cytosolic system, where the NADPH/NADP ratio is high, the rate-limiting C-reaction is stimulated by NADPH analogs, and presumably by NADPH as well, but technical difficulties prevent a direct test. The 10-CHO-$H_4PteGlu_n$ is 100% channeled for reduction to 5,10-CH_2-$H_4PteGlu$. In mitochondria, the NADH/NAD ratio is low, favoring the oxidative reaction and the conversion of 5,10-CH_2-$H_4PteGlu_n$ to 10-CHO-$H_4PteGlu_n$ which is not stimulated by nucleotides. Both cytosolic and mitochondrial DC activities are carried out at a single active site.

In contrast with cytosolic trifunctional NADP-dependent DCS, where high activity is found widely distributed among various tissues, the NAD-dependent system is usually not detectable in most tissues of adult animals, but its cognate mRNA is detectable (81). NAD-dependent DC activity is found in embryonic tissue and in most all transformed cultured cells.

The affinity of the DC complexes for folate substrates is not greatly enhanced by increasing the polyglutamate chain length. Monoglutamate forms function in substrate channeling as well as polyglutamates. This contrasts with the formiminotetrahydrofolate transferase-formiminotetrahydrofolate cyclodeaminase system involved in histidine catabolism, in which affinity and channeling are enhanced with polyglutamate substrates.

The 10-CHO-$H_4PteGlu_n$ synthetase domain of cytoplasmic DCS catalyzes the formation of 10-CHO-$H_4PteGlu_n$ from formate and $H_4PteGlu_n$ accompanied by the hydrolysis of MgATP to MgADP. In contrast with DC activities, S has a very high affinity for its polyglutamate substrate. The K_m value for $H_4PteGlu_5$ for the rabbit liver enzyme is 0.1 μM and the binding of $H_4PteGlu_n$ and MgATP enhance the binding of formate. The activity of S from bacteria and mammals is stimulated by K^+ or by NH_4^+, but Na^+ and Li^+ have no effect (82). Spermine stimulates S from *Lactobacillus arabinosus* and *L. casei* by lowering the K_m of $H_4PteGlu_1$ (83). This observation is noteworthy because spermine reduces the amount of thymidine required to reverse the inhibition of growth of *L. arabinosus* by aminopterin and other antifolates (84). Therefore, spermine might play a regulatory role at the formyl level as well as at the methyl level mentioned above. Both of these stimulations could benefit growing cells by stimulating the formation of single-carbon units for methionine, thymidylate, and purine nucleotide synthesis.

In vitro kinetic studies with rabbit liver DCS coupled to SHMT suggest that the two proteins interact to facilitate the conversion of formate to serine (76). DCS plus SHMT provide an estimated in vivo concentration of 25 μM folate active sites, which indicates that most of the folate coenzymes in cells are protein bound.

Specific antifolate inhibitors of the DCS activities have not been reported.

5. 10-FORMYLTETRAHYDROFOLATE DEHYDROGENASE

10-Formyltetrahydrofolate dehydrogenase (FDH) is a homotetrameric cytosolic enzyme with a subunit molecular mass of 99 kDa (85). The rat enzyme has been cloned, sequenced, and expressed (86,87). Each subunit has three domains: an N-terminal domain (310 amino acids) that resembles glycinamide ribonucleotide formyltransferase, a

C-terminal domain (500 amino acids) that resembles aldehyde dehydrogenase, and a connecting peptide of 100 amino acids. It is likely that the major function of FDH is to catalyze the oxidation of the formyl group of 10-CHO-H_4PteGlu$_n$ to CO_2 using NADP as the hydrogen acceptor. This would provide egress of single-carbon units from the cellular one-carbon pool as well as providing NADPH for reductive reactions (Fig. 6). This function requires the appropriate juxtaposition of the NH_2-terminal and COOH-terminal domains provided by the connecting peptide. In addition, the NH_2-terminal domain catalyzes the hydrolysis of 10-CHO-H_4PteGlu$_n$ to H_4PteGlu$_n$ and formate. This activity, combined with that of C1THF synthase, leads to a futile cycle for the production and reincorporation of formate. The isolated COOH-terminal domain has aldehyde dehydrogenase activity and serves this function in the conversion of 10-CHO-H_4PteGlu$_n$ to CO_2 and H_4PteGlu$_n$ by FDH, the 10-CHO group corresponding to the aldehyde portion of formic acid.

FDH has a very high affinity (K_d = 20 nM) for both 10-CHO-H_4PteGlu$_5$ and H_4PteGlu$_5$, the latter being the product of both the dehydrogenase and hydrolase activities and a likely product inhibitor *(88)*. Both SHMT and C1THF synthase discharge H_4PteGlu$_5$ from FDH, thus FDH could serve as a distribution point for 10-CHO-H_4PteGlu$_5$ and H_4PteGlu$_5$.

In rat and rabbit liver FDH accounts for 1.2% of the soluble protein. This is equivalent to a concentration of FDH subunits of 42 μM in vivo *(88)*. Adding this to the concentration of folate-binding sites provided by SHMT plus C1THF synthase (26 μM) yields 68 μM. This reinforces the suggestion that most all the folate coenzymes, whose concentration in rabbit liver is estimated at 26 μM, are enzyme bound in vivo especially since the estimate of 68 μM for folate-binding sites does not include other folate enzymes or GNMT.

Since the N-terminal portion of FDH shows homology with GARFT, the GARFT inhibitors DDATHF (5,10-dideazatetrahydrofolate) and 5, DACTHF (a folate analog lacking the tetrahydropyrazine ring) were tested as inhibitors of rat liver FDH *(89)*. DDATHF showed an IC$_{50}$ of 48 μM but 5-DACTHF showed no inhibition at 340 μM. Polyglutamate derivatives were not tested, but this work opens the possibility of influencing FDH activity, and thus one-carbon metabolism, with folate analogs. In this connection it is of interest to consider mice that are totally lacking FDH *(90)*. Although these mice are able to grow and reproduce, their breeding time is greatly extended. The liver folates of these animals were compared with those of normal mice and 10-CHO-H_4PteGlu went from 2.8 nmol/g in normal mice to 7.3 nmol/g in the FDH-deficient mice, whereas H_4PteGlu went from 19.0 nmol/g in normals to 4.4 nmol/g in the deficient strain. Levels of 5-CHO-H_4PteGlu and 5-CH_3-H_4PteGlu were unchanged. These results are compatible with the loss of FDH in that the increase in 10-CHO-H_4PteGlu could be because of diminished ability to metabolize the CHO group and the decrease in H_4PteGlu could be caused by the loss of a major liver H_4PteGlu-binding protein.

6. 5,10-METHENYLTETRAHYDROFOLATE SYNTHETASE

5,10-methenyltetrahydrofolate synthetase (MTHFS) (formerly 5-formyltetrahydrofolate cyclodehydrase) catalyzes the irreversible MgATP-dependent conversion of 5-CHO-H_4PteGlu$_n$ to 5,10-CH-H_4PteGlu$_n$ *(91)*. As discussed above, 5-CHO-H_4PteGlu$_n$ is formed from 5,10-CH-H_4PteGlu$_n$ in a reaction catalyzed by SHMT. The reactions catalyzed by SHMT and MTHFS therefore constitute a futile cycle (Fig. 6) that is proposed to regulate cellular levels of 5-CHO-H_4PteGlu$_n$ an inhibitor of SHMT *(47)* and AICARFT *(49)*. MTHFS is the only known enzymatic reaction capable of returning 5-CHO-H_4PteGlu$_n$ to the major pathways of one-carbon metabolism and therefore is a key enzyme in the clinical uses of 5-CHO-H_4PteGlu for prevention of methotrexate toxicity and for enhancing the antitumor activity of fluorouracil.

Human MTHFS has been cloned, sequenced, and expressed *(91,92)*. It is a cytosolic 23-kDa protein with little homology to other folate enzymes except for an SLLP sequence found in most enzymes having 10-CHO-H_4PteGlu$_n$ as a substrate. It is highly homologous to rabbit liver MTHFS which was chemically sequenced earlier *(93)*. Some MTHFS has been found in human mitochondria *(91)*, but none in rabbit liver mitochondria *(92)*, which is surprising because 5-CHO-H_4PteGlu$_n$ is probably formed in vivo by rabbit liver mSHMT and would require a mechanism to re-enter the pool of mitochondrial folate coenzymes. However, folate polyglutamates can leave mitochondria *(4)*, which might replace the need for a mitochondrial MTHFS.

Human cytosolic and mitochondrial MTHFS have similar molecular weights and substrate affinities. Both forms show a much higher affinity for 5-CHO-H_4PteGlu$_5$ than for 5-CHO-H_4PteGlu$_1$, as does the rabbit liver cytosolic enzyme. A cDNA isoform for MTHFS encoding a mitochondrial signal sequence has not been reported.

5-CHO-H_4 homofolate (having an additional methylene group between the 9 and 10 positions of H_4PteGlu) is a competitive inhibitor of MTHFS. The K_i values are 0.1 μM for the rabbit enzyme *(94)* and 1.4 μM for human cytosolic enzyme *(91)*. 5-CHO-H_4 homofolate also behaves as a poor substrate for the reaction. The inhibition of MTHFS by 5-CHO-H_4 homofolate in MCF-7 cells provided important evidence that 5-CHO-H_4PteGlu$_n$ inhibits AICARFT in vivo as well as in vitro *(49)*.

7. GLYCINAMIDE RIBONUCLEOTIDE FORMYLTRANSFERASE (GARFT)

The *de novo* pathway for purine nucleotide biosynthesis consists of 10 enzyme-catalyzed reactions starting from 5-phosphoribosyl-1-pyrophosphate, leading to inosinic acid, the precursor of AMP and GMP *(95)*. Two reactions in this pathway, the third and the ninth, require 10-CHO-H_4PteGlu$_n$ as a formyl donor: glycinamide ribonucleotide formyltransferase and aminoimidazolecarboxamide ribonucleotide formyltransferase (AICARFT) (Fig. 7). The gene for mouse and human GARFT encodes a trifunctional protein of 110 kDa, the GARFT activity residing in the carboxy-terminal 29-kDa portion *(96)*. The other two activities on the trifunctional protein catalyze the second and fifth steps on the purine biosynthetic pathway, synthesis of glycinamide ribonucleotide and aminoimidazole ribonucleotide, respectively. The genes for both mouse and human trifunctional protein have been cloned and expressed and a fully functional 23-kDa human GARFT segment has been expressed as well *(95–97)*. The mouse and human genes are very similar.

10-formyl-5,8-dideazafolate and its polyglutamate derivatives are usually employed as substrates in enzymatic studies because they are more stable than the natural substrate, 10-CHO-H_4PteGlu$_n$. 10-formyl-5,8-dideazaPteGlu$_6$ binds to mouse GARFT 10 times more tightly than the monoglutamate *(98)*. These substrate analogs, their deformylated products, as well as the corresponding derivatives of the inhibitor, 5-10-dideazatetrahydrofolate (DDATHF), all bind to the enzyme very tightly with dissociation constants in

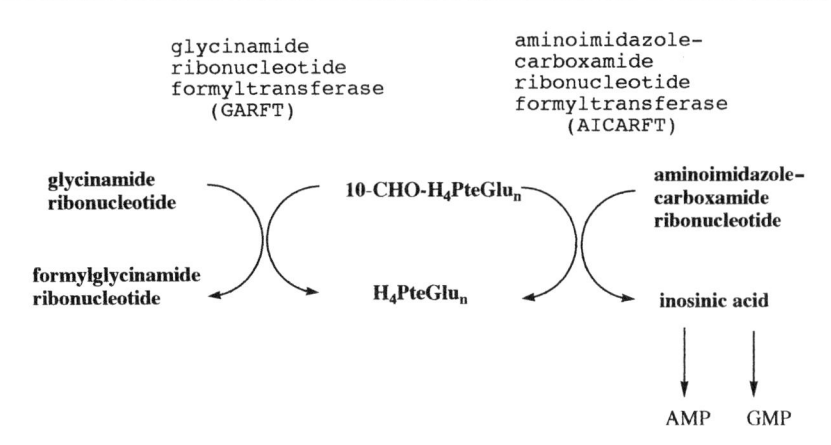

Fig. 7. Folate enzymes involved in purine nucleotide synthesis.

the nanomolar range. Therefore K_i values determined under the standard assay conditions do not reflect true dissocation constants. These studies (98) also show that the order of binding of the folate and GAR substrates is random sequential rather than ordered sequential, with the folate substrate binding first as was suggested by studies carried out under the standard conditions (97).

Site-directed mutagenesis studies have identified putative residues for the binding of the polyglutamate chain (99). These residues are located on the opposite lobe of GARFT from that which binds the pteridine portion of the cofactor. The polyglutamate substrate therefore appears to span the active site cleft of the enzyme.

8. AMINOIMIDAZOLECARBOXAMIDE RIBONUCLEOTIDE FORMYLTRANSFERASE (AICARFT)

The ninth and tenth steps on the pathway of the conversion of 5-phospho-ribosyl-1-pyrophosphate to inosinic acid are catalyzed by a bifunctional protein having AICARFT and inosine monophosphate cyclohydrolase (IMPCH) activity, respectively (Fig. 7). The human 64-kDa AICARFT has been cloned, sequenced, and expressed and the two activities have been expressed separately, a 39-kDa carboxy-terminal fragment containing AICARFT activity and a 25-kDa amino-terminal fragment containing IMPCH activity (100). Although both AICARFT and GARFT utilize 10-CHO-H_4PteGlu$_n$ as the formyl donor, there is very little sequence homology between the two enzymes. However, there is a high degree of homology between AICARFT/IMPCH amino acid sequences from different sources.

Polyglutamate forms of coenzymes and inhibitors are more effective with AICARFT than the monoglutamate forms. For example, methotrexate plus four glutamate residues is more than 2000-fold more inhibitory than methotrexate for AICARFT from MCF-7 cells with 10-CHO-H_4PteGlu$_1$ as substrate (101). With 10-CHO-H_4PteGlu$_5$ as substrate, however, the methotrexate polyglutamate was only sixfold more inhibitory than methotrexate. The true K_d values for folate and antifolate polyglutamates with AICARFT have not been determined as they have for GARFT (98). 10-CHO-5,8,10-trideazapteroic acid (102) is reported to be an effective inhibitor of human AICARFT (103).

9. METHIONYL tRNA$_f^{met}$ FORMYLTRANSFERASE

In animal mitochondria and in prokaryotes, the initiation of protein synthesis utilizes formyl tRNA$_f^{met}$ *(104)*. The tRNA$_f^{met}$ formyltransferase of animal mitochondria has not been studied extensively. 10-CHO-H$_4$PteGlu$_n$ is the formyl donor for the reaction for the *E. coli* enzyme which has a strong structural resemblence to *E. coli* GARFT *(105)*. An alternative system to initiate protein synthesis in mammalian mitochondria must be available since cultured cells grow in folate-free RPMI 1640 medium supplemented with thymidine and inosine. The human dietary requirement for folate therefore results from in vivo metabolite deficiencies.

10. FORMIMINOTRANSFERASE-CYCLODEAMINASE

The two activities of this protein serve to catalyze the conversion of the formimino group, arising as formiminoglutamic acid in histidine catabolism, to formimino H$_4$PteGlu$_n$ and then to 5,10-CH-H$_4$PteGlu$_n$. The porcine enzyme has been cloned, sequenced, and expressed *(106)*. It is a 480-kDa tetramer of dimers that channels formiminoH$_4$PteGlu$_5$ between the formiminotransferase and cyclodeaminase sites. Both activities require the formation of specific subunit interfaces *(107)*.

11. GLYCINE CLEAVAGE SYSTEM

The glycine-cleavage system is a tetrafunctional enzyme complex found in mitochondria that converts glycine to CO$_2$, NH$_3$, and 5,10-CH$_2$-H$_4$PteGlu$_n$ *(37,40)*. In the first step, P-protein, a pyridoxal phosphate enzyme, catalyzes the decarboxylation of glycine to CO$_2$ and an enzyme-bound methylamine group. In the second step, the enzyme-bound methylamine is transfered to lipoic acid (S-S) attached to H-protein. During this transfer, the lipoic acid is reduced to the SH level with the methylamine group still attached. In the third step, T-protein catalyzes the conversion of the attached methylamine to NH$_3$ and 5,10-CH$_2$-H$_4$PteGlu$_n$. The fourth step, the reoxidation of reduced lipoic acid by NAD is catalyzed by L-protein, which is dihydrolipoyl dehydrogenase, an enzyme shared among several mitochondrial α-keto acid dehydrogenases *(108,109)*. The four protein components, P,H,T, and L can be separated from one another by molecular-sieve chromatography.

The glycine cleavage system is the principle route for the catabolism of glycine in mammals and the system is stimulated by glucagon in rat hepatocytes *(110)*. Metabolic leisons in the glycine cleavage system are associated with nonketotic hyperglycinemia, a condition causing severe neurological symptoms in neonates *(111)*. It is suggested that the glycine cleavage system plays a role in regulating glycine levels near N-methyl-D-aspartate (NMDA) receptors in the central nervous system *(112)* that contain a glycine-specific site. Deficiency of the glycine cleavage system leads to increased levels of D-serine in mammalian brain. D-serine occurs naturally in mammalian brain and binds to the glycine site of NMDA receptors *(112)*.

cDNA clones encoding the P, H, T, and L components of the human glycine cleavage system have been isolated and their primary structures determined *(111)*. Lipoylated bovine H-protein has been expressed in *E. coli (108)*.

12. DIMETHYLGLYCINE DEHYDROGENASE AND SARCOSINE DEHYDROGENASE

These two mitochondrial enzymes provide a pathway for the conversion of the methyl groups of choline, betaine, and methionine to 5,10-CH_2-$H_4PteGlu_n$. Both rat liver enzymes contain covalently bound FAD, have kDa values near 100 and, as isolated, contain $H_4PteGlu_5$ *(113)*. Whereas sarcosine dehydrogenase is very specific for sarcosine, dimethylglycine dehydrogenase shows activity with many N-methyl compounds including sarcosine *(113)*. In the absence of $H_4PteGlu_n$ or if the folate site is blocked chemically, both enzymes continue to oxidize methyl groups unabated, yielding free formaldehyde stoichiometrically *(114,115)*. Dimethylglycine dehydrogenase from rat liver and from rabbit liver bind both $H_4PteGlu_1$ and $H_4PteGlu_5$ very tightly with K_d values < 1 µM *(44,115)*. Rat liver dimethylglycine dehydrogenase has been cloned *(116)*. The enzyme is present in highest amounts in liver and kidney, but low levels are found in many tissues *(117)*. FAD spontaneously binds covalently to rat dimethylglycine dehydrogenase and this binding aids in protein folding and mitochondrial import *(118)*. Sarcosinemia is found in mice lacking sacrcosine dehydrogenase *(119)*.

13. FOLYLPOLY-γ-GLUTAMATE SYNTHETASE

Folylpoly-γ-glutamate synthetase (FPGS) catalyzes the MgATP and K^+-dependent attachment of glutamate residues to the γ-position of folates and folate analog *(4)*. Cells lacking this enzyme cannot retain folates after their transport through the cell membrane and therefore cannot grow. FPGS activity in cells controls the level of folate polyglutamates in cells as well as the glutamate-chain length. Most folate enzymes have a higher affinity for polyglutamate forms of folate coenzymes and folate analogs. FPGS is found in the mitochondria and in the cytosol. Mitochondrial folate accumulation and cytosolic folate accumulation require the activity of mFPGS and cFPGS, respectively. However, pteroyltriglutamates synthesized in mitochondria can move to the cytoplasm and function there, whereas the reverse does not occur, indicating a unidirectional flow of mitochondrial folate triglutamates. Cells lacking mFPGS can synthesize thymidylate and purine nucleotides in the cytoplasm but require glycine for growth. Cells lacking cFPGS require thymine and purines for growth (methionine is routinely added to tissue-culture media) because the mitochondrial Glu chain lengths are longer than three and cannot pass into the cytosol. FPGS activity is increased in proliferating tissues and activity as well as mRNA levels increase after mitogen stimulation and decline during differentiation.

The 60-kDa human FPGS has been cloned, sequenced, and expressed. A single gene with an alternative splice site codes for cytosolic and mitochondrial FPGS, the mitochondrial transcript coding for a 42-residue amino-terminal leader sequence *(120–123)*. $H_4PteGlu_n$ and 10-CHO-$H_4PteGlu_n$ are much better substrates than the corresponding PteGlu, 5-CHO-$H_4PteGlu$, and 5-CH_3-$H_4PteGlu$ derivatives *(121)*. Thus, under conditions in which methionine synthase activity is low, 5-CH_3-$H_4PteGlu_1$ the major circulating form of folate produced in the liver is poorly polyglutamylated and is not retained after entering cells, leading to folate coenzyme deficiency.

Lowered expression of FPGS is associated with resistance to polyglutamylatable antifolates *(124)*.

14. GLUTAMYL HYDROLASE

γ-Glutamyl hydrolase (GH) catalyzes the hydrolytic cleavage of γ-linked polyglutamates *(125)*. A role for GH in regulating the levels of ptereoylpolyglutamates in cells is indicated since cells expressing high levels of this enzyme show resistance to the polyglutamylatable antifolate DDATHF *(126,127)*. The levels of methotrexate polyglutamates in human blast cells in vivo can be related to their sensitivity to treatment with methotrexate *(128)*. The extent of accumulation of methotrexate polyglutamates has been attributed to the relative activities of FPGS and GH *(129)*.

The gene encoding human GH has been cloned, sequenced, and expressed *(130)*. The 35-kDa protein product has four potential asparagine-containing glycoyslation sites and is a glycoprotein when purified from tissues. Human GH shows 74% homology with rat GH. However the two enzymes show a different pattern of polyglutamate products with $4\text{-}NH_2\text{-}10\text{-}CH_3PteGlu_5$ as a substrate. Human GH behaves like an exopeptidase, yielding a series of products containing from one to four Glu residues, whereas the rat enzyme is an endopeptidase yielding $4\text{-}NH_2\text{-}10\text{-}CH_3PteGlu_1$ (methotrexate) as the product. GH is found in lysosomes that have a transport system for methotrexate polyglutamates *(131)*. GH is also excreted from tumor cells *(132)*. Prostate-specific membrane antigen has GH activity *(133)*.

15. CONCLUSIONS

Advances in studies of the genes encoding folate enzymes are empowering investigators with knowledge of the expression of these genes in specific tissues, and tumors, during the cell cycle and during development. Further development of mathematical models of folate and antifolate transport and metabolism will aid in predicting the consequences of inhibiting a given enzyme or combination of enzymes. The interaction of folate enzymes with messenger RNA, the phosphorylation of TS, the potential role of polyamines as regulators, mechanisms of antifolate-induced apoptosis, and levels of DNA methylation are examples of exciting phenomena that could aid the understanding of antifolate selectivity. We eventually should be able to address such problems as:

1. Why do the target cells involved in methotrexate treatment of psoriasis or of rheumatoid arthritis not become resistant to methotrexate?
2. What is the metabolic basis of methotrexate selectivity in the treatment of choriocarcinoma?
3. What is the metabolic basis of the effect of diurnal rhythms on antifolate sensitivity?
4. What is the basis of lipophilic, nonpolyglutamylatable antifolate antitumor selectivity?
5. Why is methotrexate toxic to the liver where cells are not dividing?
6. What folate system is particularly sensitive to folate deprivation in the genesis of neural tube defects?
7. How can agents superior to methotrexate be designed based on knowledge of folate and antifolate metabolism, enzymes, and pharmacology?
8. Are there combinations of folates and antifolates that can maintain cytotoxicity and improve selectivity?

ACKNOWLEDGMENTS

The author is grateful to the following investigators for their helpful suggestions: R. Banerjee, G. P. Beardsley, R. J. Cook, A. Jackman, R. E. MacKenzie, F. Maley, R. Moran, M. G. Nair, V. Schirch, F. M. Sirotnak, P. Stover, and C. Wagner.

REFERENCES

1. Farber S, Diamond LK, Mercer RD, Sylvester RF, Jr, Wolff JA. Temporary remissions in acute leukemia in children produced by folic acid antagonist, 4-aminopteroyl-glutamic acid (aminopterin) *New Engl J Med* 1948;238:787–793.
2. Blakley RL, Benkovic, SJ (eds.). *Folates and Pterins,* vol. 1, John Wiley & Sons, NY, 1984.
3. Kisliuk RL. The biochemistry of folates, in Sirotnak FM, Burchall JJ, Ensminger WD, Montgomery JA, eds. Folate Antagonists as Therapeutic Agents. vol 1 Academic Press, Orlando, 1984, pp. 1–68.
4. Shane B. Folylpolyglutamate synthesis and role in the regulation of one-carbon metabolism. *Vitam Horm* 1989;45:263–235.
5. Wagner C. Biochemical role of folate in cellular metabolism, in Bailey LB (ed.) Folate in Health and Disease. Marcel Dekker, New York, 1995, pp. 23–42.
6. Refsum H, Ueland PM, Nygard O, Vollset SE. Homocysteine and cardiovascular disease. *Annu Rev Med* 1998;49:31–62.
7. Green R, Jacobsen DW. Clinical implications of hyperhomocysteinemia, in Bailey LB (ed.) Folate in Health and Disease. Marcel Dekker, New York, 1995, pp. 75–122.
8. Wang H, Yoshizumi M, Lai K, Tsai JC, Perrella MA, Haber E, Lee ME. Inhibition of growth and p21ras methylation in vascular endothelial cells by homocysteine but not cysteine. *J Biol Chem* 1997;272:25,380–25,385.
9. Scott JM, Wier DG, Kirke PN. Folate and neural tube defects, in Bailey, LB (ed.) *Folate in Health and Disease* Marcel Dekker, New York, 1995, pp. 329–360.
10. Sunden SLF, Renduchintala MS, Park EI, Miklasz SD, Garrow TA. Betaine-homocysteine methyltransferase expression in porcine and human tissues and chromosomal localization of the human gene. *Arch Biochem Biophys* 1997;345:171–174.
11. Green JM, Ballou DP, Matthews RG. Examination of the role of methylenetetrahydrofolate reductase in incorporation of methyltetrahydrofolate into cellular metabolism. *FASEB J* 1988;2:42–47.
12. Donaldson KO, Keresztesy JC. Enzymatic conversion of methylenetetrahydrofolate to methyltetrahydrofolate. *J Biol Chem* 1962;237:1298–1304.
13. Herbert V, Sullivan LW, Streiff RR, Friedkin M. Failure of menadione to affect folate utilization in vitamin B_{12}-deficient human beings. *Nature* 1964;201:196–197.
14. Ma J, Stampfer MJ, Hennekens CH, Frosst P, Selhub J, Horsford J, Manilow MR, Willet WC, Rozen R. Methylenetetrahydrofolate reductase polymorphism, plasma folate, homocysteine, and risk of myocardial infarction in US physicians. *Circulation* 1996;94:2410–2416.
15. Sheppard AC, Matthews RG. Studies on a mutant methylenetetrahydrofolate reductase that is associated with cardiovascular disease in humans. *Pteridines* 1997;8:68.
16. Li YN, Gulati S, Baker PJ, Brody LC, Banerjee R, Kruger WD. Cloning, mapping and RNA analysis of the human methionine synthase gene. *Hum Mol Genet* 1996;5:1851–1858.
17. Leclerc D, Campeau E, Goyette P, Adjalla CE, Christensen B, Ross M, Eydoux P, Rosenblatt DS, Rozen R, Gravel RA. Human methionine synthase: cDNA cloning and identification of mutations in patients of the cbl/G complementation group of folate/cobalamin disorders. *Hum Mol Genet* 1996;1867–1874.
18. Chen LH, Liu M-L, Hwang H-Y, Chen L-S, Korenberg J, Shane B. Human methionine synthase. *J Biol Chem* 1997;272:3628–3634.
19. Ludwig ML, Matthews RG. Structure-based perspectives on B_{12}-dependent enzymes. *Annu Rev Biochem* 1997;66:269–313.
20. Gulati S, Chen, ZQ, Brody LC, Rosenblatt DS, Banerjee R. Defects in auxiliary redox proteins lead to functional methionine synthase deficiency. *J Biol Chem* 1997;272:19,171–19,175.
21. Abels J, Kroes ACM, Ermens AAM, van Kapel J, Schoester M, Spijkers LJM, Lindemans J. Antileukemic potential of methyl-cobalamin inactivation by nitrous oxide. *Am J Hematol* 1990;34:128–131.

22. Fiskerstrand T, Ueland PM, Refsum H. Response of the methionine synthase system to short-term culture with homocysteine and nitrous oxide and its relation to methionine dependence. *Int J Cancer* 1997;72:301–306.
23. Fiskerstrand T, Ueland PM, Refsum H. Folate depletion induced by methotrexate affects methionine synthase activity and its susceptibility to inactivation by nitrous oxide. *J Pharm Exp Ther* 1997;282:1305–1311.
24. Banerjee RV, Matthews RG. Cobalamin-dependent methionine synthase. *FASEB J* 1990; 4:1450–1459.
25. McLean GR, Pathare PM, Wilbur DS, Morgan AC, Woodhouse CS, Schrader JW, Ziltener HJ. Cobalamin analogues modulate the growth of leukemia cells *in vitro*. *Cancer Res* 1997; 57:4015–4022.
26. Aposhian HV. Enzymatic, methylation of arsenic species and other new approaches to arsenic toxicity. *Annu Rev Pharmacol* 1997;37:397–419.
27. Bartolomei MS, Tilghman SM. Genomic imprinting in mammals. *Annu Rev Genetics* 1997; 31:493–526.
28. Capdevila A, Decha-Umphai W, Song, KH, Borchardt RT, Wagner C. Pancreatic exocrine secretion is blocked by inhibitors of methylation. *Arch Biochem Biophys* 1997;345:47–55.
29. Krupenko NI, Wagner G. Transport of rat liver glycine-N-methyltransferase into rat liver nuclei. *J Biol Chem* 1997;272:27,140–27,146.
30. Pogribny IP, Miller BJ, James SJ. Alterations in hepatic p53 gene methylation patterns during tumor progression with folate/methyl deficiency in the rat. *Cancer Lett* 1997;115:31–38.
31. Kim YI, Pogribny IP, Basnakian AG, Miller JW, Selhub J, James SJ, Mason JB. Folate deficiency in rats induces DNA strand breaks and hypomethylation within the p53 tumor suppressor gene. *Am J Clin Nutr* 1997;65:46–52.
32. Ruan H, Shantz LM, Pegg AE, Morris DR. The upstream open reading frame of the mRNA encoding S-adenosylmethionine decarboxylase is a polyamine-responsive translational control element. *J Biol Chem* 1996;271:29,576–29,582.
33. Kenyon SH, Nicolaou A, Ast T, Gibbons WA. Stimulation *in vitro* of vitamin B_{12}-dependent methionine synthase by polyamines. *Biochem J* 1996;316:661–665.
34. Kramer DL, Fogel-Petrovic M, Diegelman P, Cooley JM, Bernacki RJ, McManis JS, Bergerson RJ, Porter CW. Effects of novel spermine analogues on cell cycle suppression and apoptosis in MALME-3M human melanoma cells. *Cancer Res* 1997;57:5521–5527.
35. Houghton JA, Harwood FG, Tillman DM. Thymineless death in colon carcinoma cells is mediated via Fas signalling. *Proc Natl Acad Sci USA* 1997;94:8144–8149.
36. O'Dwyer PJ, King SA, Hoth DF, Leyland-Jones B. Role of thymidine in biochemical modulation. *Cancer Res* 1987;47:3911–3919.
37. Schirch V. Folates in serine and glycine metabolism. In *Folates and Pterins*, vol. 1 (Blakley RL, Benkovic SJ, eds) Wiley, New York, 1984, pp. 399–432.
38. Santi DV, Danenberg PV. Folates in pyrimidine nucleotide biosynthesis, in *Folates and Pterins*, vol. 1, (Blakley RL, Benkovic SJ, eds.) Wiley, New York, 1984;345–398.
39. Blakley RL. Dihydrofolate reductase, In (Blakley RL, Benkovic SJ, eds) *Folates and Pterins*. vol. 1 Wiley, New York, 1984, pp. 191–254.
40. Hayasaka K, Nano K, Takada G, Okamura-Ikeda K, Motokawa Y. Isolation and sequence determination of cDNA encoding human T-protein of the glycine cleavage system. *Biochem Biophys Res Commun* 1993;192:766–771.
41. Garrow TA, Brenner AA, Whitehead VM, Chen X-N, Duncan RG, Korenberg JR, Shane B. Cloning of human cDNAs encoding mitochondrial and cystosolic serine hydroxymethyltransferases and chromosomal localization. *J Biol Chem* 1993;268:11,910–11,916.
42. Stover PJ, Chen LH, Suh JR, Stover DM, Keyomarsi K, Shane B. Molecular cloning, characterization, and regulation of the human mitochondrial serine hydroxymethyltransferase gene. *J Biol Chem* 1997;272:1842–1848.
43. Matthews RG, Ross J, Baugh CM, Cook JD and Davis L. Interactions of pig liver serine hydroxymethyltransferase with methyltetrahydropteroylpolyglutamate inhibitors and with tetrahydropteroylpolyglutamate substrates. *Biochemistry* 1982;21:1230–1238.
44. Strong WB, Cook R, Schirch V. Interaction of tetrahydropteroylpolyglutamates with two enzymes from mitochondria. *Biochemistry* 1989;28:106–114.
45. Stover P, Schirch V. Serine hydroxymethyltransferase catalyzes the hydrolysis of 5, 10-methenyltetrahydrofolate to 5-formyltetrahydrofolate. *J Biol Chem* 1990;265:14,227–14,233.

46. Stover P, Schirch V. Enzymatic mechanism for the hydrolysis of 5,10-methenyltetrahydropteroylglutamate to 5-formyltetrahydropteroylglutamate by serine hydroxymethyltransferase. *Biochemistry* 1992;31:2155–2164.
47. Stover P, Schirch V. 5-Formyltetrahydrofolate polyglutamates are slow tight binding inhibitors of serine hydroxymethyltransferase. *J Biol Chem* 1991;266:1543–1550.
48. Friedkin M, Plante LT, Crawford EJ, Crumm M. Inhibition of thymidylate synthetase and dihydrofolate reductase by naturally occurring oligoglutamate derivatives of folic acid. *J Biol Chem* 1975;250:5614–5621.
49. Bertrand R, Jolivet J. Methenyltetrahydrofolate synthetase prevents the inhibition of phosphoribosyl 5-aminoimidazole 4-carboxamide ribonucleotide formyltransferase by 5-formyltetrahydrofolate polyglutamates. *J Biol Chem* 1989;264:8843–8846.
50. Stover P, Schirch V. The metabolic role of leucovorin. *Trends Biochem Sci* 1993;18:102–106.
51. Girgis S, Suh JR, Jolivet J, Stover PJ. 5-Formyltetrahydrofolate regulates homocysteine remethylation in human neuroblastoma. *J Biol Chem* 1997;272:4729–4734.
52. Wang EA, Kallen R, Walsh C. Mechanism-based inactivation of serine transhydroxymethylases by D-fluoroalanine and related amino acids. *J Biol Chem* 1981;256:6917–6926.
53. Webb HK, Matthews RG. 4-Chlorothreonine is substrate, mechanistic probe and mechanism-based inhibitor of serine hydroxymethyltransferase. *J Biol Chem* 1995;270:17,204–17,209.
54. Carreras CW, Santi DV. The catalytic mechanism and structure of thymidylate synthase. *Annu Rev Biochem* 1995;64:721–762.
55. Elcock AH, Potter MJ, Matthews DA, Knighton DR, McCammon JA. Electrostatic channeling in the bifunctional enzyme dihydrofolate reductase-thymidylate synthase. *J Mol Biol* 1996;262:370–372.
56. Davisson VJ, Sirawaraporn W, Santi DV. Expression of human thymidylate synthase in *Escherichia coli*. *J Biol Chem* 1989;264:9145–9148.
57. Pedersen-Lane J, Maley GF, Chu E, Maley F. High-level expression of human thymidylate synthase. *Protein Expression Purification* 1997;10:256–262.
58. Schiffer CA, Clifton IJ, Davisson VJ, Santi DV, Stroud RM. Crystal structure of human thymidylate synthase: a structural mechanism for guiding substrates into the active site. *Biochemistry* 1995;34:16,279–16,287.
59. Samsonoff WA, Reston J, McKee M, O'Connor B, Galivan J, Maley G, Maley F. Intracellular location of thymidylate synthase and its state of phosphorylation. *J Biol Chem* 1997;272:13,281–13,285.
60. Chu E, Voeller DM, Jones KL, Takechi T, Maley GF, Maley F, Segal S, Allegra CJ. Identification of a thymidylate synthase ribonucleoprotein complex in human colon cancer cells. *Mol Cell Biol* 1994;14:207–213.
61. Horie N, Takeishi K. Identification of functional elements in the promoter region of the human gene for thymidylate synthase and nuclear factors that regulate the expression of the gene. *J Biol Chem* 1997;272:18,375–18,381.
62. Ladner RD, Caradonna SJ. The human dUTPase gene encodes both nuclear and mitochondrial isoforms. *J Biol Chem* 1997;272:19,072–19,080.
63. Mol CD, Harris JM, Mcintosh EM, Tainer JA. Human dUTP pyrophosphatase: uracil recognition by a β-hairpin and active sites formed by three separate subunits. *Structure* 1996;4:1077–1092.
64. Blakley RL. Eukaryotic dihydrofolate reductase. *Adv Enzymol Mol Biol* 1995;70:23–102.
65. Davies JF, II, Delcamp TJ, Prendergast NJ, Ashford VA, Freisheim JH, Kraut J. Crystal structures of recombinant human dihydrofolate reductase complexed with folate and 5-deazafolate. *Biochemistry* 1990;29:9467–9479.
66. Stockman BJ, Nirmala NR, Wagner G, Delcamp TJ, De Yarman MT, Freisheim JH. Sequence-specific 1H and 15N resonance assignments for human dihydrofolate reductase in solution. *Biochemistry* 1992;31:218–229.
67. Spencer HT, Sleep SEH, Rehg JH, Blakley RL, Sorrentino BP. A gene transfer strategy for making bone marrow cells resistant to methotrexate. *Blood* 1996;87:2579–2587.
68. Zhao SC, Banerjee D, Mineshi S, Bertino JR. Post-transplant methotrexate administration leads to improved curability of mice bearing a mammary tumor transplanted with marrow transduced with a mutant human dihydrofolate reductase cDNA. *Hum Gene The* 1997;8:903–909.
69. Kumar P, Kisliuk RL, Gaumont Y, Freisheim JH, Nair MG. Inhibition of human dihydrofolate reductase by antifolyl polyglutamates. *Biochem Pharmacol* 1989;38:541–543.
70. Rosowsky A, Galivan J, Beardsley GP, Bader H, O'Conner BM, Rusello O, Moroson BA, DeYarman MT, Kerwar SS, Freisheim JH. Biochemical and biological studies on 2-desamino-2-methyl-

aminopterin, an antifolate the polyglutamates of which are more potent than the monoglutamate against three key enzymes of folate metabolism. *Cancer Res* 1992;52:2148–2155.

71. Chu E, Takimoto CH, Voeller D, Grem JI, Allegra CJ. Specific binding of human dihydrofolate reductase protein to dihydrofolate reductase messenger RNA *in vitro*. *Biochemistry* 1993;32:4756–4760.

72. Erican-Abali EA, Banerjee D, Waltham MC, Skacel N, Scotto KW, Bertino JR. Dihydrofolate reductase protein inhibits its own translation by binding to dihydrofolate reductase mRNA sequences within the coding region. *Biochemistry* 1997;36:12,317–12,322.

73. Fry CJ, Slansky JE, Farnham PJ. Position-dependent transcriptional regulation of the murine dihydrofolate reductase promoter by the E2F transactivation domain. *Mol Cell Biol* 1997;17:1966–1976.

74. MacKenzie RE. Biogenesis and interconversion of substituted tetrahydrofolates, in (Blakley RL, Benkovic SJ, eds) *Folates and Pterins* vol. 1 Wiley, New York, 1984, pp. 256–306.

75. Hum DW, Mackenzie RE. Expression of active domains of a human folate-dependent trifunctional enzyme in *Escherichia coli*. *Protein Eng* 1991;4:493–500.

76. Strong WB, Schirch V. In vitro conversion of formate to serine: effect of tetrahydropteroylpolyglutamates and serine hydroxymethyltransferase on the rate of 10-formyltetrahydrofolate synthetase. *Biochemistry* 1989;28:9430–9439.

77. Pelletier JN, Mackenzie RE. Binding and interconversion of tetrahydrofolates at a single site in the bifunctional methylenetetrahydrofolate dehydrogenase/cyclohydrolase. *Biochemistry* 1995;34:12,673–12,680.

78. Pawelek PD, MacKenzie RE. Methenyltetrahydrofolate cyclohydrolase is rate limiting for the enzymatic conversion of 10-formyltetrahydrofolate to 5,10-methylenetetrahydrofolate in bifunctional dehydrogenase-cyclohydrolase enzymes. *Biochemistry* 1998;37:1109–1115.

79. Pawelek PD, MacKenzie RE, Methylenetetrahydrofolate dehydrogenase-cyclohydrolase from *Photobacterium phosphoreum* shares properties with a mammalian mitochondrial homologue. *Biochim. Biophys Acta* 1996;1296:47–54.

80. Yang X, MacKenzie RE. NAD-dependent methylenetetrahydrofolate dehydrogenase-methenyltetrahydrofolate cyclohydrolase is the mammalian homolog of the mitochondrial enzyme encoded by the yeast MIS1 gene. *Biochemistry*, 1993;32:11,118–11,123.

81. Peri KG, Belanger C, MacKenzie RE. Nucleotide sequence of the human NAD-dependent methylenetetrahydrofolate dehydrogenase-cyclohydrolase. *Nucleic Acids Res* 1989;17:8853.

82. Paukert JL, D'Ari Straus L, Rabinowitz JC. Formyl-methenyl-methylenetetrahydrofolate synthetase-(combined). *J Biol Chem*, 1976;251:5104–5111.

83. Turner RB, Lansford EM Jr., Ravel JM, Shive W. A metabolic relationship of spermine to folinic acid and thymidine. *Biochemistry* 1963;2:163–167.

84. Lansford EM, Jr., Turner RB, Weathersbee CJ, Shive W. Stimulation by spermine of tetrahydrofolate formylase activity. *J Biol Chem* 1964;239:497–501.

85. Krupenko SA, Wagner C, Cook RJ. Recombinant 10-formyltetrahydrofolate dehydrogenase catalyzes both dehydrogenase and hydrolase reactions utilizing the synthetic substrate 10-formyl-5,8-dideazafolate. *Biochem J* 1995;306:651–655.

86. Krupenko SA, Wagner C, and Cook RJ. Expression, purification and properties of the aldehyde dehydrogenase homologous carboxyl-terminal domain of rat 10-formyltetrahydrofolate dehydrogenase. *J Biol Chem* 1997;272:10,266–10,272.

87. Krupenko SA, Wagner C, Cook RJ. Domain structure of rat 10-formyltetrahydrofolate dehydrogenase. *J Biol Chem* 1997;272:10,273–10,278.

88. Kim DW, Huang T, Schirch D, Schirch V. Properties of tetrahydropteroylpentaglutamate bound to 10-formyltetrahydrofolate dehydrogenase. *Biochemistry* 1996;35:15,772–15,783.

89. Cook RJ, Wagner C. Enzymatic activities of rat liver cytosol 10-formyltetrahydrofolate dehydrogenase. *Arch Biochem Biophys*, 1995;321:336–344.

90. Champion KM, Cook RJ, Tollaksen SL, Glometti CS. Identification of a heritable deficiency of the folate-dependent enzyme 10-formyltetrahydrofolate dehydrogenase in mice. *Proc Natl Acad Sci USA* 1994;91:11,338–11,342.

91. Jolivet J. Human 5,10-methenyltetrahydrofolate synthetase. *Methods Enzymol* 1997;281:162–170.

92. Dayan A, Bertrand R, Beauchemin M, Chahla D, Mamo A, Filion M, Skup D, Massie B, Jolivet J. Cloning and characterization of the human 5,10-methenyltetrahydrofolate synthetase-encoding cDNA. *Gene* 1995;165:307–311.

93. Maras B, Stover P, Valiante S, Barra D, Schirch V. Primary structure and tetrahydropteroylglutamate binding site of rabbit liver cytosolic 5,10-methenyltetrahydrofolate synthetase. *J Biol Chem* 1994;269:18,429–18,433.
94. Huang T, Schirch V. Mechanism for the coupling of ATP hydrolysis to the conversion of 5-formyltetrahydrofolate to 5,10-methenyltetrahydrofolate. *J Biol Chem* 1995;270:22,296–22,230.
95. Rowe PB. Folates in the biosynthesis and degradation of purines, in *Folates and Pterins,* vol. 1 (Blakley, RL, Benkovic SJ, eds) Wiley, New York, 1984, pp. 329–344.
96. Kan JL, Moran RG. Intronic polyadenylation in the human glycinamide ribonucleotide formyltransferase gene. *Nucleic Acids Res* 1997;25:3118–3123.
97. Caperelli CA, Giroux EL. The human glycinamide ribonucleotide transformylase domain: purification, characterization and kinetic mechanism. *Arch Biochem Biophys* 1997;341:98–103.
98. Sanghani S, Moran RG. Tight binding of folate substrates and inhibitors to recombinant mouse glycinamide ribonucleotide formyltransferase. *Biochemistry* 1997;36:10506–10516.
99. Pouliot JM, Beardsley GP, Almassey RJ. The polyglutamate binding region of human glycinamide ribonucleotide formyltransferase (hGARFT) spans the putative active site cleft. *Pteridines* 1997;8:129.
100. Rayl EA, Moroson BA, Beardsley GP. The human purH gene product, 5-aminoimidazole-4-carboxamide ribonucleotide formyltransferase/IMP cyclohydrolase. Cloning, sequencing, expression, purification, kinetic analysis and domain mapping. *J Biol Chem* 1996;271:2225–2233.
101. Allegra CJ, Drake JC, Jolivet J, Chabner BA. Inhibition of phosphoribosylaminoimidazolecarboxamide transformylase by methotrexate and dihydrofolic acid polyglutamates. *Proc Natl Acad Sci USA* 1985;82:4881–4885.
102. Liu L, Nair MG, Kisliuk RL. Novel nonclassical inhibitors of glycinamide ribonucleotide formyltransferase: 10-formyl and 10-hydroxymethyl derivatives of 5,8,10-trideazapteroic acid. *J Mol Recognition* 1996;9:169–174.
103. Gunn K, Beardsley GP, Worland S, Davies J, Nair MG. Identification of the substrate binding and catalytic sites of the 5-aminoimidazolecarboxamide ribonucleotide (AICAR) formyltransferase activity in the human *pur* H gene product. *Pteridines* 1997;8:130.
104. Staben C, Rabinowitz JC. Formation of formylmethionyl-tRNA and initiation of protein synthesis, in *Folates and Pterins*, vol. 1 (Blakley, RL, Benkovic SJ, eds.) Wiley, New York, 1984, pp. 457–495.
105. Schmitt E, Blanquet S, Mechulam Y. Structure of crystalline *Escherichia coli* methionyl-tRNAfmet formyltransferase: comparison with glycinamide ribonucleotide formyltransferase. *EMBO J* 1996;15:4749–4758.
106. Murley LL, Mejia NR, MacKenzie RE. The nucleotide sequence of porcine formiminotransferase cyclodeaminase. Expression and purification from *Escherichia coli. J Biol Chem* 1993;268:22820–22824.
107. Murley LL, MacKenzie RE. The two monofunctional domains of octameric formiminotransferase-cyclodeaminase exist as dimers. *Biochemistry* 1995;34:10,358–10,364.
108. Fujiwara K, Okamura-Ikeda K, Packer L, Motokawa Y. Synthesis and characterization of selenolipoylated H-protein of the glycine cleavage system. *J Biol Chem* 1997;272:19,880–19,883.
109. Johnson M, Yang HS, Johanning GL, Patel MS. Characterization of the mouse dihydrolipoamide dehydrogenase (Dld) gene: genomic structure, promoter sequence, and chromosomal localization. *Genomics* 1997;41:320–326.
110. Mabrouk GM, Bronsan JT. Activation of the hepatic glycine cleavage system by glucagon and glucagon-related peptides. *Can J Physiol Pharmacol* 1997;75:1096–1100.
111. Kure S, Tada K, Narisawa K. Nonketotic hyperglycinemia: biochemical molecular and neurological aspects. *Jpn J Hum Genet* 1997;42:13–22.
112. Iwama I, Takahashi K, Kure S, Hayashi F, Narisawa K, Tada K, Mizoguchi M, Takashima S, Tomita U, Nishikawa T. Depletion of cerebral D-serine in non-ketotic hyperglycinemia: possible involvement of glycine cleavage system in control of endogenous D-serine. *Biochem Biophys Res Commun* 1997;231:793–796.
113. Wittwer AJ, Wagner C. Identification of the folate-binding proteins of rat liver mitochondria as dimethylglycine dehydrogenase and sarcosine dehydrogenase. *J Biol Chem* 1981;256:4102–4108, 4109–4115.
114. Wagner C, Briggs WT, Cook RJ. Covalent binding of folic acid to dimethylglycine dehydrogenase. *Arch Biochem Biophys* 1984;233:457–461.

115. Porter DH, Cook RJ, Wagner C. Enzymatic properties of dimethylglycine dehydrogenase and sarcosine dehydrogenase from rat liver. *Arch Biochem Biophys* 1985;243:396–407.
116. Lang H, Polster M, Brandsch R. Rat liver dimethylglycine dehydrogenase: flavinylation of the enzyme in hepatocytes in primary culture and characterization of a complementary DNA clone. *Eur J Biochem* 1991;198:793–800.
117. Lang R, Minaian K, Freudenberg N, Hoffman R, Brandsch R. Tissue specificity of rat mitochondrial dimethyglycine dehydrogenase expression. *Biochem J* 1994;299:393–398.
118. Otto A, Stoltz M, Sailer H-P, Brandsch R. Biogenesis of the covalently flavinylated mitochondrial enzyme dimethylglycine dehydrogenase. *J Biol Chem* 1996;271:9823–9829.
119. Brunialti AL, Harding CO, Wolff JA, Guenet JL. The mouse mutation sarcosinemia (sar) maps to chromosome 2 in a region homologous to human 9q33–q34. *Genomics* 1996;36:182–184.
120. Garrow TA, Admon A, Shane B. Expression cloning of a human cDNA encoding folylpoly(γ-glutamate) synthetase and determination of its primary structure. *Proc Natl Acad Sci USA* 1992;89:9151–9155.
121. Chen L, Qi H, Korenberg J, Garrow TA, Choi Y-J, Shane B. Purification and properties of human cytosolic folypoly-γ-glutamate synthetase and organization, localization, and differential splicing of its gene. *J Biol Chem* 1996;271:13,077–13,087.
122. Freemantle SJ, Taylor SM, Krystal G, Moran RG. Upstream organization of and multiple transcripts from the human folylpoly-γ-glutamate synthetase gene. *J Biol Chem* 1995;270:9579–9584.
123. Freemantle SJ, Moran RG. Transcription of the human folylpoly-γ-glutamate synthetase gene. *J Biol Chem* 1997;272:25,373–25,379.
124. Roy K, Egan MG, Sirlin S, Sirotnak FM. Posttranscriptionally mediated decreases in folypolyglutamate synthetase gene expression in some folate analogue resistant variants of the L1210 cell. Evidence for an altered cognate mRNA in the variants affecting the rate of de novo synthesis of the enzyme. *J Biol Chem* 1997;272:6903–6908.
125. McGuire JJ, Coward JK. Pteroylpolyglutamates: biosynthesis, degradation and function, in *Folates and Pterins,* vol. 1 (Blakley RL, Benkovic SJ, vol. 1). Wiley, New York, 1984, pp. 135–190.
126. Samuels LL, Goutas LJ, Priest DG, Piper JR, Sirotnak FM. Hydrolytic cleavage of methotexate γ-polyglutamates by folylpolyglutamate hydrolase derived from various tumors and normal tissues of the mouse. *Cancer Res.* 1986;46:2230–2235.
127. Yao R, Rhee MS, Galivan J. Effects of γ-glutamyl hydrolase on folyl and antifolylpolyglutamates in cultured H35 hepatoma cells. *Mol Pharmacol* 1995;48:505–511.
128. Whitehead VM, Vuchich MJ, Lauer SJ, Mahoney D, Carroll AJ, Shuster JJ, Esseltine DW, Payment C, Look AT, Akabutu J, Bowen T, Taylor LD, Camitta B, Pullen DJ. Accumulation of high levels of methotrexate polyglutamates in lymphoblasts from children with hyperdiploid (> 50 chromosomes) B-lineage acute lymphoblastic leukemia: a pediatric oncology group study. *Blood* 1992; 80: 1316–1323.
129. Longo GSA, Gorlick R, Tong WP, Lin SL, Steinherz P, Bertino JR. γ-Glutamyl hydrolase and folylpolyglutamate synthetase activities predict polyglutamylation of methotrexate in acute leukemias. *Oncol Res* 1997;9:259–263.
130. Yao R, Schneider E, Ryan TJ, Galivan J. Human γ-glutamyl hydrolase: cloning and characterization of the enzyme expressed *in vitro. Proc Natl Acad Sci USA* 1996;93:10,134–10,138.
131. Barrueco JR, O'Leary DF, Sirotnak FM. Facilitated transport of methotrexate polyglutamates into lysosomes derived from S180 cells. *J Biol Chem* 1992;267:19,986–19,991.
132. Yao R, Nimec Z, Ryan TJ, Galivan J. Identification, cloning, and sequencing of a cDNA coding for rat γ-glutamyl hydrolase. *J Biol Chem* 1996;271:8525–8528.
133. Heston WD. Characterization and glutamyl preferring carboxypeptidase function of prostate specific membrane antigen: a novel folate hydrolase. *Urology* 1997;49:104–112.

3   Clinical Pharmacology and Resistance to Dihydrofolate Reductase Inhibitors

Richard Gorlick and Joseph R. Bertino

CONTENTS

INTRODUCTION
MECHANISM OF METHOTREXATE ACTION
CLINICAL PHARMACOLOGY OF METHOTREXATE
RESISTANCE MECHANISMS TO METHOTREXATE IN EXPERIMENTAL
  TUMORS
INTRINSIC RESISTANCE TO METHOTREXATE
ACQUIRED RESISTANCE TO METHOTREXATE
TUMOR-SUPPRESSOR GENES AND DRUG RESISTANCE
STRATEGIES TO OVERCOME OR EXPLOIT METHOTREXATE
  RESISTANCE
REFERENCES

1. INTRODUCTION

It has been almost 50 years since aminopterin, the first drug capable of inducing complete remissions in children with acute lymphoblastic leukemia (ALL), was first tested *(1)*. Methotrexate (MTX), also an antifolate inhibitor of dihydrofolate reductase (DHFR), soon after replaced aminopterin in the clinic and is used widely not only for the treatment of various forms of cancer, such as lymphoma, germ-cell tumors, breast cancer, and head and neck cancer but also for the treatment of autoimmune diseases such as rheumatoid arthritis, psoriasis, and for the prevention of graft-vs-host disease *(2)*. Although dramatic responses and even cures are observed in some malignancies with MTX treatment alone or in combination, in the majority of tumors, intrinsic resistance limits effectiveness. In malignancies that are initially sensitive to therapy, e.g., ALL, acquired resistance may develop, contributing to treatment failure and relapse *(3)*.

During the past decade, application of new discoveries have made it possible to identify and study the changes associated with intrinsic and acquired resistance to MTX in

From: *Anticancer Drug Development Guide: Antifolate Drugs in Cancer Therapy*
Edited by: A.L. Jackman © Humana Press Inc., Totowa, NJ

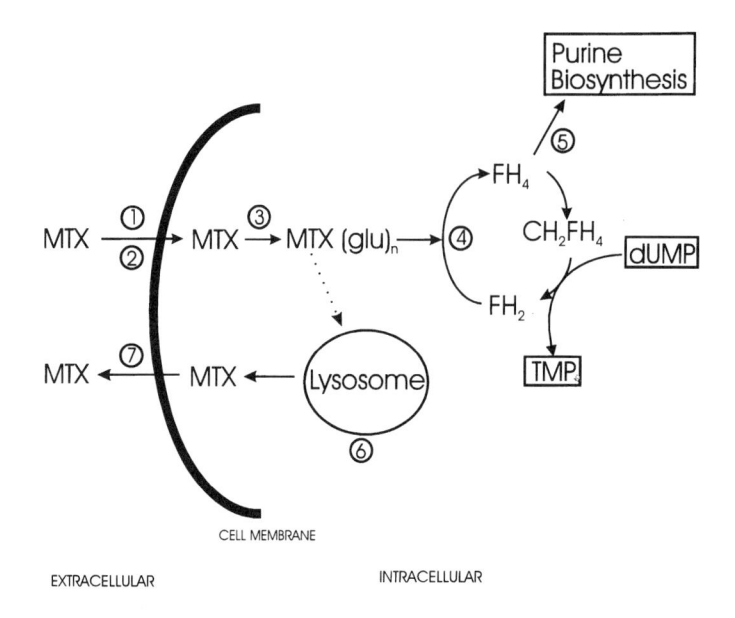

Fig. 1. MTX metabolism and action: MTX is taken up by mammalian cells by the reduced folate carrier (1) and by an endocytic pathway activated by a folate receptor (2). Once inside the cell, MTX is polyglutamylated by the enzyme FPGS (3). Both MTX and MTX(glu)$_n$ act as potent inhibitors of DHFR (4) and by depleting cells of tetrahydrofolate (FH$_4$) inhibits thymidylate synthesis. By inhibition of FH$_4$ formation as well as by direct inhibition of GAR and AICAR transformylase, MTX inhibits purine biosynthesis (5). MTX polyglutamates are transported into and hydrolyzed in the lysosome to monoglutamate forms by the enzyme GGH (6). Free MTX is rapidly effluxed (7).

tumors from patients. Sensitive molecular techniques have been increasingly applied to these studies as many of the genes involved in folate and antifolate metabolism have been recently cloned. In particular, the study of ALL presents a unique opportunity to determine mechanisms of acquired resistance to MTX, as relatively pure populations of blast cells can be obtained before treatment and at relapse. Acute myeloid leukemia (AML) blasts, soft tissue sarcoma, and epidermoid cancers have been investigated as examples of malignancies intrinsically resistant to this agent.

2. MECHANISM OF METHOTREXATE ACTION

Although MTX action is now understood in considerable detail, we continue to learn more about this drug in relation to folate metabolism (Fig. 1). MTX enters cells through an active carrier transport mechanism used by reduced folates or by binding to folate receptors (FR) and entering through an endocytic pathway *(4–6)*. Once inside the cell, MTX is polyglutamylated, i.e., additional glutamates (up to five) are added via linkage to the γ-carboxyl of glutamate. MTX polyglutamates are retained for longer periods in cells compared to MTX, thus the level of MTX polyglutamates achieved in tumor cells after MTX administration is an important determinant of cytotoxicity *(7)*. MTX and MTX polyglutamates bind tightly to the enzyme DHFR, thus inhibiting tetrahydrofolate formation, required for thymidylate biosynthesis. In addition MTX polyglutamates as well as dihydrofolate polyglutamates (the latter accumulated because of DHFR inhibition) inhibit the enzymes of purine synthesis, including 5'-phosphoribosylglycinamide (GAR) and aminoimidazole carboxamide ribonucleotide (AICAR) transformylases *(8,9)*. Recent findings regarding MTX action and resistance mechanisms are reviewed in the following sections.

2.1. Methotrexate Transport

Folates are transported into cells via the reduced folate carrier (RFC) or by an endocytic mechanism termed potocytosis, which requires binding to glycosylphosphatidylinositol anchored FR in cell membranes *(10,11)*. The FR and RFC are expressed at different levels in different tissues, with some cells, such as leukemic blasts expressing both proteins *(12)*. The RFC transport pathway has a high turnover number and has a higher affinity for MTX and reduced folates (approx 1–5 µM) than for folic acid (100–200 µM) *(12)*. The cDNA for the RFC has been recently identified in hamster, mouse, and human cells *(13–18)*. In contrast to the RFC the FR, are low capacity transporters with a high affinity for folic acid (1 nM) and the reduced folates 5-formyl and 5-methyltetrahydrofolate (10–40 nM) and a lower affinity for MTX and other 4-amino-antifolates (0.15–1.7 µM) *(12)*. The distribution of this protein(s) as studied by immunohistochemistry is limited to a few normal tissues that include the kidney tubules and the choroid plexus *(19)*. Its function may be to conserve or partition folates in specific tissues. Certain tumors, especially ovarian cancer, have high levels of this protein *(20)*. In cell lines expressing both the FR and the RFC, overall drug sensitivity to MTX and certain other folate antagonists appeared to correlate with differential efficacy of drug transport via the RFC rather than by the FR *(21)*.

2.2. Methotrexate Polyglutamylation

Intracellular MTX polyglutamates are generated by the enzyme folylpolyglutamate synthetase (FPGS), whereas catabolism of MTX polyglutamates is dependent on the rates of entry of polyglutamates into lysosomes, and hydrolysis by the lysosomal enzyme gamma-glutamyl hydrolase (GGH) (Fig. 1). Mammalian FPGS is well characterized enzymatically and catalyzes the addition of glutamates to all naturally occurring folates as well as many folate analogs including MTX *(22)*. The cDNA encoding this gene has been identified *(23)*. Recent studies have further elucidated the genomic organization of the gene encoding this enzyme and have identified numerous splice variants in the mouse and human FPGS gene *(24–26)*. Recent studies suggest that there may be differences in the kinetic properties of FPGS in different cell types *(27)*.

Compared to FPGS, less is known about GGH. Whereas it is generally accepted that the predominant lysosomal enzyme form is the most important in regulation of folate and antifolate polyglutamate chain length, the content and specificity of the enzyme varies markedly across cell types, tissues, and different species *(28)*. For example, GGH from rodent cultured cells is primarily an endopeptidase *(29,30)*, whereas the enzyme from human sarcoma cells (HT-1080) displays almost exclusive exopeptidase activity under identical conditions *(31)*. The recent identification of the cDNA for rat and human GGH will allow a determination of the role of GGH *(32,33)*. Glutamine antagonists that are inhibitors of human GGH, such as 6-diazo-5-oxo-L-norleucine (DON) have been identified and will aid in elucidating the role of GGH in MTX metabolism *(31)*.

2.3. Translational Autoregulation

Administration of MTX to patients leads to an increase in the level of DHFR protein (mostly bound to MTX) in both normal and leukemic leukocytes as well as in erythrocytes within hours to days *(34)*. Studies carried out in vitro using a lymphoblastoid cell line showed that an increase in DHFR protein was not inhibited by actinomycin D but was abrogated by cycloheximide treatment, suggesting that the increase was not caused by increased transcription. The rapid increase in DHFR observed after MTX treatment could not be explained by either protection of DHFR from degradation by bound MTX and/or dihydrofolate, or to an increase in translation of this enzyme *(34)*. An increase in thymidylate synthase (TS) activity has also been reported to occur in tumor cells after 5-fluorouracil treatment, and it has been suggested that this increase may be caused by regulation at a translational level *(35)*. Using a rabbit reticulocyte translation system our laboratory has found that DHFR protein inhibits its own synthesis *(36)*. The reversal of this inhibition by MTX or dihydrofolate may partially explain the observed increase of DHFR activity in normal and leukemic cells after MTX treatment *(36)*. Recent experiments have revealed that a small region toward the 3' end of its coding region may be involved in the binding *(37)*. The relationship between this increase of DHFR protein after MTX administration and resistance to MTX is not clear.

3. CLINICAL PHARMACOLOGY OF METHOTREXATE

3.1. Pharmacokinetics (for reviews, see refs. 38,39)

MTX can be absorbed orally through a saturable active transport system but its uptake is unpredictable and relatively poor *(40,41)*. Absorption decreases with increasing dosage, but even at low doses ($< 15 mg/m^2$) absorption may be less than 50% *(38)*. Peak plasma concentrations occur 1 to 5 h after a dose but food, nonabsorbable antibiotics, and a decreased intestinal transit time will decrease the rate and extent of MTX absorption *(38,42)*.

After iv administration, MTX distributes with a volume that approximates that of total body water following an initial distribution phase *(39)*. MTX binding to plasma proteins is approx 50% *(43)*. The entry of MTX into the cerebrospinal fluid is poor and cytocidal concentrations in the cerebrospinal fluid are not achieved with conventional systemic doses *(44)*. MTX penetrates and exits slowly from peritoneal and pleural fluid collections *(45)*. This can lead to prolonged elevations of serum MTX concentrations, which can be problematic when high drug doses are employed. It may be advisable to evacuate these fluid collections prior to drug administration or alternatively, plasma concentrations of MTX should be monitored closely with prolonged leucovorin (LV) rescue administered in these cases *(38,39)*.

The bulk of drug administered, is excreted in the urine in the first 12 h following administration *(39,46)*. This initial phase of drug disappearance from the plasma has a half life of three to four h and is almost entirely determined by the rate of renal excretion *(47)*. A second phase of drug disappearance is also observed with a longer half life of 6 to 20 h and represents reabsorption in the gut and secondary excretion *(38,42)*. When high dose MTX ($> 6 g/m^2$) is administered, rapid drug excretion may lead to high concentrations of MTX in the urine. Particularly, if the urine is acidic the solubility of the drug can be exceeded which may lead to intrarenal precipitation and renal failure. Administration of vigorous hydration and alkalinization of the urine are therefore recommended for high dose MTX therapy *(39,48)*.

MTX undergoes uptake and metabolism in the liver. MTX is transported into hepatocytes and converted to polyglutamate forms that can persist for several months following administration *(39,49)*. Following iv MTX administration, from 6.7 to 20% of the administered dose will enter the biliary tract. Less than 10% of administered MTX will be eliminated in the feces, consistent with other experiments demonstrating that enterohepatic circulation of MTX occurs *(38,50)*.

The major pathway of metabolic inactivation of MTX is hydroxylation by hepatic aldehyde oxidase to 7-hydroxy MTX. This compound is only 1% as potent of a DHFR inhibitor, as compared to MTX *(51–53)*. A second pathway of metabolic inactivation occurs in the intestine where bacteria hydrolyze MTX to 4-amino-4-deoxy-N10-methyl pteroic acid (dAMPA) and glutamic acid *(54)*. Both this metabolite and 7-hydroxy MTX are less water soluble than MTX. The role of these compounds in producing MTX toxicity is unclear but their lack of solubility suggests they may contribute to the renal toxicity observed frequently following high dose MTX therapy *(38,53)*.

Several drugs used in cancer patients may increase toxicity of MTX if administered concomitantly. Fatal reactions have occurred with the simultaneous use of MTX and nonsteroidal anti-inflammatory agents, particularly naproxen and ketoprofen *(55,56)*. This may be secondary to decreased renal elimination secondary to competition. Increased toxicity has also been reported when trimethoprim is used together with MTX. Trimethoprim also an antifolate presumably lowers folate stores making bone-marrow cells more susceptible to MTX-induced toxicity *(57)*.

3.2. Methotrexate Toxicity

The primary toxic effects of DHFR inhibitors are on self-renewing cell populations, particularly bone marrow and the gastrointestinal tract, resulting in myelosuppression and gastrointestinal toxicity, in particular mucositis *(38,39)*. The incidence of these toxicities depends on the dose, schedule, and route of drug administration *(39)*. Myelosuppression affects bone marrow progenitors of all lineages, but predominantly results in neutropenia which recovers rapidly in 14 to 21 d following a nadir approx 10 d after administration of a single dose of methotrexate. The effects on marrow are dose related but a large intrapatient variability is observed *(38)*.

Mucositis is a common side effect of MTX treatment and occurs approx 3–5 d following a dose of the drug. More severe gastrointestinal toxicity is manifested by diarrhea that can become bloody. Nausea and vomiting with MTX is mild to moderate and rarely requires the use of antiemetics *(38)*.

Severe renal toxicity can be observed following the administration of high-dose MTX. This toxicity is believed to be the result of MTX precipitation in the renal tubules as well as a direct drug effect *(38,39,53)*. The incidence of this toxicity has been significantly reduced by vigorous hydration and alkalinization of the urine, following high-dose MTX administration *(38,39,48)*. The guidelines for LV rescue and hydration for some of the high-dose MTX regimens in current use are presented in Table 1. Occasional patients, despite hydration and alkalinization, develop significant renal impairment. In these patients, prolonged LV rescue or alternatively thymidine rescue will ameliorate toxicity *(58,59)*. Recent studies have demonstrated the value of carboxypeptidase G1, an

Table 1
Regimens for High-Dose Methotrexate (MTX) Therapy

Hydration and Urinary Alkalinization

MTX Dose (g/m^2)	Infusion Duration (h)	Leucovorin (LV) Rescue	Onset of LV Rescue (h after MTX start)	Onset of MTX level monitoring (h after MTX start)
0.5–3.0	0.3–0.5	15 mg/m²q 6 hr × 6 doses	24	24
8–12	4	10 mg q 6h × 10 doses	24	24
1.2–6	6	15 mg/m² q 6 hr × 7 doses	8	48
1–1.5	24–36	25 mg/m²q 6 hr × 7 doses	36	48

Administer 2.5–3.5 L/m²/d of iv fluids starting 12 h prior to MTX infusion. The fluid should contain 45–100 mEq/L sodium bicarbonate to ensure urine pH is greater than 7.0 at the time of drug infusion.

Drug Monitoring

MTX	Leucovorin Dose
$5 \times 10^{-7} M$	15 mg/m² q 6 hr × 8 doses
$1 \times 10^{-6} M$	100 mg/m² q 6 hr × 8 doses
$2 \times 10^{-6} M$	200 mg/m2 q 6 hr × 8 doses

In general MTX levels of greater than $1 \times 10^{-5} M$ at 24 h and levels of greater than $5 \times 10^{-7} M$ at 48 h after the start of MTX infusion require additional LV rescue. General guidelines for leucovorin rescue are presented below.

MTX drug levels should be repeated every 24 h and the dose of leucovorin adjusted until the MTX level is less than $5 \times 10^{-6} M$.

Adapted from refs. *38,39*.

enzyme capable of cleaving the peptide bond in MTX resulting in its metabolic inactivation, in reducing elevated MTX blood levels and decreasing toxicity *(60)*.

Elevations of the liver transaminases (SGOT, SGPT) are common several days following the administration of high-dose methotrexate, but rapidly return to normal *(61)*. Chronic, low-dose, continuous treatment with MTX has been associated with portal fibrosis and cirrhosis. Alcohol and other hepatotoxic drugs should be avoided in patients receiving chronic MTX as it increases the frequency of hepatotoxicity *(38)*.

The most common side effect of intrathecal MTX administration is a chemical arachnoiditis that is manifested by headache, fever, meningismus, vomiting, and cerebrospinal fluid pleocytosis *(38,39)*. More serious neurotoxicity includes motor paralysis, cranial nerve palsies, seizure, and coma and this usually occurs subacutely, during the second or third week of intrathecal therapy *(38,39)*. A severe chronic demyelinating encephalopathy has also been observed with intrathecal MTX, usually in association with cranial irradiation. These patients develop dementia, motor spasticity, and coma, months to years after therapy *(38,39)*. A rare transient cerebral dysfunction syndrome (paresis, aphasia, seizure) has also been reported in patients receiving systemic MTX and usually physical signs resolve within 2 to 3 d *(38,39,62)*.

Other toxicities observed with MTX include pneumonitis, cutaneous rashes, and teratogenic effects. The pneumonitis is extremely uncommon and self limited, manifesting as cough, tachypnea, fever, and hypoxemia *(63,64)*. Skin toxicity is observed in 5 to 10% of patients and consists of an erythematous, pruritic rash usually involving the neck and upper trunk. When MTX toxicity is severe, the rash can progress to bullae formation and desquamation. Cutaneous photosensitivity is also observed following MTX treatment *(65)*. MTX is a potent abortifacient and has been used therapeutically for that purpose *(66)*.

3.3. Clinical Uses of Methotrexate

MTX has been administered utilizing a variety of different dose schedules both orally and parenterally. High-dose MTX therapy is administered with LV rescue. The regimen used varies based on the specific tumor being treated as well as the other antineoplastic agents being utilized. Schedule as well as dose may be important determinants of efficacy *(3,38,39)*. MTX has been shown to be synergistic in combination with many other chemotherapeutic agents including 5-fluorouracil, L-asparaginase, cytosine arabinoside, 6-thioguanine, and 6-mercaptopurine. MTX is used in the treatment of a variety of malignancies. It is a major component of the maintenance phase of chemotherapy for ALL in the majority of current protocols. In ALL it is also administered intrathecally for CNS prophylaxis. MTX is a major component of many protocols for treating lymphoma (M-BACOD, COMLA) including large-cell and Burkitt's types. High doses of MTX are also used to treat central nervous system lymphoma, as doses above 0.5 g/m^2 result in cytotoxic levels of MTX in the cerebrospinal fluid *(38,39)*. A recent study explored the use of high-dose MTX with peripheral administration of the inactivating enzyme carboxypeptidase G *(67)*. MTX is employed either singly or in combination to treat choriocarcinoma, breast cancer, osteogenic sarcoma, and head and neck cancer *(38,39,68)*.

4. RESISTANCE MECHANISMS TO METHOTREXATE IN EXPERIMENTAL TUMORS

The knowledge of the mechanisms of MTX action has allowed the elucidation of various mechanisms by which cells acquire resistance to MTX. Two common mechanisms of MTX resistance found in experimental tumors are a decrease in transport and an increase in the enzyme activity of DHFR because of gene amplification. Less commonly, a decrease in retention of MTX because of defective polyglutamylation, an increase in breakdown of MTX polyglutamates, or a decrease in binding of MTX to DHFR, because of point mutations resulting in amino acid changes in DHFR have been observed *(23,69)*. With an understanding of the mechanism of action of MTX and resistance mechanisms in experimental systems, as well as sensitive techniques to measure these events, attention has now focused on tumor samples from patients to determine the mechanisms of acquired and intrinsic resistance to MTX.

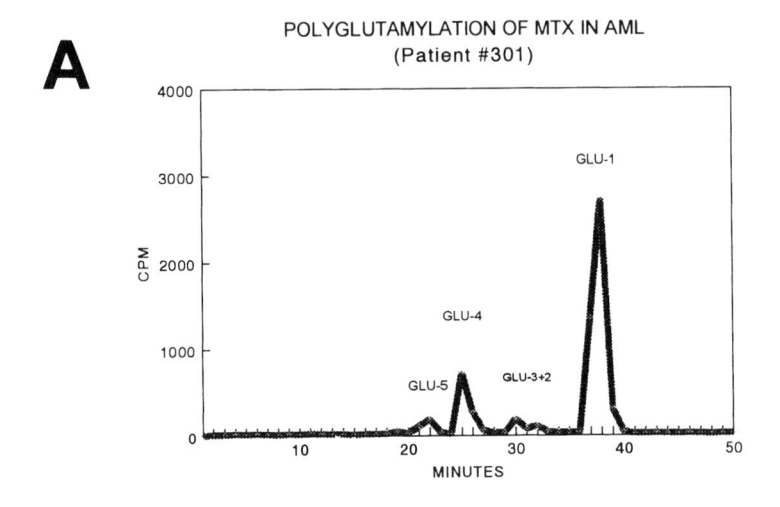

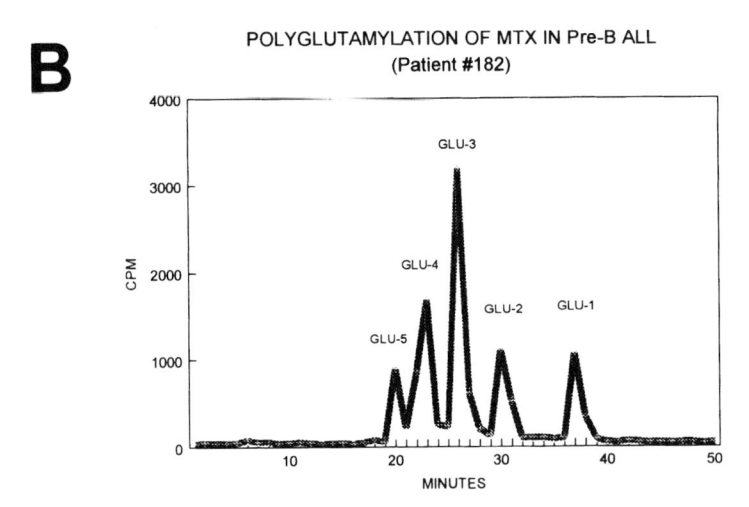

Fig. 2. MTX polyglutamate formation in blasts from two patients with leukemia. (**A** and **B**) depict HPLC separations of MTX polyglutamates obtained after a 24-h in vitro incubation with 10FM [^{3}H]-MTX. (**A**) Blasts obtained from an AML patient; (**B**) blasts from an ALL patient.

5. INTRINSIC RESISTANCE TO METHOTREXATE

Leukemic blast cells obtained from patients with untreated AML and its subtypes provide an opportunity to investigate mechanisms of intrinsic resistance. After an in vitro 24-h incubation with 10 μM [^{3}H]-MTX, MTX polyglutamates were measured by high-pressure liquid chromatography (HPLC) in blasts from 43 patients with AML and the results compared to blasts from 34 patients with pediatric pre-B ALL, a disease that is intrinsically sensitive to MTX. The AML blasts as compared to the ALL blasts were less able to form long-chain polyglutamates (Figs. 2, 3) (summarized from refs. *70–72* and unpublished observations). Studies were also performed with these blast cells to detect other possible mechanisms of MTX resistance. Transport resistance was found to be uncommon in AML and no evidence for either increases in DHFR activity or alterations in

MTX Polyglutamate Formation

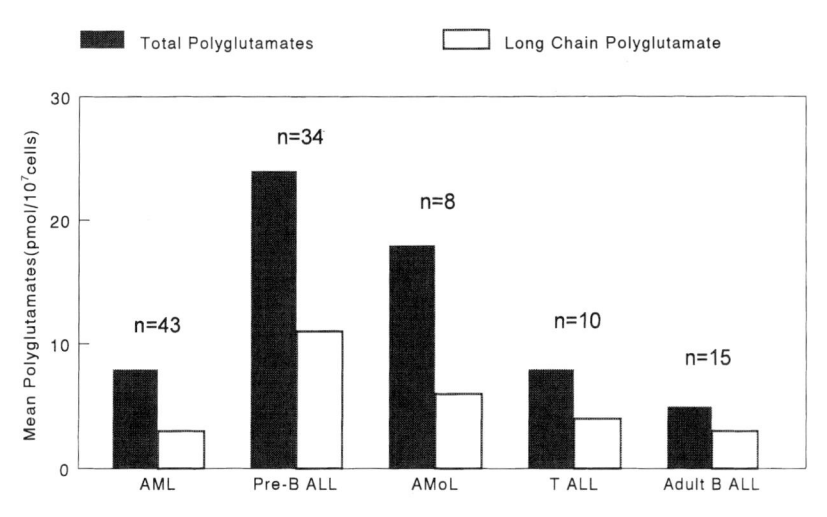

Fig. 3. Total MTX polyglutamates and long-chain MTX polyglutamates (glu_{3-6}) in leukemic blasts obtained from untreated patients with AML, pediatric pre-B ALL, AMoL, T-cell ALL, and adult B-cell ALL.

DHFR were found. The basis for the intrinsic resistance of AML to MTX therefore appears to be predominantly impaired polyglutamylation. This conclusion supports a previous study from this laboratory that showed that there was no difference in inhibition of DNA biosynthesis in AML vs ALL cells by MTX, after short-term incubations with this drug (73). However, polyglutamylation defects are noted if the cells are then washed free of extracellular MTX, and inhibition of thymidylate or DNA synthesis is measured several hours later (74).

Intrinsic methotrexate resistance was studied in soft-tissue sarcoma and epidemoid carcinoma and in most samples may result from impaired polyglutamylation. In a study of 15 soft-tissue sarcoma samples, 10 of the 12 that were resistant to MTX had markedly decreased long-chain polyglutamate formation. Intrinsic defects in MTX transport were not observed but in contrast to AML, DHFR amplification was observed in four of the eight samples tested (75). In a study of cervical and head and neck squamous-cell carcinoma cell lines, intrinsic resistance to MTX was found to be secondary to impaired polyglutamylation. No alterations in MTX transport or DHFR levels were observed (76,77).

The ability of blasts to form significant amounts of long-chain MTX polyglutamates has been identified as an important determinant of outcome of treatment of ALL. Adult T lineage as well as adult B lineage ALL were compared to pediatric B lineage ALL and both adult groups were found to accumulate lower amounts of long-chain polyglutamates, correlating with prognosis (71). Pediatric T lineage ALL blasts compared to B lineage ALL blasts were found to accumulate significantly less long-chain polyglutamates (71,78). Hyperdiploid B lineage blasts were also found to accumulate significantly more long-chain polyglutamates once again correlating with a favorable outcome (79). The ability of leukemia blasts to accumulate MTX and MTX polyglutamates was tested as a prognostic factors at diagnosis in childhood ALL. Children whose lymphoblasts accumulated both high MTX and high MTX polyglutamate levels together had a significantly better event-free survival than those who accumulated either low MTX or low MTX polyglutamates or both (65 ± 15% vs 22 ± 9%, $p = 0.010$). These correlations were observed only in "good," not "poor risk" subgroups *(80)*. This study demonstrated that even in "good risk" ALL patients, there may be some whose blasts form low levels of MTX polyglutamates, and may have a poor prognosis. However, to date, polyglutamylation of MTX, as an independent variable has not been evaluated.

Of interest is that two subsets of AML (FAB classifications—M5 and M7 subtypes) have been found to accumulate MTX polyglutamates following in vitro exposure to [^{3}H]-MTX to almost the same levels as childhood ALL blasts *(72,81)*. It may be worthwhile testing MTX for efficacy in these AML subtypes as the value of this drug to treat these AML subsets may have been overlooked because of the relative rarity of these diseases.

Studies are beginning to clarify the relative contributions that alterations of FPGS and GGH activities and transport of MTX polyglutamates into lysosomes provide to MTX resistance because of decreased polyglutamate accumulation. Studies have shown higher FPGS activities in B lineage ALL as compared to T lineage ALL blasts, consistent with the differences observed in intracellular levels of MTX polyglutamates measured after incubation with tritiated MTX *(78,82)*. These studies failed to show a direct correlation between FPGS activity and MTX polyglutamylation. Recent studies have shown that the ratio of FPGS/GGH enzyme activity correlates with MTX polyglutamylation *(83)*. It is therefore a combination of both activities that likely determines the level of MTX polyglutamylation in a cell. The recent cloning of the cDNA's encoding GGH and FPGS will allow quantitation of the expression of these genes; a quantitative PCR methodology for measuring FPGS mRNA expression in leukemic blasts has recently been developed *(23,33,84)*.

Another potential basis for the differences in polyglutamylation between intrinsically MTX-sensitive and MTX-resistant tumors, which requires further study, is the possibility that different isoforms of FPGS are expressed in different tissues. A recent study by our laboratory has shown a twofold difference in the affinity (K_m) for MTX between AML and ALL cell lines and blast samples *(27)*. A previous study of soft-tissue sarcoma cell lines had also shown a difference in the K_m of FPGS for MTX in resistant as compared to MTX-sensitive cell lines *(85)*. Expression of different splice variants selectively in different tissues may explain this observation, but further studies will be necessary to determine if different isoforms of FPGS are expressed in different cell types.

6. ACQUIRED RESISTANCE TO METHOTREXATE

6.1. Transport Defects

Standard radiolabeled transport assays have played a limited role in the assessment of transport defects in the clinical setting because of the inability to obtain an adequate sample size and difficulty interpreting data accurately because of heterogeneity within the sample. In an effort to overcome these limitations, a competitive displacement flow-cytometric assay utilizing the fluorescent lysine analog of MTX, N^α-(4-amino-4-deoxy-N^{10}-methylpteroyl)-N^ϵ-(4'-fluoresceinthiocarbamyl)-L-lysine or PT-430, was developed as a sensitive method of detection of transport resistance to MTX in blast cells obtained from leukemia patients *(86)*. The essential component of the assay, PT-430, is rapidly taken up into blasts utilizing an alternate mechanism for transport than MTX and binds directly to DHFR, thus making it an effective intracellular marker. After achievement of steady-state levels of intracellular PT-430, subsequent incubation with the competitors, MTX and trimetrexate (TMTX) which differ in the mode of carrier transport, produce characteristic displacement patterns of PT-430 distinguishing MTX transport defective blasts from those with normal transport *(86)*. MTX transport was examined in 27 patients with untreated ALL and 31 patients with relapsed ALL using this assay. Only 13% of untreated patients were considered to have impaired MTX transport, whereas more than 70% of relapsed patients had evidence of impaired MTX transport, indicating that decreased transport is a common acquired-resistance mechanism to MTX in relapsed ALL *(86,87)*. Of interest, in newly diagnosed AML patients analyzed by this assay, a heterogenous pattern was observed with variable displacement seen with MTX as well as TMTX. A subset of patients were found to have minimal uptake of TMTX, suggesting resistance to this agent. A possible explanation for this observation is the expression of p-glycoprotein the product of the multidrug resistance (MDR) gene in these cells, which has been described in newly diagnosed patients with AML and can result in the efflux of trimetrexate *(87)*.

The availability of cDNA clones encoding the human RFC has allowed studies of the molecular basis of impaired MTX transport. A quantitative RT-PCR methodology was developed to measure RFC mRNA expression. Of nine transport-defective ALL samples, five had decreased and one had no detectable RFC expression. In the remaining three samples, the basis of the impaired transport was unclear, and may be caused by mutations in the RFC gene. Mutations in the RFC gene resulting in decreased MTX transport have been described in mouse and human leukemia cell lines *(87–89)*.

6.2. DHFR Gene Amplification

A common mechanism of resistance to MTX in many experimental tumors is an increase in DHFR activity secondary to gene amplification *(90)*. Resistance to MTX in mouse, hamster, and human cell lines grown in sequentially increased MTX concentrations has been shown in most cases to be caused by increased DHFR synthesis and a proportional increase in DHFR gene copy number *(91,92)*. Four case reports appeared subsequently in the literature, one from our laboratory, indicating that low-level gene amplification occurs in tumor cells from patients treated with MTX, consistent with the expectation that a low-level amplification would be sufficient to cause clinical resistance to this drug *(69)*. Based on these findings, leukemic blasts from 29 patients with relapsed ALL who had been treated with MTX were analyzed using a sensitive dot blot assay; low level (2–4 copy number) DHFR gene amplification was detected in approx 30% of samples (9 of 29 samples). In contrast gene amplification was present in only 4 of 38 samples of leukemic blasts obtained from patients with newly diagnosed ALL and in 1 of 53 samples of leukemic blasts obtained from patients with newly diagnosed AML. The results of the dot blot assays were confirmed by Southern and Northern analyses, as well as DHFR enzyme activity in several cases *(93)*. DHFR gene amplification is a frequent mechanism of acquired resistance to MTX, occurring in approx 20–30% of relapsed ALL patients. In some patient samples, as has been obtained in experimental tumors made resistant to MTX, both impaired transport and increased DHFR activity were observed.

The amount and heterogeneity of expression of DHFR in ALL blast cells has also been analyzed at diagnosis and relapse in ALL samples by other investigators, utilizing a PT-430 assay *(94)*. At initial diagnosis 30 of 45 T-cell ALL samples (78%) exhibited dual blast populations with one population exhibiting higher levels of DHFR as measured by higher levels of PT-430 fluorescence. In B-cell ALL specimens, 17 of 36 samples (47%) exhibited dual populations *(94)*. Heterogeneous DHFR expression therefore correlated more closely with a T-cell ALL phenotype, which has been associated with a worse prognosis. For patients with low white blood cell counts ($< 50,000$) at presentation with ALL, the presence of DHFR overexpression was associated with a decreased event-free survival ($p < 0.016$), a relationship not observed in patients with high white blood cell counts at presentation *(64)*. At relapse 11 of 14 samples exhibited dual blast populations *(94)*. This study suggests that marked heterogeneity exists in leukemic blasts for DHFR levels, and high levels of DHFR at diagnosis and relapse may be an important and clinically relevant mechanism of intrinsic and acquired resistance to MTX in ALL *(94)*. This study conflicts with the prior study that demonstrated defective transport as the major mechanism of acquired resistance in ALL. This may reflect either methodologic differences or a difference in the study populations.

6.3. DHFR Mutations

Mutations in the DHFR gene, resulting in an altered DHFR protein with reduced affinity for MTX have been observed in multiple cell lines following (in most cases) exposure to sequentially increased doses of the drug *(95–98)*. In order to determine if mutations in DHFR occur in patients, we have tested blast samples from over 20 patients for alterations in the binding of MTX to DHFR using an enzyme-level MTX-binding assay and sequenced the complete DHFR cDNA from blasts of eight patients; six ALL (four relapsed and two untreated) and two patients with untreated AML (unpublished observations). Although this represents only a small number of patient samples, we did not detect decreased MTX binding at the protein level, nor alterations in the coding region of the DHFR cDNA from any of these samples. Other investigators have sequenced the cDNA for DHFR from 17 patients with relapsed ALL who had been treated with MTX and they also did not identify any mutations *(99)*. Thus, it seems unlikely that mutations in DHFR are a frequent mechanism of acquired resistance in patients exposed to MTX, although further studies seem warranted. It is of interest that the evolution of altered DHFR in the organism *Plasmodium falciparum* has rendered the use of the DHFR inhibitor, pyrimethamine, ineffective as a malaria prophylactic in regions of the world where it saw widespread use *(100)*.

7. TUMOR-SUPPRESSOR GENES AND DRUG RESISTANCE

Loss of functional retinoblastoma protein (pRb) may also contribute to antimetabolite resistance as cells lacking pRb may have increased levels of enzymes associated with proliferation (e.g., DHFR, TS) as a consequence of increased levels of free E2F, a transcription factor (Fig. 4) that is normally quenched by hypophosphorylated pRb. When cells begin to move out of G1 and into S phase, pRb becomes hyperphosphorylated and releases the bound E2F, which then enhances the transcription of genes involved in DNA synthesis *(101)*. The E2F-4 member of the E2F family of transcription factors has been most closely associated with the increase in DHFR transcription *(102)*. A human os-

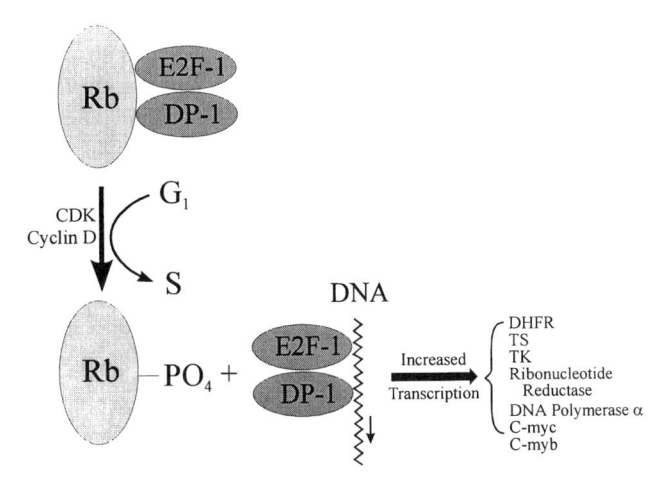

Fig. 4. Proposed mechanism of increased DHFR activity in cells lacking the retinoblastoma protein. At the G1 to S transition, Rb is hyperphosphorylated by cyclin D and E kinases. As a result, free E2F is generated (at least five family members of the E2F transcripts factor have been identified. $E2F_1$, $E2F_2$, and $E2F_3$ have been shown to bind to pRB). E2F bound to DP-1 increases transcription of several genes involved in DNA replication, including DHFR.

teosarcoma cell line SaOS-2 that lacks pRb is intrinsically resistant to MTX as compared to lines with pRb present. This cell line has a higher level of DHFR and the increase in this activity is attributable to increased transcription of the DHFR gene. When the cDNA encoding pRb was reintroduced into this cell line, sensitivity to MTX was restored. Other human sarcoma-cell lines established in the laboratory that lack pRb also show a similar level of resistance to MTX *(103)*.

Since free or unbound E2F levels increase when pRb is hyperphosphorylated, activation of regulators of pRb phosphorylation such as the cyclin-dependent kinase system (cyclin D1-CDK4) may also cause an increase in DHFR transcription and hence MTX resistance. Transfection of cyclin D1 into HT-1080 human sarcoma-cell line resulted in an increase in MTX resistance in clones that expressed high levels and not in clones that expressed low levels of the gene, suggesting a direct relationship between the level of cyclin D1 expression and DHFR transcription *(104)*. As certain tumors have been shown to express high levels of cyclin D1, MTX sensitivity may be decreased in these tumors. It is becoming increasingly clear that deregulation of cell-cycle genes may have a profound effect on antimetabolite resistance.

In cell lines with mutated p53, a tumor-suppressor gene, amplification of genes occurs more readily *(105,106)*. Mutations in the p53 gene were found in seven of nine ALL blast samples associated with DHFR amplification. In contrast, only 2 of 26 ALL blast samples without DHFR gene amplification had p53 mutations *(93)*. Patients with p53 mutations had a poor outcome. Studies performed by other investigators, have also shown that p53 mutations are associated with a poor outcome in ALL *(107)*.

8. STRATEGIES TO OVERCOME OR EXPLOIT METHOTREXATE RESISTANCE

An understanding of the mechanisms underlying cellular resistance to MTX has directed the development of new therapeutic strategies that include the design of new

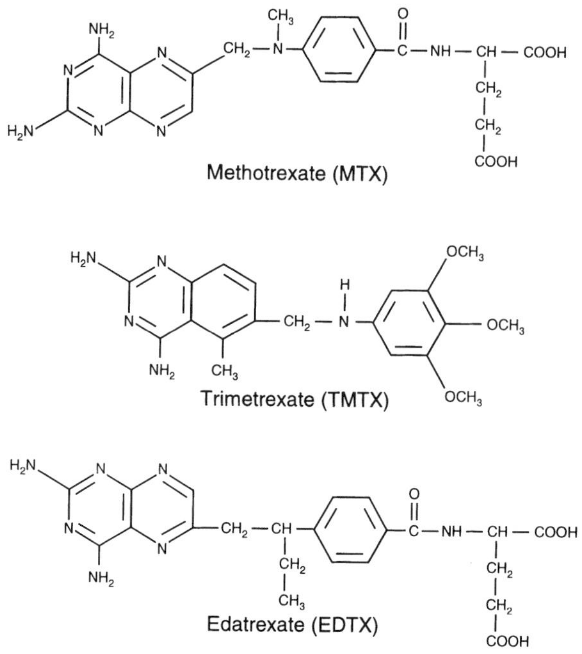

Fig. 5. Chemical structures of antifolate inhibitors of dihydrofolate reductase.

agents and the rediscovery of older agents that avoid resistance, and strategies in which agents selectively target resistant cells.

8.1 New Agents

Several new antifolate inhibitors of DHFR have been synthesized with attributes that may overcome or advert the causes of intrinsic and acquired resistance to MTX. That is, drugs that either are more efficiently converted to polyglutamate forms may not require polyglutamylation for retention and efficacy, and/or do not require the reduced folate carrier for cell entry. In addition, an older agent, aminopterin has been rediscovered as having some of these properties. Aminopterin and two newer agents are described below (Fig. 5).

Aminopterin, an antifolate inhibitor of DHFR, was first clinically tested in the 1940s and was the first drug capable of inducing complete remissions in children with ALL *(1)*. Aminopterin was largely replaced by MTX based on studies in tumor-bearing animals that showed similar efficacy with decreased toxicity *(108,109)*. Since MTX has become widely used, there has been limited clinical interest in aminopterin *(110)*. Some recent studies of leukemic blasts in vitro suggest aminopterin may have improved uptake and polyglutamylation as compared to MTX *(109)*. Based on these observations, clinical trials of aminopterin have been initiated.

Trimetrexate (TMTX), a lipophilic analog of MTX, has been studied extensively in recent years, and appears to have the advantage of not being dependent on the reduced folate carrier for cell entry and in some cells, is retained at high concentrations despite its inability to be polyglutamylated *(111)*. TMTX with LV has shown clear benefit for the treatment of *Pneumocystis carinii* pneumonia *(112)*. Clinically, TMTX has had limited activity as a single agent in phase II clinical trials. Response rates of 5 to 15% in breast cancer, 14 to 19% in nonsmall-cell lung cancer, 26% in head and neck cancer, and 17% in bladder cancer have been observed *(113–115)*. Only limited and transient responses have been observed in acute leukemia (though mainly in patients refractory to MTX) *(116,117)*. In most clinical trials, the dose-limiting toxicity has been myelosuppression *(113)*. In the trials for leukemia, the major dose-limiting toxicity was severe mucositis precluding dose intensification *(116,117)*. The major promise of TMTX may be in combination with other agents. TMTX in combination with 5-fluorouracil and LV has been shown in vitro to have more activity than MTX in combination with the same agents *(118)*. The regimen of TMTX/5-fluorouracil/LV has produced a response rate of 20% in patients with gastrointestinal cancer who have previously been treated, *(119)* and a 50% response rate in a phase II trial in previously untreated patients with colorectal cancer *(120)*. A phase III trial comparing this regimen with 5-fluorouracil and LV is in progress. The combined use of this agent with simultaneous LV in the treatment of acute leukemia is discussed further in the next section.

Edatrexate (EDTX), another MTX analog is taken up and retained at higher concentrations than MTX in leukemic cells primarily because of its superior cellular import and better substrate activity for FPGS *(113,121)*. However, as this drug also requires the reduced folate carrier for cell entry and it also targets DHFR, some cross resistance to this drug in MTX-resistant blasts may be expected *(113,122)*. EDTX had promising activity as a single agent in phase II clinical trials. Response rates of 17 to 41% in breast cancer, 7 to 32% in nonsmall-cell lung cancer, 24 to 41% in head and neck cancer, 27% in non-Hodgkin's lymphoma, and 14% in sarcomas (five of seven with malignant fibrous histiocytoma responded) have been observed *(113,122,123)*. Phase III trials of EDTX in the treatment of sarcoma are anticipated in the near future. No responses have been observed in prostate cancer, colorectal cancer, or melanoma *(113,122)*. The toxicities of EDTX are similar to that observed with MTX, with mucositis and stomatitis being the dose-limiting toxicities *(113)*. Limited clinical studies have been performed to date on EDTX for the treatment of leukemias. Based on the studies of Mauritz et al. *(124)*, this drug may not only be better than MTX for the treatment of newly diagnosed ALL, but also deserving of a clinical trial in patients with AML.

8.2. Drug-Resistant Cells as Targets for Chemotherapy

The finding that defective transport of MTX is a common resistance mechanism to MTX in relapsed ALL has led to an interest in drugs such as TMTX that do not utilize the reduced-folate carrier for cell entry. In addition, leukemic cells that are resistant to MTX on the basis of transport are collaterally sensitive to TMTX, possibly because of decreased uptake of folates *(125)*.

The combination of TMTX and LV is very active and nontoxic for the treatment of *Pneumocystis carinii* infections in acquired immunodeficiency syndrome (AIDS) patients *(112)*. The basis of this selectivity is that TMTX is transported by passive diffusion in this parasite, and LV can not rescue this organism because of lack of LV transport. With this combination, the side effects of TMTX on the host are eliminated as normal host cells are protected by LV. We have applied this strategy to selectively target leukemia cells that developed resistance to MTX on the basis of transport. In vitro cytotoxicity studies showed that CCRF-CEM cells resistant to MTX because of defective transport are not protected from the cytotoxic effects of TMTX by LV. Severe combined immunodeficiency mice bearing MTX-resistant, transport-defective CCRF-CEM ALL cells were then tested with the combination of TMTX and LV, and marked tumor regression occurred without toxicity *(126)*. These studies have prompted a study using. TMTX with LV protection (not rescue) in relapsed ALL patients that demonstrate resistance to MTX associated with impaired uptake of this drug.

REFERENCES

1. Farber S, Diamond LK, Mercer RD, Sylvester RF Jr, Wolff JA. Temporary remissions in acute leukemia in children produced by folic acid antagonist, 4-aminopteroyl-glutamic acid (aminopterin). *N Engl J Med* 1948;238:787–793.
2. Gorlick R, Goker E, Trippett T, Waltham M, Banerjee D, Bertino JR. Intrinsic and acquired resistance to methotrexate in acute leukemia. *N Engl J Med* 1996;335:1041–1048.
3. Bertino JR. Ode to methotrexate. *J Clin Oncol* 1993;11:5–14.
4. Goldman ID, Lichenstein WS, Oliveiro VT. Carrier-mediated transport of the folic acid analog methotrexate in the L1210 leukemia cell. *J Biol Chem* 1968;243:5007–5017.
5. Sirotnak FM, Goutas LJ, Mines LS. Extent of requirement for folate transport by L1210 cells for growth and leukemogenesis in vivo. *Cancer Res* 1985;45:4732–4734.
6. Antony AC. The biological chemistry of folate receptors. *Blood* 1992;79:2807–2820.
7. Pizzorno G, Mini E, Coronnello M, McGuire JJ, Moroson BA, Cashmore AR, Dreyer RN, Lin JT, Mazzei T, Periti P, Bertino JR. Impaired polyglutamylation of methotrexate as a cause of resistance in CCRF-CEM cells after short-term, high-dose treatment with this drug. *Cancer Res* 1988;48:2149–2155.
8. Allegra CJ, Chabner BA, Drake JC, Lutz R, Rodbard D, Jolivet J. Enhanced inhibition of thymidylate synthase by methotrexate polyglutamates. *J Biol Chem* 1985;260:9720–9726.
9. Allegra CJ, Drake JC, Jolivet J, Chabner BA. Inhibition of phosphoribosylaminoimidazole carboxamide transformylase by methotrexate and dihydrofolic acid polyglutamates. *Proc Natl Acad Sci USA* 1985;82:4881–4885.
10. Anderson RG, Kamen BA, Rothberg KG, Lacey SW. Potocytosis: sequestration and transport of small molecules by caveolae. *Science* 1992;255:410–411.
11. Lacey SW, Sanders JM, Rothberg KG, Anderson RG, Kamen BA. Complementary DNA for the folate binding protein correctly predicts anchoring to the membrane by glycosyl-phosphatidylinositol. *J Clin Invest* 1989;84:715–720.
12. Spinella MJ, Brigle KE, Sierra EE, Goldman ID. Distinguishing between folate receptor mediated transport and reduced folate carrier mediated transport in L1210 leukemia cells. *J Biol Chem* 1995;270:7842–7849.
13. Williams FMR, Murray RC, Underhill TM, Flintoff WF. Isolation of a hamster cDNA clone coding for a function involved in methotrexate uptake. *J Biol Chem* 1994;269:5810–5816.
14. Dixon KH, Lampher BC, Chiu J, Kelley K, Cowan KH. A novel cDNA restores reduced folate carrier activity and methotrexate sensitivity to transport deficient cells. *J Biol Chem* 1994;269:17–20.
15. Williams FMR, Flintoff WF. Isolation of a human cDNA that complements a mutant hamster cell defective in methotrexate uptake. *J Biol Chem* 1995;270:2987–2992.
16. Moscow JA, Gong M, He R, Sgagias MK, Dixon KH, Anzick SL, Meltzer PS, Cowan KH. Isolation of a gene encoding a human reduced folate carrier (RFC1) and analysis of its expression in transport-deficient methotrexate-resistant human breast cancer cells. *Cancer Res* 1995;55:3790–3795.
17. Wong SC, Proefke SA, Bhushan A, Matherley LH. Isolation of human cDNAs that restore methotrexate sensitivity and reduced folate carrier activity in methotrexate transport-defective Chinese hamster ovary cells. *J Biol Chem* 1995;270:17,468–17,475.
18. Prasad PD, Ramamoorthy S, Leibach FH, Ganapathy V. Molecular cloning of the human placental folate transporter. *Biochem Biophys Res Commun* 1995;206:681–687.
19. Weitman SD, Lark RH, Coney LR, Fort DW, Frasca V, Zurawski VR, Kamen BA. Distribution of the folate receptor GP38 in normal and malignant cell lines and tissues. *Cancer Res* 1992;52:3396–3401.

20. Campbell IG, Jones TA, Foulkes WD, Trowsdale J. Folate-binding protein is a marker for ovarian cancer. *Cancer Res* 1991;51:5329–5338.
21. Westerhof GR, Rijnbout S, Schomagel JH, Pinedo HM, Peters GJ, Jansen G. Functional activity of the reduced folate carrier in KB, MA104 and IGROV-1 cells expressing folate-binding protein. *Cancer Res* 1995;55:3795–3802.
22. Mcguire JJ, Hsieh P, Coward JK, Bertino JR. Enzymatic synthesis of folylpolyglutamates. Characterization of the reaction and its products. *J Biol Chem* 1980;255:5776–5788.
23. Garrow TA, Admon A, Shane B. Expression cloning of a human cDNA encoding folylpoly (γ-glutamate) synthetase and determination of its primary structure. *Proc Natl Acad Sci USA* 1992;89:9151–9155.
24. Chen L, Qi H, Korenberg J, Garrow TA, Choi YJ, Shane B. Purification and properties of human cytosolic folylpoly-—glutamate synthetase and organization, localization, and differential splicing of its gene. *J Biol Chem* 1996;271:13,077–13,087.
25. Roy K, Mitsugi K, Sirotnak FM. Organization and alternate splicing of the murine folylpolyglutamate synthetase gene. *J Biol Chem* 1996;271:23,820–23,827.
26. Roy K, Mitsugi K, Sirotnak FM. Additional organizational features of the murine folylpolyglutamate synthetase gene. *J Biol Chem* 1997;272:5587–5593.
27. Longo GSA, Gorlick R, Tong WP, Ercikan E, Bertino JR. Disparate affinities of antifolates for folylpolyglutamate synthetase from human leukemia cells. *Blood* 1997;90:1241–1245.
28. Galivan J, Johnson T, Rhee M, McGuire JJ, Priest D, Kesevan V. The role of folylpolyglutamate synthesis and gamma-glutamyl hydrolase in altering cellular foly- and antifolypolyglutamates. *Adv Enz Reg* 1987;26:147–55.
29. Wang Y, Dias JA, Nimec Z, Rotundo RM, O'Connor BM, Freisheim J, Galivan J. The properties and function of gamma-glutamyl hydrolase and poly-gamma-glutamate. *Adv Enz Reg* 1993;33:207–218.
30. Samuels LL, Goutas LJ, Priest DG, Piper JR, Sirotnak FM. Hydrolytic cleavage of methotrexate gamma-polyglutamates by folylpolyglutamyl hydrolase derived from various tumors and normal tissues of the mouse. *Cancer Res* 1986;46:2230–2235.
31. Waltham MC, Li WW, Gritsman H, Tong WP, Bertino JR. γ-Glutamyl hydrolase from human sarcoma HT-1080 cells: Characterization and inhibition by glutamine antagonists. *Molec Pharmacol* 1997;51:825–832.
32. Yao R, Nimec Z, Ryan TJ, Galivan J. Identification, cloning, and sequencing of a cDNA coding for rat γ-glutamyl hydrolase. *J Biol Chem* 1996;271:8525–8528.
33. Yao R, Schneider E, Ryan TJ, Galivan J. Human gamma-glutamyl hydrolase: cloning and characterization of the enzyme expressed in vitro. *Proc Acad Sci USA* 1996;93:10,134–10,138.
34. Bertino JR, Donohue DM, Simmons B, Gabrio BW, Silber R, Huennekens FM. The induction of dihydrofolate reductase in leukocytes and erythrocytes of patients treated with methotrexate. *J Clin Invest* 1963;42:466–475.
35. Chu E, Koeller DM, Casey JL, Drake JC, Chabner BA, Elwood PC, Zinn S, Allegra CA. Autoregulation of human thymidylate synthase messenger RNA translation by thymidylate synthase. *Proc Natl Acad Sci USA* 1991;88:8977–8981.
36. Hillcoat BL, Swett V, Bertino JR. Increase of dihydrofolate reductase activity in cultured mammalian cells after exposure to methotrexate. *Proc Natl Acad Sci USA* 1967;58:1632–1637.
37. Ercikan-Abali E, Banerjee D, Waltham MC, Skacel N, Scotto KW, Bertino JR. Dihydrofolate reductase protein inhibits its own translation by binding to dihydrofolate reductase mRNA sequences within the coding region. *Biochemistry* 1997;36:12317–12322.
38. Bertino JR, Kamen B, Romanini A. Folate antagonists, in *Cancer Medicine,* vol. 1 (Holland JF, Frei E, Bast RC, Kufe DW, Morton DL, Weichselbaum RR, eds.) Williams & Wilkins, Baltimore, 1997, pp. 907–921.
39. Chu E, Allegra CJ. Antifolates, in (Chabner BA, Longo DL, eds.) *Cancer Chemotherapy and Biotherapy.* Lippincott-Raven, Philadelphia, 1996, pp. 109–14.
40. Chungi VS, Bourne DW, Dittert LW. Drug absorption VIII: kinetics of GI absorption of methotrexate. *J Pharm Sci* 1978;67:560–561.
41. Balis FM, Savitch JL, Bleyer WA. Pharmacokinetics of oral methotrexate in children. *Cancer Res* 1983;43:2342–2345.
42. Steinberg SE, Campbell CL, Bleyer WA, Hillman RS. Enterohepatic circulation of methotrexate in rats in vivo. *Cancer Res* 1982;42:1279–1282.

43. Steele WH, Lawrence JR, Stuart JF, McNeill CA. The protein binding of methotrexate by the serum of normal subjects. *Eur J Clin Pharmacol* 1979;15:363–366.
44. Shapiro WR, Young DF, Mehta BM. Methotrexate: distribution in cerebrospinal fluid after intravenous ventricular and lumbar injections. *N Eng J Med* 1975;293:161–166.
45. Wan SH, Huffman DH, Azarnoff DL, Stephens R, Hoogstraten B. Effect of route and administration and effusions on methotrexate pharmacokinetics. *Cancer Res* 1974;34:3487–3491.
46. Calvert AH, Bondy PK, Harrap KR. Some observations on the human pharmacology of methotrexate. *Cancer Treat Rep* 1977;61:1647–1656.
47. Kristensen LO, Weismann K, Hutters L. Renal function and the rate of disappearance of methotrexate from serum. *Eur J Clin Pharmacol* 1975;8:439–444.
48. Romolo JL, Goldberg NH, Hande KR, Rosenberg SA. Effect of hydration on plasma-methotrexate levels. *Cancer Treat Rep* 1977;61:1393–1396.
49. Gewirtz DA, White JC, Randolph JK, Goldman ID. Transport, binding and polyglutamation of methotrexate in freshly isolated rat hepatocytes. *Cancer Res* 1980;40:573–578.
50. Creaven PJ, Hansen HH, Alford DA, Allen LM. Methotrexate in liver and bile after intravenous dosage in man. *Bri J Cancer* 1973;28:589–591.
51. Sonneveld P, Schultz FW, Nooter K, Hahlen K. Pharmacokinetics of methotrexate and 7-hydroxymethotrexate in plasma and bone marrow of children receiving low-dose oral methotrexate. *Cancer Chemother Pharmacol* 1986;18:111–116.
52. Stewart AI, Margison JM, Wilkinson PM, Lucas SB. The pharmacokinetics of 7-hydroxymethotrexate following medium dose methotrexate therapy. *Cancer Chemother Pharmacol* 1985;14:165–167.
53. Jacobs SA, Stoller RG, Chabner BA, Johns DG. 7-Hydroxymethotrexate as a urinary metabolite in human subjects and rhesus monkeys receiving high dose methotrexate. *J Clin Invest* 1976;57:534–538.
54. Valerino DM, Johns DG, Zaharko DS, Oliverio VT. Studies of the metabolism of methotrexate by intestinal flora. I. Identification and study of biological properties of the metabolite 4-amino-4-deoxy-N 10-methylpteroic acid. *Biochem Pharmacol* 1972;21:821–831.
55. Daly H, Boyle J, Roberts C, Scott G. Interaction between methotrexate and non-steroidal anti-inflammatory drugs. *Lancet* 1986;1:557.
56. Singh RR, Malaviya AN, Pandey JN, Guleria JS. Fatal interaction between methotrexate and naproxen. *Lancet* 1986;1:1390.
57. Maricic M, Davis M, Gall EP. Megaloblastic pancytopenia in a patient receiving concurrent methotrexate and trimethoprim-sulfamethoxazole treatment. *Arthritis Rheum* 1986;29:133–135.
58. Pinedo HM, Zaharko DS, Bull JM, Chabner BA. The reversal of methotrexate cytotoxicity to mouse bone marrow cells by leucovorin and nucleosides. *Cancer Res* 1976;36:4418–4424.
59. Howell SB, Ensminger WD, Krishan A, Frei E. Thymidine rescue of high-dose methotrexate in humans. *Cancer Res* 1978;38:325–330.
60. Widemann BC, Balis FM, Murphy RF, Sorensen JM, Montello MJ, O'Brien M, Adamson PC. Carboxypeptidase-G2, thymidine and leucovorin rescue in cancer patients with methotrexate-induced renal dysfunction. *J Clin Oncol* 1997;15:2125–2134.
61. Weber BL, Tanyer G, Poplack DG, Reaman GH, Feusner JH, Miser JS, Bleyer WA. Transient acute hepatotoxicity of high dose-methotrexate therapy during childhood. *Natl Cancer Inst Monogr* 1987;5:207–212.
62. Jaffe N, Takue Y, Anzai T, Robertson R. Transient neurologic disturbances induced by high-dose methotrexate treatment. *Cancer* 1985;56:1356–1360.
63. Clarysse AM, Cathey WJ, Cartwright GE, Wintrobe MM. Pulmonary disease complicating intermittent therapy with methotrexate. *JAMA* 1969;209:1861–1868.
64. Sostman HD, Matthay RA, Putman CE, Smith GJ. Methotrexate-induced pneumonitis. *Medicine* 1976;55:371–378.
65. Doyle LA, Berg C, Bottino G, Chabner B. Erythema and desquamation after high-dose methotrexate. *Ann Int Med* 1983;98:611–612.
66. Hausknecht RU. Methotrexate and misoprostol to terminate early pregnancy. *N Engl J Med* 1995;333:537–540.
67. DeAngelis LM, Tong WP, Lin S, Fleisher M, Bertino JR. Carboxypeptidase G2 rescue after high-dose methotrexate. *J Clin Oncol* 1996;14:2145–2149.
68. Jolivet J, Cowan KH, Curt GA, Clendeninn NJ, Chabner BA. The pharmacology and clinical use of methotrexate. *N Engl J Med* 1983;309:1094–1104.

69. Schweitzer BI, Dicker AP, Bertino JR. Dihydrofolate reductase as a therapeutic target. *FASEB J* 1990;4:2441–2452.
70. Lin JT, Tong WP, Trippett TM, Niedzwiecki D, Tao Y, Tan C, Steinherz P, Schweitzer BI, Bertino JR. Basis for natural resistance to methotrexate in human acute non-lymphocytic leukemia. *Leukemia Res* 1991;15:1191–1196.
71. Goker E, Lin JT, Trippett T, Elisseyeff Y, Tong W, Niedzwiecki D, Tan C, Steinherz P, Schweitzer BI, Bertino JR. Decreased polyglutamylation of methotrexate in acute lymphoblastic leukemia blasts in adults compared to children with this disease. *Leukemia* 1993;7:1000–1004.
72. Goker E, Kheradpour A, Waltham M, Banerjee D, Tong WP, Elisseyeff Y, Bertino JR. Acute monocytic leukemia: a myeloid subset that may be sensitive to methotrexate. *Leukemia* 1995;9:274–276.
73. Hryniuk WM, Bertino JR. Treatment of leukemia with large doses of methotrexate and folinic acid: clinical-biochemical correlates. *J Clin Invest* 1969;48:2140–2155.
74. Rodenhuis S, Mcguire JJ, Narayanan R, Bertino JR. Development of an assay system for the detection and classification of methotrexate resistance in fresh human leukemia cells. *Cancer Res* 1986;46:6513–6519.
75. Li WW, Lin JT, Tong WP, Trippett TM, Brennan MF, Bertino JR. Mechanisms of natural resistance to antifolates in human soft tissue sarcomas. *Cancer Res* 1992;52:1434–1438.
76. Barakat RR, Li WW, Lovelace C, Bertino JR. Intrinsic resistance of cervical cell carcinoma cell lines to methotrexate (MTX) as a result of decreased accumulation of intracellular MTX polyglutamates. *Gynecol Oncol* 1993;93:2255–2262.
77. Pizzorno G, Chang YM, McGuire JJ, Bertino JR. Inherent resistance of human squamous carcinoma cell lines to methotrexate as a result of decreased polyglutamylation of this drug. *Cancer Res* 1989;49:5275–5280.
78. Barredo JC, Synold TW, Laver J, Relling MV, Pui CH, Priest DG, Evans WE. Differences in constitutive and post-methotrexate folypolyglutamate synthetase activity in B-lineage and T-lineage leukemia. *Blood* 1994;84:564–569.
79. Synold TW, Relling MV, Boyett JM, Rivera GK, Sandlund JT, Mahmoud H, Crist WM, Pui CH, Evans WE. Blast cell methotrexate-polyglutamate accumulation in vivo differs by lineage, ploidy, and methotrexate dose in acute lymphoblastic leukemia. *J Clin Invest* 1994;94:1996–2001.
80. Whitehead VM, Rosenblatt DS, Vuchich MJ, Shuster JJ, Witte A, Beaulieu D. Accumulation of methotrexate and methotrexate polyglutamates in lymphoblasts at diagnosis of childhood acute lymphoblastic leukemia: a pilot prognostic factor analysis. *Blood* 1990;76:44–49.
81. Argiris A, Longo GSA, Gorlick R, Tong W, Steinherz P, Bertino JR. Increased methotrexate polyglutamylation in acute megakaryocytic leukemia (M&) compare to other subtypes of acute myelocytic leukemia. *Leukemia* 1997;11:886–889.
82. Galpin AJ, Schuetz JD, Masson E, Yanishevski Y, Synold TW, Barredo JC, Pui CH, Relling MV, Evans WE. Differences in folylpolyglutamate synthetase and dihydrofolate reductase expression in human B-lineage versus T-lineage leukemic lymphoblasts: mechanisms for lineage differences in methotrexate polyglutamylation and cytotoxicity. *Molec Pharmacol* 1997;52:155–163.
83. Longo GSA, Gorlick R, Tong WP, Lin S, Steinherz P, Bertino JR. γ-Glutamyl hydrolase and folypolyglutamate synthetase activities predict polyglutamylation of methotrexate in acute leukemias. *Onc Res* 1997;9:259–263.
84. Lenz HJ, Danenberg K, Schnieders B, Goker E, Peters GJ, Garrow T, Shane B, Bertino JR, Danenberg PV. Quantitative analysis of folylpolyglutamate synthetase gene expression in tumor tissues by the polymerase chain reaction: marked variation of expression among leukemia patients. *Oncol Res* 1994;6:329–335.
85. Li WW, Lin JT, Scweitzer BI, Tong WP, Niedzwiecki D, Bertino JR. Intrinsic resistance to methotrexate in human soft tissue sarcoma cell lines. *Cancer Res* 1992;52:3908–3913.
86. Trippett T, Schlemmer S, Elisseyeff Y, Goker E, Wachter M, Steinherz P, Tan C, Berman E, Wright JE, Rosowsky A. Defective transport as a mechanism of acquired resistance to methotrexate in patients with acute leukemia. *Blood* 1992;80:1158–1162.
87. Gorlick R, Goker E, Trippett T, Steinherz P, Elisseyeff Y, Mazumdar M, Flintoff WF, Bertino JR. Defective transport is a common mechanism of acquired methotrexate resistance in acute lymphocytic leukemia and is associated with decreased reduced folate carrier expression. *Blood* 1997;89:1013–1018.

88. Brigle KE, Spinella MJ, Sierra EE, Goldman ID. Characterization of a mutation in the reduced folate carrier in a transport defective L1210 murine leukemia cell line. *J Biol Chem* 1995;270:22,974–22,979.
89. Gong M, Yess J, Connolly T, Ivy SP, Ohnuma T, Cowan KH, Moscow JA. Molecular mechanism of antifolate transport-deficiency in a methotrexate-resistant MOLT-3 human leukemia cell line. *Blood* 1997;89:2494–2499.
90. Schimke RT. Gene amplification in cultured cells. *J Biol Chem* 1988;263:5989–5992.
91. Srimatkandada S, Medina WD, Casnmore AR, Whyte W, Engel D, Moroson BA, Franco CT, Dube SK, Bertino JR. Amplification and organization of dihydrofolate reductase genes in a human leukemia cell line, K-562, resistant to methotrexate. *Biochemistry* 1983;22:5774–5781.
92. Stark GR, Debatisse M, Guilotto E, Wahl GM. Recent progress in understanding mechanisms of mammalian DNA amplification. *Cell* 1989;57:901–908.
93. Goker E, Waltham M, Kheradpour A, Trippett T, Mazumdar M, Elisseyeff Y, Schnieders B, Steinherz P, Tan C, Berman E, Bertino JR. Amplification of the dihydrofolate reductase gene is a mechanism of acquired resistance to methotrexate in patients with acute lymphocytic leukemia and is correlated with p53 gene mutations. *Blood* 1995;86:677–684.
94. Matherly LH, Taub JW, Wong SC, Simpson PM, Ekizian R, Buck S, Williamson M, Amylon M, Pullen J, Camitta B, Ravindranath Y. Increased frequency of expression of elevated dihydrofolate reductase in T-cell versus B-precursor acute lymphoblastic leukemia in children. *Blood* 1997;90:578–589.
95. Haber DA, Beverly SM, Kiely ML, Schimke RT. Properties of an altered dihydrofolate reductase encoded by amplified genes in cultured mouse fibroblasts. *J Biol Chem* 1981;256:9501–9510.
96. Srimatkandada S, Schweitzer BI, Moroson BA, Dube S, Bertino JR. Amplification of a polymorphic dihydrofolate reductase gene expressing an enzyme with a decreased binding to Methotrexate in a human colon carcinoma cell line, HCT-8R4, resistant to this drug. *J Biol Chem* 1989;264:3524–3528.
97. Melera PW, Davide JP, Hession CA, Scotto KW. Phenotypic expression in Escherichia coli and nucleotide sequence of two Chinese hamster lung cDNAs encoding different dihydrofolate reductases. *Mol Cell Biol* 1984;4:38–48.
98. Dicker AP, Volkenandt M, Schweitzer BI, Banerjee D, Bertino JR. Identification and characterization of a mutation in the dihydrofolate reductase gene from methotrexate-resistant Chinese hamster ovary cell line Pro-3 Methotrexate RIII. *J Biol Chem* 1990;265:8317–8321.
99. Spencer HT, Sorrentino BP, Pui CH, Chunduru SK, Sleep SEH, Blakley RL. Mutations in the gene for human dihydrofolate reductase: an unlikely cause of clinical relapse in pediatric leukemia patients after therapy with methotrexate. *Leukemia* 1996;10:439–446.
100. Hyde JE. The dihydrofolate reductase-thymidylate synthetase gene in the drug resistance of malaria parasites. *Pharmacol Therapeutics* 1990;48:45–59.
101. Nevins JR. E2F: a link between the Rb tumor suppressor protein and viral oncoproteins. *Science* 1992;258:424–429.
102. Wells JM, Illenye S, Magae J, Wu, CL, Heintz NH. Accumulation of E2F-4-DP-1 DNA binding complexes correlates with induction of dhfr gene expression during the G_1 to S phase transition. *J Biol Chem* 1997;272:4483–4492.
103. Li WW, Fan J, Hochhauser D, Banerjee D, Zielenski Z, Almasan A, Yin Y, Kelly R, Wahl GM, Bertino JR. Absence of functional retinoblastoma protein mediates increased resistance to antimetabolites in human sarcoma cell lines. *Proc Natl Acad Sci USA* 1995;92:10,436–10,440.
104. Hochhauser D, Schnieders B, Ercikan-Abali E, Gorlick R, Muise-Helmericks R, Li WW, Fan J, Banerjee D, Bertino JR. Effect of cyclin D1 overexpression on drug sensitivity in a human fibrosarcoma cell line. *J Natl Cancer Inst* 1996;88:1269–1275.
105. Livingstone LR, White A, Sprouse J, Livanos E, Jacks T, Tlsty TD. Altered cell cycle arrest and gene amplification potential accompany loss of wild-type p53. *Cell* 1992;70:923–935.
106. Yin Y, Tainsky MA, Bischoff FZ, Strong LC, Wahl GM. Wild-type p53 restores cell cycle control and inhibits gene amplification in cells with mutant p53 alleles. *Cell* 1992;70:937–948.
107. Hecker S, Sauerbrey A, Volm M. p53 expression and poor prognosis in childhood acute lymphoblastic leukemia. *Anticancer Res* 1994;14:2759–2761.
108. Goldin A, Venditi JM, Humphreys SR, Dennis D, Mantel N, Greenhouse SW. A quantitative comparison of the antileukemic effectiveness of two folic acid antagonists in mice. *J Natl Cancer Inst* 1955;15:1657–1664.

109. Smith A, Hum M, Winick NJ, Kamen BA. A case for the use of aminopterin in treatment of patients with leukemia based on metabolic studies of blasts in vitro. *Clin Cancer Res* 1996;2:69–73.
110. Glode LM, Pitman SW, Ensminger WD, Rosowsky A, Papathanasopoulos N, Frei E. A phase 1 study of high doses of aminopterin with leucovorin rescue in patients with advanced metastatic tumors. *Cancer Res* 1979;39:3707–3714.
111. Kamen BA, Eibl B, Cashmore A, Bertino JR. Uptake and efficacy of trimetrexate (TMQ, 2,2-diamino-5-methyl-6-[(3,4,5-trimethoxyanilino)methyl] quinazoline), a non-classical antifolate in methotrexate-resistant leukemia cells in vitro. *Biochem Pharmacol* 1984;33:1697–1699.
112. Allegra CJ, Chabner BA, Tuazon CU, Ogata-Arakaki D, Baird B, Drake JC, Simmons JT, Lack EE, Shelhamer JH, Balis F. Trimetrexate for the treatment of pneumocystis carinii pneumonia in patients with the acquired immunodeficiency syndrome. *N Engl J Med* 1987;317:978–985.
113. Takimoto CH, Allegra CJ. New antifolates in clinical development. *Oncol* 1995;9:649–656.
114. Seitz DE. Trimetrexate: A critical appraisal of the phase II clinical trial experience: evidence of drug discovery-clinical development disjunction. *Cancer Invest* 1994;12:657–661.
115. Pappo AS, Vats T, Williams TE, Bernstein M, Kamen BA. Phase I trial of trimetrexate in pediatric solid tumors: a Pediatric Oncology Group study. *Med Ped Oncol* 1993;21:280–282.
116. Pappo A, Dubowy R, Ravindranath Y, Alvarado C, Rao S, Whitehead VM, Vega R, Kamen B, Vietti T. Phase II trial of trimetrexate in the treatment of recurrent childhood acute lymphoblastic leukemia: a Pediatric Oncology Group study. *J Natl Cancer Inst* 1990;82:1641–1642.
117. Kheradpour A, Berman E, Goker E, Lin JT, Tong WP, Bertino JR. A phase II study of continuous infusion of trimetrexate in patients with refractory leukemia. *Cancer Invest* 1995;13:36–40.
118. Romanini A, Li WW, Colofiore JR, Bertino JR. Leucovorin enhances cytotoxicity of trimetrexate/fluorouracil, but not methotrexate/fluorouracil in CCRF-CEM cells. *J Natl Cancer Inst* 1992;84:1033–1038.
119. Conti JA, Kemeny N, Seiter K, Goker E, Tong W, Andre M, Ragusa K, Bertino JR. Trial of sequential trimetrexate, fluorouracil and high-dose leucovorin in previously treated patients with gastrointestinal carcinoma. *J Clin Oncol* 1994;12:695–700.
120. Blanke CD, Kasimis B, Schein P, Capizzi R, Kurman M. Phase II study of trimetrexate, fluorouracil, and leucovorin for advanced colorectal cancer. *J Clin Oncol* 1997;15:915–920.
121. Sirotnak FM, Schmid FA, Samuels LL, Degraw JI. 10-Ethyl-10-deaza-aminopterin: structural design and biochemical, pharmacological, and antitumor properties. *Natl Cancer Inst Monographs* 1987;5:127–131.
122. Grant SC, Kris MG, Young CW, Sirotnak FM. Edatrexate: an antifolate with antitumor activity: a review. *Cancer Invest* 1993;11:36–45.
123. Casper ES, Christman KL, Schwartz GK, Johnson B, Brennan MF, Bertino JR. Edatrexate in patients with soft tissue sarcoma. Activity in malignant fibrous histiocytoma. *Cancer* 1993;72:766–770.
124. Mauritz R, Bekkenk M, Pieters R, Veerman AJP, Peters GJ, Jansen G. Resistance to methotrexate and sensitivity for novel antifolates in different types of childhood leukemia. *Blood* 1994;84:45a.
125. Jackson RC, Fry DW, Boritzki TJ, Besserer JA, Leopold WR, Sloan BJ, Elslager EF. Biochemical pharmacology of the lipophilic antifolate, trimetrexate. *Adv Enz Reg* 1984;22:187–206.
126. Lacerda JF, Goker E, Kheradpour A, Dennig D, Elisseyeff Y, Jagiello C, O'Reilly RJ, Bertino JR. Selective treatment of SCID mice bearing methotrexate-transport-resistant human acute lymphoblastic leukemia tumors with trimetrexate and leucovorin protection. *Blood* 1995;85:2675–2679.

4 Development of Nonpolyglutamatable DHFR Inhibitors

Andre Rosowsky

CONTENTS

    INTRODUCTION
    COMPOUNDS WITH MONOCARBOXYLIC ACID SIDE CHAINS
    COMPOUNDS WITH AMINOMALONATE OR ASPARTATE SIDE CHAINS
    COMPOUNDS WITH OTHER AMINOALKANEDIOIC ACID SIDE CHAINS
    COMPOUNDS WITH POLAR SUBSTITUTION ON THE GLUTAMATE MOIETY
    BRANCHED-CHAIN GLUTAMATE ANALOGS
    ANALOGS WITH A BLOCKED γ-CARBOXYL GROUP
    γ-SULFONIC AND γ-PHOSPHONIC ACID ANALOGS
    γ-TETRAZOLE ANALOGS
    δ-HEMIPHTHALOYLORNITHINE ANALOGS
    NONPOLYGLUTAMATABLE ANALOGS WITH A GLUTAMATE SIDE CHAIN
    CONCLUSION
    ACKNOWLEDGMENT
    REFERENCES

1. INTRODUCTION

Inhibitors of the enzyme dihydrofolate reductase (DHFR) first came into use as anticancer drugs in 1948 when aminopterin (AMT, **1**) and methotrexate (MTX, **2**) were found to induce temporary remission in children with acute leukemia *(1,2)*. In the five decades that followed this landmark in the history of chemotherapy *(3)*, the term "antifolate" or "antifol" has come to refer not only to inhibitors of DHFR but also to inhibitors of other enzymes of one-carbon metabolism *(4)*, especially thymidylate synthase (TS) and the two key players of *de novo* purine biosynthesis, GAR formyltransferase and AICAR formyltransferase.

From: *Anticancer Drug Development Guide: Antifolate Drugs in Cancer Therapy*
Edited by: A.L. Jackman © Humana Press Inc., Totowa, NJ

AMT (**1**, R = H)
MTX (**2**, R = CH$_3$)

Pyrimethamine (**3** : R = C$_2$H$_5$, n = 0, Z = 4'-Cl
Trimethoprim (**4**) : R = H, n = 1, Z = 3',4',5'-(OMe)$_3$
Metoprine (DDMP, **5**) : R = CH$_3$, n = 0, Z = 3',4'-Cl$_2$

Triazinate (**6**, 'Baker's antifol')

Trimetrexate (**7**) : X = CH, Y = CH$_2$NH, Z = 3',4',5'-(OMe)$_3$
Piritrexim (**8**) : X = N, Y = CH$_2$, Z = 2',5'-(OMe)$_2$

Though this was of course not known at the time of their discovery, MTX and AMT differed in a fundamental way from another large group of DHFR inhibitors that lacked an amino acid side chain and thus were predominantly lipophilic rather than hydrophilic. These lipophilic antifols, a well-known example of which is pyrimethamine (**3**), originally came to light because of their activity against tropical diseases such as malaria *(5)*. Other members of this class, also referred to in the literature as small-molecule antifols, lipid-soluble antifols, and nonclassical antifols *(6–8)*, likewise proved to have a high degree of antibacterial activity, leading to the development of the broad-spectrum agent trimethoprim (**4**) *(9)*. With the recognition that the high basicity of the 2,4-diaminopyrimidine moiety in AMT and MTX is responsible for the exceptionally high DHFR affinity of these compounds *(10)*, it became clear that lipophilic antifols, like their classical cousins with a glutamate side chain, could be useful in cancer treatment, provided that one could achieve the same degree of tumor-vs-host therapeutic selectivity as had been obtained with pyrimethamine against malaria and trimethoprim against bacteria. A large number of lipophilic nonclassical antifolates were synthesized with this in mind, starting in the late 1950s, and several of them, notably metoprine (DDMP, **5**), triazinate (Baker's antifol, **6**), trimetrexate (**7**), and piritrexim (**8**), were evaluated in patients. However, as reviewed elsewhere *(8,11–13)*, the clinical success of these drugs has proved to be somewhat limited, owing in part to their low water solubility, difficulty of pharmaceutical formulation, low therapeutic selectivity, and in some cases (e.g., DDMP), neurotoxicity.

Once the important role of polyglutamation in the biochemical pharmacology of MTX began to be appreciated in the early and mid-1980s (reviewed in refs. *14,15)*, it became apparent that the traditional terminology classifying DHFR inhibitors as classical or lipophilic might not be entirely adequate from a mechanistic perspective, since there are in the literature a substantial number of inhibitors that have a classical structure (i.e., they retain a polar amino acid side chain), but are *functionally* more akin to lipophilic

Polyglutamatable Inhibitors	Historically termed 'classical' antifolates, this group would include aminopterin and methotrexate analogues modified in the B-ring, the bridge, and/or the para-aminobenzoic acid (PABA) moiety, but with an intact L-glutamate side chain as required for FPGS substrate activity.
Nonpolyglutamatable Inhibitors (Type A)	Traditionally called 'nonclassical' or 'small-molecule' antifolates, this group would include very lipophilic drugs like metoprine, trimetrexate, and piritrexim, which are not substrates for the reduced folate carrier (RFC) system utilized by classical antifolates, and are presumably taken up by passive and/or facilitated diffusion.
Nonpolyglutamatable Inhibitors (Type B)	This group would consist of compounds that are more polar than those of Type A and retain most of the basic structural motifs of classical antifolates, including the α-carboxyl group of the side chain. However they cannot form polyglutamates because the γ-carboxyl is blocked or the distal end of the side chain is otherwise modified. Mechanistically these 'hybrid' inhibitors may be viewed as nonclassical antifolates, though they differ from Type A inhibitors in that they are water-soluble, are cleared rapidly, and enter cells via the RFC system. Moreover, in contrast to certain of the Type A inhibitors (e.g., trimetrexate), their activity is not influenced by P-glycoprotein overexpression.

Fig. 1. Proposed mechanistic/structural classification scheme for antifolates.

antifolates by virtue of the fact that the side chain is not amenable to polyglutamation. Thus, it seems appropriate to categorize DHFR inhibitors according to a slightly expanded classification scheme (Fig. 1) which divides nonpolyglutamatable DHFR inhibitors into two distinct groups—type A and type B—according to certain mechanistic/structural criteria. In principle the same scheme can also be used to differentiate among antifolates targeted against other enzymes of one-carbon metabolism, such as TS.

This chapter will present an overview of the type B nonpolyglutamatable DHFR inhibitors, and will include: (1) analogs synthesized prior to the time that the important role of polyglutamation in the therapeutic action of MTX and other classical antifolates first began to be appreciated, and (2) more contemporary examples whose rationale was inspired, at least in part, by the idea that qualitative or quantitative differences in polyglutamation—i.e., the net effect of the opposing activities of the enzymes folyl γ-polyglutamate synthetase (FPGS) and folyl γ-polyglutamyl hydrolase (FPGH)—between tumors and normal tissues might provide a logical framework for drug design.

No attempt will be made to survey the voluminous literature on type A nonpolyglutamatable DHFR inhibitors, for which several excellent reviews already exist *(7,8,11–13)*. However it is worth noting that a key distinction between the type A and type B inhibitors lies in their potential therapeutic application. Thus, the single most important feature of type A inhibitors is their ability to overcome MTX resistance based on defective transport. In contrast, the type B inhibitors have the potential—as yet largely untested in the clinic—to redress the selectivity disadvantage that might be expected to arise when polyglutamation of a classical antifolate is less efficient in a tumor than in dose-limiting normal tissues such as the marrow and gut epithelium.

It has been a longstanding tenet in the antifolate field that when AMT, MTX, and other classical DHFR inhibitors have good antitumor activity at tolerated dosages—

	Therapeutic Selectivity		
Tumor Polyglutamation Efficiency	Polyglutamatable Antifolates	Nonpolyglutamatable Antifolates	Leucovorin Rescue
High	Favorable	No difference	Unfavorable
Low	Unfavorable	No difference	Favorable

Fig. 2. Schematic representation of the predicted selectivity of polyglutamatable vs nonpolyglutamatable antifolates as a function of the polyglutamation efficiency of a tumor relative to dose-limiting tissues.

whether in animal models or in the clinic—this is not the result of intrinsic differences in binding affinity between the enzyme from tumor cells and the enzyme from normal cells, as is the case in the treatment of parasitic or bacterial infections with lipophilic antifolates like trimethoprim. Instead, therapeutic selectivity is considered to be based on differential uptake and retention in tumor vs host tissue, leading to greater depletion of tetrahydrofolate cofactor pools and ultimately selective killing of tumor cells due to lack of recovery of scheduled DNA synthesis. Because MTX and other classical antifolates do not penetrate cells passively except at very high concentrations, their uptake depends on the availability of a membrane-associated active transport system, the RFC. However, even when this system is functional, influx is not by itself sufficient to ensure preferential accumulation in one type of cell vs another. Thus, prolonged inhibition of one-carbon metabolism and DNA synthesis in tumor cells after treatment with a bolus dose of MTX can occur only when these cells are able to efficiently convert the parent drug to its γ-polyglutamated forms, whose multiple negative charge at physiologic pH prevents efflux regardless of the concentration of parent drug in the extracellular space.

Although this model is consistent with the ability of MTX and other classical DHFR inhibitors to selectively retard the growth of certain kinds of malignancy in laboratory animals and patients, it is known that many solid tumors are inherently not very sensitive to these drugs. Moreover, even MTX-sensitive tumors (e.g., leukemias) may relapse and fail to respond to further treatment, including dose intensification. A number of laboratory studies have shown that the principal biochemical phenotype in both types of resistance (i.e., inherent and acquired) is a low capacity by the tumor cells to form γ-polyglutamyl conjugates relative to cells of dose-limiting tissues. Thus host toxicity intervenes before a therapeutically effective drug exposure can be achieved in the tumor. Furthermore, using a more efficiently polyglutamated analog would not alter the outcome unless it were polyglutamated more selectively in the tumor in comparison with MTX.

Whether nonpolyglutamatable DHFR inhibitors can play a role in the treatment of patients whose tumors have a polyglutamation defect can be considered in the context of   which compares the treatment outcome one might predict for polyglutamatable vs nonpolyglutamatable DHFR inhibitors, assuming all other things (e.g., DHFR activity, transport via the RFC pathway, salvage capacity, and rate of recovery of DNA synthesis) to be equal. According to this paradigm, tumors that are *more* efficient than the normal proliferative tissues in converting a classical inhibitor like MTX to polyglutamates are expected to respond favorably, with manageable toxicity to the host. Conversely, patients with tumors that are *less* efficient in forming polyglutamates than the normal proliferative tissues are predicted to fail, since hematopoietic and gastrointestinal toxicity would take precedence over antitumor activity. In contrast, a nonpolyglutamatable (i.e., nonclassical) inhibitor should have about the same therapeutic effect regardless of the ability, or inability, of tumor cells to form polyglutamates in comparison with normal cells. In other words, treatment with a nonpolyglutamatable inhibitor would at least allow the contest to be played on a more level field.

As indicated in Fig. 2, the effect of leucovorin as a rescue agent would be predicted to work in precisely the opposite direction as that of a classical antifolate. That is, more efficient replenishment of the polyglutamated reduced folate pools would be expected in a tumor with high polyglutamation activity than in a tumor with low polyglutamation activity relative to host tissues. Thus, for tumors with low polyglutamation activity, ideal selectivity would be achieved by using a nonpolyglutamatable inhibitor to attack the tumor and leucovorin to rescue the host. Although leucovorin in combination with a type B nonpolyglutamatable inhibitor has not yet been tested in the clinic, use of the type A inhibitor DDMP in this context has been reported to give objective clinical responses in patients with advanced solid tumors *(16)*. Combined use of the type A inhibitor trimetrexate with leucovorin has recently also been advocated *(17–19)*.

Evidence of defective polyglutamation as a phenotype associated with resistance has been obtained in rodent tumor cell lines *(20–22)* and in human leukemia *(23–28)*, breast carcinoma *(29,30)*, head and neck squamous-cell carcinoma *(31–34)*, osteogenic *(35)* and soft tissue *(36,37)* sarcoma, small-cell lung carcinoma *(38,39)*, and cervical carcinoma *(40)* cell lines with inherent or acquired resistance to classical antifolates. In a number of instances, substantial differences in polyglutamation are noted among cell lines established from individual patients with a given type of tumor. Although FPGS downregulation may be a general self-defense mechanism by which cells protect themselves from the lethal action of classical antifolates, it is important to keep in mind that decreased formation of polyglutamates can occur not only via a decrease in the amount of enzyme but also via a decrease in availability of the substrate due to inefficient uptake. Thus merely analyzing the polyglutamate distribution only gives a simplified picture. Furthermore, recent evidence suggests that resistance to classical antifolates may actually result from a combination of decreased FPGS activity and increased FPGH (hydrolase) activity *(41–43)*. However, regardless of the precise reason(s) for inefficient polyglutamation in tumors vs normal tissues, the concept of using leucovorin in combination with a nonpolyglutamatable antifolate to treat these tumors appears to potentially have a wide scope.

2. COMPOUNDS WITH MONOCARBOXYLIC ACID SIDE CHAINS

As a matter of historical interest, it is worth noting that nonpolyglutamatable analogs of AMT made their appearance in the literature as early as 1949, when the Lederle group *(44)* briefly reported the synthesis of AMT analogs with a DL-alanine (**9**), DL-valine (**10**), DL-isoleucine (**11**), DL-serine (**12**), DL-threonine (**13**), L-phenylalanine (**14**), or L-tryptophan (**15**) side chain. The 3',5'-dichloro derivatives **16** and **17** of **10** and **11**, respectively, were also synthesized for comparison with the corresponding L-glutamate analogs *(45)*. Antifolate activity was assayed only against *Streptococcus faecalis,* the organism in routine use for this purpose at the time. The purity of the test samples was not specified and the reported assay data were sparse. However, where a comparison was possible, it was obvious that replacement of the glutamate moiety with a neutral amino acid led to significant loss of potency. Subsequently, MTX analogs with a DL-alanine (**18**), DL-valine (**19**), DL-isoleucine (**20**), L-leucine (**21**), or L-phenylalanine (**22**) side chain were also described *(46)*, as was an AMT analog (**23**) with a glycine side chain *(47)* and most recently an MTX analog (**24**) with an L-histidine side chain *(48)*.

None of the monocarboxylic acids showed anything like the activity of the parent dicarboxylic acids. For example, in tests against L1210 murine leukemia *(46)*, compounds **9–15** were well tolerated at a single doses in the 100–1000 mg/kg range, but extended

	R^1	R^2	X		R^1	R^2	X
9,18	H, CH_3	CH_3	H	14,22	H, CH_3	$CH_2C_6H_5$	H
10,19	H, CH_3	CH_2CH_3	H	15	H	CH_2(indol-3-yl)	H
11,20	H, CH_3	$CH_2CH(CH_3)CH_2CH_3$	H	16	H	CH_2CH_3	3',5'-Cl_2
21	CH_3	$CH_2CH_2CH(CH_3)_2$	H	17	H	$CH_2CH(CH_3)CH_2CH_3$	3',5'-Cl_2
12	H	CH_2OH	H	23	H	H	H
13	H	$CH(CH_3)CH_2OH$	H	24	CH_3	CH_2(imidazol-4-yl)	H

survival by < 25%. In the most detailed mechanistic study on this group of analog *(47)*, **23** was found to be 42-fold weaker than AMT as an inhibitor of partially purified pigeon liver DHFR, which was often used for this purpose at the time. In assays against human KB epithelial carcinoma cells in culture, **23**, had an IC_{50} of 240 μM (AMT: 0.0068 μM) *(47)*. This 35,000-fold loss of molar potency was taken to indicate that the effect of deleting the CH_2 CH_2 COOH moiety from the side chain was mainly on uptake, though our contemporary interpretation would be that the lack of concordance between DHFR inhibition and cell growth inhibition most likely reflects not just influx but also the inability of **23** to form polyglutamates. In agreement with these in vitro results, **23** was well tolerated at doses of up to 80 mg/kg (qd × 9) in mice with L1210 leukemia, but there was no antitumor activity. Not surprisingly, the analogs of MTX in which the side chain was β-alanine, sarcosine, 2-aminobutanoic acid, or 4-aminobutanoic acid, all of which lacked a carboxyl at the α-position, were likewise inactive against the L1210 tumor *(46)*. However, a 40–60% tumor growth delay of Walker 256 rat sarcoma was obtained with the 4- and 2-aminobutanoic acid analogues at doses of 8 and 60 mg/kg (qd × 14), respectively *(46)*. Interestingly, **22** inhibited the growth of the rat tumor by 58% at 40 mg/kg (qd × 9), but was inactive against the L1210 leukemia at 45 mg/kg (qd × 10). It thus appears that these monocarboxylic acids may be taken up differently by Walker 256 carcinoma.

The histidine analog **24** *(48)* was novel in that the pK_a of the imidazole NH is slightly acidic. Thus this compound may be viewed as a diacid even though it contains only one carboxyl group. Not surprisingly, **24** was not an FPGS substrate (nor was it an inhibitor at pH 7.9 or 8.5). It was also not a very effective DHFR inhibitor, with an IC_{50} of 1300 nM (MTX: 73 nM) in an *in situ* tritium release assay indirectly measuring the ability of dihydrofolate to support the synthesis of dTMP in intact L1210 cells *(49)*.

3. COMPOUNDS WITH AMINOMALONATE OR ASPARTATE SIDE CHAINS

Among the compounds originally described by the Lederle group were the aminomalonate analogs **25** and **26** *(44,45)* and the L-aspartate analogs **27** and **28** *(45,50)*. Then, in a landmark paper in 1970 *(51)*, chemists at Parke-Davis described the synthesis of a series of AMT analogs with a quinazoline ring in place of pteridine, among which were the aminomalonates **29–31**, along with the corresponding L-aspartates **32–34** and L-glutamates **35–37**. In addition, because it was not precisely known at that time how the stereochemical configuration of the α-carbon might affect DHFR binding and cellular uptake, the D-aspartate and D-glutamate analog **32A** and **35A** were also prepared. The pteridine malonate analogs **25** and **26** showed very weak activity in the *S. faecalis* screen and were not deemed to be of further interest. Presumably for the same reason (though no assay data can be found in the literature), the quinazoline **29–31** were likewise discarded.

Because the L-aspartate analog **27**, unlike **25** and **26**, showed some antifolate activity, detailed studies of its biochemical and pharmacologic properties were performed *(50)*. These studies were the groundwork for much of the subsequent thinking about the rela-

	X	Y	R	n		X	Y	R	n	
25	N	N	H	0	32	CH	CH	H	1	
26	N	N	CH₃	0	32A	CH	CH	H	1	(D-isomer)
27	N	N	H	1	33	CCH₃	CH	H	1	
28	N	N	CH₃	1	34	CCl	CH	H	1	
29	CH	CH	H	0	35	CH	CH	H	2	
30	CCH₃	CH	H	0	35A	CH	CH	H	2	(D-isomer)
31	CCl	N	H	0	36	CCH₃	CH	H	2	
					37	CCl	CH	H	2	

tionship between structure and biological activity in classical antifolates. Spectrophotometric analysis of the kinetics of inhibition of murine DHFR by **27** gave a K_i of 2 nM. Since a K_i of 0.03 nM had been reported earlier for MTX under identical assay conditions *(10)*, it appeared that shortening of the side chain in MTX by one CH_2 resulted in a 67-fold decrease in binding. This was consistent with experiments comparing the effect of **27** and MTX on *de novo* purine biosynthesis as measured by [^{14}C]formate incorporation into the acid-insoluble fraction of L1210 tumor cells in mice. Thus, the dose of **27** needed to bring about a 50% decrease in ^{14}C incorporation was 40- to 50-fold higher than that of MTX. In experiments comparing the effect of the drugs on liver DHFR activity in mice, a single 10 mg/kg dose of MTX decreased activity by 83%, whereas with **27** even 40 mg/kg given in four daily injections only produced a decrease of only 15%. While this indicated that **27** would probably be better tolerated than MTX, the effect of this analog on survival in L1210 leukemic mice was unimpressive, with a dose of 50 mg/kg (qd × 9) giving an increase in lifespan (ILS) of only 45% (MTX: 400% ILS at 0.78 mg/kg). It is now known, of course, that in addition to weaker DHFR binding, an important reason for the low potency of **27** is likely to be its very low substrate activity for FPGS, which is <1% of that of folic acid *(52)*.

In the quinazoline series, the L-aspartate analogs **32–34**, which were eventually assigned the generic names quinaspar, methasquin, and chlorasquin, were potent inhibitors of the growth of an MTX-sensitive L1210 line (L1210/TC$_2$) in culture *(53,54)*, and in fact were more active than MTX even though they contained an L-aspartate side chain. Subsequently, greater activity was likewise reported by another group for methasquin against murine neuroblastoma cells *(55)*. The IC$_{50}$ values of **32–34** against L1210/TC$_2$ cells after 7-d treatment were 40, 9.4, and 24 n*M* (**35–37**: 6.4, 2.8, and 6.4 n*M;* MTX: 70 n*M*). Moreover, these compounds showed good activity even against a more MTX-resistant L1210 line (L1210/TC$_1$), giving IC$_{50}$ values of 52, 68, and 79 n*M* (**35–37**: 8.6, 10.5, and 12.4 n*M;* MTX: 237 n*M*). However, the L-aspartates were three- to sixfold less active than the corresponding L-glutamates, indicating that shortening of the side chain was somewhat unfavorable, though not disastrously so. Curiously, the D-aspartate analog **32A**, with an IC$_{50}$ of 49 n*M,* was almost as active as the L-enantiomer. This contrasted with the D-glutamate analog **35A**, whose activity was five- to 10-fold lower than that of the L-glutamate. Since there is no published information on the DHFR binding, transport, or kinetics of interaction of **32A** with FPGS, the reason for this unexpected difference is unclear.

A most interesting observation in this early study was that resistance developed more slowly in vivo to **32** than to MTX. In retrospect, this can perhaps be seen as the earliest indication in the literature that nonpolyglutamatable DHFR inhibitors might have a clinical advantage over polyglutamatable inhibitors in the context of acquired drug resistance associated with a decrease in the ability of a tumor to form polyglutamates in comparison with dose-limiting host tissues.

To examine whether there was a correlation between cell-growth inhibition and DHFR inhibition, the IC$_{50}$ values of **32–34** against partly purified mammalian enzyme from rat liver was determined spectrophotometrically and found to be 1.7, 0.4, and 6.4 n*M* (**35–37**: 3.4, 6.9, and 7.5 n*M*) *(56)*. Thus the glutamates were more toxic even though they were bound slightly less tightly to DHFR. This was consistent with an earlier study in Chinese hamster cells, which showed that **32–34** were better inhibitors than MTX or AMT, but that their growth-inhibitory effects were less readily prevented by dihydrofolate *(57)*. Given what is now known about polyglutamation, the lower toxicity of the L-aspartate analogs, as well as the greater ability of dihydrofolate to effect rescue, was presumably because they cannot be metabolized to polyglutamates. Since polyglutamation can increase DHFR binding two- to threefold in diaminopteridine antifolates *(58,59)*, it is possible that a small loss in binding affinity on replacement of L-aspartate by L-glutamate in diaminoquinazoline antifolates would likewise be offset by a compensatory increase in binding by polyglutamation. On the other hand, it should be noted that, in other experiments comparing K_i rather IC$_{50}$ values among these compounds, the K_i of **32–34** against DHFR from L1210 cells was found to be 13, 0.9, and 0.3 pM (**35–37**: 0.6, 0.4, and 0.1 pM) *(60)*. Thus, when more rigorous kinetic analysis was performed, the glutamate analogs appeared to be superior, at least against the murine enzyme.

In vivo antitumor assays comparing the L-aspartates **32–34** with the L-glutamates **35–37** were performed at the Sloan-Kettering Institute in the late 1960s using L1210 leukemic mice *(54)*. Compound **32** gave a 150% ILS at a dose of 6 mg/kg (q2d × 8), and was more effective and less toxic than the corresponding L-glutamate **35**, which at its highest tolerated dose of 0.2 mg/kg (q2d × 8) gave an ILS of only 63%, as did the D-aspartate **32A**. That **32A** was less effective than **32** in vivo even though it had shown comparable potency culture suggested that there might be differences in the clearance rate of the two enantiomers. The 5-methyl analog **33** gave a 186% ILS at 3 mg/kg (qd × 8), and thus was slightly more active than **32**; however the 5-chloro analog **34** was only as good as **32**. Interestingly, **33** was also more toxic to the host animal than MTX, **32**, or **34**. Thus, the LD$_{50}$ of **33** on a qd × 5 schedule was 0.4 mg/kg (MTX: 3–4 mg/kg). For single-dose treatment these values were 47 mg/kg for **33**, 92 mg/kg for MTX, and 170–190 mg/kg for **32** and **34**. In addition, the toxicity of **32** was less easily reversed with leucovorin (LV) than that of MTX, and the optimal timing of rescue was different for the two drugs. Thus, simultaneous treatment with 12 mg/kg of MTX plus 20 mg/kg of LV daily for 5 d completely abrogated both antitumor activity (survival) and host toxicity (weight loss), whereas delaying LV by 16 h afforded a 175% ILS and prevented weight loss. In contrast, treatment with 3 mg/kg of **32** plus 20 mg/kg of LV, given either simultaneously or 16 h later, gave a lower ILS (only 75%) and failed to prevent weight loss, suggesting that with the nonpolyglutamated drug, LV protects the tumor better than the host. It was speculated that the poorer ability of LV to protect host tissues from **32** was caused by the latter's very tight DHFR binding, though different kinds of in vivo association were not ruled out.

Comparative studies of the K_m for influx into L1210 cells, and of the rate constant for efflux of drug from cells after treatment with a large excess of drug, have shed further light on the reason for the lower toxicity of **32–34** relative to MTX despite their strong binding to DHFR. The kinetically determined K_m for competitive inhibition of [^{3}H]MTX uptake for these compounds was in the 24–38 μM range (**35–37**: 2.8–6.7 μM; MTX: 4.4 μM; AMT: 1.4 μM) *(60,61)*. The rate constants for efflux were 0.017–0.019/min for **32–34**, 0.011–0.034/min for **35–37**, and 0.24 and 0.20/min for AMT and MTX *(61)*. Thus, whereas the transport capacity of the RFC for the quinazolines was one-log lower for the L-aspartates than for the L-glutamates, the difference in rate of efflux was relatively insignificant. As a result, when the intracellular/extracellular ratio of free drug concentration at equilibrium was calculated for the quinazolines, it was found to be in the 10–70 range for the L-glutamates and only the 3–10 range for the L-aspartates, MTX, and AMT. Thus, at equilibrium, the amount of free drug in excess of that needed to just saturate DHFR was greater with the L-glutamates than with the L-aspartates.

A novel and as yet unexplained finding was also made in this study with regard to the D-aspartate **32A** *(61)*. Whereas the transport K_m was 38 μM and the first-order constant for efflux was 0.019/min for the **32**, these were 7.7 μM and 0.053/min for **32A**. Since the difference in K_m between the two compounds was greater than the difference in efflux of nonbound drug, the ratio of free intracellular drug relative to extracellular drug at equilibrium was higher for the enantiomer with the unnatural side chain, which was consistent with its greater toxicity in cell culture. Oddly enough, the D- and L-glutamates **35** and **35A** did not show this very unusual feature.

The issue of the tissue selectivity of nonpolyglutamated vs polyglutamated DHFR inhibitors was addressed in a study comparing the extent and duration of DHFR inhibition and DNA synthesis inhibition in tumor cells, gut epithelium, and liver from mice treated with an approximately equimolar bolus dose (3 mg/kg) of MTX, AMT, the L-aspartate **33**, or the L-glutamate **37** *(62)*. Tumors included leukemias (P288, P388, L1210), sarcoma 180, and Ehrlich carcinoma, all implanted intraperitoneally in the ascites form. The peak level of free (i.e., exchangeable) **33** and **37** in L1210 cells was 50- to 100-fold greater than the DHFR level by 1 h, whereas for MTX this level was only half as high. By 24 h, only the level of nonbound quinazolines still exceeded that of the enzyme. Interestingly, the persistence of free drug in L1210 cells was longer for **33** than for MTX, even though only the latter can form polyglutamates. In small intestine, the peak level of exchangeable **33** at 1–2 h only exceeded the DHFR level fivefold and was lower than that of MTX. Moreover free **33** declined to the DHFR level in just 18 h in intestinal cells, whereas in the tumor cells it remained above this level for about twice as long. Interestingly, free **33** in the intestinal cells appeared to persist for a much shorter time than **37**, suggesting that **33** would be less likely to cause the mucositis which is dose-limiting for AMT in mice. The overall pattern for the other tumors was similar, although the peak level tended to be lower and the time for exchangeable drug to decline to the DHFR level tended to be shorter. There was an excellent correlation between the kinetics of cellular drug accumulation and the onset of, and recovery from, DNA synthesis inhibition as measured by [^{3}H]uridine incorporation. Synthesis was inhibited for a longer time in the tumor cells than in the small intestine (24 h for **33** and MTX, 16 h for AMT and **37**) than in the small intestine (approx 12 h for all four drugs). The results, which were similar to those obtained in an earlier paper comparing **33** with MTX and AMT *(63)*, suggested that a greater level of discrimination between tumor cells and intestinal cells might be possible with the nonpolyglutamatable L-aspartate analog **33** than with AMT or the polyglutamatable L-glutamate analog **37**.

Since the conclusion of the preclinical studies was that **33** was the most promising of the quinazoline analogs, a phase I clinical trial was conducted *(64)*, but the drug's effects in humans proved to be not very different from those of AMT, and it was decided that the pharmacological rationale was not compelling enough to justify further clinical evaluation. This came at the time of a major paradigm change, when intense interest arose in targeting enzymes of folate metabolism other than DHFR. Although the decision to abandon methasquin as an anticancer drug was perhaps unfortunate, this compound offered many important lessons and was a milestone in the history of antifolates.

4. COMPOUNDS WITH OTHER AMINOALKANEDIOIC ACID SIDE CHAINS

Nonpolyglutamable AMT and MTX analogs with a side chain consisting of a dicarboxylic amino acid other than aminomalonic, aspartic, or glutamic acid have been synthesized, and have been tested in vitro and in vivo with a view to assessing the effect of increasing the distance between the carboxyl groups.

The AMT analog **38** *(47)* inhibited pigeon liver DHFR with an IC$_{50}$ of 13 nM (MTX,

AMT: 26 n*M*), suggesting that the introduction of an additional carbon atom was not detrimental to binding and might in fact enhance it slightly. However, in cytotoxicity as-

	R	n	α-configuration
38	H	3	not specified
39–46	Me	3–10	L
47–49	H	6,9,10	L

says against KB cells, the IC_{50} was 25 n*M* (AMT: 3 n*M*; MTX: 4 n*M*) (note that these are IC_{50} rather than K_i values, which would be in the picomolar range). In mice with L1210 leukemia, an optimal 20 mg/kg (qd × 9) dose of **38** gave only a 57% ILS (MTX: 74% at 0.67 mg/kg). Similar findings were reported *(65)* for the MTX analogs **39–41**, which were specified to have the natural L-enantiomeric configuration. The IC_{50} of these compounds against murine DHFR was in the 35–40 n*M* range (MTX: 32 n*M*), and their IC_{50} values against L1210 cells in culture ranged from 30 n*M* (**39**) to 6.3 n*M* (**41**) (MTX: 20 n*M*). In vivo against L1210 leukemia, **40** and **41** both gave a 133% ILS at 40 mg/kg (qd × 9), whereas **39** required a larger dose of 60 mg/kg to produce the same effect (MTX: 133% ILS at only 6 mg/Kg). Overall it appeared that the therapeutic effect of these chain-extended analogs was comparable to that of MTX, but the dose needed to achieve this effect was consistently higher. The results were taken to mean that the chain-extended analogs were not taken up as efficiently as MTX. However it was also speculated that these results might reflect the fact that **39–41** were not polyglutamatable and thus were acting solely as DHFR inhibitors. Furthermore it was proposed that the inability of these compounds to form polyglutamates had a potential therapeutic advantage in certain situations. This concept was articulated for the first time in the following sentence (ref. *65,* page 1720): "Lack of polyglutamation is potentially a therapeutic asset, because in the treatment of MTX-resistant tumors with a *capacity for polyglutamation that is low in comparison with normal proliferative tissue,* dose escalation should be tolerated better with nonpolyglutamatable compounds than with MTX." The very low efficiency of **39–41** as FPGS substrates in comparison with MTX was subsequently demonstrated, though **40** actually seemed to have some low-level substrate activity (20% relative to folic acid) *(66)*. It was speculated that the $(CH_2)_n$ chain could adopt a conformation allowing the terminal CO_2H to fit properly into FPGS active site when *n* was 2 or 4, but not when *n* was 3 or 5.

The question of whether chain-extended MTX and AMT analogs utilize the RFC pathway was examined by comparing the ability of LV and **39** to inhibit influx of [^{3}H]MTX in CCRF-CEM human leukemic lymphoblasts *(67)*. Although competitive inhibition kinetics by **39** were observed, indicating that it is taken up at least in part via the RFC, **39** ($K_i = 15$ μ*M*, $K_i/K_m = 11$) was a sevenfold poorer inhibitor than LV ($K_i = 2.1$ μ*M*, $K_i/K_m = 1.5$).

In a later study extending this work, D,L-2-aminoalkanedioic acid analogs of MTX and AMT with up to ten CH_2 groups (**42–49**), were synthesized and tested *(68)*. All of these chain-lengthened analogs were good DHFR inhibitors, with IC_{50} values ranging from 23 to 34 n*M* for the MTX analogs **42–46** and 54 to 67 n*M* for the AMT analogs **47–49**. None of the longer-chain compounds were FPGS substrates, and indeed, at equimolar concentration, inhibited the FPGS-catalyzed reaction of folic acid by

40–60%. In growth inhibition assays against L1210 cells, the IC_{50} ranged from 1.2 to 26 nM for the MTX analogs **42–46** (MTX: 4.6 nM) and from 0.65 to 20 nM for the AMT analogs **47–49** (AMT: 2 nM). The best member of the series, **48** ($n = 9$), was three times more active than AMT. If most of this effect was due to the L-enantiomer, the activity ratio relative to AMT could be as high as 6:1; however, given the data reported for the L- and D-aspartates **32** and **32A** (*see* above), the validity of this assumption still needs to be formally shown.

In vivo against L1210 leukemia, the best MTX analog was **46** ($n = 10$), giving a 137% ILS at a dose of 20 mg/kg (qd × 9) (MTX: 95% ILS at 4 mg/Kg). The AMT analog **49**, with same number of CH_2 groups, was therapeutically less effective, giving only a 57% ILS at 12.5 mg/kg. At 25 and 50 mg/kg there were toxic deaths. Thus MTX analogs, but not AMT analogs, with a chain-extended side chain seemed to be more active than the parent drug on the same qd × 9 schedule even though they were not FPGS substrates.

Two other nonpolyglutamatable analogs containing a nonbranched dicarboxylic acid side chain are worth noting briefly. The DL-3-aminoglutaric acid analog **50**, in which the position of attachment of the pteroyl moiety has been moved down the chain by one carbon *(69)*, was found to be a surprisingly good DHFR inhibitor, with an IC_{50} against the murine enzyme of 10 nM (MTX: 3.5 nM). However **50** had < 0.01% of the substrate activity of folic for murine FPGS *(52,66)*, and it is therefore not surprising that, when it was given to mice with L1210 leukemia, this compound gave an ILS of only 18% at 100 mg/kg (qd × 9) (MTX: 54% at 2 mg/kg). The DL-2-amino-3-*trans*-hexenedioic acid analogs **51** and **52** were likewise good inhibitors of mouse DHFR, with IC_{50} values of 46 and 32 nM *(70)*. However, whereas the AMT analog **51** was reasonably active against cultured L1210 cells, with an IC_{50} of 31 nM, the activity of the MTX analog **52** (IC_{50} = 350 nM) was 10-fold lower (unpublished data provided by J.H. Freisheim). This was in agreement with the results for a number of other nonpolyglutamatable AMT and MTX analogs described elsewhere in this chapter, which suggest that, as a general rule, a CH_2NH bridge is preferable to a CH_2NMe bridge when polyglutamation is not possible.

Other interesting recent examples of DHFR inhibitors with an aminoadipic acid side chain are compounds **53–55**, which were developed as potential antiarthritic agents with the rationale that their inability to undergo polyglutamation might decrease toxicity to normal proliferative tissues *(71,72)*. Although drugs against arthritis are not within the scope of this review, it is worth noting that type B nonpolyglutamatable DHFR inhibitors may one day prove useful in the treatment of diseases other than cancer.

53 : X = CH$_2$
54 : X = CH$_2$O
55 : X = CH$_2$S

5. INHIBITORS WITH POLAR SUBSTITUTION ON THE GLUTAMATE SIDE CHAIN

The first example of this category to be investigated as a nonpolyglutamatable DHFR inhibitor was γ-fluoroMTX, whose synthesis and properties as a mixture of DL-*erythro* and DL-*threo* diastereomers (**56–59**) were described in preliminary fashion in 1983 *(73)*, and were reported again recently with full details *(74)*. An independent account of the synthesis of the four-diastereomer mixture has also appeared *(75,76)*, as well as stereospecific syntheses of the DL-*erythro* mixture **56/57** and the DL-*threo* mixture **58/59** from purified DL-*erythro*- and DL-*threo*-γ-fluoroglutamic acid precursors, followed by HPLC resolution of the individual diastereomers *(77)*. A method of chemical synthesis of the pure *threo*-γ-fluoroMTX (**59**) which avoids the need for resolution has also been developed *(74)*. In addition, syntheses of β,β-difluoroMTX (**60**) *(74)* and γ,γ-difluoro-MTX (**61**) *(78)*, both as DL mixtures, have been reported.

	A	B	C	D	E	F	Stereochemistry	
56	H	COOH	H	H	F	H	L-*threo*	(2S,4S)
57	COOH	H	H	H	H	F	D-*threo*	(2R,4R)
58	H	COOH	H	H	H	F	L-*erythro*	(2S,4R)
59	COOH	H	H	H	F	H	D-*erythro*	(2R,4S)
60 {	H	COOH	H	H	H	F	L (2S)	
	COOH	H	H	H	H	F	D (2R)	
61 {	H	COOH	H	H	F	H	L (2S)	
	COOH	H	H	H	F	H	D (2R)	
62	H(COOH)	COOH(H)	H	H	OH(H)	H(OH)	Mixture	
63	H(COOH)	COOH(H)	H	H	SCH$_3$(H)	H(SCH$_3$)	Mixture	
64	H(COOH)	COOH (H)	H	H	CN(H)	H(CN)	Mixture	
65	H(COOH)	COOH(H)	OH(H)	H(OH)	H	H	Mixture	

The ability of the mono- and difluorinated MTX analogs **56–61** to inhibit mammalian DHFR is similar to MTX, though there appear to be some very minor differences depending on the number and location of the fluorine atom(s) and the stereochemistry of the α-carbon. Thus, in direct spectrophotometric assays against partly purified DHFR from CCRF-CEM cells, for example, L-*threo*-γ-fluoroMTX (**56**) had an IC$_{50}$ of 0.62 nM, whereas L-*erythro*-γ-fluoroMTX (**58**), in which the α-carboxyl group and γ-fluorine atom have a gauche orientation, had an IC$_{50}$ of 0.50 nM *(77)*. The same order of activity was obtained in assays comparing DL-*threo*-γ-fluoroMTX with DL-*erythro*-γ-fluoroMTX, except that the IC$_{50}$ values were higher (1.35 and 1.0 nM, respectively), implying that the D-isomer was more tightly bound than the L-isomer in each case; the IC$_{50}$ of DL-MTX was 1.18 nM vs variously given values in the 0.6–0.9 nM range for L-MTX *(74,77,80,81)*. These results were also consistent with earlier data from competitive [^{3}H]MTX displacement assays *(73)*. In transport experiments using CCRF-CEM cells, the K_m for **56** was found to 65 μM ($V_{max}/K_m = 0.13$) vs 9.3 μM ($V_{max}/K_m = 0.8$) for **58** and 6–10 μM ($V_{max}/K_m = 1.4$–1.7) for MTX, indicating considerable preference by the RFC system for the *erythro* configuration *(77)*. Inhibition of the transport of **56** and **58** by MTX obeyed competitive kinetics, and both compounds effluxed at about the same rate as MTX. An unexpected finding was that γ-fluoro substitution in the mixed diastereomers decreased, but did not abolish, the ability to form γ-glutamyl adducts. Moreover the product of γ-monoglutamation of the mixed diastereomers **56–59**, whatever its diastereomeric composition, resisted degradation by γ-glutamyl hydrolase *(79)*. Thus, to the extent that the γ-monoglutamyl adduct of **56** were taken up into cells, it could be viewed as another type of nonpolyglutamatable MTX analog.

Reflecting its stronger DHFR binding and more efficient accumulation, **56** (IC$_{50}$ = 37 nM) was a little more active than **58** (IC$_{50}$ = 102 nM) as an inhibitor of CCRF-CEM cell growth after 120 h of incubation. However the difference in potency between **56** and MTX (IC$_{50}$ = 15 nM) under these rather prolonged conditions of exposure was less than threefold. It had been noted at the outset of this work that there is a dramatic difference in IC$_{50}$ between the mixture **56–59** and MTX as a function of drug exposure, ranging from 2300-fold after a 2-h incubation to 12-fold after a 72-h incubation *(73)*. Thus the relatively small difference in potency between **56** and MTX after 120 h of treatment was not surprising.

Although in vivo data have thus far been reported only for the four-diastereomer mixture **56–59** *(76)*, it appears that introduction of a strongly electron withdrawing γ-fluoro substituent does not alter the therapeutic benefit as measured by survival, but does lead to considerable loss of potency. Thus, whereas MTX gave a 241% ILS (5/7 mice living >30 d) in L1210 leukemic mice treated with at a dose of 10 mg/kg (qd × 5), the mixture of γ-fluoro derivatives gave an ILS of >221% (3/7 mice living >30 d), but this required a dose of 640 mg/kg. Although the pure L-*threo* diastereomer **56** would very likely have shown greater potency than the mixture, it appears even from these limited results that γ-fluoro substitution does not offer an advantage over the other nonpolyglutamatable DHFR inhibitors described above.

Bioassay results reported for the DL-γ,γ-difluoro and DL-β,β-difluoro analogs **60** and **61** are generally consistent with those for γ-monofluoro substitution. Thus, in spectrophotometric assays of DHFR activity in extracts of CCRF-CEM cells, **60** gave an IC$_{50}$ of 1.53 nM (MTX: 0.72 nM), the IC$_{50}$ for inhibition of [^{3}H]MTX uptake was approximately twice that of nonradioactive L-MTX *(78)*, and substrate activity for FPGS from CCRF-CEM cells was virtually nil. With **61** the IC_{50} against DHFR was 1.34 nM (MTX: 0.60 nM), indicating little difference between β,β- and γ,γ-difluoro substitution as far as DHFR binding was concerned *(74)*. Interestingly, **61** was a better inhibitor of [³H]MTX uptake than **60** and, unlike **60**, showed very good FPGS substrate activity, with a K_m of 5.4 μM (V_{max}/K_m = 0.16) against the human enzyme and 3.1 μM (V_{max}/K_m = 0.25) against the rat enzyme, assuming that only the L-enantiomer was active *(80)*. The K_m for MTX as the substrate for the two enzymes was 47 μM (V_{max}/K_m = 0.022) and 19 μM (V_{max}/K_m = 0.053), respectively. It should be noted, however, that the γ-L-glutamyl adduct of **61**, like that of **60**, is not a substrate for FPGS and thus may be viewed as another nonpolyglutamatable γ-substituted MTX analog. Consistently with its DHFR binding and cellular uptake properties, **61** was a potent inhibitor of the growth of CCRF-CEM cells, with an IC_{50} (120 h) of 16.3 nM (MTX: 14.6 nM). Recalling that **61** is racemic, it is very likely that the IC_{50} for the L-enantiomer under these long-exposure conditions could be as low as 8.2 nM (i.e., roughly one-half the IC_{50} of MTX). On the other hand it is also likely that, in shorter-term exposures, **61**, like the diastereomeric mixture **56–59**, would be less active than MTX even though it can be partially converted to a γ-glutamyl dipeptide.

In addition to being tested against human enzymes and cells as discussed above, the fluorinated MTX analogs, either as mixtures of diastereomers or as single isomers, were tested as substrates for FPGS from H35 rat hepatoma cells, as well as for the ability to inhibit the growth of these cells and several MTX-resistant H35 sublines *(73,77,80,81)*. In general, the results obtained with rat and human FPGS were quite similar, as were the results with wild-type H35 cells and CCRF-CEM cells. The original publications should be consulted for details.

The possibility that other polar, but less electronegative groups might be superior to a γ-fluoro substituent has been addressed, albeit in very limited fashion, by the Shionigi Laboratories group, which, in addition to the diastereomeric mixture of γ-fluoro analogs *(75)*, also synthesized the γ-hydroxy analog **62** and the γ-methylthio analog **63**, in both cases as mixtures of stereoisomers in various ratios *(79)*. The IC_{50} values of these compounds against bovine DHFR and avian DHFR were found to quite similar to that of MTX. In vivo, the γ-methylthio analog **63**, as 2.3:1 mixture of structurally unspecified stereoisomers, gave a 99% ILS when given at a dose of 100 mg/kg (qd × 5), but it is unclear whether this was the highest tolerated dose or merely the highest dose tested. The γ-hydroxy analog **62**, with an ILS of <60%, was much less active, and no follow-up data have appeared. Another nonpolyglutamatable analog with a polar group in the side chain, the γ-cyano derivative **64**, has been synthesized and tested *(82)*. The IC_{50} of **64**, as a mixture of diastereomers, against murine DHFR was 57 nM (MTX: 25 nM), and its IC_{50} (48 h) against cultured L1210 cells was 18 nM (MTX: 4.6 nM). Assuming that one of the four diastereomers is mainly responsible for these activities, it seems likely that the active species may have about the same potency as MTX despite the presence of γ-substituent.

In addition to the γ-substituted analogs **62–64**, the synthesis and biological properties of β-hydroxyMTX (**65**), as a mixture of diastereomers, have been reported *(83)*. The IC_{50} for inhibition of human DHFR by **65** was 5.9 nM (MTX: 5.2 nM), and there was negligible substrate activity for human FPGS. Some activity was obtained in culture against a human B-cell lymphoma (Manca), with an IC_{50} (72 h) of 29 nM (MTX: 6 nM). Activity was also obtained against H35 and H35R rat hepatoma cells, the latter of which are a MTX-resistant subline with defective transport. It thus appeared that introduction of a polar group in the side chain could yield an active nonpolyglutamatable inhibitor of cell growth even when the substituent was on the β-carbon rather than the γ-carbon.

To summarize this section, introduction of polar substituents at the β- or γ-position seems to offer no advantage over lengthening the distance between carboxyl groups as a strategy for the design of type B nonpolyglutamatable DHFR inhibitors.

6. BRANCHED-CHAIN GLUTAMATE ANALOGS

Two examples of branched-chain MTX analogs with an α-substituent have been described, α-methylMTX (**66**) and α-difluoromethylMTX (**67**) *(76)*. Although these compounds were DHFR inhibitors, with an IC_{50} only a little higher than that of MTX, they were inactive (ILS <25%) against L1210 leukemia in mice at doses up to 400 mg/kg (qd × 5) *(75)*. Though experiments were not carried out to address this point, it seems likely that sterically bulky α-substitution is unfavorable for binding to the RFC and may also prevent FPGS substrate activity. In contrast to these results, mixtures of the diastereomers of **68** (γ-methylMTX) were found to bind reasonably well to bovine and avian DHFR, and gave a 90–100% ILS in mice with L1210 leukemia when given at a dose of 40 mg/kg (qd × 5) *(76)*. Lower ILS values were obtained at higher doses, suggesting that the compound may be toxic.

66,67 : X = NCH$_3$; R^1 = CH$_3$, CHF$_2$; R^2 = R^3 = H (diastereomer mixture)
68 : X = NCH$_3$; R^2 = CH$_3$; R^1 = R^3 = H (diastereomer mixture)
69,70 : X = NH, NCH$_3$; R^1 = H; R^{2}R^3 = CH$_2$ (racemic)
71 : X = CH$_2$, R^1 = H, R^{2}R^3 = CH$_2$
72 : X = CH(C$_2$H$_5$), R^1 = H, R^{2}R^3 = CH$_2$ (diastereomer mixture)

Several nonpolyglutamatable γ-methylene analogs of classical DHFR inhibitors have likewise been synthesized and tested *(82–84)*. An obvious advantage of γ-methylene derivatives is that they contain only one chiral center. In general the biological properties of the γ-methyleneglutamates proved comparable to those of analogs with a tetrahedral rather than trigonal carbon at the γ-position. Thus, γ-methyleneAMT (**69**), as a mixture of D- and L-enantiomers, inhibited murine DHFR with an IC_{50} of 88 nM (MTX: 25 nM) and inhibited the growth of L1210 cells with an IC_{50} (48 h) of 29 nM (MTX: 4.6 nM) *(82)*. Similarly, racemic γ-methyleneMTX (**70**) inhibited human DHFR with an IC_{50} of 6.4 nM (MTX: 4 nM) and inhibited the growth of CCRF-CEM cells with an IC_{50} (72 h) of 30 nM (MTX: 10 nM) *(83)*.

The γ-methylene-10-deaza derivatives, **71** and **72,** were potent inhibitors of human DHFR with IC$_{50}$ values of 8.8 and 5.8 nM (10-DAM and 10-EDAM: 3.9 nM) *(83),* but substrate activity for human FPGS was negligible, as in the case of **69** and **70**. The IC$_{50}$ (72 h) for CCRF-CEM cell-growth inhibition was 13 nM for **71** and 7.4 nM for **72** (MTX: 14 nM) *(84)*. Thus, γ-methylene substitution led to about the same modest decrease in binding with 10-DAM and 10-EDAM as it did with AMT and MTX, and the ability to inhibit cell growth during 72-h exposure was retained despite loss of FPGS substrate activity. Growth inhibition data were also obtained against Manca human lymphoma cells, as well as H35 and H35R rat hepatoma cells. The γ-methylene derivatives were active against the H35 cells but failed to overcome resistance in the H35R cells. In assays against the National Cancer Institute in vitro solid tumor panel, **71** and **72** gave IC$_{50}$ values that were generally in the 0.1–1.0 nM range, well below the IC$_{50}$ of MTX *(84)*.

In experiments to assess in vivo antitumor efficacy *(84)*, **72** was administered in slow-release pellet form to leukemic mice with at doses of 5–30 mg/kg/d for 15 d starting 1 d after tumor implantation. The results were rather disappointing, in that the ILS at 30 mg/kg/d was only 43% against L1210 leukemia and 69% against P388 leukemia. However, when a 100 mg/kg loading dose was added, the ILS against P388 leukemia increased to 97%. Neither results with 10-EDAM nor results with other regimens were reported. Given the excellent activity of **72** against human solid-tumor cell lines in culture, it is possible that better in vivo results could be obtained in xenograft models.

73 : R^1 = R^2 = H(COOH); R^3 = COOH(H) (two D,L pairs)
74 : R^1 = CH$_3$; R^2 = H(COOH); R^3 = COOH(H) (two D,L pairs)

In addition to the compounds with a β- or γ-substituted glutamate side chain described above, two novel nonpolyglutamatable AMT and MTX analogs (**73,74**) have been reported in which the side chain is a conformationally rigid β,γ-disubstituted glutamate analog, *trans*-γ-(2-carboxycyclopropyl)glycine *(85)*. Each compound was tested as a mixture of diastereomers, each of which could in principle have different affinities for DHFR and the RFC. Not surprisingly, neither compound was a substrate for murine FPGS, but both were good inhibitors of murine DHFR, with IC$_{50}$ values of 22 and 28 nM (AMT, MTX: 25 nM). Since the pair of isomers with the D-configuration at the α-carbon would presumably not bind as well as the pair with the L-configuration, one of the diastereomers with L-configuration may actually bind better than AMT and MTX. Despite their good activity against DHFR, **73** and **74** were very poor inhibitors of cell growth, with an IC$_{50}$ (48 h) in the 1000–2000 nM range against L1210 cells (MTX: 4.6 n$M;$ AMT: 2 nM) and 300–600 nM range against WI-L2 human leukemic lymphoblasts (MTX: 13 nM; AMT: 7.1 nM). Thus, even after making allowance for the fact that only one diastereomeric form of each compound is responsible for activity, this particular modification of the side chain seemed most unpromising, perhaps because of the conformational rigidity inherent in the cyclopropane ring.

7. ANALOGS WITH A BLOCKED γ-CARBOXYL GROUP

7.1 γ-Esters

A mechanistically obvious approach to the design of type B nonpolyglutamatable DHFR inhibitors is to convert the terminal carboxyl of the glutamate side chain to a stable ester or amide and leave the α-carboxyl free to allow tight binding to DHFR and utilization of the RFC pathway for cellular uptake. The literature contains many such compounds, though in most cases they were not synthesized for this purpose.

75: $R^1 = CH_3, R^2 = t\text{-Bu}$
76: $R^1 = H, R^2 = t\text{-Bu}$
77: $R^1 = CH_3; R^2 = CH_3, C_2H_5, C_4H_9\text{-n}, C_8H_{17}\text{-n}, C_{12}H_{25}\text{-n}, C_{16}H_{33}\text{-n}$

Because of the lability of straight-chain alkyl esters to nonspecific serum esterases, these γ-blocked derivatives are better viewed as prodrugs than as drugs in their own right. In contrast, tertiary alkyl esters such as γ-t-butylMTX (**75**) *(86,87)* and γ-t-butyl-AMT (**76**) *(87)* are sterically hindered and resistant to esterase cleavage. Although a number of straight-chained MTX γ-esters (**77**, R = O-alkyl), have been described *(88,89)*, they are potentially cleavable by esterases and thus will not be discussed further here.

The IC_{50} of **75** against purified murine DHFR was found to be 55 nM (MTX: 67 nM) *(87)*. This confirmed that a free γ-carboxyl group is not required for tight binding to DHFR. Against cultured CCRF-CEM and L1210 cells, however, **75** had an IC_{50} (48 h) of 620 and 56 nM (MTX: 32 and 2 nM). Against a panel of three human head-and-neck squamous-cell carcinoma (SCC) lines, the IC_{50}s of **75** were in the 0.3–0.5 nM range (MTX: 0.01–0.03 nM). Thus, in addition to preventing polyglutamation *(52)*, blocking of the γ-carboxyl group probably diminished cellular uptake. However it was of interest, in terms of the potential utility of nonpolyglutamatable DHFR inhibitors in the treatment MTX-resistant tumors, that full growth-inhibitory activity was retained against a 210-fold MTX-resistant cell line, CEM/MTX *(90)*, whose RFC was so impaired that there was negligible polyglutamation even when the extracellular MTX concentration was 100 μM *(91)*. Moreover, there was only partial cross-resistance to **75** in two MTX-resistant L1210 and three MTX-resistant SCC sublines. The AMT analog gave similar overall results *(87)*.

In comparative kinetic studies of influx into CCRF-CEM cells *(92)*, **75** gave K_m and V_{max} values of approx 3.4 μM and 0.06 pmol/min/mg protein (V_{max}/K_m = 57), whereas with MTX these values were 4.7 and 0.40 (V_{max}/K_m = 12). Thus, influx into the parental cell line was approx fivefold more efficient with **75** even though the γ-carboxyl was blocked. When the kinetics of influx were analyzed for each drug in CEM/MTX cells, the K_m and V_{max} were found to be almost the same as in CCRF-CEM cells. However there were significant differences in the rate of drug efflux after a 2-h preloading period (during which at least some polyglutamation would be expected to occur): the $t_{1/2}$ of **75** was 4.3 min from both cells (MTX: 11 min from CCRF-CEM cells, 1.6 min from CEM/MTX cells). Rapid efflux of MTX from CEM/MTX cells was consistent with their inability to form polyglutamates. It thus appeared that inefficient MTX uptake associated with defective transport and polyglutamation could be overcome through the use of a nonpolyglutamatable MTX analog with a lipophilic moiety in the γ-terminal region.

When tested against L1210 leukemia in mice, **75** at its highest tolerated dose of 80 mg/kg/injection (bid × 10, total dose 1600 mg) gave an 80% ILS (**76**: 69% at 12 mg/kg; MTX: 78% at 0.5 mg/kg; AMT: 75% at 0.12 mg/kg) *(87)*. Thus, when the two esters and two acids were compared at roughly equiactive doses, each ester was approx 100-fold less potent than the corresponding acid. Curiously, treatment with **76** at 80 mg/kg (qd × 9, total dose 720 mg) gave a similar ILS of 89%. Thus, somewhat suprisingly in view of earlier work on other analogs with a modified side chain *(65,86,93,94)*, the twice-daily regimen in this case was not superior to once-a-day treatment.

The low in vivo activity of **75** and **76** relative to MTX and AMT was consistent with the working hypothesis that, in order for nonpolyglutamatable DHFR inhibitors to be as potent as MTX or AMT (or more potent) in vivo as well as in vitro, they have to be much more efficiently transported into cells, much more tightly bound to the enzyme, or both. The t-butyl esters, perhaps because they are not lipophilic enough, apparently failed to adequately meet these criteria.

7.2. γ-Amides

A number of these γ-blocked nonpolyglutamatable compounds have been described in the literature, including MTX and AMT derivatives of general structure **78** (R = alkyl, aralkyl, aryl) *(95–101)* and very recently an extensive series of γ-amide derivatives of general structure **79** *(102,103)*. The latter were designed by the Takeda Chemical Industries group as nonpolyglutamatable versions of their novel 2,4-diaminopyrrolo[2,3-*d*]pyrimidine antifolates with a two- to four-carbon bridge *(102–105)*. Similar γ-amide derivatives of other classical 2,4-diamino antifolates with a glutamate side chain have not been studied to date. Because of the large number of congeners in each of the above series, the biological properties of only a few representative examples will be reviewed here.

MTX γ-(benzylamide) (**78**, R = CH_3, X = $NHCH_2C_6H_5$) inhibited murine DHFR with a K_i of 3.6 pM (MTX: 4.3 pM) *(97)*, and was predictably not a substrate for FPGS *(52)*. In experiments measuring competitive inhibition of [^{3}H]MTX influx, the amide had a K_i of 3.8 μM (nonradioactive MTX: 3.5 μM). The first-order rate constant for efflux from cells 24 h after preloading was 0.19/min (MTX: 0.23/min). Thus, even though it prevented the ability to form polyglutamates, this structure modification produced

78

R	X	References
CH_3	NHOH	95
CH_3	$NHNH_2$, NHC_4H_9-n, $CH_2C_6H_5$,	96
CH_3	NH_2, $NHCH_3$, $N(CH_3)_2$, $NH(CH_2)_4CH_3$, $NHCH_2C_6H_5$	97
CH_3	NH_2, $NHCH_3$, NHC_2H_5, NHC_3H_7-n, NH(cyclohexyl), piperidino, morpholino	98,99
CH_3	NHC_6H_3(3,4-methylenedioxy), NH(3,4-dihydroxyphenyl)	100
CH_3	NHC_6H_4COOH-m, $NHC_6H_4B(OH)_2$-m	101
H	NHC_4H_9-t, NH(1-adamantyl), $NHCH_2C_6H_5$, $NHCH_2C_6H_3$(3,4-Cl_2), $NHCH_2C_6H_3$(2,6-Cl_2), NHC_6H_5, NHC_6H_3(3,4-methylenedioxy), NH(3,4-dihydroxyphenyl)	100
H	NHC_6H_4COOH-m	101

79

n	R	References
2	C_6H_5, C_6H_4[3-$B(OH)_2$], C_6H_4(2-, 3-, 4-CO_2H), C_6H_4(2-, 3-, 4-CN), C_6H_4(2-, 3-, 4-tetrazolyl), C_6H_4(2-, 3-, 4-OH), C_6H_4(3-CH_2CO_2H), C_6H_4(3-CO_2H-4-OH), C_6H_4(3-CO_2H-6-F), C_6H_3(3,4-OCH_2O), C_6H_4(3-$SCH_2C_6H_5$), (3-, 4-, 5-carboxy-2-naphthyl), (5-benzotriazolyl), (5-carboxy-2-pyridyl), (5-carboxy-3-pyridyl), (1H-tetrazol-5-yl), (4-carboxymethylthiazol-2-yl)	102,103
3	C_6H_5, C_6H_4[3-$B(OH)_2$], C_6H_4(3-CO_2H), (1H-tetrazol-5-yl), (4-carboxymethylthiazol-2-yl)	102,103

only minor changes in DHFR binding and cellular accumulation. The IC_{50} (72 h) of the amide against H.Ep.2 cells was found to be 210 nM (MTX: 2.4 nM). Against this particular cell line abolition of FPGS substrate activity led to a 100-fold decrease in biological activity. Interestingly, when the amide was tested against L1210 cells rather than H.Ep.2 cells, it was found to have an IC_{50} of 30 nM, a value close to that of MTX *(96)*. However when tested in vivo against L1210 leukemia in mice *(97)*, it gave only a 33% ILS at 100 mg/kg (qd × 9) (MTX: 48% at 1.3 mg/kg, a 76-fold difference in potency). The reasons for the divergent results between H.Ep.-2 and L1210 cells in vitro and between L1210 leukemia in vitro and in vivo are unknown.

The γ-(benzylamide) of AMT (**78**, R = H, X = $NHCH_2C_6H_5$) has also been studied *(100)*. Its binding to purified DHFR from L1210 cells was approx fourfold weaker than that of AMT, and its IC_{50} against L1210 cells in culture was 5 nM (AMT: 2 nM). Against L1210 leukemia in mice at a dose of 80 mg/kg (qd × 9), there was a 56% ILS (AMT: 122% ILS at 1 mg/kg, an 80-fold difference in potency). Thus the overall results with the MTX and AMT amide were quite similar.

The most active γ-amide of this series against L1210 cells in culture was AMT γ-(3,4-methylenedioxyanilide) (**78**, R = H, X = NHC_6H_3[3,4-OCH_2O]) *(100)*, with an IC_{50} (48 h) of 0.4 nM (AMT: 2 nM). When it was tested in vivo against L1210 leukemia this aromatic amide gave a 56% ILS at 20 mg/kg (qd × 9). Thus, a similar outcome was obtained as with the γ-benzylamide but at a fourfold lower dose. Unfortunately, doses of the 3,4-methylenedioxyanilide greater than 20 mg/kg were not tolerated, indicating that this modification increased not only antitumor activity but also toxicity to host tissues. In the in vivo experiments, the best compound of this group proved to be AMT γ-(3,4-

dichlorobenzyl)amide, with an ILS of 110% at 70 mg/kg. Interestingly this compound was 100-fold less active than the 3,4-methylenedioxyanilide against L1210 cells in culture, attesting to the imprecision of in vitro vs in vivo correlation as a guide to analog design.

Among the more than 30 different γ-amides from the Takeda group, the best DHFR inhibitors were those in which the γ-substituent contained an aromatic ring and a carboxyl group *(102,103)*. For example, the γ-(m-carboxyanilide) inhibited beef liver DHFR with an IC_{50} of 8.2 nM vs 370 nM for TNP-351, the parent drug with a free γ-carboxyl. Against CCRF-CEM cells, the IC_{50} (72 h) of this analog was 4 nM (MTX: 10 nM). Against the murine solid tumor cell line Meth A, the IC_{50} (72 h) was only 0.8 nM. In vivo against the Meth A tumor in mice, 4 mg/kg of the m-carboxyanilide every other day gave a 50% greater tumor growth delay than 8 mg/kg of TNP-351. Similar results were obtained against the Colon 26 tumor. By way of comparison, it may be noted that in an earlier paper on the γ-(m-carboxyanilides) of MTX and AMT, the IC_{50} of these derivatives against cultured L1210 cells were reported to be 1.6 and 0.7 nM, respectively (MTX: 4.6 nM; AMT: 2.0 nM) *(101)*. Almost all the other γ-amides of TNP-351 were tight-binding DHFR inhibitors and had IC_{50} values in the 1–10 nM range against Meth A sarcoma cells. Thus there was reasonable literature precedent for the design of analogs with two acid groups and a hydrophobic aromatic ring in the side chain. To date, however, the heterocyclic ring system exemplified by TNP-351 is the only one in which this type of glutamate modification has been systematically examined.

A most interesting observation in the context of the development of type B nonpolyglutamable DHFR inhibitors was that the aromatic γ-amides of TNP-351 were able to overcome MTX resistance in human leukemic cells whose principal phenotypic change involved transport *(90)* or polyglutamation *(24)*. Whereas the IC_{50} of MTX against these resistant sublines were 2000 and 9.6 nM, respectively, the corresponding values for TNP-351 γ-(m-carboxylanilide) were 100 and 1.6 nM. Thus the amide was substantially more active than the free acid against both cells, just as it was against the parental MTX-sensitive CCRF-CEM cells (*see* above). In fact the IC_{50} of this compound against the polyglutamation-defective cells was lower than that of MTX against the parental line, an SAR feature which, until then, had been observed only with PT523, a molecule with a side chain that similarly contains an aromatic acid moiety *(106)*. The properties of PT523 are detailed in a later section of this chapter.

7.3 γ-Peptides

A member of this class of nonpolyglutamable γ-substituted MTX analogs, of which the literature contains only scattered examples, is MTX-γ-L-aspartic acid (MTX-γ-L-Asp, **80**, R = CH_3, X = CH_2COOH) *(97,107)*. MTX-γ-glycine (**80**, R = CH_3, X = H), described in the same work, was of less interest. The K_i of MTX-γ-L-Asp against DHFR from L1210 cells was 2.8 nM (MTX: 4.3 nM; MTX-γ-L-Glu [i.e., the first product of the FPGS reaction with MTX], 3.7 nM). However both the K_m for influx and the IC$_{50}$ (48 h) for growth inhibition of L1210 cells were approx 100-fold higher than those of MTX, suggesting major loss of recognition by the RFC transport system. In vivo against the L1210 tumor, however, MTX-γ-L-Asp gave a 65% ILS at 5 mg/kg (qd × 9) (MTX: 48% at 1.3 mg/kg). Since the γ-peptide was resistant to the action of liver γ-glutamyl carboxypeptidase, its considerable in vivo activity was somewhat surprising unless metabolism by this enzyme to free MTX is more extensive in vivo than in vitro, or is catalyzed by another enzyme. An interesting prodrug application of this compound involved encapsulation in antibody-targeted liposomes *(108)*. Since the IC$_{50}$ of liposomal MTX-γ-L-Asp and liposomal MTX as inhibitors of the growth of the targeted cells (L929 or BalbC 3T6) were about the same, and only a little higher than the IC$_{50}$ of nonencapsulated MTX, the peptide was assumed to be capable of being selectively degraded lysosomally in the targeted cell.

Whereas MTX-γ-L-Asp was obviously of little value as a nonpolyglutamatable antifolate because of its highly unfavorable uptake characteristics, the possibility that other, much more lipophilic γ-peptides would succeed in this regard has not been excluded.

8. ANALOGS WITH γ-SULFONIC OR γ-PHOSPHONIC ACID GROUPS

Replacement of the γ-carboxyl group in MTX and AMT by γ-sulfonic or γ-phosphonic acid groups, as in **81–84**, has led to potent FPGS inhibitors *(93,94,109–111)*. Thus, in addition to being DHFR inhibitors, these compounds have the potential to interfere with cellular one-carbon metabolism by preventing efficient reutilization of endogenous reduced folates. However in order for such self-potentiation to occur it would be necessary for a cell to take up an amount of the dual DHFR-FPGS inhibitor greater than the K_i for *both enzymes*. Since the K_i of **81–84** as FPGS inhibitors is much higher than their K_i as DHFR inhibitors, it is unlikely that this mechanism contributes significantly to their effect on cells. Effective dual inhibitors, with similar K_i values for DHFR and FPGS, remain to be developed; in fact, as is discussed later in the section on analogs with a basic side chain (subheading 10), the best dual inhibitor discovered to date has a K_i for FPGS which is still three orders of magnitude higher than its K_i for DHFR. Thus it is appropriate to view **81–84** as type B nonpolyglutamatable DHFR inhibitors in the context of this review, but their role as dual inhibitors is at the moment mainly heuristic. The L-cysteic acid analogs of MTX and AMT (**85,86**), as well as the phosphonic acid analogs **87–89** of AMT, the latter as racemic mixtures, were also made and tested as inhibitors *(93,94,109–111)*. Likewise studied in this series were analogs of **82, 84**, and **86–89** from which the α-carboxyl was deleted *(112)*. Predictably, all of these compounds were DHFR inhibitors, but none were FPGS substrates. Thus, they qualified to be viewed as type B nonpolyglutamatable DHFR inhibitors. In general, however, they tended to have less antitumor activity in vitro than **81–84** and therefore will not be discussed further.

The MTX and AMT analogs with a γ-sulfonate group *(81,82)* inhibited murine DHFR with IC$_{50}$s of 41 and 63 nM (MTX: 50 nM; AMT: 40 nM), but were only weak competitive inhibitors of murine FPGS, with K_is of 198 and 59 μM (and zero substrate

81: n = 2, R = CH$_3$, X = SO$_2$OH (DL, L)
82: n = 2, R = H, X = SO$_2$OH (L)
83: n = 2, R = CH$_3$, X = PO(OH)$_2$ (DL)
84: n = 2, R = H, X = PO(OH)$_2$
85, 86: n = 1; R = CH$_3$, H; X = SO$_2$OH (L)
87–89: n = 1, 3, 4; R = H; X = PO(OH)$_2$ (DL)

activity) *(93)*. Interestingly, racemic **81** and the L-isomer had about the same K_i, suggesting that the L-stereochemistry may not be critical for binding. In another study, the K_i of **81** and **82** against FPGS from human liver was 131 and 35 µM, as would be the case if the active site of the human and murine enzymes were similar *(111)*. Against L1210 cells in culture, the IC$_{50}$ (48 h) was 180 nM for **81** (MTX: 12 nM) and 31 nM for **82** (AMT: 3.1 nM). Thus the AMT analog was sixfold more potent than the MTX analog even though both compounds bound almost equally well to DHFR. Since polyglutamation could obviously play no part, the higher potency of the AMT analog was presumably caused by more efficient cellular accumulation. In vivo against L1210 leukemia in mice, **81** gave a 144% ILS at 32 mg/kg (bid × 10) (MTX: 133% at 1 mg/kg, a 30-fold difference in potency), whereas **82** gave a 138% ILS at 2 mg/kg (AMT: 138% at 0.24 mg/kg, a 10-fold difference). Thus, just as AMT was more potent than MTX, **82** was more potent than **81**. The therapeutic outcome on the bid × 10 schedule was about the same with all four drugs, though a higher dose of each nonpolyglutamatable analog had to be administered. It is worth noting that **82**, at least on this schedule, was nearly equivalent to MTX in terms of both potency and prolongation of survival. The effect of more frequent dosing (e.g., constant infusion) would have been of interest but was not investigated.

The phosphonic acid analogs **83** and **84** inhibited purified DHFR from L1210 cells with an IC$_{50}$ of 6.5 and 6.0 nM (MTX, AMT: 4.0 nM) *(109,110)*. Assuming that the L-enantiomer is probably responsible for most of the effect of the DL-mixture, these results suggested that substitution of a PO(OH)$_2$ group for the COOH group at the γ-position, like that of an SO$_2$OH group, was well tolerated at the active site. Against murine FPGS, the K_is of **83** and **84** were 195 and 8.4 µM, respectively *(109,110)*, whereas against the enzyme from human liver these values were 83 and 1.9 µM *(111)*. Thus the MTX γ-phosphonate and γ-sulfonate had similar binding activity, whereas the AMT γ-phosphonate was significantly better in each case than the AMT γ-sulfonate. There was, however, a qualitative difference between **83** and **84**; the latter obeyed competitive kinetics, whereas the former gave mixed kinetics consistent with binding to more than one site. In cell-culture assays against L1210 cells, the IC$_{50}$ (48 h) of **83** was 190 nM (MTX: 12 nM) and that of **84** was 35 nM (AMT: 3.1 nM), in good agreement with the γ-sulfonates. The tenfold lower cytotoxic potency of these compounds relative to MTX and AMT, like that of **81** and **82**, could not be explained by differences in DHFR binding, and thus had to be caused by less efficient cellular uptake. In vivo antitumor assays with **83** and **84** were not carried out.

9. γ-TETRAZOLE ANALOGS

An innovative approach to blocking polyglutamation while only slightly altering the bioisosteric character of the γ-terminal region in MTX and AMT was taken by replacing the γ-carboxyl group with a tetrazole ring as in structures **90** and **91** *(113)*. The pK_a of the tetrazole NH is similar to that of a carboxyl, and the tetrazole ring is often viewed as bioisosteric surrogate for this group. Not suprisingly, analysis of the crystalline ternary complex between **90** NADPH, and human DHFR showed this compound to be in virtually exact alignment with MTX in the active site *(114)*.

90,91: R = CH$_3$, H

The IC$_{50}$ of **90** against DHFR from CCRF-CEM cells was 0.89 nM (MTX: 0.92 nM), and that of **91** was 0.60 nM (AMT: 0.70 nM). Thus, in agreement with other types of changes in the γ-terminal region reviewed above, this modification did not significantly alter DHFR binding, at least insofar as could be assessed from IC$_{50}$ as opposed to K_i values. In assays using FPGS from the same cells and AMT as the substrate, **90** was a noncompetitive inhibitor (K_{is} 51 μM, K_{ii} 321 μM), whereas **91** was more potent and obeyed competitive kinetics (K_{is} 50 μM). Not surprisingly, neither compound was a substrate. Both compounds appeared to utilize the RFC for transport, inasmuch as their growth-inhibitory effect was prevented by leucovorin and they were almost as active as MTX and AMT as inhibitors of [^{3}H]MTX influx and accumulation in CCRF-CEM cells. Thus these compounds not only had the desired characteristics for a type B nonpolyglutamatable DHFR inhibitor—i.e., good DHFR binding and efficient transport—but also had at least the possibility of functioning as self-potentiating antifolates as had been proposed originally for other dual inhibitors of DHFR and FPGS *(93,94,109,110)*.

Regardless of whether or not there is in fact a self-potentiation mechanism for **90** and **91**, these compounds were potent inhibitors of cell growth, with IC$_{50}$ values that were slightly lower than those of MTX and AMT *(113)*. Thus, against CCRF-CEM cells treated with drug for the first 24 h of a 120-h incubation, the IC$_{50}$ of **90** was 1.6 nM (MTX: 5 nM) and that of **91** was 0.9 nM (AMT: 1.5 nM). Similar results were obtained against K562 myeloblastic leukemia cells. Not surprisingly in view of their inability to form polyglutamates, the effect of **90** and **91** was highly schedule-dependent. Thus, when the cells were only exposed to drug for only the first 6 h, the IC$_{50}$ was >20,000 nM (MTX: 525 nM; AMT: 67 nM). This appears to be an inherent feature of nonpolyglutamatable DHFR inhibitors, and presumably relates to how quickly reduced folate pools are depleted in the face of dTMP synthesis inhibition and how long cells have to remain in G1/S arrest before undergoing apoptosis and death.

10. COMPOUNDS WITH AN AMINO GROUP AT THE END OF THE SIDE CHAIN

A special category of type B nonpolyglutamatable MTX and AMT analogs are those in which the glutamate moiety is replaced by a basic amino acid, as in structures **92–96** *(115–121)* and the related deazapteridines **97–100** *(122–124)*. Like the other types of compounds discussed so far, these molecules are structurally prevented from forming polyglutamates. More significantly, however, they are the most potent FPGS inhibitors known to date and thus are logical candidates one could use to test the self-potentiation hypothesis, provided that a high enough intracellular concentration of drug is achieved. Most recently the γ,γ-difluoro analog **101**, as a DL mixture, was also reported, but although it resembled **92–100** in not forming polyglutamates, it differed markedly (and unexpectedly) in being an extremely poor FPGS inhibitor *(125)*. Compound **101** is of particular interest because the pK_a of the terminal amino group is estimated to be only 6.9, whereas that of **94** is about four units higher. The MTX and AMT analogs **92–95** have been used as scaffolds for the introduction of a fluorescent moiety *(126–128)* or electrophilic haloacetyl group *(116,129)* on the terminal nitrogen. These derivatives can themselves be viewed as type B nonpolyglutamatable DHFR inhibitors.

	X	Y	R	n	References
92	N	N	CH$_3$	4	115-119
93-95	N	N	CH$_3$	1-3	110,118-120
96	N	N	H	3	110,118
97,98	CCl,CH	CH	H	3	121-123
99,100	CH,N	N,CH	H	3	123,124
101	N	N	H	3 (γ,γ-F$_2$)	125

In comparative assays of their ability to inhibit purified DHFR from murine L1210/R81 cells *(118)*, the MTX analogs **92–95** and the AMT analog **96** had IC$_{50}$ values in the 65–180 nM range (MTX, AMT: 35 nM). The compound with the same number of CH$_2$ groups as MTX was **94**, with an IC$_{50}$ of 120 nM. Lower IC$_{50}$ values, ranging from 2.5 nM (**95**) to 18 nM (**93**) (MTX: 1 nM) were obtained in another study using enzyme from CCRF-CEM and K562 cells *(119)*. In this case the IC$_{50}$ of **94** was 5.7 and 7.5 nM, respectively (MTX: 1 nM). Thus, other things being equal, introduction of an amino group (positively charged at physiologic pH) resulted in a loss of binding of up to eightfold depending on the enzyme. In assays to assess the interaction of these compounds with FPGS partially purified from different sources, the ornithine analogs **95** and **96** turned out to be excellent competitive inhibitors, with a K_i in the 3–5 μM range for **95** *(118–121)* and 0.15 μM for **96** *(118)*. However **92–96** proved to be weakly cytotoxic in culture, indicating that the positive charge on the end of the side chain interfered with transport. Thus, the IC_{50} (48 h) of **95** against CCRF-CEM cells was 740 nM (MTX: 11 nM), whereas that of **96** against L1210 cells was even higher, 1300 nM (AMT: 2 nM). Interestingly, when the effects of **95** and MTX on the growth of transport-defective CEM/MTX cells were compared, the two compounds were essentially equitoxic, with IC_{50} values of 3700 and 2700 nM, respectively. On the other hand, even though all the IC_{50} values were quite high, **96** (32 μM) was more toxic than AMT (84 μM) or MTX (220 μM) against the transport-defective L1210/R81 cell line *(118)*. This subline of L1210 leukemia is much more resistant than the CEM/MTX cells. However, while the results against resistant cells were interesting, the low activity of this group of nonpolyglutamatable analogs against wild-type tumor cells in tissue culture argued against their being tested in vivo.

The IC_{50} of the γ,γ-difluoro analog **101** against DHFR from CCRF-CEM cells was 1.2 nM (**92**: 2.5 nM; MTX: 1 nM), but surprisingly, whereas the IC_{50} of **94** against FPGS from these cells was 33 μM, that of **101** was >300 μM *(125)*. Thus, this nonpolyglutamatable compound cannot function via self-potentiation. Nevertheless, the IC_{50} of **101** against CCRF-CEM cells (93 nM; MTX: 11 nM) was eightfold lower than that of **94** (740 nM), suggesting that γ,γ-difluoro substitution may improve uptake even though it is unfavorable for FPGS binding. An interpretation of these results is that binding to the FPGS active site requires protonation of the terminal amino group, whereas for efficient transport a nonprotonated nitrogen is preferred.

In assays of the ability of B-ring analogs of **96** to inhibit purified DHFR (from WI-L2/M4 human leukemic lymphoblasts), **98–100** had IC_{50} values in the 16–35 nM range (**96**: 72 nM; MTX: 20 nM) *(123)*. Thus, deletion of either or both ring nitrogens was well tolerated, and even afforded a slight increase in binding, though this would have to be confirmed by rigorous K_i measurement. These compounds were also potent inhibitors of mouse liver FPGS, with K_is of 0.46 μM (**95**), 0.018 μM (**96**), and 0.072 μM (**98**) *(124)*. However when these analogs were tested against cultured L1210 cells, their potency was again found to be quite low. The best member of this group, **98**, with an IC_{50} (48 h) of 280 nM, was tenfold less active than MTX or AMT despite its very similar DHFR binding *(123)*. It may be noted that the 5-chloro-5,8-dideaza analog **97** is reported to bind to human DHFR with an IC_{50} of 30 nM (MTX: 4 nM) and to FPGS with a remarkably low K_i of just 0.17 nM *(122)*, but cytotoxicity data for this compound have unfortunately not been reported. Given its exceptionally strong binding to FPGS, it would be of interest to examine the effects of this compound on endogenous reduced folate cofactor pools.

To summarize this section, AMT and MTX analogs with a positively charged amino group at the end of the side chain are another type of type B nonpolyglutamatable DHFR inhibitors as defined in this chapter. However the compounds studied to date suffer from an obvious transport disadvantage relative to those in which the side chain is negatively charged or neutral. Thus membrane permeant prodrugs of these amino compounds might be of interest.

11. δ-HEMIPHTHALOYLORNITHINE ANALOGS

A highly potent member of this group, N^α-(4-amino-4-deoxypteroyl)-N^δ-hemiphthaloyl-L-ornithine (PT523, **102**), was discovered at the Dana-Farber Cancer Institute as part of a study of N^δ-acyl derivatives of the nonpolyglutamatable AMT analog **96** as possible prodrugs *(106,130)*. Five other amides (**103–107**) were also synthesized and tested as DHFR inhibitors and cell growth inhibitors in the same study. Three similar compounds (**108–110**) related to the nonpolyglutamatable MTX analogs **93–95** had been studied earlier at the Southern Research Institute *(117)*. Four ureido derivatives (**111–114**) were also synthesized *(117)*, but there is no indication in this work that either the amides or the ureas were intended to be prodrugs. PT523 was tested against some MTX-resistant cell lines, whereas **108–114** were tested only against MTX-sensitive cells. This was important because, as will be discussed below, the resistant cells were not cross-resistant to PT523, and in fact *were more sensitive to PT523 than the parent cells were to MTX* (i.e., they were collaterally sensitive).

	n	R^1	R^2
102-107	3	H	COC_6H_4(2-COOH), $COCH_3$, $COCH_2CH_2COOH$, COC_6H_5, COC_6H_4(4-Cl), COC_6H_3(3,4-Cl_2)
108-110	1-3	CH_3	COC_6H_4(4-Cl)
111, 112	1,2	CH_3	$NHCONH_2$
113, 114	1	CH_3	$NHCONHCH_3$, $NHCH(COOH)CH_2CH_2COOH$

All three chain-homologous amides **108–110** were similar to MTX as DHFR inhibitors, with K_i values in the 5–7 pM range, and two of them (**109,110**) had essentially the same K_i values of 4 to 5 μM as competitive inhibitors of [^{3}H]MTX transport in L1210 cells (MTX: 4.6 μM), though interestingly all three compounds effluxed somewhat faster from the cells than MTX *(117)*. In cell culture against L1210 cells, the chain homolog with the best activity by a factor of at least 10 was **110**, with an IC_{50} (72 h) of 1.7 nM (MTX: 3.3 nM). This was rather surprising in view of the DHFR and transport data, and suggested that the in vitro potency of this nonpolyglutamatable analog relative to MTX might involve something other than tighter DHFR binding or better uptake. However, further preclinical development was not pursued because, in vivo on a q2d × 5 schedule against L1210 leukemia, **110** gave a 104% ILS at 768 mg/kg vs 173% with MTX at 12 mg/kg, a rather discouraging 64-fold difference in the optimal dose.

The N^{10}-unsubstituted analogs **102–107** were all better inhibitors of murine DHFR than **96** and had similar IC_{50} values in the 30–50 nM range (AMT: 35 nM) *(106)*. However there were substantial differences among these compounds in their activity against cultured L1210 cells, though all of them were much more potent than **96**. The most active were PT523 and **105**, with IC_{50} (48 h) values of 0.75 and 0.90 nM against L1210 cells (MTX: 4.6 nM; AMT: 2.0 nM) and 4.3 and 6.6 nM against CCRF-CEM cells (MTX: 32 nM). Even more interestingly, the IC_{50} (48 h) values of PT523 against the transport- and polyglutamation-defective CEM/MTX cell line was 0.42 μM (MTX: 6.7 μM). Thus these 210-fold-resistant cells were only partially cross-resistant to PT523. Qualitatively similar results were obtained against the CEM/MTX cells with **105**. Moreover, incomplete cross-resistance was observed even with the more highly resistant L1210/R81 cell line, against which PT523 gave an IC_{50} (48 h) of 52 μM (MTX: 200

μM). However the most striking results were obtained with two pairs of MTX-sensitive and MTX-resistant human head-and-neck squamous carcinoma cell lines (SCC15, SCC15/R1; SCC25, SCC25/R1). The resistance phenotype of the SCC15/R1 line was known to involve defective MTX transport and polyglutamation, whereas that of the SCC25/R1 line was normal for MTX transport and polyglutamation, but featured higher DHFR expression due to gene amplification *(31,32)*. The IC$_{50}$ of PT523 against SCC15 and SCC15/R1 cells in a 2-wk assay of colonies in monolayer culture was 1.1 nM and 4.0 nM (MTX: 38 and 580 nM, 15X resistance), and against SCC25 and SCC25/R1 cells these values were 0.96 and 1.3 nM (MTX: 7.5 and 150 nM, 20X resistance). Thus, PT523 could overcome not only resistance associated with defective transport and polyglutamation but also resistance due to an increase in DHFR binding capacity. Moreover, in a finding for which there was little or no precedent, the IC$_{50}$ of PT523 against the MTX-resistant cells was lower than that of MTX against the MTX-sensitive cells, suggesting that PT523 might find clinical use for the treatment of MTX-resistant tumors. It was speculated that, since polyglutamation is obviously not needed for this drug to kill cells, resistance might not develop so easily to PT523 as it does to MTX.

Potent in vitro antitumor activity exceeding that of MTX has also been observed with PT523 against cells other than those mentioned above. For example, against the human fibrosarcoma HT-1080 and four human soft-tissue sarcoma cell lines with a phenotype featuring MTX resistance because of defective polyglutamation (HS-42, HS-16, HS-30, HS-18) *(37)*, PT523 had an IC$_{50}$ for inhibition of TS activity (^{3}H-release from [^{3}H]dUrd after 3 h) ranging from 2.3 to 160 nM, whereas for MTX against the same cells these values were 18–580 nM (unpublished data from J. R. Bertino, Memorial Sloan-Kettering Institute). Soft-tissue sarcomas are clinically not very responsive to MTX. Not surprisingly, when intracellular free drug was allowed to efflux for 4 h prior to *in situ* measurement of TS activity, the increase in IC$_{50}$ was greater for PT523 than for MTX. However, even under these conditions, PT523 had an IC$_{50}$ close to, or lower than, that of MTX, suggesting that at nonexchangeable levels the two drugs are similar when the cells have a low ability to convert MTX to polyglutamates.

Activity comparable to, or exceeding that of, MTX and 10-EDAM has likewise been observed for PT523 against several established human squamous-cell carcinoma lines and against blast cells from children with ALL, using the *in situ* TS assay *(131)*.

An indication of the potency of PT523 relative to other antifolates of current interest, all of which can form polyglutamates, has been obtained with CCRF-CEM cells *(132)* and L1210 cells *(133)*. Against both cell lines, the IC$_{50}$ of PT523 was at least as low as, or lower than, three well-known DHFR inhibitors (MTX, AMT, 10-EDAM), two TS inhibitors (1843U89, D1694), and a GAR formyltransferase inhibitor (DDATHF) *(132,134)*. The potency difference between PT523 and 10-EDAM was only twofold, whereas for DDATHF this difference was as much as 20-fold.

A broad spectrum of in vitro antitumor activity has also been obtained with PT523 against the cell lines in the NCI solid tumor panel *(135,136)*. Thus, against a group of 23 nonsmall cell lung, colon, ovarian, and renal carcinomas, melanomas, and CNS cell lines for which data were available from at least two experiments on different days, the IC$_{50}$ (48 h) of PT523 was in the 0.1–1.0 nM range for 4 of 23 cell lines (17%), the 1.0–10 nM range for 15 of 23 (65%), the 10–100 nM range for 2 of 23 (9%), and >100 nM for 4 of 23 (17%). By contrast, the IC$_{50}$ (48 h) of MTX was >10 nM against all 23 cell lines, and in several instances (5 of 23, 22%) this value exceeded 1000 nM. Notably, when four of the most highly MTX-resistant cell lines (IC$_{50}$ > 100 nM) were exposed to PT523 for 144 instead of 72 h, low nanomolar values were obtained for the IC$_{50}$, attesting to the importance of long drug exposure (C × t) for nonpolyglutamatable compounds such as PT523. An even better illustration of this was provided in a clonogenicity assay using SCC25 head-and-neck squamous carcinoma cells, in which the IC$_{50}$ varied over a 600-fold range as drug exposure was lengthened from 24 to 96 h *(137)*. These results suggested that in vivo effects of PT523 on both tumors and host tissues ought to be very schedule-dependent.

With regard to the mechanism of action of PT523, all evidence to date points to DHFR inhibition as the primary target. Thus, H35 rat hepatoma cells exposed to a concentration of PT523 that blocks DNA synthesis by at least 90% were protected by leucovorin or a combination or dThd and hypoxanthine, but not by dThd or hypoxanthine alone *(138)*. Marked expansion of the dihydrofolate pool was observed, along with a decrease in the combined pool of tetrahydrofolate and 10-formyltetrahydrofolate, as is typical with other DHFR inhibitors such as MTX and trimetrexate. A decrease in the tetrahydrofolate cofactor pool (using 5,10-methylenetetrahydrofolate as a surrogate) was also shown in vivo in the tumor, marrow, and gut of mice with subcutaneously implanted SCC VII squamous-cell carcinoma *(139)*. The duration of depletion of the methylenetetrahydrofolate pool, which was not followed beyond 2 h in these preliminary experiments, would obviously be helpful in designing an optimal dose schedule for therapeutic efficacy. Not surprisingly in view of these results, PT523 was found to give greater than additive cytotoxicity in vitro as well as in vivo when used in combination with etoposide *(137)*. The basis for this drug interaction is presumably that DNA repair is inhibited when ATP pools become depleted downstream as a result of *de novo* purine synthesis inhibition. A similar interaction of etoposide has been noted with MTX *(140)* and with trimetrexate *(141)*. Although depletion of ATP pools by PT523 has not yet been shown directly, the fact that PT523 potentiates etoposide very much like MTX and trimetrexate is suggestive of such an effect. As with the other newer antifolates with which it has been compared in this chapter, it is not unreasonable to think that the most efficacious use of PT523 in the clinic might be in a multidrug regimen with nonantifolates.

Intracellular cleavage of PT523 would give the nonacylated ornithine analog **96**, which in principle could exert a self-potentiation effect because of its ability to inhibit both DHFR and FPGS. This possibility was examined by treating H35 cells or CCRF-CEM cells first with PT523 for 2 h and then with [^{3}H]MTX for 4 or 24 h, followed by analysis of the [^{3}H]MTX polyglutamate distribution pattern *(138)*. No significant difference was seen between the cells treated with PT523 and [^{3}H]MTX and those treated with [^{3}H]MTX alone, suggesting that PT523 was not in fact a prodrug of **96**.

Since PT523 cannot be polyglutamated, its potent cytotoxicity was suspected to be caused by tighter binding to DHFR, more efficient uptake, or both. Although initial estimates of DHFR binding based on IC$_{50}$ comparisons vs MTX did not suggest much difference between the two compounds in their binding affinity for the enzyme *(106)*, more recent comparison of K_i rather than IC$_{50}$ values has revealed that PT523 actually binds 15-fold more tightly than MTX to human DHFR (PT523: 0.35 ± 0.13 pM; MTX: 5.19 ± 0.45 pM) *(142,143)*. To the extent that slower dissociation from the enzyme would make it easier to maintain >99% inhibition of dihydrofolate reduction, and thus shut down cellular dTMP synthesis *(144)*, this 15-fold difference in DHFR binding is not inconsequential. According to a compilation of the literature data for human DHFR inhibition by MTX, the range of reported K_i values for this compound is 3.4–7.3 pM *(145)*. The K_i of 10-EDAM is 1.0 pM *(146)* and that of MTX+Glu$_4$ is 1.3 pM, an increase in binding of < threefold in comparison with MTX itself *(145)*. Thus, PT523 compares very favorably with classical diaminopteridine antifolates, even when slight enhancement in binding after polyglutamation is taken into account. To date, the only polyglutamatable or type B nonpolyglutamatable inhibitors with a DHFR binding affinity comparable to that of PT523 are the diaminoquinazoline **35–40**, of which the two most potent members, at least against mouse enzyme, are **37** (K_i = 0.3 pM) and **40** (K_i = 0.1 pM) *(147)*.

While the 15-fold increase in DHFR affinity of PT523 relative to MTX is substantial, it does not by itself suffice to explain its 100-fold greater potency against many human tumor-cell lines in culture. However, it turns out that in addition to being a more powerful DHFR inhibitor, PT523 is also more efficiently transported into cells. An early indication that PT523 uptake occurs, at least in part, via the RFC pathway came from the finding that it inhibits the uptake of [^{3}H]MTX and [^{3}H]leucovorin in H35 rat hepatoma cells while having no effect on [^{3}H]folic acid uptake *(138)*. Subsequently PT523 was also shown to inhibit the uptake of [^{3}H]MTX in SCC25 human head-and-neck squamous carcinoma cells with an IC$_{50}$ of 0.17 μM (MTX: 2.9 μM) *(148)*. An even more favorable trend was obtained for PT523 vs MTX against two resistant sublines, SCC25/R1 (PT523: 0.17 μM; MTX: 3.0 μM) and SCC25/CP (PT523: 0.046 μM; MTX 1.1 μM) *(148)*. Resistance to MTX in SCC25/R1 cells is due to increased DHFR activity, whereas in SCC25/CP cells MTX resistance is attributed to decreased polyglutamation. PT523 has also been shown to be superior to MTX and several other polyglutamatable antifolates as an inhibitor of [^{14}C]lometrexol uptake in wild-type CCRF-CEM cells and the transport- and polyglutamation-defective subline CEM/MTX *(132)*. The K_i values for PT523, assumed to be equivalent to the K_m for transport via the RFC, were found to be 0.65 μM (MTX: 4.5 μM) and 0.44 μM (MTX: 9.7 μM), respectively. These values were comparable to those obtained for 10-EDAM (CCRF-CEM: 0.64 μM; CEM/MTX: 2.0 μM), D1694 (CCRF-CEM: 1.1 μM; CEM/MTX: 1.6 μM), 1843U89 (CCRF/CEM: 0.21 μM; CEM/MTX: 1.4 μM), and DDATHF (CCRF-CEM: 0.68 μM; CEM/MTX: 0.17 μM) *(132,134)*. The low K_m of DDATHF in CEM/MTX cells may reflect increased uptake via folic acid membrane receptors, for which it is a 100-fold better substrate than MTX *(133)*. Slightly greater affinity of PT523 relative to MTX, AMT, 10-EDAM, D1694, and 1843U89 has likewise been observed in the RFC-overproducing cell line CEM-7A *(133)*. In the case of PT523 vs MTX the difference was approx 10-fold. Thus, if one assumes that multiplying the increase in transport efficiency (10X) by the increase in DHFR-binding affinity (15X) will give an approximation of the increase in cytotoxicity, the 100-fold greater potency of PT523 over MTX against many cell lines can be explained reasonably well. These results also showed that a glutamate side chain is not required for efficient utilization of the RFC.

Not surprisingly in view of its exceptionally high DHFR affinity, efficient cellular transport, and potent activity in cell culture, PT523 has proved to be quite toxic in mice, and it is by no means clear what the optimal in vivo schedule should be to maximize antitumor efficacy while minimizing host toxicity. In dose-finding experiments done to date at the Dana-Farber Cancer Institute using mice with SCC VII squamous carcinoma, PT523 and MTX were compared on two schedules, bid × 10 and 5-d constant infusion *(136,142)*. The maximum tolerated dose (MTD) of PT523 given bid × 10 was 1.1 mg/kg or a total of 22 mg/kg (MTX: 1.0 mg/kg, total 20 mg/kg). In contrast, when PT523 was infused over 5 d the MTD was only 0.16 mg/kg/d × 5, or a total of 0.80 mg/kg (MTX: 0.96 mg/kg/d, total 4.8 mg/kg). Thus on the bid × 10 schedule the two drugs were equally well tolerated, whereas in a constant infusion setting the PT523 dosage had to be decreased sixfold. In terms of tumor size, in mice treated with 0.16 mg/kg/d × 5 of PT523 there was a 90% decrease on the day that controls reached a mean diameter of 10 mm (approx. 500 mm^3), whereas with MTX at 0.96 mg/kg/d × 5 this decrease was only 50%. When the results were expressed as a tumor growth delay (i.e., the time for both treated and control tumors to reach 10 mm), the T/C of PT523 was 157% whereas that of MTX was only 112%. Tumor shrinkage was also seen with both drugs on the bid × 10 schedule, but the effect was smaller than in the 5-d infusions. It should be noted that (1) these experiments only compared two schedules, (2) the optimal schedule for polyglutamatable and nonpolyglutamatable drugs is not necessarily be the same, (3) the SCC VII tumor is not very responsive to MTX and thus may not respond well to other DHFR inhibitors, and (4) an inherent drawback to using murine preclinical models to predict clinical activity is that plasma folates and plasma dThd levels are both 10-fold higher in mice than in humans. A possible approach to this problem is to use mice kept on a folate-free diet for 1–2 wk prior to treatment, or use a tumor that cannot efficiently salvage dThd. These strategies have been used in the laboratory with other potent clinical candidates including D1694 *(149)*, DDATHF *(150, 151)*, and 1843U89 *(152)*. Very recently, PT523 at a dose of 1.1 mg/kg (bid × 5) was independently reported to produce statistically significant delay of the growth of subcutaneously implanted Colon 26A carcinoma in BalbC mice kept for 2 wk on a folate-free diet prior to treatment *(131)*.

Although it was obvious that the superior affinity of PT523 for DHFR had to be due to the hemiphthaloylornithine moiety, it was of some importance to investigate the structural basis for this effect using physical methods. Accordingly, the structure of the PT523-NADPH-DHFR ternary complex was examined in the solid state by X-ray crystallography at 2.5Å resolution *(153,154)* and in solution by high-field protein ^{1}H-NMR *(143)*. The major results of the two studies were generally consistent, albeit with certain differences between the solid-state and solution structures, as might be expected. Interestingly, the ternary complex was obtained in two discrete crystal types, monoclinic (space group C2) and orthorhombic (space group P2$_1$2$_1$2$_1$), the latter of which had not been seen previously with DHFR. A key finding was that, when PT523 becomes bound to the active site, certain hydrophobic residues in the distal region of the active site appear to occupy an altered position relative to the ternary complex with MTX or MTX γ-tetrazole (TMTX). Moreover, several energetically similar conformers and/or rotamers of PT523 appear to co-exist in solution as well as in the crystal lattice, perhaps contributing entropically to tight binding. For example, in one of the major conformers inferred from the monoclinic C2 crystal structure, the carboxyl group on the phthaloyl ring forms an intramolecular hydrogen bond to the adjacent amide nitrogen and the ring lies in a compact hydrophobic pocket involving Phe-31, Pro-26, Pro-61, and the p-aminobenzoyl moiety. In another conformer the carboxyl group appears to be able to make hydrogen bond contacts through an intervening water molecule to Arg-28 and Arg-32. In both the solid-state model and the solution model the entrance to the active site appears to be narrower than it is the MTX ternary complex, suggesting that the protein has adapted to the shape of the ligand so as to generate additional contact points and make dissociation more difficult than when the side chain is a glutamate (or even an oligoglutamate) moiety.

Two important structural questions with regard to PT523 were how biological activity is affected by modification of the hemiphthaloylornithine side chain and how activity is affected by modification of the B-ring or p-aminobenzoyl moiety. A number of second-generation analogues of PT523 have been synthesized in order to address these questions. Compounds in which the side chain is altered include, to date, the lysine, diaminobutanoic acid, and diaminopropanoic acid analogs (**115–117**) *(132,136)* and the isophthaloyl, terephthaloyl, and 4,5-dichlorophthaloyl analogues (**118–120**) *(136)*. The chain-lengthened and chain-shortened analogues **115** and **116** were both substantially less cytotoxic than PT523. Against cultured SCC25 human head-and-neck squamous carcinoma cells, for example, the IC_{50} (72 hr) of **115** and **116** was 18 and 13 nM respectively (PT523 control: 1.0 nM). Lower activity was likewise obtained with these compounds against SCC VII murine squamous cell carcinoma and MCF-7 human breast carcinoma cells, indicating that three CH_2 groups, as in PT523, are optimal. In a different experiment using SCC25 cells the IC_{50} (72 h) of **118** was 2.9 nM, that of **119** was 72 nM, and that of **120** was 18 nM (PT523 control: 0.3 nM). Thus, moving the carboxyl group from the *ortho* to the *meta* or *para* position was deleterious, as was the introduction of the two chlorine atoms in the hemiphthaloyl moiety. Substitution *para* to the amide bond, as in **119** and **120** seemed to have an especially strong effect. Interestingly, when **115** and **116** were tested as DHFR inhibitors, they seemed more potent than PT523, at least at the IC_{50} level, whereas **118–120** seemed less potent. However the differences in IC_{50} were < twofold, suggesting that differences in cellular uptake among these compounds might be more important than differences in DHFR binding as determinants of cytotoxicity.

	n	W	X	Y	Z		n	W	X	Y	Z
115	4	N	N	H	2-COOH	121	3	CH	N	H	H
116	2	N	N	H	2-COOH	122	3	CCH_3	N	H	H
117	1	N	N	H	2-COOH	123	3	N	CH	H	H
118	3	N	N	H	3-COOH	124	3	CH	CH	H	H
119	3	N	N	H	4-COOH	125	3	CCH_3	CH	H	H
120	3	N	N	H	2-COOH-4,5-Cl_2	126	3	CCl	CH	H	H
						127	3	N	N	3',5'-Cl_2	H

A number of B-ring analogs have also been synthesized, including the 5-deaza compounds **121** and **122**, the 8-deaza compound **123**, and the 5,8-dideaza analogs **124–126** *(142)*. In addition, the first example of a substituted p-aminobenzoyl analog (**127**) has been made *(142)*. This compound was slightly less active than PT523 against SCC25

Chapter 4 / Nonpolyglutamatable DHFR Inhibitors

cells, with an IC$_{50}$ (72 h) of 2.5 nM (PT523 control: 1.0 nM), but appeared to be a slightly better DHFR inhibitor. On the basis of the preliminary data obtained thus far, it appears that all the B-ring analogs of PT523 are at least as active as PT523, both as inhibitors of DHFR and as inhibitors of cell growth. Thus the K_is of 5-deazaPT523 (**121**) and 5-methyl-5-deazaPT523 (**122**) as DHFR inhibitors were 0.48 ± 0.23 and 0.32 ± 0.13 pM, and those of 5,8-dideazaPT523 (**124**) and 5-chloro-5,8-dideazaPT523 (**126**) were 0.09 ± 0.03 and 0.11 ± 0.05 pM. By comparison, the K_i of PT523 was 0.35 ± 0.23 pM, suggesting that deletion of both B-ring nitrogens favors binding. In cytotoxicity assays against SCC25 cells, **121, 122, 124,** and **126** all showed slightly greater potency than PT523, with IC$_{50}$ (72 h) values in the 0.2–0.4 nM range (PT523 control: 0.80 nM) *(142)*. Thus replacement of B-ring nitrogens by carbon was well tolerated, and cell-growth inhibition correlated reasonably well with DHFR inhibition. However, while PT523 and its B-ring analogs clearly represent an interesting group of type B nonpolyglutamatable DHFR inhibitors, it would be premature at this stage to say that any of the second-generation analogs are better clinical candidates than PT523 itself.

12. NONPOLYGLUTAMATABLE ANALOGS WITH A CLASSICAL GLUTAMATE SIDE CHAIN

Although a large number of type B nonpolyglutamatable DHFR inhibitors with side chains other than glutamic acid are now known, the possibility cannot be ruled out that some compounds might be good DHFR inhibitors and at the same time be *nonsubstrates for FPGS even though they contain a glutamate side chain*. The best embodiment of this hypothesis described to date are the naphthalene analogs **128–134** *(155)* all of which inhibit murine DHFR with a K_i in the 3.0–6.0 pM range (MTX: 4.8 pM) and inhibit L1210 cell growth with an IC$_{50}$ in the 2.0–9.0 μM range (MTX: 9.0 μM) even though their V_{max} for polyglutamation by murine FPGS is 20- to 60-fold lower than that of MTX.

	R	X	Y
128	H	N	N
129	CH$_3$	N	N
130	H	CH	N
131	CH$_3$	CH	N
132	H	CCH$_3$	N
133	CH$_3$	CCH$_3$	N
134	H	CH	CH

Another example is N-[4-[2-(2,4-diamino-5,6,7,8-tetrahydropyrido[4,3-*d*]pyrimidin-6-yl)ethyl]benzoyl]-L-glutamic acid (**135**) *(156)*, which is a rather poor FPGS substrate, but whose activity as a DHFR inhibitor and cell growth inhibitor is similar to that of MTX. The first-order rate constant k' (i.e., K_m/rel.V_{max}) for addition of the first glutamate residue to **135** by mouse liver FPGS is approx sixfold lower than that of MTX, and yet the two compounds have essentially the same IC$_{50}$ against murine DHFR (**135**:

38 n*M*; MTX: 46 n*M*) and as inhibitors of L1210 cell growth in culture (**135**: 38 n*M*; MTX: 46 n*M*). Other compounds that are 10- to 20-fold poorer FPGS substrates than folic acid even though they contain a glutamate side chain are the diaminopyrimidines **136–138** *(157,158)*.

Further examples are **139** and **140**, which were designed intentionally to minimize toxicity when used against rheumatoid arthritis *(72)*. Because of their lack of ability to accumulate in liver and other tissues during long-term therapy, it has been suggested that nonpolyglutamatable DHFR inhibitors might be safer to use than MTX or other classical antifolates in the treatment of patients with severe autoimmune disease who do not tolerate or respond well to steroids and other standard antiinflammatory agents.

11. CONCLUSION

Many more type B nonpolyglutamatable DHFR inhibitors than have been described in this chapter can undoubtedly be designed. Moreover some of the older DHFR inhibitors with a glutamate side chain that have never tested as FPGS substrates might be worth revisiting in this context. Reasonable possibilities could include for example the 10-thia and 10-oxa analogs of AMT and homoAMT, all of which are potent DHFR inhibitors and are toxic to cultured cells, but whose activity as FPGS substrates is unknown *(159–162)*. On the other hand, it should be noted that the development of nonpolyglutamatable DHFR inhibitors with a glutamate side chain would have two inherent problems. In the first place, in order for this approach to be as effective as the use of analogs with nonglutamate side chains it would be necessary to achieve *zero* substrate activity for FPGS, and not just a partial reduction in activity. Given the well-known structural promiscuity of this enzyme, it is somewhat counterintuitive to think that nonpolyglutamation would be as easy with a glutamate as it is with a nonglutamate side chain. Furthermore, even if the addition of a second glutamate to the side chain were slow, it is still possible that further elongation of the side chain would occur quickly. Thus, while it would be an instructive exercise in medicinal chemistry, this strategy would probably not be as attractive as the others reviewed in this chapter.

ACKNOWLEDGMENT

This chapter is written in celebration of the fiftieth anniversary of the founding of the Dana-Farber Cancer Institute.

REFERENCES

1. Farber S, Diamond LK, Mercer RD, Sylvester RF, Jr., Wolff JA. Temporary remissions in acute leukemia in children produced by folic acid antagonist, 4-aminopteroyl-glutamic acid (aminopterin). *N Engl J Med* 1948;238:787–793.
2. Farber S, Diamond LK, Mercer RD, Sylvester RF, Wolff J, Lenz GG. Effect of chemotherapeutic agents on acute leukemia; folic acid antagonists. *Am J Dis Child* 1948;78:961–962.
3. Jukes TH. Searching for magic bullets: early approaches to chemotherapy—antifolates, methotrexate—the Bruce F. Cain Memorial Award Lecture. *Cancer Res* 1987;47:5528–5536.
4. Kisliuk RL. The biochemistry of folates, In *Folate Antagonists as Therapeutic Agents*, vol. 1 (Sirotnak FM, Burchall JJ, Ensminger WD, Montgomery JA, eds.) Academic, New York, 1984, pp. 1–68.
5. Falco EA, Goodwin LG, Hitchings GH, Rollo IM, Russell PB. 2,4-Diaminopyrimidines—a new series of antimalarials. *Br J Pharmacol* 1951;6:185–200.
6. Hitchings GH, Burchall JJ. Inhibition of folate biosynthesis and function as a basis for chemotherapy. *Adv Enzymol* 1965;27:417–468.
7. Werbel LM. Design and synthesis of lipophilic antifols as anticancer agents. *Folate Antagonists as Therapeutic Agents*, vol. 1. Sirotnak FM, Burchall JJ, Ensminger WD, Montgomery JA, eds. Academic, New York, 1984, pp. 261–287.
8. Berman EM, Werbel LM. The renewed potential for folate antagonists in contemporary cancer chemotherapy. *J Med Chem* 1991;34:479–485.
9. Roth B, Falco ER, Hitchings GH, Bushby SRM. 5-Benzyl-2,4-diaminopyrimidines as antibacterials agents. I. Synthesis and antibacterial activity *in vitro*. *J Med Pharm Chem* 1962;5:1103–1123.
10. Werkheiser WC. Specific binding of 4-amino folic acid analogues by folic acid reductase. *J Biol Chem* 1961;236:888–893.
11. Laszlo J, Iland HJ, Sedwick WD. Overcoming methotrexate resistance by a lipophilic antifolate (BW 301U): from theory to models in practice. *Adv Enz Regul* 1986;24:357–373.
12. Fry DW, Jackson RC. Biological and biochemical properties of new anticancer folate antagonists. *Cancer Metastasis Rev* 1987;5:251–270.
13. Roth B, Cheng CC. Recent progress in the medicinal chemistry of 2,4-diaminopyrimidines. *Prog Med Chem* 1989;19:269–331.
14. Goldman ID, Chabner BA, Bertino JR, eds. *Folyl and Antifolyl Polyglutamates*. Plenum, New York, 1983.
15. Goldman ID, ed. *Proceedings of the Second Workshop on Folyl and Antifolyl Polyglutamates*. Praeger, New York, 1985.
16. Alberto P, Peytreman R, Modenica R, Beretta-Piccoli M. Initial clinical experience with a simultaneous combination of 2,4-diamino-5-(3',4'-dichlorophenyl)-6-methylpyrimidine (DDMP) with folinic acid. *Cancer Chemother Pharmacol* 1978;1:101–105.
17. Li W-W, Bertino JR. Inability of leucovorin to rescue a naturally methotrexate-resistant human soft tissue sarcoma cell line from trimetrexate cytotoxicity. *Cancer Res* 1992;52:6866–6870.
18. Lacerda JF, Göker E, Kherdapour A, Dennig D, Elisseyeff Y, Jagiello C, O'Reilly RJ, Bertino JR. Selective treatment of SCID mice bearing methotrexate-transport resistant human acute lymphoblastic leukemia tumors with trimetrexate and leucovorin protection. *Blood* 1995;85:2675–2679.
19. Kheradpour A, Berman E, Göker E, Lin JT, Tong WP, Bertino JR. A Phase II study of continuous infusion of trimetrexate in patients with refractory acute leukemia. *Cancer Investig* 1995;13:36–40.
20. Galivan J. Transport and metabolism of methotrexate in normal and resistant cultured rat hepatoma cells. *Cancer Res* 1979;39:735–743.

21. Rumberger BG, Schmid FA, Otter G, Sirotnak FM. Preferential selection during therapy in vivo by edatrexate compared to methotrexate of resistant L1210 cell variants with decreased folylpolyglutamate synthetase activity. *Cancer Commun* 1990;2:305–310.
22. Roy K, Mitsugi K, Sirlin S, Shane B, Sirotnak FM. Different antifolate-resistant L1210 cell variants with either increased or decreased folylpolyglutamate synthetase gene expression at the level of mRNA transcription. *J Biol Chem* 1995;270:26918–26922.
23. Koizumi S. Impairment of methotrexate (MTX)-polyglutamate formation of MTX-resistant K562 cell lines. *Gann* 1988;79:1230–1237.
24. Pizzorno G, Mini E, Coronnello M, McGuire JJ, Moroson BA, Cashmore AR, Dreyer RN, Lin JT, Mazzei T, Periti P, Bertino JR. Impaired polyglutamylation of methotrexate as a cause of resistance in CCRF-CEM cells after short-term, high-dose treatment with this drug. *Cancer Res* 1988;48:2149–2155.
25. Whitehead VM, Rosenblatt DS, Vuchich M-J, Suster JJ, Witte A, Beaulieu D. Accumulation of methotrexate and methotrexate polyglutamates in lymphoblasts at diagnosis of childhood acute lymphoblastic leukemia: a pilot prognostic factor analysis. *Blood* 1990;76:44–49.
26. McCloskey DE, McGuire JJ, Russell CA, Rowan BG, Bertino JR, Pizzorno G, Mini E. Decreased folylpolyglutamate synthetase activity as a mechanism of methotrexate resistance in CCRF-CEM human leukemia sublines. *J Biol Chem* 1991;266:6181–6187.
27. Göker E, Lin JT, Trippett T, Elisseyeff Y, Tong WP, Niedzwicki D, Tan C, Steinherz P, Schweitzer BI, Bertino JR. Decreased polyglutamylation of methotrexate in acute lymphoblastic leukemia blasts in adults compared to children with this disease. *Leukemia* 1993;7:1000–1004.
28. Barredo JC, Synold TW, Laver J, Relling MV, Pui C-H, Priest DG, Evans WE. Differences in constitutive and post-methotrexate folylpolyglutamate synthetase activity in B-lineage and T-lineage leukemia. *Blood* 1994;84:564–569.
29. Jolivet J, Schilsky RL, Bailey BD, Drake JC, Chabner BA. Synthesis, retention, and biological activity of methotrexate polyglutamates in cultured human breast cancer cells. *J Clin Invest* 1982;70:351–360.
30. Cowan KH, Jolivet J. A methotrexate-resistant human breast cancer cell line with multiple defects, including diminished formation of methotrexate polyglutamates. *J Biol Chem* 1984;259:10793–10800.
31. Frei E III, Rosowsky A, Wright JE, Cucchi CA, Lippke JA, Ervin TJ, Jolivet J, Haseltine WA. Development of methotrexate resistance in a human squamous cell carcinoma of the head and neck in culture. *Proc Natl Acad Sci USA* 1984;81:2873–2877.
32. Rosowsky A, Wright JE, Cucchi CA, Lippke JA, Tantravahi R, Ervin TJ, Frei E III. Phenoptyic heterogeneity in cultured human head and neck squamous cell carcinoma lines with low-level methotrexate resistance. *Cancer Res* 1985;45:6205–6212.
33. Pizzorno G, Chang Y-M, McGuire JJ, Bertino JR. Inherent resistance of human squamous carcinoma cell lines to methotrexate as a result of decreased polyglutamylation of this drug. *Cancer Res* 1989;49:5275–5280.
34. Braakhuis BJM, Jansen G, Noordhuis P, Kegel A, Peters GJ. Importance of pharmacodynamics in the in vitro antiproliferative activity of the antifolates methotrexate and 10-ethyl-10-deazaaminopterin against human head and neck squamous cell carcinoma. *Biochem Pharmacol* 1993;46:2155–2161.
35. Samuels LL, Feinberg A, Moccio DM, Sirotnak FM, Rosen G. Detection by high-performance liquid chromatography of methotrexate and its metabolites in tumor tissue from osteosarcoma patients treated with high-dose methotrexate/leucovorin rescue. *Biochem Pharmacol* 1984;33:2711–2714.
36. Li W-W, Lin JT, Tong WP, Trippett TM, Brennan MF, Bertino JR. Mechanisms of natural resistance to antifolates in human soft tissue sarcomas. *Cancer Res* 1992;52:1434–1438.
37. Li W-W, Lin JT, Schweitzer BI, Tong WP, Niedzwicki D, Bertino JR. Intrinsic resistance to methotrexate in human soft tissue sarcoma cell lines. *Cancer Res* 1992;52:3908–3913.
38. Curt GA, Jolivet J, Bailey BD, Carney DN, Chabner BA. Synthesis and retention of methotrexate polyglutamates by human small cell lung cancer. *Biochem Pharmacol* 1984;33:1682–1685.
39. Curt GA, Jolivet J, Carney DN, Bailey BD, Drake JC, Clendeninn NJ, Chabner BA. Determinants of the sensitivity of human small-cell lung cancer cell lines to methotrexate. *J Clin Invest* 1985;76:1323–1329.
40. Barakat RR, Li W-W, Lovelace C, Bertino JR. Intrinsic resistance of cervical squamous cell carcinoma cell lines to methotrexate (MTX) as a result of decreased accumulation of intracellular MTX polyglutamates. *Gynecol Oncol* 1993;51:54–60.

41. Rhee MS, Wang Y, Nair MG, Galivan J. Acquisition of resistance to antifolates caused by enhanced γ-glutamyl hydrolase activity. *Cancer Res* 1993;53:2227–2230.
42. Yao R, Rhee MS, Galivan J. Effects of γ-glutamyl hydrolase on folyl and antifolylpolyglutamates in cultured H35 hepatoma cells. *Mol Pharmacol* 1995;48:505–511.
43. Rots MG, Pieters R, Noordhuis P, van Zantwijk CH, Peters GJ, Veerman AJP, Jansen G. Role of folylpolyglutamate synthetase (FPGS) and folylpolyglutamate hydrolase (FPGH) in methotrexate (MTX) polyglutamylation in childhood leukemia. *AACR Proc* 1997;38:162.
44. Wright WB Jr, Cosulich DB, Fahrenbach MJ, Waller CW, Smith JM Jr, Hultquist ME. Analogs of pteroylglutamic acid. IV. Replacement of glutamic acid by other amino acids. *J Am Chem Soc* 1949;71:3014–3017.
45. Cosulich DB, Seeger DR, Fahrenbach MJ, Roth B, Mowat JH, Smith JM, Jr, Hultquist ME. Analogs of pteroylglutamic acid. VI. 3', 5'-Dihalopteroyl derivatives. *J Am Chem Soc* 1951;73:2554–2557.
46. Suster DC, Tarnauceanu E, Ionescu D, Dobre V, Niculescu-Duvaz I. Potential anticancer agents. 16. Methotrexate analogues with a modified peptide side chain. *J Med Chem* 1978;21:1162–1165.
47. Montgomery JA, Piper JR, Elliott RD, Temple C Jr, Roberts EC, Shealy YF. Analogues of methotrexate. *J Med Chem* 1979;22:862–868.
48. Mao Z, Pan J, Kalman TI. Design and synthesis of histidine analogues of folic acid and methotrexate as potential folylpolyglutamate synthetase inhibitors. *J Med Chem* 1996;39:4340–4344.
49. Harvison PJ, Kalman TI. Synthesis and biological activity of novel folic acid analogues: pteroyl-S-alkylhomocysteine sulfoximines. *J Med Chem* 1992;35:1227–1233.
50. Mead JAR, Greenberg NH, Schrecker AW, Seeger DR, Tomcufcik AS. The pharmacology and biochemical activity of 4-amino-4-deoxy-10-methylpteroylaspartic acid. *Biochem Pharmacol* 1965;14:105–114.
51. Davoll J, Johnson AM. Quinazoline analogues of folic acid. *J Chem Soc (C)* 1970;997–1002.
52. Moran RG, Colman PD, Rosowsky A, Forsch RA, Chan KK. Structural features of 4-amino antifolates required for substrate activity with mammalian folylpolyglutamate synthetase. *Mol Pharmacol* 1985;27:156–166.
53. Hutchison DJ. Quinazoline antifolates: biologic activities. *Cancer Chemother Repts Part 1* 1968;52:697–705.
54. Hutchison DJ, Shimoyama M, Schmid F. Quinazoline antifolates: dosage schedules and toxicity. *Cancer Chemother Repts Part 1* 1971;55:123–132.
55. Carlin SC, Rosenberg RN, Vande Venter L, Friedkin M. Quinazoline antifolates as inhibitors of growth, dihydrofolate reductase, and thymidylate synthase of mouse neuroblastoma cells in culture. *Mol Pharmacol* 1974;10:194–203.
56. Hynes JB, Eason DE, Garrett CM, Colven PL Jr, Shores KE, Freisheim JH. Quinazolines as inhibitors of dihydrofolate reductase. 4. Classical analogues of folic and isofolic acid. *J Med Chem* 1977;20:588–591.
57. Albrecht AM, Biedler JL, Hutchison DJ. Two different species of dihydrofolate reductase in mammalian cells differentially resistant to amethopterin and methasquin. *Cancer Res* 1972;32:1539–1546.
58. Kumar P, Kisliuk RL, Gaumont Y, Nair MG, Baugh CM, Kaufman BT. Interaction of polyglutamyl derivatives of methotrexate, 10-deazaaminopterin, and dihydrofolate with dihydrofolate reductase. *Cancer Res* 1986;46:5020–5023.
59. Kumar P, Kisliuk RL, Gaumont Y, Freisheim JH, Nair MG. Inhibition of human dihydrofolate reductase by antifolyl polyglutamates. *Biochem Pharmacol* 1989;38:541–543.
60. Sirotnak FM, Donsbach RC. Comparative studies on the transport of aminopterin, methotrexate, and methasquin by the L1210 leukemia cell. *Cancer Res* 1972;32:2120–2126.
61. Sirotnak FM, Donsbach RC. Stereochemical characteristics of the folate-antifolate transport mechanism in L1210 leukemia cells. *Cancer Res* 1974;34:371–377.
62. Sirotnak FM, Donsbach RC. Further evidence for a basis of selective activity and relative responsiveness during antifolate therapy of murine tumors. *Cancer Res* 1975;35:1737–1744.
63. Philips FS, Sirotnak FM, Sodergren JE, Hutchison DJ. Uptake of methotrexate, aminopterin, and methasquin and inhibition of dihydrofolate reductase and of DNA synthesis in mouse small intestine. *Cancer Res* 1973;33:153–158.
64. Etcubanas E, Tan C, Go SC, Krakoff IH. Preliminary clinical trials of the quinazoline antifolate methasquin. *AACR Proc* 1972;13:48.
65. Rosowsky A, Forsch R, Uren J, Wick M, Kumar AA, Freisheim JH. Methotrexate analogues. 20. Re-

placement of glutamate by longer-chain amino diacids: effects on dihydrofolate reductase inhibition, cytotoxicity, and in vivo antitumor activity. *J Med Chem* 1983;26:1719–1724.
66. Moran RG, Colman PD, Rosowsky A. Structural requirements for the activity of antifolates as substrates for mammalian folylpolyglutamate synthetase. *NCI Monogr* 1987;5:133–138.
67. Browman GP, Spiegl P, Booker P, Rosowsky A. Comparison of leucovorin protection from a variety of antifolates in human lymphoid cell lines. *Cancer Chemother Pharmacol* 1985;15:111–114.
68. Rosowsky A, Bader H, Kohler W, Freisheim JH, Moran RG. Methotrexate analogues. 34. Replacement of the glutamate moiety in methotrexate and aminopterin by long-chain 2-aminoalkanedioic acids. *J Med Chem* 1988;31:1338–1344.
69. Lee WW, Martinez AP, Goodman L. Folic acid antagonists. Methotrexate analogs containing spurious amino acids. Dichlorohomofolic acid. *J Med Chem* 1974;17:326–330.
70. Rosowsky A, Bader H, Forsch RA, Moran RG, Freisheim JH. Methotrexate analogues. 31. Meta and ortho isomers of aminopterin, compounds with a double bond in the side chain, and a novel analogue modified at the α-carbon: chemical and in vitro biological studies. *J Med Chem* 1988;31:763–768; cf. erratum in *J Med Chem* 1989;32:2582.
71. Matsuoka H, Kato N, Tsuji K, Maruyama N, Suzuki H, Mihara M, Takeda Y, Yano K. Antirheumatic agents. 1. Novel methotrexate derivatives bearing an indoline moiety. *Chem Pharm Bull* 1996;44:1332–1337.
72. Matsuoka H, Ohi N, Mihara M, Suzuki H, Miyamoto K, Maruyama N, Tsuji K, Kato N, Akimoto T, Takeda Y, Yano K, Kuroki T. Antirheumatic agents: novel methotrexate derivatives bearing a benzoxazine or benzothiazine moiety. *J Med Chem* 1987;40:105–111.
73. Galivan J, Inglese J, McGuire JJ, Nimec Z, Coward JK. γ-Fluoromethotrexate: synthesis and biological activity of a potent inhibitor of dihydrofolate reductase with greatly diminished ability to form poly-γ-glutamates. *Proc Natl Acad Sci USA* 1985;82:2598–2602.
74. Hart BP, Haile WH, Licato NJ, Bolanowska WE, McGuire JJ, Coward JK. Synthesis and biological activity of folic acid and methotrexate analogues containing L-*threo*-(2S,4S)-4-fluoroglutamic acid and DL-3,3-difluoroglutamic acid. *J Med Chem* 1996;39:56–65.
75. Tsushima T, Kawada K, Shiratori O, Uchida N. Fluorine-containing amino acids and their derivatives. 5. Synthesis of novel fluorinated analogues of the antitumor agent, methotrexate. *Heterocycles* 1985;23:45–49.
76. Tsushima T, Kawada K, Ishihara S, Uchida N, Shiratori O, Higaki J, Hirata M. Fluorine-containing amino acids and their derivatives. 7. Synthesis and antitumor activity of α- and γ-substituted methotrexate analogs. *Tetrahedron* 1988;44:5375–5387.
77. McGuire JJ, Graber M, Licato N, Vincenz C, Coward JK, Nimec Z, Galivan J. Biochemical and growth inhibitory effects of the *erythro* and *threo* isomers of γ-fluoromethotrexate, a methotrexate analogue defective in polygluatmylation. *Cancer Res* 1989;49:4517–4525.
78. Tsukamoto T, Kitazume T, McGuire JJ, and Coward JK. Synthesis and biological evaluation of DL-4,4-difluoroglutamic acid and DL-γ,γ-difluoromethotrexate. *J Med Chem* 1996;39:66–72.
79. Licato NJ, Coward JK, Nimec Z, Galivan J, Bolanowska WE, McGuire JJ. Synthesis of N-[N-(4-deoxy-4-amino-10-methylpteroyl)-4-fluoroglutamyl]-γ-glutamate , an unusual substrate for folylpoly-γ-glutamate synthetase and γ-glutamyl hydrolase. *J Med Chem* 1990;33:1022–1027.
80. McGuire JJ, Hart BP, Haile WH, Magee KJ, Rhee M, Bolanowska WE, Russell C, Galivan J, Paul B, Coward JK. Biological properties of fluoroglutamate-containing analogs of folates and methotrexate with altered capacities to form poly (γ-glutamate) metabolites. *Biochem Pharmacol* 1996;52:1295–1303.
81. McGuire JJ, Bolanowska WE, Coward JK, Sherwood RF, Russell CA, Felschow DM. Biochemical and biological properties of methotrexate analogs containing D-glutamic acid or D-erythro,threo-4-fluoroglutamic acid. *Biochem Pharmacol* 1991;42:2400–2403.
82. Rosowsky A, Bader H, Freisheim JH. Analogues of methotrexate and aminopterin with γ-methylene and γ-cyano substitution of the glutamate side chain: Synthesis and in vitro biological activity. *J Med Chem* 1991;34:203–208.
83. Abraham A, McGuire JJ, Galivan J, Nimec Z, Kisliuk RL, Gaumont Y, Nair MG. Folate analogues. 34. Synthesis and antitumor activity of non-polyglutamatable inhibitors of dihydrofolate reductase. *J Med Chem* 1991;34:222–227.
84. Abraham A, Nair MG, McGuire JJ, Galivan J, Kisliuk RL, Vishnuvajjala BR. Antitumor efficacy of

classical non-polyglutamatable antifolates that inhibit dihydrofolate reductase. *Adv Exptl Biol Med* 1993;338:663–667.
85. Rosowsky A, Forsch RA, Moran RG, Freisheim JH. Synthesis and in vitro biological evaluation of β,γ-methano analogues of methotrexate and aminopterin. *Pteridines* 1990;2:133–139.
86. Rosowsky A, Forsch R, Uren J, Wick M. Methotrexate analogues. 14. New γ-substituted derivatives as dihydrofolate reductase inhibitors and potential anticancer agents. *J Med Chem* 1981;24:1450–1455.
87. Rosowsky A, Freisheim JH, Bader H, Forsch RA, Susten SS, Cucchi CA, Frei E III. Methotrexate analogues. 25. Chemical and biological studies on the γ-*tert*-butyl esters of methotrexate and aminopterin. *J Med Chem* 1985;28:660–667.
88. Rosowsky A, Beardsley GP, Ensminger WD, Lazarus H, Yu CS. Methotrexate analogs. 11. Unambiguous chemical synthesis and in vitro biological evaluation of α- and γ-monoesters as potential prodrugs. *J Med Chem* 1978;21:380–386.
89. Rosowsky A, Forsch RA, Yu CS, Lazarus H, Beardsley GP. Methotrexate analogues. 21. Divergent influence of alkyl chain length on the dihydrofolate reductase affinity and cytotoxicity of methotrexate monoesters. *J Med Chem* 1984;27:605–609.
90. Rosowsky A, Lazarus H, Yuan GC, Beltz WR, Mangini L, Abelson HT, Modest EJ, Frei E III. Effects of methotrexate esters and other lipophilic antifolates on methotrexate-resistant human leukemic lymphoblasts. *Biochem Pharmacol* 1980;29:648–652.
91. Wright JE, Rosowsky A, Waxman DJ, Trites D, Cucchi CA, Flatow J, Frei E III. Metabolism of methotrexate and γ-*tert*-butyl methotrexate by human leukemic cells in culture and by hepatic aldehyde oxidase in vitro. *Biochem Pharmacol* 1987;36:2209–2214.
92. Wright JE, Rosowsky A, Cucchi CA, Flatow J, Frei E III. Methotrexate and γ-*tert*-butyl methotrexate transport in CEM and CEM/MTX human leukemic lymphoblasts. *Biochem Pharmacol* 1993;46:871–876.
93. Rosowsky A, Forsch RA, Freisheim JH, Moran RG, Wick M. Methotrexate analogues. 19. Replacement of the glutamate side chain in classical antifolates by L-homocysteic acid and L-cysteic acid: effect on enzyme inhibition and antitumor activity. *J Med Chem* 1984;27:600–604.
94. Rosowsky A, Moran RG, Forsch R, Colman P, Wick M. Methotrexate analogues. 17. The antitumor activity of 4-amino-4-deoxy-N^{10}-methylpteroyl-D,L-homocysteic acid and its dual inhibition of dihydrofolate reductase and folylpolyglutamate synthetase. *Biochem Pharmacol* 1984;33:155–162.
95. Rosowsky A, Yu CS, Uren J, Lazarus H, Wick M. Methotrexate analogues. 13. Chemical and pharmacologic studies on amide, hydrazide, and hydroxamic acid derivatives of the glutamate side-chain. *J Med Chem* 1981;24:559–567.
96. Rosowsky A, Forsch R, Uren J, Wick M. Methotrexate analogues. 14. Synthesis of new γ-substituted derivatives as dihydrofolate reductase inhibitors and potential anticancer agents. *J Med Chem* 1981;24:1450–1455.
97. Piper JR, Montgomery JA, Sirotnak FM, Chello PL. Syntheses of α- and γ-substituted amides, peptides, and esters of methotrexate and their evaluation as inhibitors of folate metabolism. *J Med Chem* 1982;25:182–187.
98. Antonjuk DJ, Boadle DK, Cheung HTA, Tran TQ. Synthesis of monoamides of methotrexate from L-glutamic acid monoamide t-butyl esters. *J Chem Soc Perkin Trans 1* 1984:1989–2003.
99. Antonjuk DJ, Birdsall B, Cheung HTA, Clore GM, Feeney J, Gronenborn A, Roberts GCK, Tran TQ. A ^{1}H n.m.r. study of the role of the glutamate moiety in the binding of methotrexate to *Lactobacillus casei* dihydrofolate reductase. *Br J Pharmacol* 1984;81:309–315.
100. Rosowsky A, Bader H, Radike-Smith M, Cucchi CA, Wick MM, Freisheim JH. Methotrexate analogues. 28. Synthesis and biological evaluation of new γ-monoamides of aminopterin and methotrexate. *J Med Chem* 1986;29:1703–1709.
101. Rosowsky A, Bader H, Freisheim JH. Synthesis and biological activity of methotrexate analogues with two acid groups and a hydropobic aromatic ring in the side chain. *J Med Chem* 1991;34:574–579.
102. Itoh F, Russello O, Akimoto H, Beardsley GP. Novel pyrrolo[2,3-*d*]pyrimidine antifolate TNP-351: cytotoxic effect on methotrexate-resistant CCRF-CEM cells and inhibition of transformylases of de novo purine biosynthesis. *Cancer Chemother Pharmacol* 1994;34:273–279.
103. Itoh F, Yoshioka Y, Yukishige K, Yoshia S, Wajima M, Ootsu K, Akimoto H. Nonglutamate type

pyrrolo[2,3-*d*]pyrimidine antifolates. II. Synthesis and antitumor activity of N^5-substituted glutamine analogs. *Chem Pharm Bull (Tokyo)* 1996;44:1498–1509.
104. Miwa T, Hitaka T, Akimoto H, Nomura H. Novel pyrrolo[2,3-*d*]pyrimidine antifolates: synthesis and antitumor activities. *J Med Chem* 1991;34:555–560.
105. Miwa T, Hitaka T, Akimoto H. A novel synthetic approach to pyrrolo[2,3-*d*]pyrimidine antifolates. *J Org Chem* 1993;58:1696–1701.
106. Rosowsky A, Bader H, Cucchi CA, Moran RG, Kohler W, Freisheim JH. Methotrexate analogues. 33. N^δ-Acyl-N^α-(4-amino-4-deoxypteroyl)-L-ornithine derivatives: synthesis and in vitro antitumor activity. *J Med Chem* 1988;31:1332–1337.
107. Sirotnak FM, Chello PL, Piper JR, Montgomery JA. Growth inhibitory, transport and biochemical properties of the γ-glutamyl and γ-aspartyl peptides of methotrexate in L1210 leukemia cells *in vitro*. *Biochem Pharmacol* 1978;27:1821–1825.
108. Heath TD, Montgomery JA, Piper JR, Papahadjopoulos D. Antibody-targeted liposomes: increase in specific toxicity of methotrexate-γ-aspartate. *Proc Natl Acad Sci USA* 1983;80:1377–1381.
109. Rosowsky A, Moran RG, Forsch RA, Radike-Smith M, Colman PD, Wick MM, Freisheim JH. Methotrexate analogues. 27. Dual inhibition of dihydrofolate reductase and folylpolyglutamate synthetase by methotrexate and aminopterin analogues with a γ-phosphonate group in the side chain. *Biochem Pharmacol* 1986;35:3327–3333.
110. Rosowsky A, Moran RG, Freisheim JH, Bader H, Forsch RA, Solan VC. Synthesis and biologic activity of new side-chain-altered methotrexate and aminopterin analogs with dual inhibitory action against dihydrofolate reductase and folylpolyglutamate synthetase. *NCI Monogr* 1987;5:145–152.
111. Clarke L, Rosowsky A, Waxman DJ. Inhibition of human liver folylpolyglutamate synthetase by non-γ-glutamylatable antifolate analogs. *Mol Pharmacol* 1987;31:122–127.
112. Rosowsky A, Forsch RA, Moran RG, Kohler W, Freisheim JH. Methotrexate analogues. 32. Chain extension, α-carboxyl deletion, and γ-carboxyl replacement by sulfonate and phosphonate: effect on enzyme binding and cell growth inhibition. *J Med Chem* 1988;31:1326–1331.
113. McGuire JJ, Russell CA, Bolanowska WE, Freitag CM, Jones CS, Kalman TI. Biochemical and growth inhibition studies of methotrexate and aminopterin analogues containing a tetrazole ring in place of the γ-carboxyl group. *Cancer Res* 1990;50:1726–1731.
114. Cody V, Luft JR, Ciszak E, Kalman TI, Freisheim JH. Crystal structure determination at 2.3Å of recombinant human dihydrofolate reductase ternary complex with NADPH and methotrexate-γ-tetrazole. *Anticancer Drug Design* 1992;7:483–491.
115. Kempton RJ, Black AM, Anstead GM, Kumar AA, Blankenship DR, Freisheim JH. Lysine and ornithine analogues of methotrexate as inhibitors of dihydrofolate reductase. *J Med Chem* 1982;25:475–477.
116. Rosowsky A, Wright JE, Ginty C, Uren J. Methotrexate analogues. 15. A methotrexate analogue designed for active-site-directed irreversible inactivation of dihydrofolate reductase. *J Med Chem* 1982;25:960–964.
117. Piper JR, McCaleb GS, Montgomery JA, Schmid FA, Sirotnak FM. Synthesis and evaluation as antifolates of MTX analogues derived from 2,ω-diaminoalkanoic acids. *J Med Chem* 1985;28:1016–1025.
118. Rosowsky A, Freisheim JH, Moran RG, Solan VC, Bader H, Wright JE, Radike-Smith M. Methotrexate analogues. 26. Inhibition of dihydrofolate reductase and folylpolyglutamate synthetase activity and in vitro cell growth by methotrexate and aminopterin analogues containing a basic amino acid side-chain. *J Med Chem* 1986;29:655–660.
119. McGuire JJ, Hsieh P, Franco CT, Piper JR. Folylpolyglutamate synthetase inhibition and cytotoxic effects of methotrexate analogs containing 2,ω-diaminoalkanoic acids. *Biochem Pharmacol* 1986;35:2607–2613.
120. McGuire JJ, Piper JR, Coward JK, Galivan J. Folate analog nonsubstrates and inhibitors of folylpolyglutamate synthetase as potential cancer chemotherapy drugs. *NCI Monogr* 1987;5:139–144.
121. McGuire JJ, Bolanowska WE, Piper JR. Structural specificity of inhibition of human folylpolyglutamate synthetase by ornithine-containing analogs. *Biochem Pharmacol* 1988;37:3931–3939.
122. Patil SA, Shane B, Freisheim JH, Singh SK, Hynes JB. Inhibition of mammalian folylpolyglutamate synthetase and human dihydrofolate reductase by 5,8-dideaza analogues of folic acid and aminopterin bearing a terminal L-ornithine. *J Med Chem* 1989;32:1559–1565.
123. Rosowsky A, Forsch RA, Bader H, Freisheim JH. Synthesis and in vitro biological activity of new

deaza analogues of folic acid, aminopterin, and methotrexate with an L-ornithine side chain. *J Med Chem* 1991;34:1447–1454.
124. Rosowsky A, Forsch RA, Moran RG. Inhibition of folylpolyglutamate synthetase by substrate analogues with an ornithine side chain. *J Heterocycl Chem* 1996;33:1355–1361.
125. Tsukamoto T, Haile WH, McGuire JJ, Coward JK. Synthesis and biological evaluation of N^α-(4-amino-4-deoxy-10-methylpteroyl)-DL-4,4-difluoroornithine . *J Med Chem* 1996;39:2536–2540.
126. Rosowsky A, Wright JE, Shapiro H, Beardsley GP, Lazarus H. A new fluorescent dihydrofolate reductase probe for studies of methotrexate resistance. *J Biol Chem* 1982;257:14162–14167.
127. Kumar AA, Freisheim JH, Kempton RJ, Anstead GM, Black AM, Judge L. Synthesis and characterization of a fluorescent analogue of methotrexate. *J Med Chem* 1983;26:111–113.
128. Rosowsky A, Wright JE, Cucchi CA, Boeheim K, Frei E III. Transport of a fluorescent antifolate by methotrexate-sensitive and methotrexate-resistant human leukemic lymphoblasts. *Biochem Pharmacol* 1986;35:356–360.
129. Rosowsky A, Solan VC, Forsch RA, Delcamp TJ, Baccanari DP, Freisheim JH. Methotrexate analogues. 30. Dihydrofolate reductase inhibition and in vitro tumor cell growth inhibition by N^ϵ-haloacetyl-L-lysine and N^δ-haloacetyl-L-ornithine analogues and an acivicin analogue of methotrexate. *J Med Chem* 1987;30:1463–1469.
130. Rosowsky A, Bader H, Forsch RA. Synthesis of the folylpolyglutamate synthetase inhibitor N^α-pteroyl-L-ornithine and its N^δ-benzoyl and N^δ-hemiphthaloyl derivatives, and an improved synthesis of N^α-(4-amino-4-deoxypteroyl)-N^δ-hemiphthaloyl-L-ornithine. *Pteridines* 1989;1:91–98.
131. Peters GJ, Braakhuis BJM, Rosowsky A, Rots M, Pieters R, van der Wilt CL, Smid K, Jansen G. Preclinical activity of PT523 in relation to membrane transport in *Eleventh International Symposium on Chemistry and Biology of Pteridines,* Berchtesgaden, Germany, June 15–20, 1997, pp. 267–270.
132. Rosowsky A, Bader H, Wright JE, Keyomarsi K, Matherly LH. Synthesis and biological activity of N^ω-hemiphthaloyl-α,ω-diaminoalkanoic acid analogues of aminopterin and 3',5'-dichloroaminopterin. *J Med Chem* 1994;37:2167–2174.
133. Westerhof GR, Schornagel JH, Kathmann I, Jackman AL, Rosowsky A, Forsch RA, Hynes JB, Boyle FT, Peters GJ, Pinedo HM, Jansen G. Carrier- and receptor-mediated transport of folate antagonists targeting folate dependent enzymes: correlates of molecular structure and biological activity. *Mol Pharmacol* 1995;48:459–471.
134. Matherly LH, Angeles SM, McGuire JJ. Determinants of the disparate antitumor activities of (6R)-5,10-dideaza-5,6,7,8-tetrahydrofolate and methotrexate toward human lymphoblastic leukemia cells, characterized by severely impaired antifolate membrane transport. *Biochem Pharmacol* 1993;46:2185–2195.
135. Rosowsky A, Bader H, Frei E III. In vitro and in vivo antitumor activity of N^α-(4-amino-4-deoxypteroyl)-N^δ-hemiphthaloyl-L-or nithine (PT523), a potent side chain modified aminopterin analog that cannot form polyglutamates. *AACR Proc* 1991;32:325.
136. Rosowsky A, Vaidya CM, Bader H, Wright JE, Teicher BA. Analogues of N^α-(4-amino-4-deoxypteroyl)-N^δ-hemiphthaloyl-L-ornithine (PT523) modified in the side chain: synthesis and biological evaluation. *J Med Chem* 1997;40:286–299.
137. Holden SA, Teicher BA, Robinson MF, Northey D, Rosowsky A. Antifolates can potentiate topoisomerase II inhibitors in vitro and in vivo. *Cancer Chemother Pharmacol* 1995;36:165–171.
138. Rhee MS, Galivan J, Wright JE, Rosowsky A. Biochemical studies on PT523, a potent nonpolyglutamatable antifolate, in cultured cells. *Mol Pharmacol* 1994;45:783–791.
139. Wright JE, Pardo AM, Trites DH, Menon K, Rosowsky A. Pharmacokinetics and antifolate activity of N^α-(4-amino-4-deoxypteroyl)-N^δ-hemiphthaloyl-L-ornithine (PT523) in SCC VII murine squamous cell carcinoma. *AACR Proc* 1993;34:277.
140. Lorico A, Toffoli G, Boiocchi M, Erba E, Broggini M, Rappa G, D'Incalci M. Accumulation of DNA strand breaks in cells exposed to methotrexate or N^{10}-propargyl-5,8-dideazafolic acid. *Cancer Res* 1988;48:2036–2041.
141. Fry DW. Cytotoxic synergism between trimetrexate and etoposide: evidence that trimetrexate potentiates etoposide-induced protein-associated DNA strand breaks in L1210 cells through intracellular ATP concentrations. *Biochem Pharmacol* 1990;40:1981–1988.
142. Rosowsky A, Bader H, Chen Y-N, Forsch RA, Mota CE, Pardo J, Teicher BA, Tretyakov A, Vaidya CM, Wright JE. Potent DHFR inhibition and cytotoxicity of nonpolyglutamatable analogs of aminopterin (AMT). *AACR Proc* 1997;38:99.
143. Johnson JM, Meiering EM, Wright JE, Pardo J, Rosowsky A, Wagner G. NMR solution structure of

the antitumor compound PT523 and NADPH in the ternary complex with human dihydrofolate reductase. *Biochemistry* 1997;36:4399–4411.
144. Jackson RC, Hart LI, Harrap KR. Intrinsic resistance to methotrexate of cultured mammalian cells in relation to the inhibition kinetics of their dihydrofolate reductases. *Cancer Res* 1976;36:1991–1997.
145. Appleman JR, Prendergast N, Delcamp TJ, Freisheim JH, Blakley RL. Kinetics of the formation and isomerization of methotrexate complexes of recombinant human dihydrofolate reductase. *J Biol Chem* 1988;263:10304–10313.
146. Margosiak SA, Appleman JR, Santi DV, Blakley RL. Dihydrofolate reductase from the pathogenic fungus *Pneumocystis carinii:* catalytic properties and interaction with antifolates. *Arch Biochem Biophys* 1993;305:499–508.
147. Sirotnak FM, Chello PL, DeGraw JI, Piper JR, Montgomery JA. Membrane transport and the molecule basis for selective antitumor action of folate analogs. In: *Molecular Actions and Targets for Cancer Chemotherapeutic Agents* (Sartorelli AC, Lazo JS, Bertino JR, eds.). Academic, New York, 1981, pp. 349–384.
148. Chen G, Wright JE, Rosowsky A. Dihydrofolate reductase binding and cellular uptake of nonpolyglutamatable antifolates: correlates of cytotoxicity toward methotrexate sensitive and resistant human head and neck squamous carcinoma cells. *Mol Pharmacol* 1995;48:758–765.
149. Jackman AL, Taylor GA, Gibson W, Kimbell R, Brown M, Calvert AH, Judson IR, Hughes LR. ICI D1694, a quinazoline antifolate thymidylate synthase inhibitor that is a potent inhibitor of L1210 tumor cell growth in vitro and in vivo: a new agent for clinical study. *Cancer Res* 1991;51:5579–5586.
150. Schultz RM, Andis SL, Shackelford KA, Gates SB, Ratnam M, Mendelsohn LG, Shih C; Grindey GB. Role of membrane-associated folate binding protein in the cytotoxicity of antifolates in KB, IGROV1, and L1210A cells. *Oncol Res* 1995;7:97–102.
151. Alati T, Worzalla JF, Shih C, Bewley JR, Lewis S, Moran RG, Grindey GB. Augmentation of the therapeutic activity of lometrexol [(6-*R*)5,10-dideazatetrahydrofolate] by oral folic acid. *Cancer Res* 1996;56:2331–2335.
152. Duch DS, Banks S, Dev IK, Dickerson SH, Ferone R, Heath LS, Humphreys J, Knick B, Pendergast W, Singer S, Smith GK, Waters K, Wilson HR. Biochemical and cellular pharmacology of 1843U89, a novel benzoquinazoline inhibitor of thymidylate synthase. *Cancer Res* 1993;53:810–818.
153. Cody V, Galitsky N, Luft JR, Cotter D, Pangborn, Rosowsky A, Blakley RL. Structure of hDHFR ternary complex with the potent inhibitor, PT523. *AACR Proc* 1997;38:163.
154. Cody V, Galitsky N, Luft JR, Pangborn W, Blakley RL. Comparison of two independent crystal structure determinations of the antitumor compound PT523 and NADPH as ternary complexes with human dihydrofolate reductase. In: *Eleventh International Symposium on Chemistry and Biology of Pteridines and Folates,* Berchtesgaden, Germany, June 15–20, 1997, 403–406.
155. Piper JR, Johnson CA, Maddry JA, Malik ND, McGuire JJ, Otter GM, Sirotnak RM. Studies on analogues of classical antifolates bearing the naphthoyl group in place of benzoyl in the side chain. *J Med Chem* 1993;36:4161–4171.
156. Rosowsky A, Bader H, Moran RG, Freisheim JH. 6-Aza-5,8,10-trideaza analogues of tetrahydrofolic acid and tetrahydroaminopterin: synthesis and biological studies. *J Heterocycl Chem* 1989;26:509–516.
157. Fry DW, Werbel LM, Hung J, Besserer JA, Boritzki TJ, Leopold WR. In vivo and in vitro evaluation of 5-[4-(substituted aryl)-1-piperazinyl]-6-alkyl-2,4-pyrimidine diamines as antitumor agents. *AACR Proc* 1986;27:253.
158. Moran RG, Colman PD, Jones TR. Relative substrate activities of structurally related pteridine, quinazoline, and pyrimidine analogs for mouse liver folylpolyglutamate synthetase. *Mol Pharmacol* 1989;36:736–743.
159. Nair MG, Campbell PT, Braverman E, Baugh CM. Synthesis of thioaminopterin: a potent anti-bacterial agent. *Tetrahedron Lett* 1975;2745–2748.
160. Nair MG, Campbell PT. Folate analogues altered in the C^9-N^{10} bridge region. 10-Oxafolic acid and oxaaminopterin. *J Med Chem* 1976;19:825–829.
161. Nair MG, Chen S-Y, Kisliuk RL, Gaumont Y, Strumpf D. Folate analogues altered in the C^9-N^{10} region. 16. Synthesis and antifolate activity of 11-thiohomoaminopterin. *J Med Chem* 1980;23:899–903.
162. Nair MG, Bridges TW, Henkel TJ, Kisliuk RL, Gaumont Y, Sirotnak FM. Folate analogues altered in the C^9-N^{10} bridge regions. 18. Synthesis and antitumor evaluation of 11-oxahomoaminopterin and related compounds. *J Med Chem* 1981;24:1068–1073.

5 Fluoropyrimidines as Antifolate Drugs

G.J. Peters and C.H. Köhne

Contents
- Introduction
- Mechanism of Action
- Targets/role in Resistance
- (Anti)folate-Related Combinations
- Other Combinations
- Summary and Conclusions

1. INTRODUCTION

5 Fluorouracil (5FU) is a rationally designed antineoplastic agent *(1,2)* with distinct antifolate and antipyrimidine properties. 5FU is usually given in combination with other agents for the treatment of various types of cancer *(3–11)* such as cancers of the gastrointestinal tract, breast cancer, and head and neck cancer. For combinations of leucovorin (LV) and 5FU objective response rates between 20 and 40% have been achieved in randomized trials in patients with colorectal cancer, which means that more than 60% of the tumors are still resistant and will thereafter develop resistance. This resistance can be multifactorial (Table 1), and related to either the antipyrimidine or the antifolate properties of the drug. This also implies that many patients have an intrinsic resistance to 5FU, and since almost all patients will show a relapse, this means that in the remaining tumors acquired resistance will occur. Unfortunately the mechanism of modulation-resistance has hardly been addressed in most of these studies.

Clinical application of fluoropyrimidines is changing *(12–14)*. Generally 5FU has been administered as a bolus injection of 350–500 mg/m^2 given either weekly or daily times 5 and repeated every 28 d or weekly, respectively. LV is usually added to both regimens; for the daily schedule, a low dose of LV has a similar activity as a high dose, whereas for the weekly schedule a high dose seems preferable *(14)*. In the last decade there have been changes in the way of administration. Higher response rates have been observed by prolonging the infusion period of 5FU to 24 or 48 h, during which period

From: *Anticancer Drug Development Guide: Antifolate Drugs in Cancer Therapy*
Edited by: A.L. Jackman © Humana Press Inc., Totowa, NJ

Table 1
Mechanisms of Resistance to 5FU[a]

A. Decreased accumulation of activated metabolites
   a. decreased activation
   b. increased inactivation
   c. increased inactivation of 5FU nucleotides
B. Target-associated resistance
   a. decreased RNA effect
   b. altered effect on thymidylate synthase
      aberrant enzyme kinetics
      increased dUMP levels
      decreased FdUMP accumulation
      decreased stability of ternary complex
      depletion of intracellular folates
      decreased polyglutamylation of folates
      recovery and enhanced enzyme synthesis
      gene amplification
      enzyme kinetic variants of the enzyme
C. Pharmacokinetic resistance
   a. the drug does not reach the tumor
   b. disease state affects drug distribution
   c. increased elimination

[a]Modified from (3, 6)

very high doses of 5FU can be administered (15). Protracted infusions of up to several months are also being used increasingly. Lokich et al. (16) reported a higher response rate and less toxicity for continuous infusions in a randomized study compared to bolus administration. Although techniques to administer continuous infusions have improved considerably, it may not be widely regarded as a feasible method of 5FU administration. For that purpose alternative ways to simulate continuous infusions have been developed, such as oral administration forms of 5FU or 5FU prodrugs (Fig. 1) that release 5FU over a prolonged period, resulting in plasma concentrations of 5FU in the same range as observed with continuous infusions. However, whether the oral application of 5FU prodrugs are clinically equivalent to infusional 5FU remains to be proven. It has become evident that all these different routes of administration can have various effects on the mechanism of action of 5FU, either its incorporation into RNA or inhibition of TS.

This review will focus on relevant aspects of the mechanism of action of 5FU in clinical resistance to 5FU, with emphasis on the antifolate aspects in the various administration procedures that are used to enhance its antitumor activity and decrease side-effects.

2. MECHANISM OF ACTION

2.1. Anabolic Pathways; Which One is Important?

The complexity of the mechanism of action of 5FU, which is dependent on the type of tissue, either tumor or normal tissue, implicates the possibility of a large number of mechanisms of resistance (6,13). 5FU itself is an inert drug and has to be activated to a nucleotide (Fig. 2). Theoretically, conversion of 5FU to FUDR and subsequently to

Chapter 5 / Fluoropyrimidines

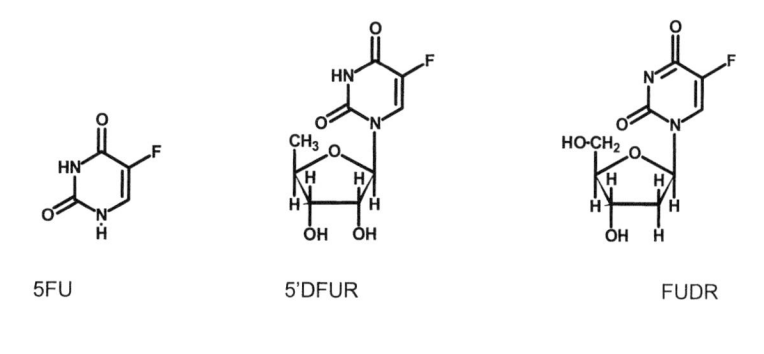

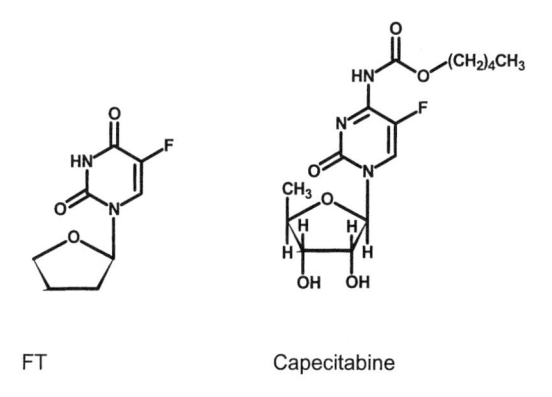

Fig. 1. Structural formulas of clinically used fluoropyrimidines: 5FU, 5-fluorouracil; FUDR, 2'-deoxy-5-fluorouridine; 5'DFUR, 5'-deoxy-5-fluorouridine (Doxifluridine); capecitabine (Xelopa); Ft, Ftorafur (Tegafur).

FdUMP is an activation pathway, but sufficient amounts of the cosubstrate deoxyribose-1-phosphate (dRib-1-P) are usually not present in tissues *(17)*. Thus, the major activation pathway of 5FU is its conversion to FUMP. This can proceed via an indirect pathway (via FUR to FUMP) or via direct phosphoribosylation (catalyzed by orotate phosphoribosyl transferase, OPRT).

Initial studies on 5FU resistance concentrated on its activation pathways. Thus it was recognized in several model systems that a low activity of uridine kinase (UK) and phosphorylase (UP) (and the channelled UP-UK) *(18–20)* and OPRT *(21,22)* were related to resistance to 5FU. In in vivo models, both high UP activity and high OPRT activity *(23,24)* were related to 5FU sensitivity. However, Ardalan et al. *(25)* observed low 5-phosphoribosyl-1-pyrophosphate (PRPP) levels in 5FU-resistant tumors and observed a higher activity of PRPP synthetase in the sensitive tumor, indicating an important role for OPRT since PRPP is the cosubstrate for this enzyme in activation of 5FU. Activation of 5FU via UP also requires the action of UK which is usually limiting *(17,26,27)*. More evidence for the importance of the OPRT pathway was obtained by Holland et al. *(28)*; injection of the UP inhibitor, benzylacyclouridine (BAU) together with 5FU resulted in the accumulation of FUR in the tumor, although no FUR was observed when 5FU was

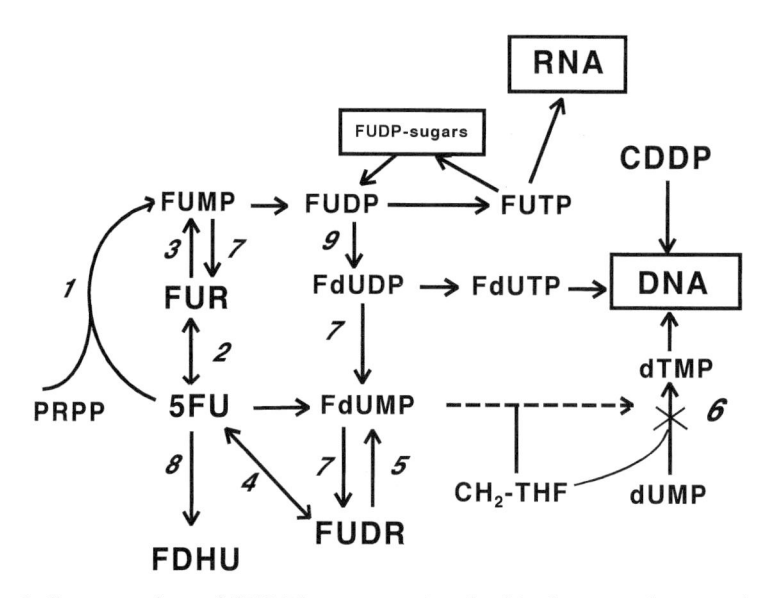

Fig. 2. Metabolic conversions of 5FU. The enzymes involved in these reactions are: 1, orotate phosphoribosyltransferase (OPRT); 2, uridine phosphorylase (UP); 3, uridine kinase (UK); 4, thymidine phosphorylase (TP); 5, thymidine kinase 1 (TK1); 6, thymidylate synthase (TS); 7,5′-nucleotidases and phosphatases; 8, dihydropyrimidine dehydrogenase (DPD); 9, ribonucleotide reductase (RR). Metabolic pathways are depicted as solid lines. The inhibition of TS by FdUMP is depicted as a broken line with a cross; CDDP can form DNA-platin adducts. FUDP-sugars are the family of nucleotide sugars such as FUDP-glucose, FUDP-galactose, and so on.

injected as a single agent. Since BAU would inhibit direct conversion of 5FU to FUR, this means that FUR should be formed as a degradation product of FUMP, which can only be synthesized from direct phosphoribosylation of 5FU to FUMP. These data also indicate the existence of a futile cycle 5FU→ FUMP→ FUR→ 5FU which can be considered as some hidden depot of 5FU in the tumor responsible for the long retention of 5FU in tissues *(29)*. By the use of several cosubstrates and precursors for these cosubstrates, it was postulated that in human tumors a high activity of the OPRT pathway is essential for 5FU activation *(17)*. In summary, the best evidence for activation of 5FU and 5FU analogs was observed for the OPRT activity *(21,24–28,30)*.

Sufficient anabolism of the FU-nucleotide FUMP to FUDP is essential for its action and its antifolate effects, since the latter nucleotide is at the branchpoint for other metabolic pathways (reviewed in refs. *6,13*). These include, conversion to FUTP which will be incorporated into RNA, but can also be converted to FUDP-sugars *(31)*; conversion to FdUMP, which is a potent tight-binding inhibitor of thymidylate synthase (TS); and conversion of FdUMP to FdUTP and subsequent incorporation into DNA *(13)*. Evidence is accumulating that an increase of the inhibition of TS, as seen in the combination chemotherapy with LV, point to the inhibition of TS as the main mechanism for antitumor activity *(32–34)*. This might, however, be schedule (bolus, continuous infusion) and tumor dependent. Insufficient inhibition of TS is now considered to be a major cause for clinical resistance to 5FU. Expression of TS is considered as a major predictive parameter for the response to 5FU-containing chemotherapy.

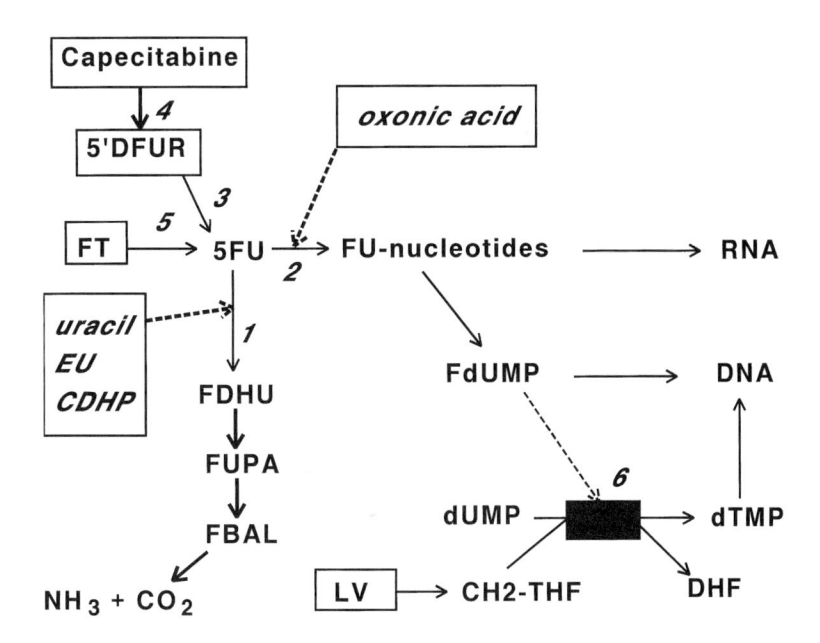

Fig. 3. The role of modulation of 5FU degradation in the metabolism of oral 5FU formulations. Enzymes involved in these reactions are: 1, DPD; 2, OPRT; 3, TP and UP; 4, carboxyl esterase; 5, cytochrome P450 2A6 (predominantly) and TP (minor). 6, TS. Inhibitory actions are depicted as broken lines: DPD by uracil, ethynyluracil (EU, GW776), and 5-chloro-2,4-dihydropyridine (CDHP); OPRT by oxonic acid; TS by FdUMP. The inhibition of DPD will lead to an enhanced bioavailability of 5FU which can be converted to FdUMP, leading to more inhibition of TS. Leucovorin (LV) acts as a precursor for CH_2-THF (5,10-methylene-tetrahydrofolate), DHF is the product of this reaction.

2.2. Relevance of the Catabolic Pathway/Oral Formulations

Dihydropyrimidine dehydrogenase (DPD) is a NADPH-dependent enzyme and catalyzes the first step in the degradation pathway of 5FU (Fig. 3). DPD has an abundant expression mainly in liver, kidney, and lung *(35)* resulting in the appearance of FDHU as the major metabolite of 5FU *(36)*; in tumor cells this enzyme is also active *(35–37)*, but further degradation to fluoroureido-propionate (FUPA) and subsequently to fluoro-β-alanine (FBAL), NH_3, and CO_2 occurs at a much lower rate and is usually undetectable. After a bolus injection, the enzymes from normal tissues such as liver will rapidly degrade 5FU to FDHU and subsequently to FUPA and FBAL *(38)*. The latter compound is predominant in the plasma and after the bolus administration still has a similar concentration after 24 h compared to 4 h. This process is of major importance since it leads to a decreased availability of 5FU to tumor tissues.

Several of the enzymes mentioned above (DPD and UP) have a circadian pattern that may affect 5FU pharmacokinetics resulting in a circadian variation of 5FU in plasma of patients *(39)* and mice *(40)* receiving continuous infusions with 5FU. Tumor and normal cells show a different circadian pattern in their sensitivity to fluoropyrimidines *(41)*, which is the basis for time-adapted administration schedules *(41)*. The importance of DPD in 5FU toxicity was shown by the observation that an absence of DPD activity in patients has been associated with severe toxicity *(42)*, since 5FU clearance is related to the activity of DPD *(43)*. Taken together these findings demonstrated that 5FU degradation, which amounts to more than 80% of its elimination, is an important factor controlling 5FU bioavailability and toxicity. It has been hypothesized that DPD activity is related not only to toxic side effects of 5FU, but also to its antitumor activity *(44,45)*.

The use of inhibitors of DPD (Fig. 3) enables 5FU (or one of its prodrugs) to be given as an oral formulation, since degradation is reduced almost completely. Such formulations of 5FU result in 5FU concentrations in the μM range. The most widely used formulation at this moment is UFT in which uracil is combined with Ftorafur (Ft) in a 4:1 molar ratio *(46)*. This formulation has been refined resulting in S-1, which is a combination of Ft-CDHP and oxonic acid in a molar ratio of 1:0.4:1 *(47)*; CDHP is a potent reversible inhibitor of DPD *(48)* and oxonic acid of OPRT; since oxonic acid accumulates specifically in normal gut, this will reduce gastrointestinal toxicity *(47)*. In another formulation 5FU is combined with ethynyluracil, a suicide inhibitor of DPD *(49)*. Capecitabine was synthesized in a series of prodrugs of 5′-deoxy-5-fluorouridine (5′-DFUR) which has to be activated to 5FU by thymidine phosphorylase *(50,51)*. All these formulations have shown clinical activity in various tumor types; representative data for colorectal cancer are summarized in Table 2. In general the antitumor activity of the oral formulation (usually with oral LV) is comparable to that found with modulated 5FU bolus schedules and probably also continuous infusions. The main advantage is the convenient oral administration of these formulations. Noticeable is the good anticancer activity of UFT and S-1 against gastric cancer of 26 and 54%, respectively *(12,60)*.

These formulations of 5FU or Ft are also suitable for combinations with other oral drugs which may affect the anticancer activity of 5FU by, e.g., enhancing the inhibition of TS, such as by LV *(12)*. However, mechanistic studies in patients in view of TS inhibition are scarce. Ichikura et al. *(61)* compared TS inhibition in patients with gastric cancer; patients receiving UFT alone for 3 d exhibit a TS inhibition of 14 to 50% and patients receiving UFT and oral LV more than 55% ($p < 0.01$). In the Amsterdam study *(62)* one patient responding to S-1 showed a 50% TS inhibition, upon relapse the total activity was increased twofold. Plasma concentrations of 5FU in these patients are in the μM range, while 5FU and FdUMP concentrations in the tumor of the responding patient were in the same range as found 24–48 h after a bolus infection *(29)*. Oral formulations of 5FU are an important feature in the administration of 5FU, but the mechanistic basis in view of TS inhibition should be investigated in more detail. Furthermore, the relative activity to infusional 5-FU regimens and their capacity to act in combination with the non-TS directed agents needs to be evaluated.

3. TARGETS/ROLE IN RESISTANCE

3.1. 5FU Incorporation into RNA vs TS Inhibition

It has been postulated that reduced 5FU incorporation into RNA could be responsible for the lower antitumor effect observed in animal model systems *(64)*. Since both in vitro and in vivo 5FU incorporation into RNA are concentration and dose dependent, respectively, it was postulated that 5FU RNA incorporation was related to the antitumor effect as the antineoplastic activity was also dose dependent *(65)*. However, the extent and duration of in vivo TS inhibition was also dose dependent *(66)*. We observed a much better antitumor activity for FUDR than for 5FU, which was not associated with a

Table 2
5FU Prodrugs Given Orally to Previously Untreated Patients with Colorectal Cancer

Drug	Dose/Schedule	LV	N Pat	CR/PR	Reference
UFT	350 mg/d × 28d	15 mg/d po × 28 d	71	15%	(52)
	300–350 mg/d × 28 d	15–150 mg/d po × 28 d	66	36%	(53)
	390 mg/m² /d × 14d	500 mg/m² iv × 1 d	177	36%	(54,55)
		30 mg/m²/d po d 2–14			
Doxifluridine	750–1200 mg/m² bid d 1–4 (5)	25 mg po d 1–5	127	25%	(56,57)
Capecitabine	1331–2510 mg/m² continuous/intermittent	—	68	24%	(58)
	1657 mg/m² intermittent	60 mg/d po +/−	33	24%	
5FU plus GW 776	20–25 mg/m²/d d 1–7	50 mg po d 2–6	23	30%	(59)
S1	50–75 mg/body × 2 d 1–28, 2 wk rest	—	30[a]	17%	(60)

[a]Pretreated and untreated patients.
Modified from Köhne (12,63).

significant increase in 5FU incorporation into RNA, but to a much longer retained inhibition of TS. In a subsequent study we determined both the inhibition of TS and the 5FU incorporation into RNA as a function of 5FU dose. The administration of uridine-diphosphoglucose (UDPG), enabled an 1.5-fold increase in 5FU dose *(67)* up to 150 mg/kg, which was associated with an enhanced antitumor activity. The higher dose of 5FU (150 mg/kg) caused a longer retained inhibition of TS than the lower dose (100 mg/kg), whereas UDPG even caused a decrease in the 5FU incorporation into RNA without affecting the TS inhibition or antitumor activity *(68)* indicating the importance of TS inhibition for the antineoplastic activity. In addition to this preclinical evidence also clinical data support the idea, that 5FU incorporation into RNA does not play a major role in the antitumor activity of 5FU. In four groups of patients who received either 5FU alone, or a combination with different schedules of LV, we measured both 5FU incorporation into RNA and TS inhibition. Whereas no difference in 5FU RNA incorporation was observed, the inhibition of TS was significantly different. Furthermore the RNA incorporation of 5FU in patients with a partial or complete response was 0.34 pmol/μg RNA, which was not significantly different from nonresponders, 0.24 pmol 5FU/μg RNA *(69)*. There is substantial evidence that the toxicity of 5FU is related to its incorporation into RNA, since a decrease of the 5FU incorporation into RNA by uridine was associated with a decreased extent of side-effects of 5FU *(70,71)*. Thus evidence is accumulating that the antitumor activity of 5FU is predominantly related to the inhibition of TS, but unlikely to its incorporation into RNA.

3.2. Thymidylate Synthase: Levels/Inhibition in Relation to Preclinical and Clinical Sensitivity

In the last decade, evidence has accumulated demonstrating that insufficient inhibition of TS by FdUMP may be a major resistance mechanism, also in patients *(32–34,69,72)*. Several alterations in TS may be responsible for resistance to 5FU (Table 1). Under physiological conditions, TS catalyzes the conversion of dUMP to dTMP, for which CH_2-THF is the limiting methyl donor (Fig. 4); the K_m for this reaction is approx 50 μM. The K_m for dUMP is approx 1–5 μM *(11,13,26,73)*. The inhibition by FdUMP (with a K_i of approx 1 nM) is mediated by the formation of a covalent ternary complex between FdUMP, TS and CH_2-THF (Fig. 4A). The stability of this ternary complex is highly dependent on the availability of CH_2-THF *(74,75)*. In the absence of CH_2-THF, an unstable binary complex is formed and in this case FdUMP acts as a weak inhibitor of TS.

LV can increase the availability of CH_2-THF (Fig. 2). After transfer across the membrane mediated by the reduced-folate carrier *(76)*, LV will be metabolized to CH_2-THF. Although intermediates of the metabolic pathway of LV to CH_2-THF can also support the formation of the ternary complex, CH_2-THF is the most active substrate *(77)*. Polyglutamates of CH_2-THF *(78)*, which are formed by the action of folyl-polyglutamate synthetase (FPGS) will enhance inhibition of TS. A decreased activity of FPGS and altered K_m values for dUMP and binding constants for FdUMP binding *(3,73,80–82)* have been associated with 5FU resistance. A high dUMP concentration or a limited FdUMP binding to TS may reduce retention of the inhibition of TS, whereas the lack of CH_2-THF or one of its polyglutamates may affect the stabilization of the ternary complex *(3,72,75,81,82)*. Disturbed folate pools *(75)* are indeed related to intrinsic resistance, re-

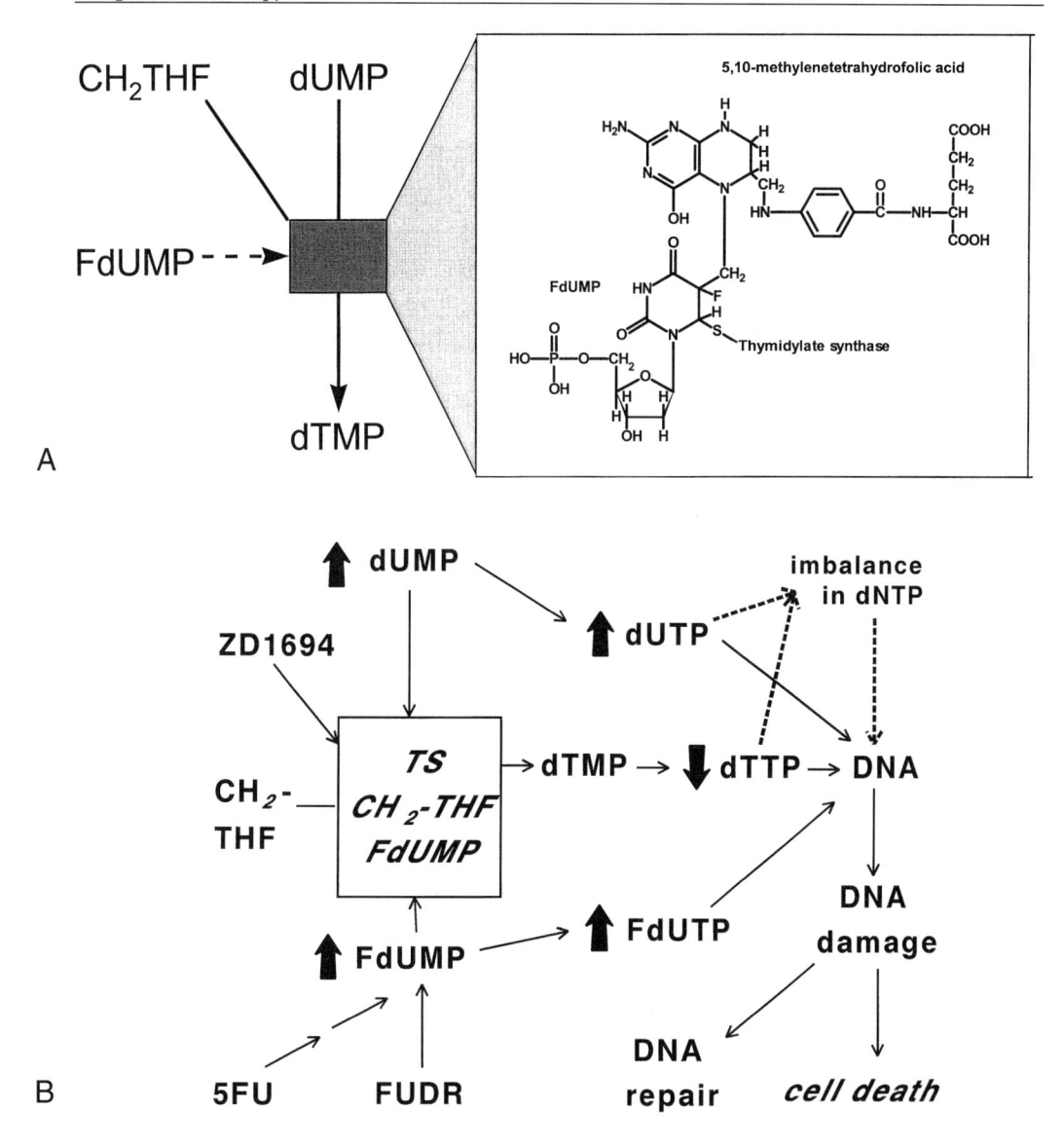

Fig. 4. Mechanism of inhibition of TS by FdUMP and the downstream effect following TS inhibition. **(A),** Inhibition of TS is mediated by ternary complex formation **(B)** depicted as a box in **(A)**. TS may also be inhibited by an unstable binary complex between FdUMP and TS. Both FdUMP-(formed either from 5FU or FUDR) and ZD1694-induced inhibition of TS will result in a depletion of dTMP and subsequently of dTTP, which may decrease the synthesis of DNA. TS inhibition also causes the accumulation of dUMP and subsequently of dUTP, which can be incorporated into DNA, and substitute dTTP, which is decreased. Similarly, FdUTP, which can be formed from FdUMP, can be incorporated into DNA and substitute dTTP. Incorporation of either dUTP or FdUTP can cause different types of DNA damage (*see* text). The increased ratio of dUTP/dTTP can cause an imbalance in other deoxyribonucleoside triphosphates (dNTP) (e.g., increased dATP and decreased dGTP) which will affect DNA synthesis, and result in DNA damage. Depending on, e.g., the p53 status (mutant, wild-type), the presence and interaction of other onco- and suppressor genes (such as bcl-2, bax, p21, mdm2, and so on), the cell will try to repair this DNA damage or undergo apoptosis.

**TS induction in colon tumors following
continuous 5FU infusion or 5FU bolus injections**

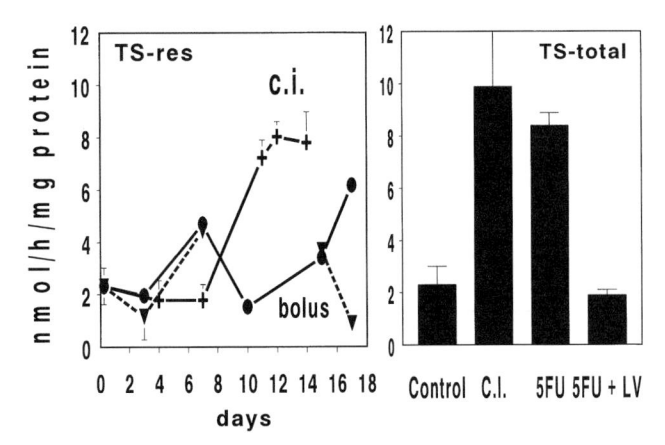

Fig. 5. Inhibition and induction of TS in Colon 26A tumors after treatment with 5FU (with or without LV). Mice bearing Colon 26A tumors were treated with continuous infusions of 5FU (solid lines, +; 10 mg/kg for 21 d released by sc-implanted pellets), bolus of 5FU without (solid lines, ●; 100 mg/kg, day 0, 7, and 14) or with LV (broken lines, ▼; 100 mg/kg, administered 1 h before and simultaneously with 5FU). TS activity was measured using 10 μM dUMP as a substrate at the indicated time points. TS levels are depicted as TS-*residual (res)*, which represents the TS-catalyzed conversion of dUMP to dTMP by unbound free enzyme. TS-bound by FdUMP is unable to convert dUMP to dTMP. Dissociation of FdUMP from TS-bound results in the presence of total TS levels, represented as bars at the time of maximal induction of TS-*res* levels. Naturally TS-*total* levels are higher than TS-*res*, indicating a substantial extent of TS induction. Tumors initially respond to 5FU (during the period when TS is below or comparable to initial levels); however, when TS levels increase, the tumors also continue to grow and do not respond to treatment, except when 5FU is combined, which also results in inhibition of TS (modified from data published in refs. *40,68,85*).

sulting in a low level of inhibition of TS. Also a high level of enzyme before treatment *(45,80,81)* is related to intrinsic resistance. Acquired resistance in FUDR-resistant sub-cell lines *(83)* was associated with gene amplification of TS. Another resistant cell line had a variant form of TS encoded by a different gene with a reduced affinity for FdUMP and CH_2-THF *(82)*. Thus changes in the TS gene at the DNA level (e.g., mutations or gene amplification) are clearly associated with acquired resistance to fluoropyrimidines.

Sobrero et al. *(84)* observed that low-dose continuous exposure to 5FU almost immediately resulted in resistant clones of the HCT-8 colon tumor-cell line, whereas short-term exposure to 5FU required a longer period to result in resistance. Cells resistant to intermittent short exposure, were sensitive to continuous exposure; but cells resistant to continuous exposure were resistant to short-term exposure. These data suggest that continuous exposure to 5FU, and consequently to FdUMP may induce resistance to 5FU more rapidly and via different mechanisms than short-term *(40,84)*.

A general form of (transient) flouropyrimidine resistance is the induction of TS upon treatment. This phenomenon has been observed in a number of model systems both in vitro and vivo, and in patients. In an in vivo murine colon tumor model *(40)*, the tumors were initially sensitive to prolonged continuous administration of 5FU, but became resistant after approx 10 d of the 21-d infusion (Fig. 5). This was associated with a rapid three- to fourfold increase in free TS levels, although plasma and tissue 5FU levels under these conditions were still comparable to levels during the first days of the infusion. We also observed a considerable increase in the amount of TS after treatment with 5FU in a relatively insensitive murine colon tumor, but treatment with LV depressed this 5FU-induced increase *(85)*. In a sensitive colon tumor, this effect was less pronounced. A similar effect was observed when 5FU was compared with FUDR; the latter compound had a much better antitumor effect than 5FU when injected as a bolus at their maximum tolerated dose. Both compounds induced a similar extent of TS inhibition, but the two- to threefold induction was observed after 7 d for 5FU and after 10 d for FUDR *(66)*.

TS induction as observed in tumors may also occur in normal tissues. In a rat model, liver TS was enhanced fivefold following local treatment (isolated liver perfusion or hepatic artery infusion) but only twofold after intraperitoneal (ip) treatment *(86)*. Also in mucosal tissue of rats a two- to threefold increase in TS levels was observed after isolated liver perfusion, but not after ip treatment. Thus, the effect on TS induction seems to be dependent on the concentration and the length of exposure to this concentration of 5FU (and consequently of FdUMP) in the tissue. Prolonged low 5FU levels seem to favor TS induction in normal tissues, whereas in the tumor, initial inhibition is followed by TS induction. Higher peak (or plateau) 5FU levels seem to favor a prolonged TS inhibition; upon decrease of 5FU levels, TS will be induced, but a new dose of 5FU can inhibit this induction when the dose is either high *(68,66)* or combined with LV *(85)*. This might favor the weekly or interval treatment. Also in patients 5FU treatment resulted in a LV-independent increase in liver TS levels *(87)*. This phenomenon seems to explain the good tolerance of 5FU in hepatic artery infusions. These data may indicate that tumors have a different (deregulated?) expression of TS than normal tissues, in which upregulation of TS seems to be some sort of protective mechanism. Thus, prolonged TS inhibition and prevention of TS-induction are of significant importance in antitumor activity of fluoropyrimidines.

This increase in TS levels is most likely explained by a deregulation of the normal TS protein synthesis. Under physiological conditions TS protein synthesis is related to the cell cycle, with a high activity during the S-phase *(88)*. The translation of the TS mRNA appears to be controlled by its endproduct, the TS protein, in an autoregulatory manner. However, when TS is bound to a ternary complex, the protein can no longer regulate its synthesis, leading to the observed increase. Thus, inhibition of TS in vitro either by the formation of the ternary complex between FdUMP, the enzyme, and $5,10$-CH_2-THF *(89,90)* or by specific TS inhibitors such as ZD1694 *(91)* disrupt the regulation of enzyme synthesis, manifested as an increase in TS protein expression (Fig. 6). This increase was not accompanied by an increase in the TS mRNA, or a change in the stability of the enzyme. Recently it was observed that the p53-mRNA translation can also be regulated by TS protein *(92)*; whereas wild-type p53 protein can also inhibit TS promotor activity *(93)*. Thus regulation of induction of TS is a very complicated process, which may even be more disrupted (more induction) in cells with mutated p53 than with wild-type p53 (low induction). The high dose 5FU and the LV-mediated prevention of the induction probably play a role in the observed enhancement of the sensitivity to 5FU and may reverse resistance to 5FU.

TS inhibition in primary human colon tumors and in liver metastases is retained for

TS as an RNA binding protein

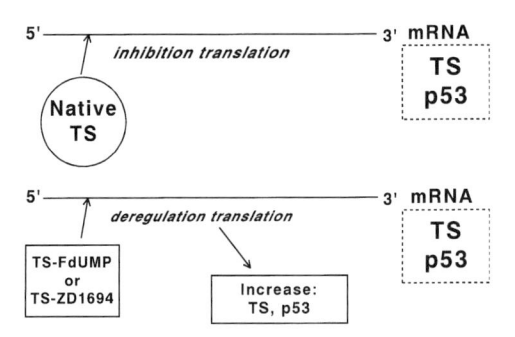

```
5'————————↑————————3' mRNA
    inhibition translation      ┌─────┐
                                 │ TS  │
   ( Native )                    │ p53 │
   (   TS   )                    └─────┘


5'————————↑————————3' mRNA
   deregulation translation     ┌─────┐
                                 │ TS  │
 ┌─────────┐      ↓              │ p53 │
 │ TS-FdUMP│   Increase:         └─────┘
 │   or    │   TS, p53
 │TS-ZD1694│
 └─────────┘
```

Fig. 6. Model of TS autoregulation and regulation of TS by p53. Under normal conditions native TS is able to bind to its own mRNA at an untranslated region at the 5´-end, resulting in inhibition of its own translation, thereby regulating its own synthesis. When cells enter the S-phase, this regulation is diminished resulting in an increased TS protein synthesis *(91)*. The ternary complex of FdUMP with TS, but also the complex of TS with TDX (tomudex, ZD1694) results in a conformational change of the enzyme, reducing the binding of the modified TS to its own mRNA, thereby deregulating TS protein synthesis, resulting in an increase of TS protein. Similarly TS protein can also bind to the p53-mRNA *(92)*. In addition wild-type p53 protein was reported to inhibit mouse TS-promotor activity *(93)*.

at least 48–72 h after a bolus injection of 500 mg/m^2 5FU *(34,69)*. In 19 patients responding to 5FU hepatic artery infusion, TS inhibition was two- to threefold higher and enzyme levels were two- to threefold lower than in 21 patients not responding. Also in breast-cancer patients, binding of FdUMP and the effect of CH$_2$-THF decreased during development of resistance *(33)*. These results demonstrate that analysis of biochemical parameters in tumor biopsies obtained at both short and longer time periods after 5FU administration gives valuable information about the in vivo mechanism of action of the drug in the tumors of patients.

The results of both in vitro and in vivo models and the initial results in patients indicate that the level of pretreatment TS might predict response to 5FU *(45)*. The large variation of both the enzyme activity levels *(94)* and at the expression of TS-mRNA *(95)* in human colorectal cancer observed in pre- and posttreatment samples *(34,69,95,96)* supported this hypothesis. Also, in patients, treatment with 5FU or 5FU-derivatives may induce TS levels *(33,34,96)* because of enhanced TS translation with no change in TS mRNA levels *(96)*. Patients with colon cancer and a low expression of TS-mRNA were more likely to respond to protracted 5FU infusions *(95)* or hepatic artery infusions *(97)* similar to patients with stomach cancer *(98)*. A high intensive immunohistochemical staining for TS was associated with a shorter survival of patients with rectal cancer *(99)*, head and neck cancer *(100)* and breast cancer *(101)* treated with (neo) adjuvant chemotherapy. For patients with metastatic colon cancer *(102)*, no relation between response and intensity of TS staining was observed, possibly because the patients were treated for advanced disease, but TS expression was measured in primary tumors. These studies indicate that pretreatment measurement of TS levels may predict whether patients are more likely to respond to fluoropyrimidine-containing treatment regimens.

3.3. Direct Effect of TS Inhibition; Deoxyribonucleotide (dNTP) Pool Imbalance and DNA Damage

Inhibition of TS will initially lead to a depletion of dTMP and dTTP, resulting in inhibition of DNA synthesis with the so-called thymine-less death as the final effect. The inhibition of TS will, however, also lead to an accumulation of dUMP and subsequently of FdUTP (Fig. 4B). In addition, FdUMP accumulation will also increase FdUTP. Both dUTP and FdUTP can be incorporated into DNA and subsequently excised, causing DNA strand breaks followed by cell death. For CB3717, a first generation antifolate TS inhibitor, it has been demonstrated that intracellular levels of dUTP can increase markedly, as measured with a sensitive radioimmunoassay *(103,104)*. This increase in dUTP pools was paralleled by growth inhibition in a dose- and time-related manner *(104)*. Depletion of dTTP pools and an increase in dUTP and FdUTP (when FdUMP is the inhibitor) pools have been shown repeatedly by several groups *(27,103–105)*. This imbalance in deoxyribonucleotides (dNTP) pools will favor either dUTP or FdUTP incorporation into DNA. Such a misincorporation has been associated with the cytotoxic effect *(106,107)*. E.g., 5FU incorporation into DNA was measured in a panel of two cell lines obtained from a patient with ovarian cancer prior to and postchemotherapy; a decreased 5FU incorporation into DNA caused by an enhanced removal from the DNA was observed in the postchemotherapy cell line that was also less sensitive to 5FU *(107)*. In mammalian cells, evidence has now been presented both supporting *(108–110)* and contradicting this theory *(111,112)*. In several studies it was also observed that the effect of 5FU on DNA damage was different from that induced by FUDR *(106,113)*. E.g., in the human colon-cancer cell line HCT-8, FUDR induced single- and double-strand breaks, whereas 5FU hardly induced DNA damage at similarly cytotoxic concentrations. Cytotoxicity by FUDR was related to this TS-inhibition-induced DNA damage since this could be reversed by thymidine *(113)*.

The prevention and repair of DNA damage induced by TS-inhibitors is mediated by two specific enzymes, dUTPase and uracil-DNA glycosylase, respectively. The first enzyme will not only degrade dUTP but also FdUTP and thus prevent their incorporation into DNA. In case either dUTP or FdUTP would still be incorporated, uracil-DNA-glycosylase is able to excise both nucleotides. The role of dUTPase in cell growth and drug cytotoxicity was studied in several model systems. Human dUTPase is highly conserved and the expression is cell-cycle dependent *(114)*. Canman et al. *(115)* used two colon-cancer cell lines that had high levels (SW620) or low levels (HT29) of dUTPase. Accumulation of dUTP after FUDR exposure was higher in SW620 cells compared to HT29 cells, which may be associated with the delayed induction of double-strand breaks in SW620 cells. Prevention of TS-inhibition-induced DNA damage can be achieved by transfecting mammalian cells with the dUTPase gene. These cells appeared to be less sensitive to CB3717 and MTX *(116)*. HT29 cells transfected with *E. coli* dUTPase had a four- to fivefold higher dUTPase level compared to the low level in the parental cells, and showed a decreased extent of DNA single-strand breaks after FUDR exposure and a lower sensitivity to the drug. The increase of dUTP incorporation into DNA can result in the formation of many small DNA fragments leading to DNA degradation resulting in apoptotic cell death. In addition, uracil-substituted DNA can interfere with protein–DNA interactions since the methyl group of thymine projects into the major groove of DNA.

Uracil DNA glycosylase can excise both the misincorporated uracil and 5FU base, which are both increased after TS inhibition. Excision of either fraudulent base results in an apyrimidinic site that is also seen in other types of DNA damage such as ionizing radiation *(114)*. A combination of these effects may contribute to the cytotoxic effect of fluoropyrimidines.

Ample evidence is now available that inhibition of TS by nucleotide analogs such as FdUMP or antifolates such as ZD1694, AG337, BW1843U89, and LY231514, will cause DNA damage *(103–106,111,112,117–121)*, which is possibly the molecular basis for growth inhibition, growth arrest, and cell death. The dose- and time-related increase in strand breaks, in both nascent and mature DNA, suggest a strong role for uracil misincorporation and excision as a mechanism of thymineless death. Also for the combination of 5FU and interferon-α (IFN-α), it has been demonstrated that increased DNA strand break formation is possibly responsible for the enhanced cytotoxic effect of the combination observed in vitro *(122)*. E.g., 5FU induced 40–25% double-strand breaks which was increased by the addition of IFN-α; interferon-γ (IFN-γ) has a different interaction with 5FU since no additional effect on DNA was observed *(123)*. The effect of IFN-α appeared to be (at least partly) independent of TS inhibition since it was only observed when 5FU was given in combination with IFN-α, but not when interferon-α was combined with a folate-based TS inhibitor *(122)*. Combination of 5FU with LV and IFN-α may further enhance the cytotoxic effect of 5FU and LV *(124,125)*. This has also been demonstrated in an animal model *(126)*. However, recent clinical results of the combination of 5FU with LV and IFN-α or of 5FU with IFN-γ in patients with colorectal cancer are variable and generally disappointing *(9,127–130)*.

Other studies that focused on the role of thymidine depletion in cellular cytotoxicity, used cell lines that were deficient in TS. Thus Ayusawa et al. *(112)* deprived TS-negative mutant FM3A cells of thymidine and observed formation of single- and double-strand breaks, the latter at specific sites in contrast to ionizing radiation, which causes double-strand breaks randomly. The process continued even after addition of thymidine to the medium. Exposure of FM3A cells to FUDR not only resulted in depletion of dTTP but also of dGTP pools, but increased the dATP pools. The imbalance in dNTP pools was accompanied by apoptotic cell death *(131)*. Also Houghton et al. *(132)* observed in human colon cancer cells GC3/cl and their TS mutant that thymidine deprivation will result in dTTP depletion and increase in dATP, which were associated with DNA damage and cytotoxicity. A subpopulation, Thy4, was isolated from the GC3/cl-TS$^-$ mutant by thymidine deprivation; Thy4 cells were resistant to commitment to thymineless death. Thymidine depletion showed a G1-arrest probably caused by an essential checkpoint at the G1-S boundary deciding whether dTTP depletion leads to cytotoxicity or cytostatic cell-cycle arrest *(133)*. Also in in vivo studies, depletion of dTTP could be achieved without the use of drugs by feeding rats a folate-deficient diet *(134)*, which led to an increased dUTP/dTTP ratio, uracil misincorporation, DNA repair-related DNA damage, and apoptosis. It can be concluded from each study that an imbalance of the dATP and dTTP pools (increased dATP/dTTP) is an early event leading to thymineless death *(131)*. An imbalance in deoxyribonucleotides seems to be a normal phenomenon after treatment with fluoropyrimidines *(135)*, and was observed in a variety of cell lines with different TS levels; the imbalance in dNTP is probably related to cell death. The exact

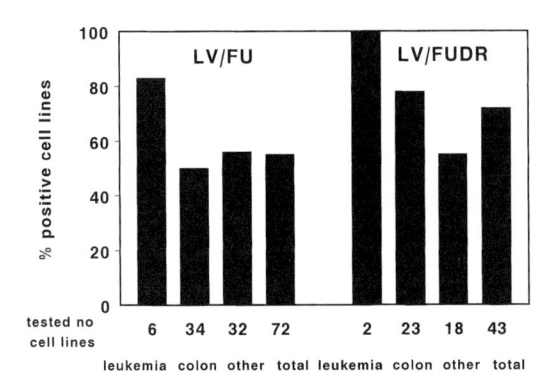

Fig. 7. Summary of published modulation studies of 5FU and FUDR by LV (data are from refs. *11,14,45*). The total number of cell lines for each tumor type (the absolute number of cell lines depicted at the bottom of the bar) was set at 100%. The bars give the number of cell lines responding to 5FU modulation by LV using a threshold potentiation factor of at least 1.5 (figure modified from ref. *45*).

nature of this interaction is still under investigation, but it is clear that several essential cell-cycle checkpoints may be affected in this process leading to apoptosis.

4. (ANTI)FOLATE-RELATED COMBINATIONS

4.1. Leucovorin Dose Scheduling

4.1.1. PRECLINICAL STUDIES

Since the initial studies by Ullman et al. *(136)*, many preclinical studies have been performed on the combination of fluoropyrimidines and LV (reviewed in refs. *6,8,10,11,13,14,45*). Following the many initially positive reports, more and more negative data have been published indicating that not all cell lines can be modulated by LV. This is in better agreement with the clinical studies that still show that more than half of patients do not respond on a schedule of 5FU in combination with LV. For the sake of clarity, only some representative data for 5FU and FUDR are presented with and without LV in a variety of colorectal cancer and some other cell lines (Fig. 7) *(11,14,45)*. FUDR was more cytotoxic than 5FU in all but three cell lines. The dose-effect curves for each drug were usually sigmoidal. Prolonged exposure of human cell lines to 5FU or FUDR greatly enhanced growth inhibition *(14,27,125,137–139)*. In general, prolonged exposure of cells also led to increased enhancement of its cytotoxicity by LV 1–10 μM *(8,14,140–142)*. Lower concentrations of LV are generally not sufficient to potentiate the effects of 5FU or FUDR, whereas higher concentrations generally do not enhance the effect *(11,45)*. The modulation of FUDR by LV was more pronounced with median factors of modulation at their IC_{50}s of 1.5 for 5FU and 2.0 for FUDR. In most (88%) of these cell lines, FUDR showed greater potentiation by LV than 5FU. Furthermore, the cytotoxicity of FUDR was enhanced by LV (potentiation factor >1.5) in relatively more cell lines, compared to 5FU by LV. Although less pronounced, the same phenomenon was observed in a panel of gastric-cancer cell lines *(141),* but in nonsmall-cell lung cancer cells neither fluoropyrimidine was modulated by LV, whereas these cell lines were resistant to fluoropyrimidines compared to colon-cancer cell lines *(141,142).* These differences between 5FU and FUDR underline the hypothesis that in cell lines 5FU can have different mechanisms (RNA and DNA incorporation or TS inhibition), which may not all be affected by LV. TS inhibition after FUDR seems to be a more general mechanism. LV seems to enhance the formation and stability of a ternary complex when FUDR is given for a short period, but this may not be the case when the duration of FUDR exposure is prolonged *(143).* Under these circumstances, the inhibition caused by the binary complex between FdUMP and TS apparently remains relatively stable with no beneficial effect of LV. For 5FU, addition of LV may also cause a shift in its mechanism of action from RNA incorporation to TS inhibition, resulting in enhanced growth inhibition in several cell lines. Evidence for this hypothesis is based on the finding that LV enhances TS inhibition, but does not affect 5FU incorporation into cellular RNA significantly in cell lines or tumor samples from mice *(68)* and patients *(69).* Thus cytotoxicity of 5FU can be optimized in a number of cell lines and tumors through LV modulation by maintenance of TS inhibition.

In vivo studies on 5FU modulation by LV are scarce and are usually limited to the description of the antitumor effect *(11)* but do not include mechanistic studies. Studies with single-agent 5FU showed a clear tumor-dependent TS inhibition *(144,145).* Ex vivo incubation of tumors with CH_2THF also indicated a difference in the extent and duration of TS inhibition in favor for incubations with the folate *(74).* We observed that the sensitive tumor Colon 38 had a lower TS activity than the 5FU-resistant tumor Colon 26-A *(85).* The potentiation of the antitumor activity of 5FU by LV given before 5FU in murine Colon 26-A and Colon 38 *(85)* was associated with a more pronounced inhibition of TS by LV plus 5FU than for 5FU alone, which only occurred after 3 wk of weekly administrations (Fig. 5) *(85)*: More importantly LV prevented the 5FU-induced increase in TS, which was seen in mice treated with 5FU alone. The importance of the time of TS measurements was revealed by studies of Iigo et al. *(146)* which also showed that 1-d measurements in the Colon 38 tumor model, were too incomplete to correlate the antitumor activity of fluoropyrimidines and LV modulation with the extent of TS inhibition. Thus, in vivo modulation of 5FU with LV seems to be related with prolonged TS inhibition and prevention of TS induction.

4.1.2. CLINICAL STUDIES

Two LV-containing bolus 5FU schedules are considered equivalent in respect to tumor response and patient survival and are frequently used as reference treatments (Tables 3,4) *(147).* Both schedules differ in their pattern of toxicity (Table 3): The monthly day 1–5 schedule (LV 20 mg/m^2 plus bolus 5FU 425 mg/m^2) (Mayo regimen) is associated with severe or sometimes even life-threatening mucositis and/or diarrhea in approx 20–25% of patients. The weekly schedule (LV 500 mg/m^2 2-h infusion plus bolus 5FU 500 mg/m^2 given in the middle of the LV infusion; the RPCI regimen) is associated with a lesser rate of severe mucositis, but with higher grades of diarrhea in approx 20–30% of patients. Some oncologists prefer the weekly schedule, because it is less toxic than the Mayo regimen and decisions to withhold or continue treatment can (and must) be made on a weekly basis according to toxicity *(153).* The Mayo regimen has been advocated

Table 3
Toxicity of Reference Regimens and High-Dose Infusional $5FU_{24h}/LV$ Given to Patients with Advanced Colorectal Cancer

Grade 3/4	Mayo (148) (n = 712)	RPC (148) (n = 581)	FU_{24h}/LV (149) (n = 90)
Nausea/vomiting	3%	4%	5%
Mucositis	18%	1%	2%
Diarrhea	19%	29%	21%
Leukopenia	10%	3%	1%
Hand-foot-syndrome[a]	0%	0%	61%

[a]Grade 1–4, Grade 3+4 8%.
Mayo: 5FU 425 mg/m² plus LV 20 mg/m² d 1–5, qw 4–5.
RPCI: 5FU 500 mg/m² plus LV 500 mg/m² weekly × 6, 2 wk rest.
Modified from Köhne (63).

Table 4
Results of Meta-Analysis in Colorectal Cancer on Combinations of 5FU with Methotrexate and Leucovorin

	n Trials	n Pat	Response (CR/PR)	p-value	Median Survival (mo)	p-value	Reference
5FU			11%		11.0		(150)
5FU/LV	9	1381	23%	<0.001	11.5	0.57	
5FU			10%		9.1		(151)
5FU/MTX	8	1178	19%	<0.001	10.7	0.024	
5FU Bolus			14%		11.3		(152)
5FU CI	6	1219	22%	<0,001	12.1	0.04	

CI, continuous infusion.
Modified from Köhne (63).

because of the lower costs because of the lower dose of LV (5). However, considering the overall costs of treatment, the potential hospital admission, and more importantly, the decrease in price of LV, this is not a major consideration anymore.

The dose of LV necessary for effective biochemical modulation continues to be under discussion. Preclinical studies indicated that concentrations of LV below 1 μM are generally not sufficient to expand intracellular folate pools, but concentrations between 1 and 10 μM seem to be essential. A 2-h infusion of 500 mg/m² LV can provide plasma concentrations in patients of above 10 μM (154), which was the background for its use in clinical protocols. However also with an iv bolus injection of 50 mg LV, plasma levels of bioactive reduced folates remain above 1 μM for 1 h, supporting the use of lower concentrations (155). Clinical trials still show contradictory results (156–158). However, in the monthly schedule in which LV is combined daily (d 1–5) with 5FU, the low dose seems sufficient to maintain folate pools in the tumor for 1 d to inhibit TS. Peters et al. *(69,159)* compared two doses of LV (500 and 25 mg/m^2) on 5FU-induced TS inhibition and clearly observed that the low dose was insufficient to maintain TS inhibition over 48 h in comparison to the high dose of LV. It is however possible that the low dose is sufficient to maintain TS inhibition for a shorter period. Reduced folate pools were not increased in the tumor after 48 h at the 25 mg/m^2 dose, but were higher with the 500 mg/m^2 dose *(69)*. The pure L-isomer L-LV did not show any advantage over DL-LV both in terms of increasing TS inhibition in tumors or being more selective in normal tissues. TS inhibition studies in normal human mucosa and liver indicated a similar extent of inhibition for the two doses of LV with 5FU or for 5FU alone *(87),* indicating that in these normal tissues reduced folate levels do not seem limiting for TS inhibition. Actually in liver tissue the total TS levels increased following 5FU treatment (either rat or human) with or without any LV schedule. These data, in combination with TS measurements in tumors, indicate that despite higher TS levels in tumor tissue, the extent and more importantly, the retention of TS inhibition is more than in normal tissues. Thus 5FU treatment seems to be selective for tumor tissue, which indicates that normal tissues have a different type of TS regulation. Thus the dose and schedule of LV seem to be more important to modulate TS inhibition in tumors, although a contribution of TS inhibition in normal (probably affected by LV) tissues can not be excluded.

Because of the short half life of 5FU *(29,66,160–162)* it is important whether "bolus" 5FU is really given as a bolus injection (in less than 5 min) as in North America or in 10–20-min or even 1–2-h infusion as frequently practiced in Europe. In a study including 203 patients with advanced colorectal cancer *(163),* a significantly higher response rate was observed for those receiving a bolus (10 min) injection (27 vs 13%, $p = 0.02$). There was also a trend for prolonged progression-free survival. This was probably related to the lower AUC for the "short" infusion compared to the "real" bolus *(164).* In case of a 2-h infusion the 5FU dose can be increased twofold compared to the bolus administration of 5FU to achieve equivalent toxicity and efficacy *(165).*

5FU has a short plasma half-life of approx 8–14 min *(29,66,160–162).* The drug is cytotoxic mainly to cells in the S-phase. Therefore, it was hypothesized that with bolus administration of 5FU, only a small proportion of cells are susceptible as compared with administration by continuous infusion (CI) of 5FU. In vitro continuous exposure is more cytotoxic than short 1-h exposure *(11,27,138,139).* Therefore, 5FU has been administered as prolonged infusions. Studies comparing CI with bolus 5FU demonstrated a high response rate with lower gastrointestinal and hematological toxicity for CI 5FU, but failed to achieve an increase in survival *(16).* Using data of six randomized trials, these were confirmed by a meta-analysis *(152)* in which an overall response rate doubling from 14 to 22% was found, but the effect on survival was small with 11.3 mo compared to a median of 12.1 mo ($p = 0.04$) for patients receiving CI (Table 4). This was very much in line with data on a preclinical mouse model, in which CI gave a good immediate antitumor effect in the first 10 d, but overall survival and tumor volume at the end of the observation period of the mice was similar *(40).* Interestingly the enhanced growth of the tumor was accompanied by a severalfold increase in TS activity (Fig. 5). A similar event in patients might be an explanation for the clinical results. It is also possible that a real bolus is a mixture between bolus and CI, since 5FU levels in tumors are much higher than in plasma *(29,66),* indicating a trapping in the tumor and thus a prolonged effect. The 5FU half-life in tumors (2–100 h) is variable, but is always much longer than in plasma *(29,66,162).* This is comparable to the half-life of 5FU-elimination out of

FU-RNA and that of total ^{18}F-FU elimination from tumors *(166)*. Thus there seems to be a depot for 5FU in tumors, enabling prolonged TS inhibition *(66)*. These data are in contrast with a general assumption based on several in vitro and in vivo studies that a bolus 5FU mainly acts by RNA incorporation, whereas infusional 5FU predominantly interferes with DNA via TS *(167,168)*. Enhanced trapping of 5FU in the tumor fits with the hypothesis that dose intensity may be important in increasing the activity of 5FU *(169)*, which can be achieved with a weekly or biweekly 24–48 h CI of 5FU. The maximum tolerated dose of weekly 24-h infusion was 2.6 g/m^2 *(170–172)*, 3.5 g/m^2 in case of weekly 48-h CI *(173)*. The superiority of various infusional 5FU schedules over bolus 5FU in terms of response rates and the effect of modulator form the basis of biochemical modulation studies of infusional 5FU (Table 4).

The 5FU continuous infusion of 300 mg/m^{2}d given for 28 d as described by Lokich et al. *(16)* is a frequently used CI regimen. Addition of LV po in a dose of 20 mg bid did not improve response rates (26 vs 29%) or survival relative to CI alone or compared to modulated bolus regimens *(174)*. This was also in agreement with preclinical data with mice that showed that none of the LV schedules (daily, weekly, infusions) enhanced the antitumor effect of CI 5FU *(40)*. Since the initial 24-h infusions were developed in combination with PALA *(171)* in two large randomized trials, PALA was used in combination with the weekly administration of 5FU 2.6 g/m^2 as 24-h infusion *(174,175)*; no improvement over the administration of high-dose 5FU alone or modulated bolus regimens was observed (response rate 21 vs 27%). The combination of 3.5 g/m^2 5FU given as a weekly 48-h CI *(176)*, 60 mg LV po every 6 h resulted in increased gastrointestinal toxicity, mainly mucositis and diarrhea *(177)* (Table 5) and the 5FU dose had to be reduced to 2 g/m^2, but did not improve the objective response rate *(178)*. High-dose 5FU alone was compared with the Mayo regimen in a randomized trial; a significantly higher response rate was observed for infusional 5FU (19 vs 30%, $p < 0.05$) *(179)*. However, up to now no improvement in the median time to progression or survival was observed. Thus oral application of LV is not sufficient to modulate 5FU effectively, similar to the 5FU bolus administration *(180)*.

In a French multicenter trial the Mayo regimen was compared with a complex bolus and CI hybrid schedule modulated by 200 mg/m^2 LV given as a 2-h infusion *(181)*. A significantly higher response was found for the rate of modulated-infusional 5FU over the Mayo regimen (33 vs 14%, $p < 0.01$) together with a longer time to progression and a longer median survival. The infusional regimen was less toxic. Because of a crossover to bolus 5FU treatment to infusional 5FU after failure to bolus 5FU, an improvement of survival may be difficult to demonstrate. It can be concluded that high-dose infusional 5FU is an effective regimen. It is however not clear from these clinical studies whether this is related to an enhanced TS inhibition compared to normal bolus 5FU.

4.2. Combinations with Interferons and Leucovorin
4.2.1. PRECLINICAL AND CLINICAL

A number of publications now report disappointing results regarding the ability of IFNs to modulate 5FU relative to 5FU alone or to 5FU/LV *(129,130,183–185)*. Only one study demonstrated increased response and time to progression, but not survival *(186)*, IFN-α did not increase the response rate, time to progression, or survival in six other studies when combined with 5FU and compared with different 5FU ± LV schedules *(63)*.

In a randomized study a weekly 24-h infusion of 5FU 2.6 g/m^2 was modulated either by Interferon (IFN-α) sc or by 500 mg/m^2 LV given as a 2-h infusion prior to 5FU or a combination of both modulators in 230 patients *(182)*. The LV-modulated arms were significantly more active in respect to response rates (38 vs 18%, $p < 0.05$), time to progression (7.1 vs 3.9 mo, $p = 0.005$) or patient survival (16.6 vs 12.7 mo, $p = 0.01$). The toxicity associated with this high-dose infusional 5FU$_{24h}$/LV schedule was similar to the weekly bolus FU/LV regimen designed by the RPCI, but less toxic than the Mayo regimen (Table 3), albeit a fivefold higher 5FU dose was delivered. This infusional schedule was not directly compared to modulated weekly or monthly bolus 5FU/LV, but these data favor LV-modulated 5FU$_{24h}$.

These reports contradict the early preclinical findings of increased 5FU cytotoxicity that provided a rationale for the clinical use of IFN-α *(11,187)*. Van der Wilt et al. *(123)* however recently reported that modulation of 5FU with either IFN-α or IFN-γ may be dependent on the folate status of the cells, with a higher extent of modulation when cells were put on low folate. Despite the lack of 5FU modulation by IFN-α or IFN-γ, IFN-α increased DNA damage caused by 5FU, similar to other studies *(122,187)*; in addition FdUMP levels, which were shown to increase in one cell line *(188)*, could not be modulated in five other colon-cancer cell lines with either IFN-α or IFN-γ *(123)*. On the other hand, these and other preclinical investigations or clinical trials did not indicate the opposite, that IFNs decrease the antineoplastic activity of 5FU (reviewed in ref. *11*). Since 5FU$_{24h}$/LV was superior to 5FU$_{24h}$/IFN-α in the above-mentioned study *(182)*, one is tempted to speculate that 5FU$_{24h}$/LV will also be superior to 5FU alone or to bolus 5FU regimens. Based on preclinical studies with high-dose 5FU *(67,68)*, one might speculate that high-dose infusional 5FU caused both a pronounced TS inhibition and that a substantial amount of 5FU is incorporated into RNA. Addition of LV *(68)* to this schedule can increase the intratumoral reduced folate pools required for a prolonged retention of TS inhibition. In a randomized clinical study by the EORTC Gastrointestinal Tract Cooperative Cancer Group (GITCCG) various schedules of infusional 5FU (+/− LV) are now compared with bolus 5FU: Patients with metastatic colorectal cancer are to receive weekly infusional 5FU$_{24h}$ alone (2600 mg/m^2), or plus LV 500 mg/m^2 (2-h infusion), or to receive the Mayo regimen (5FU 425 mg/m^2 plus LV 20 mg/m^2 given for 5 d and repeated every 4–5 wk). This trial will help to define the role of high-dose infusional 5FU, its modulation by LV, and its activity relative to bolus 5FU in the treatment of patients with advanced colorectal cancer.

4.3. Combinations with Antifolate DHFR Inhibitors

The concept of biochemical modulation is an excellent example of how translational research can be used in the right but also in the wrong way. Based on the preclinical studies, many combinations with 5FU were performed; several well-conducted studies indeed proved that the response rate of 5FU could be doubled when the correct schedule of LV was used (reviewed in refs. *5,6,8,9,11,63,151,159,168*) (Table 4). Also for MTX modulation many studies were performed; several of these were completely negative, which was actually in line with preclinical studies when a proper translation had been used *(6,64)*. In case of MTX, the time interval between both drugs is critical and MTX should be given 24 h prior 5FU *(189)*. Preclinical data also show that the presence of LV in the LV-5FU schedule can completely abrogate the modulating effect of MTX on 5FU

Table 5
Modulation of Infusional 5FU in Colorectal Cancer with LV or IFN-α

Schedule	Phase	n Pat	CR/PR	p-value	Median Survival (mo)	p-value	Reference
5FU$_{48h}$ 2000–3000 mg/m^2 weekly + LV 4 × 60 mg po	II	153	35%		15;14.5		(177,178)
5FU$_{48h}$ 3500 mg/m^2 weekly vs 5FU 425 mg/m^2 d 1–5 + LV 20 mg/m^2 d 1–5, qw 4	II,III III	244 151	33% 19%	<0.05	12 10.8	n.s.	(179)
5FU 425 mg/m^2 d 1–5 + LV 20 mg/m^2 d 1–5, qw 4 vs 5FU 400 mg/m^2 bolus 5FU 600 mg/m^2 22 h + LV 200 mg/m^2 2 h, d 1 + 2, qw 2	III	218 219	14% 33%	0.0004	14.3 15.5	0.067	(181)
5FU$_{24h}$ 2600 mg/m^2 + LV 500 mg/m^2 2 h, weekly × 6 vs 5FU$_{24h}$ 2600 mg/m^2 + IFN 3 MU sc 3×/wk, weekly × 6 vs 5FU$_{24h}$ 2600 mg/m^2 + LV + IFN, weekly × 6	III	91 90 49	44% 18% 27%	<0.05	16.2 12.7 19.6	<0.04	(182)

Modified from Köhne (63).

with an overall result of no modulation *(190,191)*. Thus LV can compete with the uptake of MTX and thus prevent any modulation by MTX. The overall net result would be at its best a modulation by LV. When high-dose, 48-h infusional 5FU (5FU 60 mg/kg, approx 2.6 g/m^2) was combined with low-dose MTX 40 mg/m^2 *(192)* and compared with infusional 5FU alone, a significantly higher response rate was observed for the combination treatment (11 vs 23%, $p = 0.025$). This indicated effective biochemical modulation of infusional 5FU through low doses of MTX without LV. However, the increase in median survival (9.3 vs 12.5 mo) was not statistically significant ($p = 0.123$) (Table 6).

A 5FU bolus regimen can be modulated more effectively by MTX, than CI *(64,168)*. Therefore a randomized trial was designed in which 5FU$_{CI}$ with LV was alternated with MTX/5FU$_{bolus}$ and compared with MTX/5FU$_{bolus}$ alone. Response rates were 34 and 12%, respectively, with an improved time to progression of 4.1 vs 6.2 mo *(193)* for the infusional arm. It is, however, possible that the 5FU-MTX arm was not optimal since it was given every 2 wk, the response in the combined arm might predominantly be related to the infusional 5FU with LV. Thus, the trial does unfortunately not proof that a schedule-specific modulation is superior over a nonschedule-specific modulation, but supports the value of infusional 5FU. Because of these variable results, the clinical interest in MTX modulation of 5FU has declined.

Trimetrexate (TMQ) is a lipophilic DHFR inhibitor *(194)*. Unlike other classic antifolates like MTX, TMQ does not use the reduced-folate transport system *(76,195,196)*, can not be polyglutamated *(196,197)*, and does not compete with LV for cellular uptake and metabolism *(76,191,196)*. Both in in vitro and in vivo model systems, the sequential use of TMQ followed by 5FU resulted in a synergistic cell kill similar to MTX and 5FU *(198,199)*. Romanini et al. *(191)* showed that LV can enhance the cytotoxicity of TMQ and 5FU metabolism intracellularly (increased 5FU activation), whereas LV can enhance TS inhibition. These results formed the basis for clinical studies on the combination of TMQ with 5FU and LV. This combination had activity in previously pretreated patients with a response rate of approx 20% *(200)*. In previously untreated patients, TMQ was combined with LV on day 1 and followed by bolus 5FU on day 2 and by 50 mg LV po *(201,202)*. In two phase II studies with 61 evaluable patients, 3 patients achieved a complete remission and 16 had a partial remission. This schedule is now being evaluated in a phase III trial. The studies are an elegant example how a proper combination can be based on preclinical studies, combining increased 5FU activation to enhance TS inhibition.

4.4. Combinations with Antifolate TS Inhibitors

Since FdUMP and the new antifolates bind at different sites of the enzyme, combination studies of 5FU with new antifolate TS inhibitors were initiated. At the molecular level Van der Wilt et al. *(203,204)* demonstrated that ZD1694, LY231514, AG337, and GW1843 could support binding of FdUMP to TS, although to a different extent. The extent of binding was dependent on the presence of a glutamate moiety; ZD1694-Glu4 and LY231514-Glu4 supported binding of FdUMP to TS at a level similar as CH$_2$THF; there was, however, a major difference: All antifolates showed a nonlinear binding with a plateau at 1 μM in contrast to the natural substrate; for GW1843-Glu4 this plateau was observed at lower concentrations. Data using double labeling (^{14}C-AG337 and ^{3}H-FdUMP) indicated that the antifolates possibly induce a structural modification of the

Table 6
Modulation of 5FU in Colorectal Cancer with MTX and TMQ

Schedule	Phase	n Pat	CR/PR	p-value	Median Survival (mo)	p-value	Reference
5FU$_{48h}$ 60 mg/kg weekly	III	156	11%	0.025	9.3	0.123	(192)
vs 5FU$_{48h}$ 60 mg/kg weekly + MTX 40 mg/m^2		154	23%		12.5		
5FU 600 mg/m^2 bolus MTX 200 mg/m^2, qw2	III	183	14%	<0.05	n.a.		(193)
vs 5FU 600 mg/m^2 bolus MTX 200 mg/m^2, qw 2 plus 5FU CI 200 mg/m^2/d 3 wk LV 10 mg/m^2 iv weekly			41%		n.a.		
TMQ 110 mg/m^2 plus LV 200 mg/m^2, d 1; plus 5FU 500 mg/m^2 and 50 mg LV po q 6 h × 7 d 2	II	61	48%				(201,202)

enzyme preventing binding of FdUMP *(205)*. The aberrant effect of GW1843 is possibly related to the fact that it binds to different amino acids in the enzyme in contrast to the other antifolates *(206)*. The concentration-dependent binding of antifolates and FdUMP to TS is possibly a major factor that should be taken in consideration when 5FU is combined with any of these antifolates. Indeed in vitro cytotoxicity experiments revealed a concentration dependence; in case 5FU concentrations were kept constant and the antifolate variable, a synergistic effect was observed at low antifolate concentrations, but only additivity was observed at higher concentrations *(121)*. This effect was also observed for the extent of *in situ* TS inhibition; the extent of *in situ* TS inhibition (5FU alone 15%, AG337, LY231514, ZD1694 10–15% inhibition; GW1843 no inhibition) was slightly higher for the combinations (all combinations of 5FU with antifolates 30–35% inhibition) in WiDr cells, but mostly additive in other cell lines. Similarly the induction of DNA damage was synergistic/additive (5FU, AG337, ZD1694 alone 25–30%; LY231514 and GW1843 alone 10–15%; combinations of antifolate with 5FU 40–60% DNA damage; additive to synergistic for LY231514, ZD1694 and GW1843). In HCT-8 human colon-cancer cells, exposure of ZD1694 for 24 h was followed by 4 h 5FU exposure and resulted in a decreased thymidine-kinase activity and mRNA level, and a high amount of incorporated 5FU into RNA compared to ZD1694 exposure alone *(207,208)*. It was postulated that this was related to the ZD1694-induced increase in dUMP leading to an increase in the incorporation of 5FU into RNA. These mechanistic aspects need further investigation. In renal-cancer cells Guimares et al. *(209)* also observed additive to slightly synergistic effects of the combination of ZD1694 and FUDR after exposure for 96 h. In initial studies with patients with colorectal cancer treated with 5FU and CB3717, no additivity was observed *(210)*. Recently, clinical phase I studies have been initiated in which a 15-min infusion of ZD1694 was followed after 24 h by a 5FU bolus injection; this scheme was tolerable and also effective in patients with prior 5FU therapy *(211)*. Together these findings should stimulate the continuation of clinical studies since additivity of the effect of two drugs would mean an improvement in the treatment of most tumors.

5. OTHER COMBINATIONS

5.1. Combinations with Natural Nucleosides

Numerous combinations of other drugs and natural agents with 5FU have been tested. Many combinations in cancer chemotherapy are based on the lack of overlapping toxicity and/or an antitumor activity of each compound in a certain disease. For 5FU many combinations have a mechanistic basis and the other compound is often used to modulate specifically one of the mechanisms of action of 5FU *(6)*. Many combinations are intended to modulate specifically one of the mechanisms of action of 5FU, such as the earlier-mentioned potentiation of TS inhibition by LV, or an increase of 5FU incorporation into RNA by channelling 5FU into RNA. Since it has been hypothesized that TS inhibition is responsible for the antitumor activity and 5FU incorporation for the toxic side effects, this offers the possibility for specific modulation of the therapeutic efficacy. Here some combinations will be summarized that were developed with this aim.

In the beginning of the 1980s it was proposed that the antitumor activity of 5FU could be increased by enhancing its incorporation into RNA *(64,212)*. For this purpose, 5FU was combined with uridine, which enabled an increase in the 5FU dose leading to an improved therapeutic efficacy *(64,70,167,213)*. Uridine did not affect the 5FU-induced inhibition of TS in cell culture *(70)* and murine tumors *(214)*. The effect of the 5FU-uridine combination could be increased even more by combination with LV *(213)*. Further studies explored the possibility of using a precursor of uridine to modulate 5FU toxicity. In mice uridine-diphosphoglucose (UDPG) can increase the concentration of UTP in liver and in intestine, but not in tumors *(215)*. The therapeutic index of 5FU could be improved by rescue with UDPG; the dose of 5FU could be increased from 100 to 150 mg/kg in mice, and this produced a better antitumor activity in several tumors *(67)*. Mechanistic studies in murine tumors using UDPG demonstrated that the higher dose of 5FU did not increase the extent of TS inhibition but prolonged the retention of TS inhibition *(68)*; thus in mice treated with standard dose 5FU, TS inhibition was retained until 7 d with a two- to threefold induction after 10 d, whereas in mice treated with the high dose of 5FU (+ UDPG) TS inhibition was retained until 10 d, the TS induction could be prevented by injection of the next dose of 5FU. Incorporation of 5FU into RNA was, however, decreased by UDPG although the antitumor effect was increased.

Clinical studies have shown that uridine can be used effectively in patients to reduce the 5FU-induced myelotoxicity. Pharmacokinetics of short-term infusions of uridine in patients resulted in plasma levels of uridine approx 2 mM *(216)*, but the rapid catabolism prevented an effective protection from 5FU toxic effects. In later studies, uridine has been administered continuously using a central venous catheter, but fever appeared to be the dose-limiting toxicity *(217,218)*; similar to animal studies. This side effect was effectively controlled using an intermittent infusion scheme consisting of alternating 3 h of infusion with a 3-h treatment-free period over a total of 72 h *(217)*. Using this schedule in combination with a weekly injection of 5FU, starting the uridine infusion 3 h after the injection of 5FU, an effective reduction of myelosuppression was obtained in patients *(219)*. Interestingly, the protective effect of uridine on myelosuppression was observed also during the following courses of 5FU, that were not combined with uridine infusion *(219)*. Also in other studies, the dose of 5FU could be increased even when 5FU was combined with different modulating agents such as PALA or methotrexate and doxorubicin (FAMTX regimen) *(220,221)*. There was a marked reduction in mucositis and myelosuppression. Also in animal-model systems, uridine administration could reduce gastrointestinal toxicity of 5FU *(67,222)*.

Intravenous infusions of uridine must be performed via a central venous catheter in order to avoid phlebitis at the site of administration. Therefore, more convenient ways of administering the drug have been explored. Preclinical data showed that with oral administration of uridine to mice it was possible to obtain plasma concentrations of approx 100 µM *(223)* that are sufficient to reduce 5FU toxicity *(224)*. Similar pharmacokinetic data have been obtained in humans *(225)*; when uridine was administered repeatedly the dose had to be lowered to 5 g/m^2 every 6 h because of the occurrence of diarrhea *(225)*. Using this schedule the myelosuppression of 5FU was reduced *(226)*. Initial studies have been performed with UDPG administration to patients; plasma uridine peak values were 40–60 µM, and a concentration of 20–25 µM was still present 8 h after the second dose (unpublished results). The studies could however not be continued. Another prodrug, PN401 (an acetylated prodrug of uridine) has also been tested (preclinically) to increase the uridine levels of 5FU. In mice, plasma concentrations of PN401 resulted in eightfold higher plasma concentrations than equimolar uridine administrations, whereas in patients 6 g PN401 gave plasma levels of approx 160 µM and 5FU doses could be escalated from 600 to 1000 mg/m² *(227)*, which is somewhat higher than with uridine *(215,225)*. Studies determining the effective dose of 5FU (with or without LV) with PN401 protection, are ongoing. It is expected that PN401 will protect both against myelosuppression and mucositis and that the use of higher 5FU doses will enable to prolong TS inhibition and thus enhance the antitumor effect of 5FU-LV bolus regimens.

Further evidence for a role of uridine in modulation of 5FU and for a difference with the specific TS inhibitor ZD1694 was obtained from studies using wild-type p53 and p53 knock-out mice. In these mice, cell death was measured as the apoptotic index in crypts of the intestine BDF-1 mice. 5FU administration induced cell death in p53 wild-type mice but not in knock-out mice, whereas p53 was also upregulated in wild-type mice. Uridine administration could prevent 5FU-induced apoptosis in p53 wild-type mice, indicating an RNA-dependent mechanism of toxicity in gut tissue. Thymidine prevented ZD1694-induced toxicity in wild-type and p53 knock-out mice *(228)*, indicating a TS-dependent mechanisms of cell death.

5.2. Platinum: An Antifolate?

Selective enhancement of the biochemical effects of fluoropyrimidines not only by LV but also by other agents might improve their therapeutic efficacy. Various strategies have been developed focusing on CDDP as modulators in several models. In Colon 26-B tumors, the antitumor effect of 5FU was enhanced by CDDP in a schedule-dependent manner, but the effect of FUDR was enhanced even more. Addition of PALA to the protocol even resulted in 100% remissions *(229,230)*. Apparently triple PALA/fluoropyrimidine/CDDP combinations might be more effective than only two of these agents. The mechanism of action of PALA in this model appears to be through reduction in pyrimidine ribo- and deoxynucleotide pools, permitting unopposed fluoropyrimidine nucleotide action and reducing repair of DNA-platin adducts. Johnston et al. *(231)* observed an increased extent of DNA damage in cells treated with the combination 5FU and CDDP compared to either drug alone. The therapeutic efficacy of 5FU could also be increased by combinations with the chemoprotector WR 2721 (ethiofos, amifostine), which reduced the platin-induced toxicity (nephrotoxicity for CDDP and myelotoxicity for carboplatin) *(232–234)*. CDDP, but not WR 2721, inhibited TS catalytic activity, whereas both compounds reduced FdUMP binding to TS, although the effect was not additive. However, the effect of CDDP and 5FU on FdUMP binding to TS was at least additive *(232)*. The effect of CDDP might be related to binding to a sulfhydryl group of TS. Reduction of TS by 5FU-CDDP treatment might offer another explanation for the synergism between fluoropyrimidines and platinum compounds *(232)*.

The mechanism of modulation by cisplatin may also be related to a block of methionine entry into tumor cells in vitro and an increase in both endogenous methionine synthesis and thymidylate synthesis activity. As a result, tumor cells may be more susceptible to injury by 5FU *(235)*. For that purpose it was postulated that continuous infusion of 5FU should be combined with low-dose daily CDDP *(236)*, permitting an interference with folate homeostasis. This indeed improved the effect in model systems *(237)*. However, in general, a lack of increased antitumor activity of chemotherapeutic regimens associating cisplatinum/5FU with or without folinic acid was observed in patients with colorectal cancer *(9)*, although some trials showed an increased response *(238)*. This is in contrast with for instance head and neck cancer, in which the combination of

5FU and CDDP is an established treatment regimen *(239)*, possibly because both drugs have single-agent activity. The contradicting results that have been found for the various combinations of 5FU and cisplatin, both preclinical (in vitro and in vivo) and clinical indicate that various mechanisms of interaction exist. Since a platinum analog in combination with 5FU may be advantageous, several new platinum derivatives were tested. Among these, oxaliplatin seems to be the best candidate to be included in a regimen for colon cancer. Oxaliplatin is a new third generation platinum complex not associated with renal toxicity and has only minimal hematological side effects. Oxaliplatin was synergistic with 5FU in preclinical studies and the combination entered clinical development *(240)*.

Oxaliplatin was first administered to patients with 5FU resistance *(241,242)* with response rates of 20–40% *(243)* for the oxaliplatin plus 5FU regimens. In first-line treatment in patients with metastatic colorectal cancer *(244,245)* (Table 7), oxaliplatin was administered every 3 wk in a single dose of 130 mg/m^2 iv over 2 h, with an objective response rate of 24% *(244)*, with disease stabilization and a median time to progression of 4 mo. In another study, 21% response rate for first-line oxaliplatin was observed. These studies indicated, that oxaliplatin is at least as effective as 5FU, but no randomized trials with 5FU regimens are available; and oxaliplatin is not indicated as first-line treatment outside clinical trials.

Levi et al. *(246)* extended their chronotherapy studies with 5FU and LV by inclusion of oxaliplatinum (Table 7). In phase II and phase III trials, very consistent objective responses of over 50% and a long median survival time exceeding 15 mo *(247–251)* were observed. This three-drug regimen showed a relatively low toxicity enabling shortened treatment intervals from 3 to 2 wk; in this schedule a response rate of over 60% was associated with a long median survival *(252,253)*. These data are very promising and stimulate the further application of oxaliplatinum. Preliminary phase III data comparing chronomodulated 5FU plus LV with or without the addition of oxaliplatin confirm the high activity of the three-drug combination but report a response rate of below 20% in patients not receiving oxaliplatin *(248)*. Additionally, the three-drug combination was associated with a high percentage of patients with severe diarrhea (grade 3/4 in 43%). Both groups had a median survival of 18 mo, but since patients not receiving oxaliplatin in first line crossed over to the three-drug regimen in second line, this could be the reason that no survival benefit could be demonstrated. These data certainly support the use of oxaliplatin in combination with 5FU and LV. It is not clear what the relative contribution of chronomodulation is, since the modulating effect might be caused by the sequential administration, which was not the case with flat infusions. No mechanistic studies accompanied these trials.

5.3. Topoisomerase Inhibitors

Topoisomerase inhibitors have been tested extensively in various tumors, following the discovery of their unique mechanism of action in the early 1980s *(254)*. The various topoisomerase inhibitors have a substantial activity in several tumors, such as irinotecan (CPT-11) for colon cancer; topotecan for ovarian, bladder cancer, and small-cell lung cancer; whereas 9-aminocamptothecin (9-AC) and GI147211 (GG-211) are in an earlier phase of development. Irinotecan is converted to SN-38, which appears to be the active compound and irinotecan thus serves as a prodrug for SN-38. The antineoplastic activ-

Table 7
Oxaliplatin-Containing Chemotherapy in Untreated Patients

Schedule	Phase	n Pat	CR/PR	Median Survival (mo)	Reference
Oxaliplatin 130 mg/m^2 2 h, qw 3	II	39	23%	n.a.	(244,245)
3 weekly					
LV 300 mg/m^2 cm d 1–5					
Oxaliplatin 25 mg/m^2 cm d 1–5					
5FU 700 mg/m^2 cm d 1–5	II, 3×III	284	55%^{a}	15, 19, 15.9, 19	(247,248,250,251)
• flat infusion	III, 2×III	140	30%^{a}	15^b, 16.9	(250,247)
• without oxaliplatin		100	16%	19	(248)
2 weekly					
LV 300 mg/m^2 cm d 1–4 oxaliplatin					
25 mg/m^2 cm d 1–4	II	103	67%	19, 21	(252,253)
5FU 700 mg/m^2 cm d 1–4					

^{a}Difference significant $p<0.05$, in three different phase III studies, compared to either flat infusion (two studies) or without oxaliplatin (one study).
^{b}In one study, significantly different from chronomodulated.
cm, chronomodulated.

ity of topoisomerase I inhibitors may or may not be S-phase restricted *(255,256)*. Several papers describe an interaction between 5FU and irinotecan in vitro and in vivo *(257–260)*. These studies indicate a clear sequence-dependent synergism between the two compounds in colon-cancer cells, irinotecan followed by 5FU was highly synergistic in the in vitro studies *(257,258,260)*, whereas simultaneous addition was additive; the reversed sequence resulted in contradicting results. Also in vivo studies with colon-cancer xenografts showed no effect/additivity at simultaneous administration *(259,260)*, but sequential administration resulted in a better antitumor effect than each compound alone. Guichard et al. *(261)* provided evidence that pretreatment with irinotecan prolonged TS inhibition, and since irinotecan induced a blockage of cells in the S-phase, the incorporation into DNA increased. 5FU given before irinotecan increased the uptake of irinotecan into HT29 cells, whereas the formation of DNA-topo I complexes was also increased. It can be concluded that there is substantial evidence that irinotecan and 5FU can be synergistic and that the effect may be TS related.

Several clinical studies investigated the combined use of irinotecan and 5FU regimens (Table 8). Alternating administration of irinotecan (once at 350 mg/m^2 or weekly at 125 mg/m$^{2)}$ with 5FU/LV resulted in a 27 or 32% *(262,263)* response rate, respectively (Table 8). Given the activity of irinotecan or 5FU/LV bolus schedules alone, the alternating schedules are probably not superior compared to the use of either regimen alone.

In several phase I studies, irinotecan was added to different 5FU schedules. A 5FU bolus of 375–500 mg/m^2 given over 5 d was combined with irinotecan, escalated from 200–350 mg/m^2; the recommended phase II doses are 300 mg/m^2 on day 0 plus 5FU 375 mg/m^2 given on day 1–5 *(264)*. A 7-d 5FU continuous infusion (400 mg/m^2) was combined with escalating doses of irinotecan on day 1, up to 200 mg/m^2 *(265)*, whereas a weekly bolus 5FU 500 mg/m^2 plus LV 20 mg/m^2 and irinotecan 100 mg/m^2 *(266)* was active in 5FU-resistant and pretreated patients. Activity was also found when irinotecan was combined on day 1 in a dose of 100–200 mg/m^2 with the schedule of bolus 5FU followed by a 22-h continuous infusion in combination with LV *(267)*, yet further dose escalation is continuing. Irinotecan (80–120 mg/m^2) was escalated in combination with LV 500 mg/m^2 and 5FU given as a 24-h continuous infusion in doses of 1800–2600 mg/m^2. Severe diarrhea was dose limiting and irinotecan 80 mg/m^2, LV 500 mg/m^2, and 5FU$_{24h}$ 2600 mg/m^2 was recommended for further use *(268)*. Although this study was intended as a phase I study in chemonaive patients, responses were observed at every dose level; with one CR and 14 PRs out of 24 patients, which resulted in a response rate of 63%. In a phase III trial, this regimen will be compared with weekly infusional high-dose 5FU plus LV alone.

It can be concluded that there is substantial preclinical evidence for a synergistic interaction of irinitecan and 5FU, which may be schedule dependent. In addition irinotecan can influence 5FU metabolism and enhance TS inhibition. The in vitro data are in agreement with in vivo data, whereas recent clinical studies provide evidence for enhanced clinical activity of the combination compared to each compound alone.

6. SUMMARY AND CONCLUSIONS

Despite its introduction into the clinic 40 yr ago, 5FU remains one of the most important anticancer agents for the treatment of gastrointestinal, breast, head and neck, and

Table 8
Irinotecan Combinations with 5FU in First-Line Treatment of Colorectal Cancer

Regimen	Phase	n Pat	CR/PR	Reference
CPT-11 alternating 5FU regimen				
CPT-11 350 mg/m^2 d 1				
LV 20 mg/m^2 d 22–26 + 5FU 425 mg/m^2 d 22–26	II	33	27%	(262)
CPT-11 125 mg/m^2 weekly × 4, 2 wk rest				
LV 20 mg/m^2 d 43–47 + 5FU 425 mg/m^2 d 43–47	II	71	32%	(263)
CPT-11 plus 5FU regimen				
CPT-11 100–200 mg/m^2 d 1				
LV 200 mg/m^2 d 1–2 + 5FU bolus 400 mg/m^2 d 1 + 2	I	30	5/20 (25%) (pretreated)	(267)
5FU$_{CI}$ 600 mg/m^2 22 h d 1 + 2, qw 2				
CPT-11 50–300 mg/m^2	I	34	5/33 (15%) (pretreated)	(265)
5FU CI 400 mg/m^2 d 1–7				
CPT-11 100 mg/m^2; LV 20 mg/m^2	I	38	6/38 (16%) (pretreated)	(266)
5FU 210–500 mg/m^2 weekly × 4, 2 wk rest				
CPT-11 80–120 mg/m^2; LV 500 mg/m^2	I	26	15/24 (62.5%) (untreated)	(268)
5FU$_{24h}$ 1800–2600 mg/m^2, weekly × 6				

Modified from Köhne (63).

also several other malignancies. However, the application and insights in the mechanisms of action of fluoropyrimidines have changed considerably. 5FU is now predominantly administered in combination with other drugs or it is given as a prodrug enabling either oral administration such as for Ft (with uracil in a ratio of 1 mol Ft and 4 moles uracil; or as S-1; a mixture of Ft, an inhibitor of DPD degradation and of 5FU activation in normal tissues), for capecitabine, or enabling local administration such as FUDR for hepatic artery infusion.

It is now clear that 5FU is metabolized differently in various tissues, enabling specific modulation of its activation; degradation predominantly takes place in liver and accounts for more than 80% of its elimination; inhibition of degradation enables an almost 100% bioavailability of the drug (administered as 5FU or as prodrug), selective activation by OPRT in tumor tissues also enables specific activation in the target tissue. There is substantial evidence that 5FU acts through inhibition of TS by its metabolite FdUMP, and the level of enzyme and the extent of inhibition predict for response to 5FU. In various model systems, 5FU induces an induction of TS levels, possibly accounting for acquired or (transient) resistance to 5FU. In model systems, it has been demonstrated that the induction can be prevented either by administration of LV, or by giving repeated high doses of the drug. A selectivity is possibly achieved through a selective higher induction in normal tissues, especially in liver. The latter phenomenon is possibly related to the relatively low extent of side effects of hepatic artery infusion, enabling administration of relatively high doses of 5FU or FUDR, resulting in good therapeutic efficacy of 5FU and FUDR when administered locally.

Modulation of the antitumor activity of 5FU can be achieved in various ways. The most widely used modulator, LV, has a schedule- and dose-dependent effect, which is also dependent on the method of administration of 5FU. Two bolus schedules show similar activity, the weekly 5FU schedule with high-dose LV, and the monthly 5FU schedule (daily times 5 with low-dose LV), but the current most active schedule seems to be a 24-h infusion of high-dose 5FU, repeated weekly. Modulation of this schedule with LV has resulted in response rate of 44%; randomized trials are ongoing.

Since the antitumor effect of 5FU can be (at least partially) attributed to inhibition of TS, several folate-based TS inhibitors have been developed and have shown substantial clinical activity against various malignancies, not only colorectal cancer but also non-small-cell lung cancer and head and neck cancer. Several preclinical studies have shown an at least additive effect of 5FU with one of these antifolates, possibly caused by additive TS inhibition resulting from a stabilization of a ternary complex between TS, FdUMP, and the antifolate.

A number of the new non-TS-directed drugs have been introduced into the clinic recently. Two of these drugs have activity in gastrointestinal malignancies, especially colorectal cancer and seem suitable for combination with 5FU. The platinum analog oxaliplatinum has been tested predominantly as part of a chronomodulated schedule with 5FU and LV, also resulting in 50–60% response rates. For the parent drug, cisplatin, an interference with folate metabolism and TS has been reported. Besides this interaction, it is not unlikely that the imbalance in the deoxyribonucleotides caused by 5FU will affect repair of DNA-platinum adducts. This mechanism may also play a role in the combinations with irinotecan, a topoisomerase I inhibitor. Irinitecan has activity in 5FU-refractory disease, and is currently investigated in combination with 5FU. A clear schedule dependence was observed in preclinical studies; some sequential combinations (irinotecan followed by 5FU/LV) also resulted in relatively high response rates.

The increased insight in 5FU metabolism, not only of its direct activation pathways and inhibition of the target TS, but also of the downstream events following TS inhibition, have resulted in the design of other potentially very active combinations. Using this approach together with the new insights in 5FU administration (high-dose infusion, oral formulations), combinations of 5FU remain an important tool for the treatment of frequently occurring malignancies, such as colorectal cancer or breast cancer. The incorporation of predictive assays may enable selective administration of 5FU in some form to patients likely to respond (a low TS level), and provide alternative therapy (chronomodulated with oxalipatinum or irinotecan combinations) to patients with an unfavorable tumor profile (high TS). It is not unlikely that in the future more active combinations with 5FU will be developed.

ACKNOWLEDGMENT

We thank A. Paalman for excellent secretarial assistance.

REFERENCES

1. Heidelberger C, Chaudhuri NK, Danneberg P, Mooren D, Crisbach L, Duschinsky R, Schnitzer RJ, Pleven E, Schreiner J. Fluorinated pyrimidines, a new class of tumor-inhibitory compounds. *Nature* 1957; 179:663–666.
2. Heidelberger C, Griesbach L, Cruz O, Schnitzer J, Crunberg E. Fluorinated pyrimidines VIII, Effects of 5-fluorouracil and 5-fluoro-2'deoxyuridine on transplanted tumors. *Proc Soc Exp Med Biol Med* 1958; 97:470–475.
3. Pinedo HM, Peters GJ. 5-Fluorouracil: biochemistry and pharmacology. *J. Clin. Oncol.* 1988; 6:1653–1664.
4. Moertel CG. Chemotherapy of gastrointestinal cancer. *New Engl J Med* 1978; 299:1049–1052.
5. Moertel CG. Chemotherapy of gastrointestinal cancer. *New Engl J Med* 1994; 330:1136–1142.
6. Peters GJ, Van Groeningen CJ. Clinical relevance of biochemical modulation of 5-fluorouracil. *Ann Oncology* 1991; 2:469–480.
7. Diasio RB, Harris BE. Clinical pharmacology of 5-fluorouracil. *Clin Pharm* 1989; 6:215–237.
8. Mini E, Trave F, Rustum YM, Bertino JR. Enhancement of the antitumor effects of 5-fluorouracil by folinic acid. *Pharmac Ther* 1990; 47:1–19.
9. Köhne-Wömpner CH, Schmoll HJ, Harstrick A, Rustum YM. Chemotherapeutic strategies in metastatic colorectal cancer—an overview of current clinical trials. *Sem Oncol* 1992; 19:105–125.
10. Weckbecker G. Biochemical pharmacology and analysis of fluoropyrimidines alone and in combination with modulators. *Pharmacol Ther* 1991; 50:367–424.
11. Van der Wilt CL, Peters GJ. New targets for pyrimidine antimetabolites for the treatment of solid tumors. Part 1, thymidylate synthase. *Pharm World Sci* 1994; 16:84–103.
12. Peters GJ, Ackland SP. New antimetabolites in preclinical and clinical development. *Expert Opin Invest Drugs* 1996; 5:637–679.
13. Peters GJ, Jansen G. Resistance to antimetabolites, in *Principles of Antineoplastic Drug Development and Pharmacology* (Schilsky RL, Milano GA, Ratain MJ, eds); Marcel Dekker, New York, 1996, pp. 543–585.
14. Van Laar JAM, Van Groeningen CJ, Ackland SP, Rustum YM, Peters GJ. Comparison of 5-fluoro-2'-deoxyuridine with 5-fluorouracil; and their role in the treatment of advanced colorectal cancer. *Eur. J. Cancer,* 1998; 34:296–306.
15. Schmoll H-J. Development of treatment for adjacent colorectal cancer: infusional 5-FU and the role of new agents. *Eur J Cancer* 1996; 32A:S18–S22.
16. Lokich JJ, Ahlgren JD, Gullo JJ, Philips JA, Fryer JG. A prospective randomized comparison of continuous infusion of fluorouracil with a conventional bolus schedule in metastatic colorectal carcinoma: a mid-Atlantic oncology program study. *J Clin Oncol* 1989; 7:425–432.

17. Peters GJ, Van Groeningen CJ, Laurensse EJ, Pinedo HM. A comparison of 5-fluorouracil metabolism in human colorectal cancer and colon mucosa. *Cancer* 1991; 68:1903–1909.
18. Sköld O. Studies on resistance against 5-fluorouracil. IV Evidence for an altered uridine kinase in resistant cells. *Biochim Biophys Acta* 1963; 76:160–162.
19. Reichard P, Sköld O, Klein G, Revesz L, Magnussen P-H. Studies on resistance against 5-fluorouracil. I Enzymes of the uracil pathway during development of resistance. *Cancer Res* 1962; 22:235–243.
20. Tezuka M, Sugiyama H, Tamemasa O, Inara M. Biochemical characteristics of a 5-fluorouracil-resistant subline of P388 leukemia. *Gann* 1982; 73:70–76.
21. Reyes P, Hall TC. Synthesis of 5-fluorouridine 5'-phosphate by a pyrimidine phosphoribosyltransferase of mammalian origin. II. Correlation between the tumor levels of the enzyme and the 5-fluorouracil-promoted increase in survival in tumor-bearing mice. *Biochem Pharmacol* 1969; 18:2587–2590.
22. Kessel D, Hall TC, Wodinsky I. Nucleotide formation as a determinant in 5-fluorouracil response in mouse leukemias. *Science* 1966; 145:911–913.
23. Schwartz PM, Moir RD, Hyde CM, Turek PJ, Handschumacher RE. Role of uridine phosphorylase in the anabolism of 5-fluorouracil. *Biochem Pharmacol* 1985; 34:3585–3589.
24. Houghton JA, Houghton PJ. Elucidation of pathways of 5-fluorouracil metabolism in xenografts of human colorectal adenocarcinoma. *Eur J Cancer Clin Oncol* 1983; 19:807–815.
25. Ardalan B, Villacorte D, Heck D, Corbett T. Phosphoribosyl pyrophosphate, pool size and tissue levels as a determinant of 5-fluorouracil response in murine colonic adenocarcinomas. *Biochem Pharmacol* 1982; 31:1989–1992.
26. Peters GJ, Laurensse E, Leyva A, Pinedo HM. Purine nucleosides as cell-specific modulators of 5-fluorouracil metabolism and cytotoxicity. *Eur J Cancer Clin Oncol* 1987; 23:1869–1881.
27. Peters GJ, Laurensse E, Leyva A, Lankelma J, Pinedo HM. Sensitivity of human, murine and rat cells to 5-fluorouracil and 5'-deoxy-5-fluorouridine in relation to drug-metabolizing enzymes. *Cancer Research* 1986; 46:20–28.
28. Holland SK, Bergman AM, Zhao Y, Adams ER, Pizzorno G. ^{19}F NMR monitoring of in vitro tumor metabolism after biochemical modulation of 5-fluorouracil by the uridine phosphorylase inhibitor 5-benzylacyclouridine. *Magnetic Resonance in Medicine* 1997; 38:907–916.
29. Peters GJ, Lankelma J, Kok RM, Noordhuis P, Van Groeningen CJ, Van der Wilt CL, Meyer S, Pinedo HM. Prolonged retention of high concentrations of 5-fluorouracil in human and murine tumors as compared with plasma. *Cancer Chemother Pharmacol* 1993; 31:269–276.
30. Peters GJ, Braakhuis BJM, de Bruijn EA, Laurensse EJ, van Walsum M, Pinedo HM. Enhanced therapeutic efficacy of 5'deoxy-5-fluorouridine in 5-fluorouracil resistant head and neck tumors in relation to 5-fluorouracil metabolizing enzymes. *Br J Cancer* 1989; 59:327–334.
31. Peters GJ, Pinedo HM, Ferwerda W, De Graaf TW, Van Dijk W. Do antimetabolites interfere with the glycosylation of cellular glycoconjugates? *Eur J Cancer* 1990; 26:516–523.
32. Spears CP, Gustavsson BG, Mitchell MS, Spicer D, Berne M, Bernstein L, Danenberg PV. Thymidylate synthase inhibition in malignant tumors and normal liver of patients given intravenous 5-fluorouracil. *Cancer Res* 1984; 44:4144–4150.
33. Swain SM, Lippman ME, Egan EF, Drake JC, Steinberg SM, Allegra CJ. Fluorouracil and high-dose leucovorin in previously treated patients with metastatic breast cancer. *J Clin Oncol* 1989; 7:890–899.
34. Peters GJ, Van der Wilt CL, Van Groeningen CJ, Meijer S, Smid K, Pinedo HM. Thymidylate synthase inhibition after administration of 5-fluorouracil with or without leucoyorin; implications for treatment with 5-fluorouracil. *J Clin Oncol* 1994; 12:2035–2042.
35. Naguib FNM, El Kouni MH, Cha S. Enzymes of uracil catabolism in normal and neoplastic human tissues. *Cancer Res* 1985; 45:5405–5412.
36. Spoelstra EC, Pinedo HM, Dekker H, Peters GJ, Lankelma J. Measurement of in vitro cellular pharmacokinetics of 5-fluorouracil in human and rat cancer cell lines and rat hepatocytes using a flow-through system. *Cancer Chemother Pharmacol* 1991; 27:320–325.
37. Etienne MC, Lagrange JL, Dassonville O, et al. (1994). Population study of dihydropyrimidine dehydrogenase in cancer patients. *J Clin Oncol* 1994; 12:2248–2253.
38. Heggie GD, Sommadossi JP, Cross DS, Huster WJ, Diasio RB. Clinical pharmacokinetics of 5-fluorouracil and its metabolites in plasma, urine and bile. *Cancer Res* 1987; 47:2203–2206.
39. Harris BE, Song R, Soong S, Diasio RB. Relationship between dihydropyrimidine dehydrogenase activity and plasma 5-fluorouracil levels with evidence for circadian variation of enzyme activity and

plasma drug levels in cancer patients receiving 5-fluorouracil by protracted continuous infusion. *Cancer Res* 1990; 50:197–201.
40. Codacci-Pisanelli G, Van der Wilt CL, Pinedo HM, Franchi F, Noordhuis P, Van Laar JAM, Braakhuis BJM, Peters GJ. Antitumor activity, toxicity and inhibition of thymidylate synthase of prolonged administration of 5-fluorouracil in mice. *Eur J Cancer* 1995; 31A:1517–1525.
41. Hrushesky WJM, Bjarnason GA. Circadian cancer therapy. *J Clin Oncol* 1993; 11:1403–1417.
42. Houyau P, Gay C, Chatelut E, Canal P, Roche H, Milano G. Severe fluorouracil toxicity in a patient with dihydropyrimidine dehydrogenase deficiency. *J Natl Cancer Instit* 1993; 85:1602–1603.
43. Fleming RA, Milano, G. Thyss A, Etienne MC, Renee N, Schneider M, Demard F. Correlation between dihydropyrimidine dehydrogenase activity in peripheral mononuclear cells and systemic clearance of fluorouracil in cancer patients. *Cancer Res* 1992; 52:2899–2902.
44. Beck A, Etienne MC, Chéradame S, et al. A role for dihydropyrimidine dehydrogenase and thymidylate synthase in tumor sensitivity to fluorouracil. *Eur J Cancer* 1994; 30A:1517–1522.
45. Peters GJ, Van der Wilt CL, Van Groeningen CJ. Predictive value of thymidylate synthase and dihydropyrimidine dehydrogenase. *Eur J Cancer* 1994; 30A:1408–1411.
46. Unemi N, Takeda S, Tajima K, et al. Studies on combination therapy with 1-(tetrahydro-2 furanyl)-5-fluorouracul plus uracil. I. Effect of coadministration of uracil on the antitumor activity of 1-(tetrahydro-2-furanyl)-5-fluorouracil and the level of 5-fluorouracil in AH 130 bearing rats. *Chemotheraphy* 1981; 29:164–175.
47. Takechi T, Nakano K, Uchida J, Mita A, Toko K, Takeda S, Unemi N, Shirasaka T. Antitumor activity and low intestinal toxicity of S-1, a new formulation of oral tegafur, in experimental tumor models in rats. *Cancer Chemother Pharmacol* 1997; 39:205–211.
48. Tatsumi K, Fukushima M, Shirasaka T, Fujii S. Inhibitory effects of pyrimidine, barbituric acid and pyridine derivatives on 5-fluorouracil degradation in rat liver extracts. *Jpn J Cancer Res (GANN)* 1987; 78:748–755.
49. Spector T, Porter DJT, Nelson DJ, et al. 5-Ethynyluracil (776C85), a modulator of the therapeutic activity of 5-fluorouracil. *Drugs Future* 1994; 19:565–571.
50. Miwa M, Ishikawa T, Eda H, Ryu M, Fujimoto K, Ninomiya Y, Umeda I, Yokose K, Ishitsuka H. Comparative studies on the antitumor and immunosuppressive effects of the new fluorouracil derivative N^4-trimethoxybenzoyl-5'-deoxy-5-fluorocytidine and its parent drug 5'-deoxy-5-fluorouridine. *Chem Pharm Bull* 1990; 38:998–1003.
51. Ninomiya Y, Miwa M, Eda H, Sahara H, Fujimoto K, Ishida M, Umeda I, Yokose K, Ishitsuka H. Comparative antitumor activity and intestinal toxicity of 5'-deoxy-5-fluorouridine and its prodrug trimethoxybenzoyl-5'-deoxy-5-fluorocytidine. *Jpn J Cancer Res* 1990; 81:188–195.
52. Pazdur R, Lassere Y, Rhodes V, et al. Phase II trial of uracil and tegafur plus oral leucovorin: an effective oral regimen in the treatment of metastatic colorectal carcinoma. *J Clin Oncol* 1994; 12:2296–2300.
53. Saltz LB, Leichman CG, Young CW, et al. A fixed-ratio combination of uracil and Ftorafur (UFT) with low doseleucovorin. An active oral regimen for advanced colorectal cancer. *Cancer* 1995; 75:782–785.
54. Gonzalez Baron M, Feliu J, de la Gandara I, et al. Efficacy of oral tegafur modulation by uracil and leucovorin in advanced colorectal cancer. A phase II study. *Eur J Cancer* 1995; 31A:2215–2219.
55. Feliu J, Gonzalez Baron M, Espinosa E, et al. Uracil and tegafur modulated with leucovorin: an effective regimen with low toxicity for the treatment of colorectal carcinoma in the elderly. Oncopaz Cooperative Group. *Cancer* 1997; 79:1884–1889.
56. Bajetta E, Di Bartolomeo M, Somma L, et al. Randomized phase II noncomparative trial of oral and intravenous doxifluridine plus levo-leucovorin in untreated patients with advanced colorectal carcinoma. *Cancer* 1996; 78:2087–2093.
57. Bajetta E, Colleoni M, Di Bartolomeo M, et al. Doxifluridine and leucovorin: an oral treatment combination in advanced colorectal cancer. *J Clin Oncol* 1995; 13:2613–2619.
58. Findlay M, Van Cutsem E, Kocha W, et al. A randomized phase II study of Xeloda™ (capecitabine) in patients with advanced colorectal cancer. *Proc Am Soc Clin Oncol* 1997; 16:227a(abstract).
59. Schilsky R, Bukowski R, Burris H, et al. A phase II study of a five day regimen of oral 5-fluorouracil (5-FU) plus GW776 (776C85) with or without leucovorin in patients with metastatic colorectal cancer. *Proc Am Soc Clin Oncol* 1997; 16:271a(abstract).

60. Horikoshi N, Mitachi Y, Sakata Y, Sugimachi K, Taguchi T. S-1, new oral fluoropyrimidine is very active in patients with advanced gastric cancer (early phase II study). *Proc. ASCO* 1996; 15:206.
61. Ichikura T, Tomimatsu S, Okusa Y, Yahara T, Uefuji K, Tamakuma S. Thymidylate synthase inhibition by an oral regimen consisting of tegafur-uracil (UFT) and low-dose leucovorin for patients with gastric cancer. *Cancer Chemother Pharmacol* 1996; 38:401–405.
62. Peters GJ, Van Groeningen CJ, Schornagel JH, Gall HE, Noordhuis P, De Vries M, Van Kuilenburg ABP, Hanauske HR. Phase I clinical and pharmacokinetic study of S-1, an oral 5-fluorouracil (5-FU) based antineoplastic agent. *Proc Am Soc Clin Oncol* 1997; 16:227a(abstract 800).
63. Köhne CH, Kretzschmar A, Wils J. First-line chemotherapy for colorectal carcinoma—we are making progress. *Onkologie,* in press.
64. Martin DS. Biochemical modulation: perspectives and objectives, In Proc. 8th Bristol-Myers Symp. on Cancer Res. *New Avenues in Developmental Cancer Chemotherapy* (Harrap KR, Connors TA, eds.) Academic, London 1987; pp 113–162.
65. Hryniuk WM, Figueredo A, Goodyear M. Applications of dose intensity to problems in chemotherapy of breast and colorectal cancer. *Sem Oncol* 1987; 14(suppl 14):3–11.
66. Van Laar, JAM, Van der Wilt, CL, Smid K, Noordhuis P, Rustum YM, Pinedo HM, Peters GJ. Therapeutic efficacy of fluoropyrimidines depends on the duration of thymidylate synthase inhibition in the murine Colon 26-b carcinoma tumor model. *Clin Cancer Res* 1996; 2:1327–1333.
67. Codacci-Pisanelli G, Kralovansky J, Van der Wilt CL, Noordhuis P, Colofiore JR, Martin DS, Franchi F, Peters GJ. Modulation of 5-fluorouracil in mice using uridine diphosphoglucose. *Clin Cancer Res* 1997; 3:309–315.
68. Codacci-Pisanelli G, Noordhuis P, Van der Wilt CL, Smid K, Franchi F, Pinedo HM, Peters GJ. Incorporation of 5FU into RNA after high-dose 5FU treatment with Uridine-diphosphoglucose (UDPG) rescue in mice is not related with antitumour activity, but thymidylate synthase (TS) inhibition is *Proc Amer Assoc Cancer Res* 1997; 38:4784(abstract 3201).
69. Peters GJ, Van der Wilt CL, Van Groeningen CJ, Priest DG, Schmitz J, Smid K, Meijer S, Noordhuis P, Hoekman K, Pinedo HM. Effect of different leucovorin formulations on 5-fluorouracil induced thymidylate synthase inhibition in colon tumors and normal tissues from patients in relation to response to 5-fluorouracil, in *Chemistry and Biology of Pteridines and Folates,* Proc. 11th International Symposium. Pfleiderer W, Rokos H, eds. Blackwell Science, Berlin, 1997; pp. 145–150.
70. Peters GJ, Van Dijk J, Laurensse E, Van Groeningen CJ, Lankelma J, Leyva A, Nadal J, Pinedo HM. *In vitro* biochemical and *in vivo* biological studies of uridine "rescue" of 5-fluorouracil. *Br J Cancer* 1988; 57:259–265.
71. Sawyer RC, Stolfi RL, Spiegelman S, Martin DS. Effect of uridine on the metabolism of 5-fluorouracil in the $CD_8 F_1$ murine mammary carcinoma system. *Pharm Res* 1984; 2:69–75.
72. Spears CP, Gustavsson BG, Berne M, Frosing R, Bernstein L, Hayes AA. Mechanisms of innate resistance to thymidylate synthase inhibition after 5-fluorouracil. *Cancer Res* 1988; 48:5894–5900.
73. Bapat AR, Zarov C, Danenberg PV. Human leukemic cells resistant to 5-fluoro-2'deoxyuridine contain a thymidylate synthase with lower affinity for nucleotides. *J Biol Chem* 1983; 258:4130–4136.
74. Houghton JA, Torrance PM, Radparvar S, Williams LG, Houghton PJ. Binding of 5-fluorodeoxyuridylate to thymidylate synthase in human colon adenocarcinoma xenografts. *Eur J Cancer Clin Oncol* 1986; 22:505–510.
75. Yin MB, Zakrzewski SF, Hakala MT. Relationship of cellular folate cofactor pools to the activity of 5-fluorouracil. *Mol Pharmacol* 1983; 23:190–197.
76. Jansen G. Receptor- and carrier-medioted transport systems for folates and antifolates: exploitation for folate-based chemotherapy and immunotherapy, in *Antifolate Drugs: Basic Research and Clinical Practice* (A. Jackman ed.), Humana Totowa, NJ, Chapter 14.
77. Van der Wilt CL, Pinedo HM, De Jong M, Peters GJ. Effect of folate diastereoisomers on the binding of 5-fluoro-2'-deoxyuridine-5'-monophosphate to thymidylate synthase. *Biochem Pharmacol* 1993; 45:1177–1179.
78. Radparvar S, Houghton PJ, Houghton JA. Characteristics of thymidylate synthase purified form a human colon adenocarcinoma. *Arch Biochem Biophys* 1988; 260:342–350.
79. Wang FS, Aschele C, Sobrero A, Chang YM, Bertino JR. Decreased folylpolyglutamate synthetase expression: a novel mechanism of fluorouracil resistance. *Cancer Res* 1993; 53:3677–3680.
80. Priest DG, Ledford SE, Doig MT. Increased thymidylate synthetase in 5-fluorodeoxyuridine resistant cultured hepatoma cells. *Biochem Pharmacol* 1980; 29:1549–1553.

81. Berger SH, Hakala MT. Relationship of dUMP and FdUMP pools to inhibition of thymidylate synthase by 5-fluorouracil. *Mol Pharmacol* 1984; 25:303–309.
82. Berger SH, Barbour KW, Berger FG. A naturally occurring variation in thymidylate synthase structure is associated with a reduced response to 5-fluoro-2'-deoxyuridine in a human colon tumor cell line. *Mol Pharmacol* 1988; 34:480–484.
83. Jenh CH, Geyer PK, Baskin F, Johnson LF. Thymidylate synthase gene amplification in fluorodeoxyuridine-resistant mouse cell lines. *Mol Pharmacol* 1985; 28:80–85.
84. Sobrero AF, Aschele C, Guglielmi AP, Mori AM, Melioli GG, Rosso R, Bertino JR. Synergism and lack of cross-resistance between short-term and continuous exposure to 5-fluorouracil in human adenocarcinoma cells. *J Natl Cancer Instit* 1993; 85:1937–1944.
85. Van der Wilt, CL, Pinedo HM, Smid K, Peters GJ. Elevation of thymidylate synthase following 5-fluorouracil treatment is prevented by the addition of leucovorin in murine colon tumors. *Cancer Res* 1992; 52:4922–4928.
86. Van der Wilt CL, Marinelli A, Pinedo HM, Cloos J, Smid K, Van de Velde CJH, Peters GJ. The effect of different routes of administration of 5-fluorouracil on thymidylate synthase inhibition in the rat. *Eur J Cancer* 1995; 31A:754–760.
87. Van der Wilt CL, Van Groeningen CJ, Pinedo HM, Smid K, Hoekman K, Meijer S, Peters GJ. 5-Fluorouracil/leucovorin-induced inhibition of thymidylate synthase in normal tissues of mouse and man. *J Cancer Res Clin Oncol* 1997; 123:595–601.
88. Navelgund LG, Rossana C, Muench AJ, Johnson LF. Cell cycle regulation of thymidylate synthetase gene expression in cultured mouse fibroblasts. *J Biol Chem* 1980; 255:7386–7390.
89. Chu E, Koeller D, Casey J. Drake J, Chabner B, Elwood P, Zinn S, Allegra C. Autoregulation of human thymidylate synthase messenger RNA translation by thymidylate synthase. *Proc Natl Acad Sci USA* 1991; 88:8977–8981.
90. Chu E, Koeller DM, Johnston PG, Zinn S, Allegra CJ. Regulation of thymidylate synthase in human colon cancer cells treated with 5-fluorouracil and interferon-gamma. *Mol Pharmacol* 1993; 43:527–533.
91. Keyomarsi K, Samet J, Molnar G, Pardee AB. The thymidylate synthase inhibitor, ICI-D1694, overcomes translational detainment of the enzyme. *J Biol Chem* 1993; 268:15142–15149.
92. Chu E, Allegra CJ. The role of thymidylate synthase as an RNA binding protein. *Bioassays* 1996; 18:191–198.
93. Lee Y, Johnson LF, Chang LS, Chen Y. Inhibition of mouse thymidylate synthase promoter activity wild-type p53 tumor suppressor protein. *Exp Cell Res* 1997; 234:270–276.
94. Peters GJ, Van Groeningen CJ, Laurensse EJ, Pinedo HM. Thymidylate synthase from untreated human colorectal cancer and colonic mucosa: enzyme activity and inhibition by 5-fluoro-2'-deoxyuridine-5'-monophosphate. *Eur J Cancer* 1991; 27:263–267.
95. Leichman L, Lenz H-J, Leichman CG, Groshen S, Danenberg K, Baranda J, Spears CP, Boswell W, Silberman H, Ortega A, Stain S, Beart R, Danenberg P. Quantitation of intratumoral thymidylate synthase expression predicts for resistance to protracted infusion 5-fluorouracil and weekly leucovorin in disseminated colorectal cancers: preliminary report from an ongoing trial. *Eur J Cancer* 1995; 31A:1306–1310.
96. Omura K, Kawakami K, Kanehira E, Nagasato A, Kawashima S, Tawaraya K, Watanabe S, Hirano K, Shirasaka T, Watanabe Y. The number of 5-fluoro-2'-deoxyuridine-5'-monophosphate binding sites and reduced folate pool in human colorectal carcinoma tissues—changes after tegafur and uracil treatment. *Cancer Res* 1995; 55:3897–3901.
97. Kornmann M, Link KH, Lenz HJ, Pillasch J, Metzger R, Butzer U, Leder GH, Weindel M, Safi F, Danenberg KD, Beger HG, Danenberg PV. Thymidylate synthase is a predictor for response and resistance in hepatic artery infusion chemotherapy. *Cancer Lett* 1997; 118:29–35.
98. Lenz H-J, Leichman CG, Danenberg KD, Danenberg PV, Groshen S, Cohen H, Crookes P, Sliberman H, Baranda J, Garcia Y, Li J, Leichman L. Thymidylate synthase mRNA level in adenocarcinoma of the stomach: a predictor for primary tumor response and overall survival. *J Clin Oncol* 1996; 14:176–182.
99. Johnston PG, Fischer KH, Rockette HE, Fischer B, Wolmark N, Drake JC, Chabner BA, Allegra CJ. The role of thymidylate synthase expression in prognosis and outcome of adjuvant chemotherapy in patients with rectal cancer. *J Clin Oncol* 1994; 12:2640–2647.

100. Johnston PG, Mick R, Recant W, Behan KA, Dolan ME, Ratain MJ, Beckmann E, Weichselbaum RR, Allegra CJ, Vokes EE. Thymidylate synthase expression and response to neoadjuvant chemotherapy in patients with advanced head and neck cancer. *J Natl Cancer Inst* 1997; 89:308–313.
101. Pestalozzi BC, Peterson HF, Gelber RD, Goldhirsch A, Gusterson BA, Trihia H, Lindtner J, Cortés-Funes H, Simmoncini E, Byrne MJ, Golouh R, Rudenstam CM, Castiglione-Gertsch M, Allegra CJ, Johnston PG. Prognostic importance of thymidylate synthase expression in early breast cancer. *J Clin Oncol* 1997; 15:1923–1931.
102. Findlay MPN, Cunningham C, Morgan G, Clinton S, Hardcastle A, Aherne GW. Lack of correlation between thymidylate synthase levels in primary colorectal tumours and subsequent response to chemotherapy. *Br J Cancer* 1997; 75:903–909.
103. Piall EM, Curtin NJ, Aherne GW, Harris AL, Marks V. The quantitation by radioimmunoassay of 2′deoxyuridine 5′triphosphate in extract of thymidylate synthase-inhibited cells. *Anal Biochem* 1989; 177:347–352.
104. Curtin NJ, Harris AL, Aherne GW. Mechanism of cell death following thymidylate synthase inhibition: 2′-deoxyuridine-5′-triphosphate accumulation, DNA damage, and growth inhibition following exposure to CB3717 and dipyridamole. *Cancer Res* 1991; 51:2346–2352.
105. Fisher TC, Milner AE, Gregory CD, Jackman AL, Aherne GW, Hartley JA, Dive C, Hickman JA. bcl-2 modulation of apoptosis induced by anticancer drugs—resistance to thymidylate stress is independent of classical resistance pathways. *Cancer Res* 1993; 53:3321–3326.
106. Lönn U, Lönn S. DNA lesions in human neoplasmatic cells and cytotoxicity of 5-fluoropyrimidines. *Cancer Res* 1986; 46:3866–3871.
107. Chu E, Lai GM, Zinn S, Allegra CJ. Resistance of a human ovarian cancer line to 5-fluorouracil associated with decreased levels of 5-fluorouracil in DNA. *Mol Pharmacol* 1990; 38:410–417.
108. Calvert AH, Newell DR, Jackman AL, Gumbrell LA, Sikora E, Grzelakowska-Sztabert B, Bishop JAM, Judson AR, Harland SJ, Harrap KR. Recent preclinical and clinical studies with the thymidylate synthase inhibitor N^{10}-propargyl-5,8-dideazafolic acid (CB 3717). *NCI Monographs* 1987; 5:213–218.
109. Sedwick WD, Kutler M, Brown OE. Antifolate-induced misincorporation of deoxyuridinemonophosphate into DNA: inhibition of high molecular weight DNA synthesis in human lymfoblastoid cells. *Proc Natl Acad Sci USA* 1981; 78:917–921.
110. Ingraham HA, Dickey L, Goulain M. DNA fragmentation and cytotoxicity form increased cellular deoxyuridylate. *Biochemistry* 1986; 25:3225–3250.
111. Fraser DC, Pearson CK. Is uracil misincorporation into DNA of mammalian cells a consequence of methotrexate treatment? *Biochem Biophys Res Commun* 1986; 135:886–889.
112. Ayasawa D, Shimizu K, Koyama H, Takeishi K, Seno T. Accumulation of DNA strand breaks during thymineless death in thymidylate synthase-negative mutants of mouse FM3A cells. *J Biol Chem* 1988; 258:12,448–12,454.
113. Yin MB, Rustum YM. Comparative DNA strand breakage induced by FUra and FdUrd in human ileocecal adenocarcinoma (HCT-8) cells: relevance to cell growth inhibition. *Cancer Commun* 1991; 3:45–51.
114. Mosbaugh DW, Bennett SE. Uracil-excision DNA repair. *Progress Nucl Acid Res Mol Biol* 1994; 48:315–371.
115. Canman CE, Lawrence TS, Shewach DS, Tang HY, Maybaum J. Resistance to fluorodeoxyuridine-induced DNA damage and cytotoxicity correlates with an elevation of deoxyuridine triphosphatase activity and failure to accumulate deoxyuridine triphosphate. *Cancer Res* 1993; 53:5219–5224.
116. Parsels LA, Loney TL, Maybaum J. Expression of E. coli dUTPase partially protects HT29 cells from DNA fragmentation and cytoxicity induced by CB3717 or methotrexate. *Proc Amer Assoc Canc Res* 1995; 36:406.
117. Yin MB, Guimaraes MA, Zhang ZG, Arredondo MA, Rustum YM. Time dependence of DNA lesions and growth inhibition by ICI-D1694, a new quinazoline antifolate thymidylate synthase inhibitor. *Cancer Res* 1992; 52:5900–5905.
118. Schober C, Gibbs JF, Yin MB, Slocum HK, Rustum YM. Cellular heterogeneity in DNA damage and growth inhibition induced by ICI D1694, thymidylate synthase inhibitor, using single cells assays. *Biochem Pharmacol* 1994; 48:997–1002.
119. Li ZR, Yin MB, Arredondo MA, Schober C, Rustum YM. Down-regulation of c-myc gene expression

with induction of high molecular weight DNA fragments by fluorodeoxyuridine. *Biochem Pharmacol* 1994; 48:327–334.
120. Rustum YM, Shousong C, Yin MB. Modulation of target enzyme associated with the action of antifolates. *Advan Enzyme Regul* 1994; 34:55–70.
121. Van der Wilt CL, Kuiper CM, Pinedo HM, Peters GJ. Combination studies of antifolates with 5-fluorouracil in colon cancer cell lines, in *Chemistry and Biology of Pteridines and Folates,* Proc. 11th International Symposium, (Pfleiderer W, Rokos H, eds.), Blackwell Science, Berlin, 1997, pp. 245–248.
122. Houghton JA, Morton CL, Adkins DA, Rahman A. Locus of the interaction among 5-fluorouracil, leucovorin, and interferon-alpha-2A in colon carcinoma cells. *Cancer Res* 1993; 53:4243–4250.
123. Van der Wilt CL, Smid K, Noordhuis P, Aherne GW, Peters GJ. Biochemical mechanisms of interferon modulation of 5-fluorouracil activity in colon cancer cells. *Eur J Cancer* 1997; 33:471–478.
124. Houghton JA, Adkins DA, Rahman A, Houghton PJ. Interaction between 5-fluorouracil, [6RS]leucovorin, and recombinant human interferon-α2a in cultured colon adenocarcinoma cells. *Cancer Comm* 1991; 3:225–231.
125. Sinnige HAM, Timmer-Bosscha H, Peters GJ, De Vries EGE, Mulder NH. Combined modulation by leucovorin and α-2a interferon of fluoropyrimidine mediated growth inhibition. *Anticancer Res* 1993; 13:1335–1340.
126. Houghton JA, Cheshire PJ, Morton CL, Stewart CF. Potentiation of 5-fluorouracil-leucovorin activity by α2a-interferon in colon adenocarcinoma xenografts. *Clin Cancer Res* 1995; 1:33–40.
127. Grem JL, Jordan E, Robson ME, Binder RA, Hamilton JM, Steinberg SM, et al. Phase-II study of fluorouracil, leucovorin, and interferon alfa-2a in metastatic colorectal carcinoma. *J Clin Oncol* 1993; 11:1737–1745.
128. Sinnige HAM, Buter J, Devries EGE, Uges DRA, Roenhorst HW, Verschueren RCJ, et al. Phase I-II study of the addition of alpha-2A interferon to 5-fluorouracil leucovorin—pharmacokinetic interaction of alpha-2A interferon and leucovorin. *Eur J Cancer* 1993; 29A:1715–1720.
129. Kocha W. Phase III randomized study of two fluorouracil combinations with advanced colorectal carcinoma. *J Clin Oncol* 1995; 13:921–928.
130. Hill M, Norman A, Cunningham D, et al. Royal Marsden phase III trial of fluorouracil with or without interferon alfa-2b in advanced colorectal cancer. *J Clin Oncol* 1995; 13:1297–1302.
131. Yoshioka A, Tanaka S, Hiraoka O, Koyama Y, Hirota Y, Ayusawa D, Seno T, Garrett C, Wataya Y. Deoxyribonucleoside triphosphate imbalance. *J Biol Chem* 1987; 262:8235–8241.
132. Houghton JA, Tillman DM, Harwood FG. Ratio of 2'-deoxyadenosin-5'-triphosphate/thymidine-5'-triphosphate influences the commitment of human colon carcinoma cells to thymineless death. *Clin Cancer Res* 1995; 1:723–730.
133. Houghton JA, Harwood FG, Houghton PJ. Cell cycle control processes determine cytostasis or cytotoxicity in thymineless death of colon cancer cells. *Cancer Res* 1994; 54:4967–4973.
134. James SJ, Miller BJ, Basnakian AG, Pogribny IP, Pogribna M, Muskhelishvili L. Apoptosis and proliferation under conditions of deoxynucleotide pool imbalance in liver of folate/methyl deficient rats. *Carcinogenesis* 1997; 18:287–293.
135. Peters GJ. Therapy related disturbances in nucleotides in cancer cells, in *Purine and Pyrimidine Metabolism in Man VIII* (Sahota A, Taylor MW, eds.) Plenum, New York, 1995, pp. 95–107. [*Adv Exp Med Biol* 1995; 370:95–107.]
136. Ullman B, Lee M, Martin DW, Santi DV. Cytotoxicity of 5-fluoro-2'-deoxyuridine; required for reduced cofactors and antagonism by methotrexate. *Proc Natl Acad Sci USA* 1978; 75:980–983.
137. Zhang ZG, Harstrick A, Rustum YM. Modulation of fluoropyrimidines: role of dose and schedule of leucovorin administration. *Sem Oncol* 1992; 19(suppl. 3):10–15.
138. Van Ark-Otte J, Peters GJ, Pizao PE, Keepers YPAM, Giaccone G. *In vitro* schedule dependency of EO9 and miltefostine in comparison to standard drugs in colon cancer cells. *Int J Oncol* 1994; 4:709–715.
139. Drewinko B, Yang LY. Cellular basis for the inefficacy of 5-FU in human colon carcinoma. *Cancer Treat Rep* 1985; 69:1391–1398.
140. Moran RG, Scanlon KL. Schedule-dependent enhancement of the cytotoxicity of fluoropyrimidines to human carcinoma cells in the presence of folinic acid. *Cancer Res* 1991; 51:4618–4623.
141. Sugimoto Y, Ohe Y, Nishio K, Ohmori T, Fujiwara Y, Saijo N. *In vitro* enhancement of fluoropyrimidine-induced cytotoxicity by leucovorin in colorectal and gastric carcinoma cell lines but not in nonsmall lung carcinoma cell lines. *Cancer Chemother Pharmacol* 1992; 30:417–422.

142. Park J-G, Collins JM, Gazdar AD, Allegra CJ, Steinberg SM, Greene RF, Kramer BS. Enhancement of fluorinated pyrimidine-induced cytotoxicity by leucovorin in human colorectal carcinoma cell lines. *J Natl Cancer Inst* 1988; 80:1560–1564.
143. Cao S, Zhang Z, Creaven PJ, Rustum YM. 5-Fluoro-2′-deoxyuridine: role of schedule in its therapeutic efficacy in *Novel Approaches to Selective Treatment of Human Solid Tumors: Laboratory and Clinical Correlation.* (Rustum YM, ed.), Plenum, New York, 1993, pp. 1–8.
144. Spears CP, Shahinian AH, Moran RG, Heidelberg C, Corbett TH. In vivo kinetics of thymidylate synthethase inhibition in 5-fluorouracil-sensitive and -resistant murine colon adenocarcinomas. *Cancer Res* 1982; 42:450–456.
145. Houghton JA, Houghton PJ. On the mechanism of cytotoxicity of fluorinated pyrimidines in four human colon adenocarcinoma xenografts maintained in immune-deprived mice. *Cancer* 1980; 45:1159–1167.
146. Iigo M, Nishikata K-I, Hoshi A. *In vivo* antitumor effects of fluoropyrimidines on colon adenocarcinoma 38 and enhancement by leucovorin. *Jpn J Cancer Res* 1992b; 83:392–396.
147. Buroker TR, O'Connell MJ, Wieand HS, et al. Randomized comparison of two schedules of fluorouracil and leucovorin in the treatment of advanced colorectal cancer. *J Clin Oncol* 1994; 12:14–20.
148. Haller DG, Lefkopoulou M, Macdonald JS, Mayer RS. Some considerations concerning the dose and schedule of 5FU and leucovorin: toxicities of two dose schedules from the intergroup colon adjuvant trial (INT-0089). *Adv Exp Med Biol* 1993; 339:51–54.
149. Köhne CH, Schöffski P, Wilke H, et al. Effective biomodulation by leucovorin of high dose infusional fluorouracil given as a weekly 24-hour infusion: results of a randomized trial in patients with advanced colorectal cancer. *J Clin Oncol* 1998; 2:1–11.
150. Advanced Colorectal Cancer Meta-Analysis Project. Modulation of fluorouracil by leucovorin in patients with advanced colorectal cancer: evidence in terms of response rate. *J Clin Oncol* 1992; 10:896–903.
151. Advanced Colorectal Cancer Meta-Analysis Project. Meta-analysis of randomized trials testing the biochemical modulation of fluorouracil by methotrexate in metastatic colorectal cancer. *J Clin Oncol* 1994; 12:960–969.
152. Anonymous. Efficacy of intravenous continous infusion of 5-Fluorouracil compared with bolus administration in advanced colorectal cancer. *J Clin Oncol* 1998; 16:301–308.
153. Petrelli N, Rustum YM. Fluorouracil and leucovorin: there is a choice [letter]. *J Clin Oncol* 1993; 11:1434.
154. Trave F, Rustum YM, Petrelli NJ, et al. Plasma and tumor tissue pharmacology of high-dose intravenous leucovorin calcium in combination with fluorouracil in patients with advanced colorectal carcinoma. *J Clin Oncol* 1988; 6:1184–1191.
155. Straw JA, Szapary D, Wynn WT. Pharmacokinetics of the diastereoisomers of leucovorin after intravenous and oral administration to normal subjects. *Cancer Res* 1984; 44:3114–3119.
156. Poon MA, O'Connell MJ, Moertel CG, et al. Biochemical modulation of fluorouracil: evidence of significant improvement of survival and quality of life in patients with advanced colorectal carcinoma. *J Clin Oncol* 1989; 7:1407–1418.
157. Petrelli N, Douglass HOJ, Herrera L, et al. The modulation of fluorouracil with leucovorin in metastatic colorectal carcinoma: a prospective randomized phase III trial. Gastrointestinal Tumor Study Group. *J Clin Oncol* 1989; 7:1419–1426.
158. Jäger E, Heike M, Bernhard H, et al. Weekly high-dose leucovorin versus low-dose leucovorin combined with fluorouracil in advanced colorectal cancer: results of a randomized multicenter trial. Study Group for Palliative Treatment of Metastatic Colorectal Cancer Study Protocol 1. *J Clin Oncol* 1996; 14:2274–2279.
159. Peters GJ, Hoekman K, Van Groeningen CJ, Van der Wilt CL, Smid K, Meyer S, Pinedo HM. Potentiation of 5-fluorouracil induced inhibition of thymidylate synthase in human colon tumors by leucovorin is dose dependent in *Chemistry and Biology of Pteridines and Folates, Adv Exp Med Biol* 338, (Ayling JE, Nair MG, Baugh CM, eds.) Plenum, New York, 1993a; pp. 613–616.
160. Grem JL, McAtee N, Murphy RF, et al. A pilot study of interferon alfa-2a in combination with fluorouracil plus high-dose leucovorin in metastatic gastrointestinal carcinoma. *J Clin Oncol* 1991; 9:1811–1820.
161. Van Groeningen CJ, Pinedo HM, Heddes J, Kok RM, De Jong APJM, Wattel E, Peters GJ, Lankelma J. Pharmacokinetics of 5-fluorouracil assessed with a sensitive mass spectrometric method in patients during a dose escalation schedule. *Cancer Res* 1988; 48:6956–6961.

162. Peters GJ, Schornagel JH, Milano GA. Clinical pharmacokinetics of antimetabolites. *Cancer Surveys* 1993; 17:123–156.
163. Berglund A, Jakobsen A, Graf W, et al. Bolus injection versus short-term infusion of 5-fluorouracil in patients with advanced colorectal cancer: a prospective randomized trial. *Eur J Cancer* 1997; 33(Suppl 8):S242(abstract).
164. Larsson PA, Carlsson G, Gustavsson B, Graf W, Glimelius B. Different entravenous administration techniques for 5-fluorouracil. *Acta Oncologica* 1996; 35:207–212.
165. Köhne CH, Hiddemann W, Schuller J, et al. Failure of orally administered dipyridamole to enhance the antineoplasticactivity of fluorouracil in combination with leucovorin in patients withadvanced colorectal cancer: a prospective randomized trial. *J Clin Oncol* 1995; 13:1201–1208.
166. Visser GWM, Van der Wilt CL, Wedzinga R, Peters GJ, Herscheid JDM. [^{18}F]-Radiopharmacokinetics of [^{18}F]-5-fluorouracil in a mouse bearing two colon tumors with a different 5-fluorouracil sensitivity: a study for a correlation with oncological results. *Nuclear Med Biol* 1996; 23:333–342.
167. Nord LD, Stolfi RL, Martin DS. Biochemical modulation of 5-fluorouracil with leucovorin or delayed uridine rescue. Correlation of antitumor activity with dosage and FUra incorporation into RNA. *Biochem Pharmacol* 1992; 43:2543–2549.
168. Sobrero AF, Aschele C, Bertino JR. Fluorouracil in colorectal cancer—a tale of two drugs: implications for biochemical modulation. *J Clin Oncol* 1997; 15:368–381.
169. Wils JA. High-dose fluorouracil: a new perspective in the treatment of colorectal cancer? *Semin Oncol* 1992; 19:126–130.
170. Ardalan B, Chua L, Tian EM, et al. A phase II study of weekly 24-hour infusion with high-dose fluorouracil with leucovorin in colorectal carcinoma. *J Clin Oncol* 1991; 9:625–630.
171. Ardalan B, Sridhar KS, Benedetto P, et al. A phase I, II study of high-dose 5-fluorouracil and high-dose leucovorin with low-dose phosphonacetyl-L-aspartic acid in patients with advanced malignancies. *Cancer* 1991; 68:1242–1246.
172. Haas NB, Hines JB, Hudes GR, Johnston N, Ozols RF, O'Dwyer PJ. Phase I trial of 5-fluorouracil by 24-hour infusion weekly. *Invest New Drugs* 1993; 11:181–185.
173. Diaz-Rubio E, Aranda E, Martin M, Gonzalez-Mancha R, Gonzalez-Larriba J, Barneto I. Weekly high-dose infusion of 5-fluorouracil in advanced colorectal cancer. *Eur J Cancer* 1990; 26:727–729.
174. Leichman CG, Fleming TR, Muggia FM, et al. Phase II study of fluorouracil and its modulation in advanced colorectal cancer: a Southwest Oncology Group Study. *J Clin Oncol* 1995; 13:1303–1311.
175. O'Dwyer PJ, Ryan LM, Valone FH, et al. Phase III trial of biochemical modulation of 5-fluorouracil by IV or oral leucovorin or by interferon in advanced colorectal cancer: an ECOG/CALGB phase III trial. *Proc Am Soc Clin Oncol* 1996; 15:207(abstract).
176. Diaz-Rubio E, Aranda E, Camps C, et al. A Phase II study of weekly 48-hour infusions with high-dose fluorouracil in advanced colorectal cancer: an alternative to biochemical modulation. *J Infusional Chemother* 1994; 4:58–61.
177. Aranda E, Cervantes A, Dorta J, et al. A phase II trial of weekly high dose continuous infusion 5-fluorouracil plus oral leucovorin in patients with advanced colorectal cancer. The Spanish Cooperative Group for Gastrointestinal Tumor Therapy (TTD). *Cancer* 1995; 76:559–563.
178. Aranda E, Cervantes A, Carrato A, et al. Outpatient weekly high-dose continuous infusion 5-fluorouracil plus oral leucovorin in advanced colorectal cancer. A phase II trial. Spanish Cooperative Group for Gastrointestinal Tumor Therapy (TTD). *Ann Oncol* 1996; 7:581–585.
179. Aranda E, Cervantes A, Anton A, et al. A phase III multicenter randomized study in advanced colorectal cancer (CRC): fluorouracil (FU) high-dose continuous infusion (CI) weekly versus fluorouracil + leucovorin (LV). Preliminary results. *Proc Am Soc Clin Oncol* 1997; 16:281a(abstract).
180. Laufman LR, Bukowski RM, Collier MA, et al. A randomized, double-blind trial of fluorouracil plus placebo versus fluorouracil plus oral leucovorin in patients with metastatic colorectal cancer. *J Clin Oncol* 1993; 11:1888–1893.
181. de Gramont A, Bosset JF, Milan C, et al. A randomized trial comparing monthly low-dose leucovorin/fluorouracil bolus with bimonthly high-dose leucovorin/fluorouracil bolus plus continuous infusion for advanced colorectal cancer: a French intergroup study. *J Clin Oncol* 1997; 15:808–815.
182. Köhne CH, Schöffski P, Wilke H, et al. Effective biomodulation by leucovorin of high dose infusional fluorouracil given as a weekly 24-hour infusion: results of a randomized trial in patients with advanced colorectal cancer. *J Clin Oncol* 1998; 2:1–11.
183. Greco FA, Figlin R, York M, et al. Phase III randomized study to compare interferon alfa-2a in com-

bination with fluorouracil versus fluorouracil alone in patients with advanced colorectal cancer. *J Clin Oncol* 1996; 14:2674–2681.
184. Kosmidis PA, Tsavaris N, Skarlos D, et al. Fluorouracil and leucovorin with or without interferon alfa-2b in advanced colorectal cancer: analysis of a prospective randomized phase III trial. Hellenic Cooperative Oncology Group. *J Clin Oncol* 1996; 14:2682–2687.
185. Seymour MT, Slevin ML, Kerr DJ, et al. Randomized trial assessing the addition of interferon alpha-2a to fluorouracil and leucovorin in advanced colorectal cancer. Colorectal Cancer Working Party of the United Kingdom Medical Research Council. *J Clin Oncol* 1996; 14:2280–2288.
186. Dufour P, Husseini F, Dreyfus B, et al. 5-Fluorouracil versus 5-fluorouracil plus alpha-interferon as treatment of metastatic colorectal carcinoma. A randomized study. *Ann Oncol* 1996; 7:575–579.
187. Wadler S, Wersto R, Weinberg V, Thompson D, Schwartz EL. Interaction of fluorouracil and interferon in human colon cancer cell lines: cytotoxic and cytokinetic effects. *Cancer Res* 1990; 50:5735–5739.
188. Schwartz E, Hoffman M, O'Connor CJ, Wadler S. Stimulation of 5-fluorouracil metabolic activation by interferon-α in human colon carcinoma cell lines. *Biochem Biophys Res Commun* 1992; 3:1231–1239.
189. Marsh JC, Bertino JR, Katz KH, et al. The influence of drug interval on the effect of methotrexate and fluorouracil in the treatment of advanced colorectal cancer. *J Clin Oncol* 1991; 9:371–380.
190. Van der Wilt CL, Braakhuis BJM, Pinedo HM, De Jong M, Smid K, Peters GJ. Addition of leucovorin in modulation of 5-fluorouracil with methotrexate: potentiating or reversing effect? *Int J Cancer* 1995; 61:672–678.
191. Romanini A, Li WW, Colofiore JR, Bertino JR. Leucovorin enhances cytotoxicity of trimetrexate/fluorouracil, but not methotrexate/fluorouracil, in CCRF-CEM cells. *J Natl Cancer Inst* 1992; 84:1033–1038.
192. Blijham G, Wagener T, Wils J, et al. Modulation of high-dose infusional fluorouracil by low-dose methotrexate in patients with advanced or metastatic colorectal cancer: final results of a randomized European Organization for Research and Treatment of Cancer Study. *J Clin Oncol* 1996; 14:2266–2273.
193. Sobrero A, Labianca R, Frassinetti GL, et al. Randomized comparison between methotrexate->fluorouracil and schedule-specific biochemical modulation in advanced colorectal cancer. *Proc Am Soc Clin Oncol* 1997; 16:272a(abstract).
194. Jackson RC, Fry DW, Boritzki TJ, et al. Biochemical pharmacology of the lipophilic antifolate, trimetrexate. *Adv Enzyme Regul* 1984; 22:187–206.
195. Kamen BA, Eibl B, Cashmore A, Bertino J. Uptake and efficacy of trimetrexate (TMQ, 2,4-diamino-5-methyl-6-[(3,4,5-trimethoxyanilino)methyl] quinazoline), a nonclassical antifolate in methotrexate-resistant leukemia cells in vitro. *Biochem Pharmacol* 1984; 33:1697–1699.
196. Westerhof GR, Schornagel JH, Kathmann I, Jackman AL, Rosowsky A, Forsch RA, Hynes JB, Boyle FT, Peters GJ, Pinedo HM, Jansen G. Carrier- and receptor-mediated transport of folate antagonists targeting folate-dependent enzymes: correlates of molecular structure and biological activity. *Mol Pharm* 1995; 48:459–471.
197. O'Dwyer PJ, DeLap RJ, King SA, Grillo Lopez AJ, Hoth DF, Leyland Jones B. Trimetrexate: clinical development of a nonclassical antifolate. *NCI Monogr* 1987; 105–109.
198. Leopold WR, Dykes DJ, Griswold DPJ. Therapeutic synergy of trimetrexate (CI-898) in combination with doxorubicin, vincristine, cytoxan, 6-thioguanine, cisplatin, or 5-fluorouracil against intraperitoneally implanted P388 leukemia. *NCI Monogr* 1987; 99–104.
199. Elliott WL, Howard CT, Dykes DJ, Leopold WR. Sequence and schedule-dependent synergy of trimetrexate in combination with 5-fluorouracil in vitro and in mice. *Cancer Res* 1989; 49:5586–5590.
200. Conti JA, Kemeny N, Seiter K, et al. Trial of sequential trimetrexate, fluorouracil, and high-dose leucovorin inpreviously treated patients with gastrointestinal carcinoma. *J Clin Oncol* 1994; 12:695–700.
201. Blanke CD, Kasimis BS, Schein P, Capizzi R, Kurman M. A phase II trial of trimetrexate (TMTX), 5-fluorouracil (%FU), and leucovorin (LCV) in patients with unresectable or metastatic colorectal cancer. *Proc Am Soc Clin Oncol* 1996; 15:198(abstract).
202. Kreuser ED, Szelenyi H, Hohenberger P, et al. A phase II trial of trimetrexate (TMTX), 5-fluorouracil (5-FU) and folinic acid (FA) in untreated patients with advanced colorectal carcinoma. *Eur J Cancer* 1997; 33(suppl 8):S169(abstract).
203. Van der Wilt CL, Pinedo HM, Kuiper CM, Smid K, Peters GJ. Biochemical basis for the combined

antiproliferative effect of AG337 or ZD1694 and 5-fluorouracil. *Proc Amer Assoc Cancer Res* 1995; 36:379(abstract 2260).
204. Peters GJ, Van der Wilt CL. Thymidylate synthase as a target in cancer chemotherapy. *Biochem Soc Trans* 1995; 23:884–888.
205. Smid K, Van der Wilt CL, Peters GJ. Effects of novel antifolates on the binding of 5-fluoro-2'-deoxyuridine-5'-monophosphate (FdUMP) to bacterial and human thymidylate synthase (TS). Proc. NCI-EORTC meeting. *Ann Oncol* 1996; 7(suppl 1):90(abstract 310).
206. Weichsel A, Montfort WR. Ligand-induced distortion of an active site in thymidylate synthase upon binding anticancer drug 1843U89. *Nature Structural Biol* 1995; 2:1095–1101.
207. Izzo J, Zielinski Z, Chang YM, Bertino JR. Molecular mechanisms of the synergistic sequential administration of D1694 (tomudex) followed by FUra in colon carcinoma cells. *Proc Am Assoc Cancer Res* 1995; 36:2272.
208. Chang YM, Zielinski Z, Izzo J. Pretreatment of colon carcinoma cells to D1694 (tomudex) markedly enhances 5-fluorouracil cytotoxicity. *Proc Am Assoc Cancer Res* 1994; 35:330.
209. Guimaraes MA, Greco WR, Slocum HK, Huben RP, Rustum YM. The combined-action of ICI-D1694, 5-fluoro-2'-deoxyuridine and 5-fluorouracil in inhibiting the growth of a human renal cell carcinoma cell line (RPMI-SE) *in vitro*. *Intern J Oncol* 1994; 4:137–141.
210. Cantwell BM, Harris AL. The efficacy of 5-fluorouracil in human colorectal cancer is not enhanced by thymidylate synthase inhibition with CB3717 (N10-propargyl-5,8 dideazafolic acid). *Br J Cancer* 1988; 58:189–190.
211. Schwartz GK, Kemeny N, Saltz L, Sugarman A, Danso D, Kelsen DK, Tong W, Bertino J. Phase I trial of sequential Tomudex^R (TOM) and 5-fluorouracil (5FU) in patients with advanced colorecal carcinoma. *Proc ASCO* 1997; 16:728.
212. Spiegelman S, Sawyer RC, Nayak R, Ritzi E, Stolfi RL, Martin DS. Improving the antitumor activity of 5-fluorouracil by increasing its incorporation into RNA via metabolic modulation. *Proc Natl Acad Sci USA* 1980; 77:4966–4970.
213. Nadal JC, Van Groeningen CJ, Pinedo HM, Peters GJ. Schedule-dependency of *in vivo* modulation of 5-fluorouracil by leucovorin and uridine rescue in murine colon carcinoma. *Invest New Drugs* 1989; 7:163–172.
214. Nord LD, Stolfi RL, Martin DS. Biochemical modulation of 5-fluorouracil with leucovorin or delayed uridine rescue. *Pharmacol Ther* 1992; 41:289–302.
215. Colofiore JR, Sawyer RC, Balis ME, Martin DS. Effect of uridine diphosphoglucose on levels of 5-phosphoribosyl pyrophosphate and uridine triphosphate in murine tissues. *Pharm Res* 1989; 6:863–866.
216. Leyva A, Van Groeningen CJ, Kraal I, Gall H, Peters GJ, Lankelma J, Pinedo HM. Phase I and pharmacokinetic studies of high-dose uridine intended for rescue from 5-fluorouracil toxicity. *Cancer Res* 1984; 44:5928–5933.
217. Van Groeningen CJ, Leyva A, Kraal I, Peters GJ, Pinedo HM. Clinical and pharmacokinetic study of prolonged administration of high-dose uridine intended for rescue from 5-fluorouracil toxicity. *Cancer Treatm Rep* 1986; 70:745–750.
218. Peters GJ, Van Groeningen CJ, Laurenssse E, Kraal I, Leyva A, Lankelma J, Pinedo HM. Effect of pyrimidine nucleosides on body temperature of man and rabbit in relation to pharmacokinetic data. *Pharmaceut Res* 1987; 4:113–119.
219. Van Groeningen CJ, Peters GJ, Leyva A, Laurenssse E, Pinedo HM. Reversal of 5-fluorouracil-induced myelosuppression by prolonged administration of high-dose uridine. *J Natl Cancer Inst* 1989; 81:157–162.
220. Seiter K, Kemeny N, Martin D, et al. Uridine allows dose escalation of 5-fluorouracil when given with N-phosphonacetyl-L-aspartate, methotrexate, and leucovorin. *Cancer* 1993; 71:1875–1881.
221. Schwartz GK, Christman K, Saltz L, et al. A phase I trial of a modified intensive FAMTX regimen (high dose 5-fluorouracil + doxorubicin + high dose metotrexate + leucovorin) with oral uridine rescue. *Cancer,* 1996; 78:1988–1995.
222. Bagrij T, Kralovanszky J, Gyergyay F, Kiss E, Peters GJ. Influence of uridine treatment in mice on the protection of gastrointestinal toxicity caused by 5-fluorouracil. *Anticancer Res* 1993; 13:789–794.
223. Klubes P, Leyland-Jones B. Enhancement of the antitumor activity of 5-fluorouracil by uridine rescue. *Pharmacol Ther* 1989; 41:289–302.
224. Martin DS, Stolfi RL, Sawyer RC. Use of oral uridine as a substitute for parenteral uridine rescue of

5-fluorouracil therapy, with and without the uridine phosphorylase inhibitor 5-bezylacyclouridine. *Cancer Chemother Pharmacol* 1989; 24:9–14.

225. Van Groeningen CJ, Peters GJ, Nadal JC, Laurensse EJ, Pinedo HM. Clinical and pharmacologic study of orally administered uridine. *J Natl Cancer Inst* 1991; 83:437–441.

226. Van Groeningen CJ, Peters GJ, Pinedo HM. Reversal of 5-fluorouracil-induced toxicity by oral administration of uridine. *Ann Oncology* 1993; 4:317–320.

227. Kelsen DP, Martin D, ONeil J, Schwartz G, Saltz L, Sung MT, vonBorstel R, Bertino J. Phase I trial of PN401, an oral prodrug of uridine, to prevent toxicity from fluorouracil in patients with advanced cancer. *J Clin Oncol* 1997; 15:1511–1517.

228. Pritchard M, Watson AJM, Potten CS, Jackman AL, Hickman JA. Inhibition by uridine but not thymidine of p53-dependent intstinal apoptosis initiated by 5-fluorouracil: evidence for the involvement of RNA perturbation. *Proc Natl Acad Sci USA* 1997; 94:1795–1799.

229. Van Laar JAM, Mayhew EG, Cao S, Durrani F, Peters GJ, Rustum YM. Modulation of the antitumor activity of cisplatin and/or 5-fluoro-2'-deoxyuridine by N-phosphonacetyl-L-aspartate in murine colon carcinoma #26. *Eur J Cancer* 1995; 31A:974–976.

230. Durrani FA, Cao S, Van Laar JAM, Rustum YM. Modulation of the antitumor activity of 5-fluorouracil and cisplatinum by *N*-phosphonacetyl-L-aspartate in the murine colon carcinoma #26. *Int J Oncol* 1994; 5:1065–1068.

231. Johnston PG, Geoffrey F, Drake J, Voeller D, Grem JL, Allegra CJ. The cellular interaction of 5-fluorouracil and cisplatin in a human colon carcinoma cell line. *Eur J Cancer* 1996; 32a:2148–2154.

232. Van der Wilt CL, Van Laar J, Gyergyay F, Smid K, Peters GJ. Biochemical modification of the toxicity and antitumour effect of 5-fluorouracil and cis-platinum by WR-2721 (ethiofos) in mice. *Eur J Cancer* 1992; 28A:2017–2024.

233. Van Laar JAM, Van der Wilt CL, Treskes M, Van der Vijgh WJF, Peters GJ. Chemoprotective effect of WR-2721 against toxicity induced by the combination of carboplatin and 5-fluorouracil. *Cancer Chemother Pharmacol* 1992; 31:97–102.

234. Treskes M, Boven E, Van de Loosdrecht AA, Wijffels JFAM, Cloos J, Peters GJ, Pinedo HM, Van der Vijgh WJF. Effects of the modulating agent WR2721 on myelotoxicity and antitumour activity in carboplatin-treated mice. *Eur J Cancer* 1994; 30A:183–187.

235. Scanlon KJ, Newman EM, Lu Y, Priest DG. Biochemical basis for cisplatin and 5-fluorouracil synergism in human ovarian carcinoma cells. *Proc Natl Acad Sci USA* 1986; 83:8923–8925.

236. Shirasaka T, Shimamoto Y, Ohshimo H, Saito H, Fukushima M. Metabolic basis of the synergistic antitumor activities of 5-fluorouracil and cisplatin in rodent tumor models in vivo. *Cancer Chemother Pharmacol* 1993; 32:167–172.

237. Kamano T, Mikami Y, Shirasaka T. Continuous infusion of 5-fluorouracil plus low-dose cisplatin in tumor-bearing mice. *Anti Cancer Drugs* 1997; 8:632–636.

238. Sagaster P, Essel R, Teich G, Fritz E, Wasilewski M, Umek H, Dünser U, Mascher H, Micksche M. Treatment of advanced colorectal cancer with folinic acid and 5-fluorouracil in combination with cis-platinum. *Eur J Cancer* 1994; 30A:1250–1254.

239. Al-Saraf M. Cisplatin combinations in the treatment of head and neck cancer. *Sem Oncol* 1994; 21(suppl 12):28–34.

240. Mathe G, Kidani Y, Segiguchi M, et al. Oxalato-platinum or 1-OHP, a third-generation platinum complex: an experimental and clinical appraisal and preliminary comparison with cis-platinum and carboplatinum. *Biomed Pharmacother* 1989; 43:237–250.

241. de Gramont A, Vignoud J, Tournigand C, et al. Oxaliplatin with high-dose leucovorin and 5-fluorouracil 48-hour continuous infusion in pretreated metastatic colorectal cancer. *Eur J Cancer* 1997; 33:214–219.

242. Machover D, Diaz Rubio E, de Gramont A, et al. Two consecutive phase II studies of oxaliplatin (L-OHP) for treatment of patients with advanced colorectal carcinoma who were resistant to previous treatment with fluoropyrimidines. *Ann Oncol* 1996; 7:95–98.

243. Schmoll HJ, Büchele T, Schöber C. The role of second-line chemotherapy in colorectal cancer. *Onkologie* 1997; 20:288–294.

244. Becouarn Y, Ychou M, Ducreux M, et al. Oxaliplatin (L-OHP) as first-line chemotherapy in metastatic colorectal cancer (MCRC) patients: preliminary activi/toxicity report. *Proc Am Soc Clin Oncol* 1997; 16:229a(abstract).

245. Diaz-Rubio E, Zaniboni A, Gastiaburu JJ, et al. Phase II multicentric trial of oxaliplatin (L-OHP) as

first line chemotherapy in metastatic colorectal cancer (MCRC). *Proc Am Soc Clin Oncol* 1996; 15:207(abstract).
246. Levi F, Giacchetti S, Adam R, Zidani R, Metzger G, Misset JL. Chronomodulation of chemotherapy against metastatic colorectal cancer. International Organization for Cancer Chronotherapy. *Eur J Cancer* 1995; 31A:1264–1270.
247. Levi F, Zidani R, Misset JL. Randomised multicentre trial of chronotherapy with oxaliplatin, fluorouracil, and folinic acid in metastatic colorectal cancer. International Organization for Cancer Chronotherapy. *Lancet* 1997; 350:681–686.
248. Giacchetti S, Zidani R, Perpoint B, et al. Phase III trial of 5-fluorouracil (5-FU), folinic acid (FA), with or without oxaliplatin (OXA) in previously untreated patients (pts) with metastatic colorectal cancer (MCC). *Proc Am Soc Clin Oncol* 1997; 16:229a(abstract).
249. Levi F, Giacchetti S, Adam R, Zidani R, Metzger G, Misset JL. Chronomodulation of chemotherapy against metastatic colorectal cancer. International Organization for Cancer Chronotherapy. *Eur J Cancer* 1995; 31A:1264–1270.
250. Levi FA, Zidani R, Vannetzel JM, et al. Chronomodulated versus fixed-infusion-rate delivery of ambulatorychemotherapy with oxaliplatin, fluorouracil, and folinic acid (leucovorin) inpatients with colorectal cancer metastases: a randomized multi-institutionaltrial. *J Natl Cancer Inst* 1994; 86:1608–1617.
251. Levi F, Misset JL, Brienza S, et al. A chronopharmacologic phase II clinical trial with 5-fluorouracil, folinic acid, and oxaliplatin using an ambulatory multichannel programmable pump. High antitumor effectiveness against metastatic colorectal cancer. *Cancer* 1992; 69:893–900.
252. Levi F, Dogliotti L, Perpoint B, et al. A multicenter phase II trial of intensified chronotherapy with xaliplatin (L-OHP), 5-fluorouracil (5-FU) and folinic acid (FA) in patients with previously untreated metastatic colorectal cancer (MCC). *Proc Am Soc Clin Oncol* 1997; 16:266a(abstract).
253. Bertheault Cvitkovic F, Jami A, Ithzaki M, et al. Biweekly intensified ambulatory chronomodulated chemotherapy with oxaliplatin, fluorouracil, and leucovorin in patients with metastatic colorectal cancer. *J Clin Oncol* 1996; 14:2950–2958.
254. Eng WK, Faucette L, Johnson RK, Sternglanz R. Evidence that DNA topoisomerase I is necessary for the cytotoxic effects of camptothecin. *Mol Pharmacol* 1988; 34:755–760.
255. Morris EJ, Geller HM. Induction of neuronal apoptosis by camptothecin, an inhibitor of DNA topoisomerase-I: evidence for cell cycle-independent toxicity. *J Cell Biol* 1996; 134:757–770.
256. Baserga R. The cell cycle: myths and realities. *Cancer Res* 1990; 50:6769–6771.
257. Erlichman C, Svingen PA, Mullany SA, Kaufmann SH. Synergistic interaction of SN-38 and 5FU/Leucovorin. *Proc Am Assoc Cancer Res* 1996; 37:294.
258. Mans DRA, Brondani da Rocha A, Vargas Schwartzbold C, Sschwartsmann G. Assessment of the efficacy of the irinotecan-5 fluorouracil combination in a panel of human colon carcinoma cell lines. *Proc Am Assoc Cancer Res* 1996; 37:291.
259. Houghton JA, Cheshire PJ, Hallman JDN, Lutz L, Luo X, Li Y, Houghton PJ. Evaluation of irinotecan in combination with 5-fluorouracil or itoposide in xenograft models of colon adenocarcinoma and rhabdomyosarcoma. *Clin Cancer Res* 1996; 2:107–118.
260. Guichard S, Cussac D, Hennebelle I, Bugat R, Canal P. Sequence dependent activity of the irinotican-5FU combination in human colon cancer model HT-29 in vitro and in vivo. *Int J Cancer* 1997; 73:729–734.
261. Guichard S, Hennebelle I, Bugat R, Canal P. Cellular interactions of 5-fluorouracil and the camptothecin analogue CPT-11 (irinotecan) in a human colorectal carcinoma cell line. *Biochem Pharmacol,* 1998; 55:667–676.
262. Barone C, Pozzo C, Starkhammar H, et al. CPT-11 alternating with 5-fluorouracil (5-FU)/folinic acid (FA): a multicentre phase II study in first-line chemotherapy (CT) of metastatic colorectal cancer (CRC). Preliminary results. *Proc Am Soc Clin Oncol* 1997; 16:270a(abstract).
263. Rothenberg ML, Pazdur R, Rowinsky E, et al. A phase II multicenter trial of alternating cycles of irinotecan (CPT-11) and 5-FU/LV in patients with previously untreated metastatic colorectal cancer (CRC). *Proc Am Soc Clin Oncol* 1997; 16:266a(abstract).
264. Benhammouda A, Bastian G, Rixe O, et al. A phase I and pharmacokinetic (PK) study of CPT-11 (C) and 5-FU (F) combination. *Proc Am Soc Clin Oncol* 1997; 16:202a(abstract).
265. Shimada Y, Sasaki Y, Sugano K, et al. Combination phase I study of CPT-11 (Irinotecan) combined with continous infusion of 5-fluorouracil (5-FU) in metastatic colorectal cancer. *Proc Am Soc Clin Oncol* 1993; 12:196(abstract).

266. Saltz LB, Kanowitz J, Kemeny NE, et al. Phase I clinical and pharmacokinetic study of irinotecan, fluorouracil, and leucovorin in patients with advanced solid tumors. *J Clin Oncol* 1996; 14:2959–2967.
267. Ducreux M, Rougier P, Ychou M, et al. Phase I/II study of escalating dose of CPT-11 in combination with LV5FU2 ("De Gramont" regimen) every two weeks in the treatment of colorectal cancer (CRC) after 5-FU failure. *Proc Am Soc Clin Oncol* 1997; 16:234a(abstract).
268. Vanhoefer U, Harstrick A, Müller C, et al. Phase I study of a weekly schedule of irinotecan (CPT-11) in combination with high-dose folinic acid and 5-fluorouracil as first-line chemotherapy in patients with advanced colorectal cancer. *Proc Am Soc Clin Oncol* 1997; 16:272a(abstract).

6 Raltitrexed (Tomudex™), a Highly Polyglutamatable Antifolate Thymidylate Synthase Inhibitor

Design and Preclinical Activity

Leslie R. Hughes, Trevor C. Stephens, F. Thomas Boyle, and Ann L. Jackman

CONTENTS

INTRODUCTION
CB3717: THE FIRST SPECIFIC ANTIFOLATE TS INHIBITOR
SECOND-GENERATION TS-INHIBITOR DESIGN
ZD1694—CELLULAR PHARMACOLOGY
IN VIVO PHARMACOLOGY
SUMMARY

1. INTRODUCTION

Folic acid has, over the past 50 yr, formed the basis of an enormous amount of medicinal chemistry aimed at finding improved anticancer agents. This stemmed from the discovery of aminopterin (AMT) and methotrexate (MTX) in the late 1940s. Several years after their discovery, they were shown to exert their antitumor activity via the inhibition of dihydrofolate reductase (DHFR). MTX is still widely prescribed today for the treatment of a number of solid tumors and leukemias (*see* Chapter 3). Over the last decade there has been a resurgence in the number of folic acid analogs entering clinical studies that has resulted from the knowledge that a number of key enzymic reactions in the *de novo* biosynthesis of nucleotides depend on folate cofactors. The cellular and in vivo pharmacology of MTX and some of its more recent analogs have been very well described in the literature and has formed a platform of knowledge for the development of the antifolate thymidylate synthase (TS) inhibitors over the last 20 yr (*see* Chapter 1). For example, it was shown that the cytotoxicity induced by the indirect inhibition of TS by MTX may be antagonized by its inhibitory effects on *de novo* purine synthesis *(1)*. The antipurine effects of MTX were also believed to contribute to the drug-induced gut

From: *Anticancer Drug Development Guide: Antifolate Drugs in Cancer Therapy*
Edited by: A.L. Jackman © Humana Press Inc., Totowa, NJ

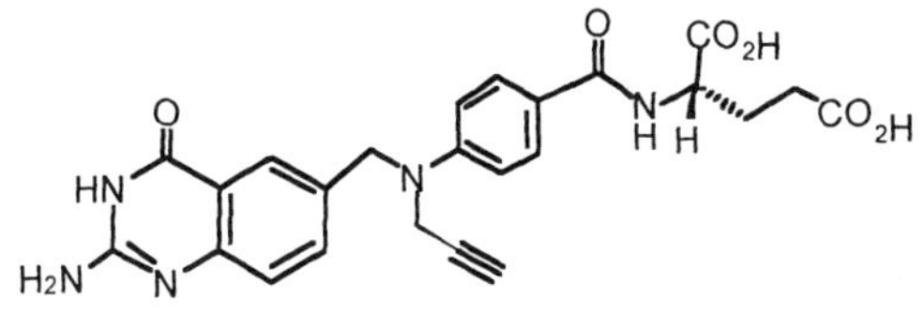

Fig. 1. Structures of CB3717 and ZD1694 (Tomudex®; Raltitrexed).

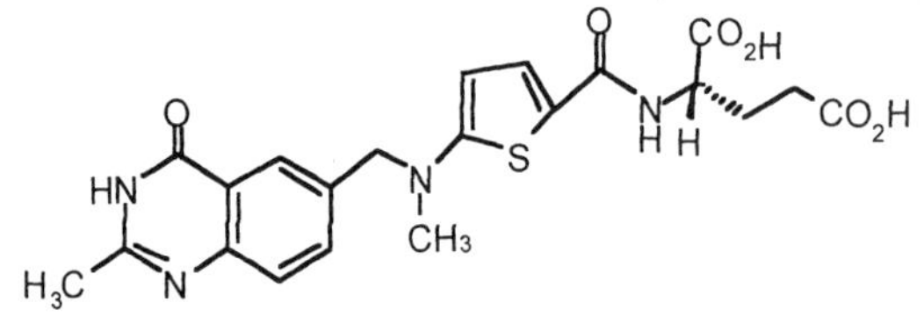

toxicity in mice *(2)*. These and other data, particularly that relating to 5-fluorouracil (5FU) metabolism and activity, argued that specific folate-based inhibitors of TS may prove to be better drugs *(3)*. Furthermore, ground-breaking research on other aspects of MTX action including drug resistance and polyglutamation substantially contributed to the acceleration of the development of TS inhibitors from basic concept through to clinical evaluation. Indeed several of the early dual inhibitors of DHFR and TS were 5,8-dideaza (quinazoline) analogs of MTX (*see* Subheading 2.1.). This chapter focuses on reviewing the medicinal chemistry path from these early compounds to the selection of Tomudex (Raltitrexed; ZD1694; Fig. 1) for clinical study. Additionally, a summary is provided of the current state of knowledge regarding the cellular and in vivo pharmacology of the drug. Readers are also advised of a recent review that may provide more detailed information on certain aspects of development *(3)*.

2. CB3717: THE FIRST SPECIFIC ANTIFOLATE TS INHIBITOR

2.1. Discovery and Preclinical Development

A range of folate-related structures have been shown to inhibit isolated TS to varying degrees. For example the 2,4-diaminopteridines, AMT and MTX, which are very potent DHFR inhibitors, are also weak inhibitors of TS *(4)*. Importantly, it was suggested that in DHFR-overproducing cells, the growth rate-limiting locus of action of high concentrations of MTX changed from DHFR to TS *(5)*. The original work of Bird et al. identified some quinazoline analogs of folic acid as potential TS inhibitors *(6, reviewed in 7)* which prompted Jones and his colleagues at the Institute of Cancer Research, UK, to investigate systematically the influence of the N^{10} substituent on TS inhibition and cytotoxicity. This work showed that the N^{10}-propargyl substituent (CB3717; Fig. 1) was optimal for inhibition of TS (K_i 1–3 nM), but that a number of other substituents were tolerated by the enzyme *(7–10)*. Although CB3717 was at least 20-fold more potent as a TS inhibitor than the original N^{10}-hydrogen compound, both compounds showed equivalent cell-growth inhibitory potency (IC$_{50}$ approx 5 µM). This was one of the first indications that the cellular pharmacology of these compounds was complex and led to refinements in the compound evaluation process that followed the discovery of CB3717.

Nevertheless, CB3717 was the most potent folate-based TS inhibitor known, had activity that was selective for TS, overcame MTX resistance caused by elevated DHFR, and showed considerable activity against a varaint tetraploid L1210 tumor in mice *(7,9,11–13)*. Preclinical mouse toxicology suggested that nephrotoxicity and possibly hepatotoxicity may be dose-limiting *(14)*.

2.2. Clinical Activity of CB3717

Several phase I/II studies were initiated in 1981 with good activity reported in solid tumors such as breast and platinum-refractory ovarian carcinomas, and hepatomas (reviewed in refs. *15,16*). Administration was by 1-h iv infusion given every three weeks. Unfortunately, sporadic nephrotoxicity, which was particularly serious when coupled with myelosuppression, curtailed further development of CB3717. Other toxicities were mainly rashes, malaise, and transient rises in liver transaminases that were self-limiting.

3. SECOND-GENERATION TS-INHIBITOR DESIGN

3.1. Rationale

The fact that the toxicities seen with CB3717 were largely confined to the liver and kidney suggested that accumulation in the excreting organs was the problem. It was known that CB3717 exhibited poor water-solubility at physiological pH and the hypothesis was advanced that this property was a contributing factor. Thus, enhanced water-solubility was considered an essential property for novel analogs. Whereas it was not certain at this stage which properties, other than TS inhibition, were responsible for the CB3717 clinical activity observed, it was decided to retain as many of the structural features of the compound as possible in any new compounds. In particular, the glutamate was seen as crucial for activity as studies were revealing the probable importance of polyglutamation in CB3717 activity *(17,18)*.

A number of options for obtaining compounds with greater water-solubility were considered: incorporating "hydrophilic water-solublizing" groupings into the molecule; making more soluble prodrugs of CB3717; and weakening of the strong intermolecular hydrogen bonds that are manifest in the crystal form by the very high melting point for CB3717. Taking these options in turn, a number of hydrophilic groups had been incorporated into the N^{10}-alkyl substituent that had either lowered TS-inhibitory potency (e.g., CH_2COOH) or not greatly enhanced solubility (e.g., $[CH_2]_3OH$) *(10)*. Whereas the addition of hydrophilic groups elsewhere in the molecule was possible, this experience with the N^{10}-substituents, as well as the fact that there were already a considerable number of hydrophilic substituents already contained in the core structure, suggested this might not be a particularly fruitful approach. The possibility of using prodrugs was ruled out as it could not circumvent the problem of parent compound excretion, only delivering slower release of the drug. Thus, it was decided to seek compounds that had lower melting points than CB3717 by virtue of decreased packing forces.

3.2. More Soluble Analogs Lacking the 2-Amino Group

Jones and colleagues believed that the polar groups at positions 1–4 of the quinazoline nucleus were capable of forming tight intermolecular hydrogen bonds which in turn would affect the crystal packing and ultimate solubility. Thus, it was decided to investi-

Table 1
In vitro Activity of 2-Desamino-2-Substituted, N^{10}-Propargyl Quinazolines

R	Inhibition of L1210 TS, IC_{50}, nM	Inhibition of L1210 cell growth, IC_{50} μM	
NH_2	20 (K_i = 3 nM)	3.4	CB3717
H	160 (K_i = 27 nM)	0.4	desamino-CB3717
CH_3	40 (K_i = 10 nM)	0.09	ICI 198583
CH_2F	100	0.37	
CF_3	570	>100	
CH_2OH	100	5.0	
OCH_3	20	2.0	
Ph	220	>100	

Examples taken from refs. *21, 22*.

gate modifications in this region of the molecule and it was found that the 2-amino could be replaced with hydrogen (desamino-CB3717) without seriously reducing TS inhibition (approx 10-fold) *(19,20)*. Surprisingly this modification resulted in an increase in TS-mediated cytotoxic potency. These results encouraged the synthesis of a range of C2-substituted analogs. A range of substituents were tolerated by the enzyme (Table 1) and only when strongly electron-withdrawing substituents, such as the trifluoromethyl, were incorporated did TS potency fall dramatically *(21,22)*. Requirements for cytotoxicity however were more stringent where large groups such as phenyl were not tolerated. In addition, compounds with similar TS potencies, for example the 2-methyl compared with 2-methoxy or 2-hydroxymethyl analogs, showed dramatically different growth inhibition IC_{50}s (0.1, 2, and 5 μM, respectively) against L1210 tumour cells under continuous exposure conditions. This differential was even more apparent in in vitro clonogenic assays using the thymidine kinase (TK) deficient L5178Y TK-/- mouse lymphoma cell line when incubation times were restricted to 4 h. Virtually no cytotoxic activity could be measured for certain compounds (e.g., C2-hydroxymethyl or C2-methoxy) at concentrations of up to 10 μM, whereas the same concentration of the C2-methyl compound inhibiting colony formation by >99.5% *(23)*. In vitro pharmacodynamic studies using a mouse L1210 cell *in situ* TS inhibition assay (^{3}H release from 5-^{3}H dUrd) demonstrated that, whereas all the compounds were capable of inhibiting TS within 4 h, only some continued to inhibit the enzyme after withdrawal of drug from the medium *(24)*, indicating that some compounds were retained (probably as polyglutamates) inside cells better than others. Supporting data for the polyglutamation hypothesis later came from direct measurement of intracellular polyglutamate metabolites of CB3717, desamino-CB3817 and the 2-desamino-2-methyl analogue (ICI 198583); and substrate activity for mouse liver FPGS *(18,20,25–27)*. Structure-activity analysis of the

Table 2
Effect of Replacement of the Para-Aminobenzoate of 2-Deasmino-2-Methyl N^{10}-Substituted Quinazolines with Thiophene or Thiazole

N^{10}	aryl ring	Inhibition of L1210 TS IC_{50}, nM	Inhibition of L1210 cell growth IC_{50}, μM	FPGS (mouse liver) K_m, μM	TK$-/-$L5178Y tumor [b](in vivo)
CH_2CCH (2-NH_2; CB717)	benzene	20	5.0	38	[c]>200
H	benzene	4500	[a]0.07	8	N.T.
CH_3	benzene	300	0.17	19	[d]>200
CH_2CH_3	benzene	170	0.27	35	[e]>200
CH_2CCH	benzene	50	0.09	43	[f]>200
H	thiazole	7100	[a]0.28	34	N.T.
CH_3	thiazole	420	0.006	0.95	approx 30
CH_2CH_3	thiazole	230	0.015	<6	25
CH_2CCH	thiazole	230	0.008	<6	250
H	thiophene	25000	[a]0.70	12	
CH_3	thiophene	670	0.009	1.3	approx 5
CH_2CH_3	thiophene	580	0.017	3.5	approx 25
CH_2CCH	thiophene	440	0.11	17	>1000

[a] Activity not completely prevented by dThd.
[b] Cultured L5178Y TK$-/-$ cells (thymidine salvage incompetent) were implanted intramuscularly into the hind legs of DBA2 mice. Compounds were administered as 2 equal ip doses 8 h apart 3 d after tumor implantation. Results are presented as the total dose (mg/kg) to give at least 3/5 cures.
[c] No activity at this dose (toxic above this).
[d] 250 mg/kg 8 hourly × 5 gave 3/5 cures.
[e] 100 mg/kg 8 hourly × 5 gave 5/5 cures.
[f] 100 mg/kg 8 hourly × 5 gave 3/5 cures.
N.T. = not tested
Some of the L1210 growth inhibition data has been updated since the original publications and represent the mean of several experiments.

effect of other N^{10}-substituents (C2-methyl) revealed a pattern of activity similar to that seen in the C2-amino series, i.e., smaller aliphatic N^{10}-substituents (e.g., hydrogen or methyl) had weaker TS inhibitory activity but no concomitant loss of growth inhibitory potency (Table 2). Furthermore, their *in situ* TS and isolated FPGS substrate activities suggested that this was because of an increased rate of their polyglutamation *(24,25,27)*.

The more highly retained/polyglutamated compounds in vitro were also those with higher antitumor activity in mice (bolus injection), particularly against the L5178Y thymidine kinase (TK)-negative tumor (unpublished data). The *in situ* TS assay was adapted for measurement of TS inhibition in ip L1210 cells removed from mice into drug-free medium at intervals after drug injection. Cells removed, for example, 2 and 12 h after injection of 250 mg/kg of the C2-methyl analog displayed a rate of ^{3}H release that was 4 and 24% of control activity, respectively. In contrast, cells removed 2 h after mice were injected with 500 mg/kg of the C2-OCH$_3$ analog had a rate comparable to controls *(28)*.

Expanded studies comparing CB3717 (2-amino) with ICI 198583 (2-methyl) confirmed that the latter was a threefold less potent TS inhibitor (K_i values = 3 and 10 nM, respectively), a comparable substrate for FPGS, but a significantly better substrate for the RFC *(26)*. The polyglutamates of both compounds were shown to be potent TS inhibitors, by 1–2 orders of magnitude, and not rapidly effluxed from cells *(18,26)*. Thus it was concluded that the faster rate of cellular, carrier-mediated uptake of ICI 198583 led, in turn, to a faster rate of polyglutamation.

As expected, desamino-CB3717 and ICI 198583 had lower melting points than CB3717, were considerably more soluble at physiological pH (at least 100-fold) and did not induce toxicity to the kidney or liver of mice at the highest dose administered (500 mg/kg) *(28)*. Furthermore, ICI 198583 was much more potent in inhibiting the growth of *in vivo* mouse tumors *(23,26)*. Parenthetically, the early results showing rapid plasma clearance of the CB3717 analogs (half-life of approx 20 min compared with 90 min for CB3717) caused some concern for their likely efficacy by bolus administration. However the emerging picture of in vivo activity and retention of polyglutamate derivatives inside tumor cells in vitro and in vivo soon led to confidence in the analog approach. Although it was appreciated that, and indeed later exploited (*see* Chapter X), continuous administration of non- or poorly polyglutamatable compounds could still provide the desired efficacy. However, a decision was made to design a highly polyglutamatable drug to be administered by bolus (or short-infusion) for clinical evaluation. The possibility also existed that some tumors may express relatively high levels of FPGS, contributing to the therapeutic efficacy of classical antifolates such as MTX *(29,30)*.

3.3. Modifications to ICI 198583

3.3.1. RATIONALE

Further chemistry involving removal of the N1 nitrogen from ICI 198583 resulted in a large reduction in TS potency as did replacement of the N3 nitrogen and C4 carbonyl *(31)*. Thus, with the exception of the C2-position, modifications of the hydrogen-bonding groups in the quinazoline ring resulted in compounds with poor activity in cells. With this knowledge, ICI 198583 was used as a starting point for further modifications. The target was a range of structurally diverse compounds that were, at least as potent as ICI 198583 as cytotoxic agents both in short and continuous exposure assays; and had antitumor activity in the L5178K TK−/− tumor by single-bolus injection. Although potent inhibition of isolated TS was not required, proof of specific, TS-mediated cytotoxicity was essential. Indeed, because an almost inverse relationship was observed between isolated TS-inhibitory and FPGS-substrate activity *(27)*, traditional enzyme inhibition-based structure-activity studies in isolation were considered particularly inappropriate.

3.3.2. PABA Ring Substitution

One synthetic avenue pursued was the addition of fluorine to the phenyl ring. Variable results in terms of inhibition of TS and cell growth through polyglutamation were obtained and are detailed elsewhere *(32–34)*. In brief, enhanced activity was observed with the 2'F or 2',6'-difluoro analogs of ICI 198583 although introduction of the fluorine in other positions gave reduced TS inhibition but often potent growth inhibition (e.g., 2',5'diF). Similarly, varying the N^{10}-substituents could also give this reversed pattern of activity. Later studies indicated, as might have been predicted, that differences in polyglutamation potential were responsible *(35)*.

3.3.3. PABA Heterocyclic Replacements

A variety of heterocycles were tolerated in terms of TS-mediated growth inhibition but the 2,5 substituted thiophenes and the 2,5 substituted thiazoles proved particularly interesting (Table 2). Compared with the equivalent compounds in the benzene series, the N^{10}-methyl and ethyl analogs displayed similar TS-inhibitory activity but the N^{10}-propargyl compounds were relatively weaker *(27,36)*. In fact the nature of the aliphatic substituent in the heterocyclic series was not critical for TS inhibition. Of particular note was the observation that, with the exception of the N^{10}-propargyl thiophene, the N^{10}-substituted heterocyclic compounds were approx 10-fold more potent inhibitors of cell growth than their benzene counterparts. Importantly, all the N^{10}-methyl and ethyl compounds, and the propargyl thiazole, were extremely potent in the L5178Y TK−/− 4 h clonogenic assay (>99% inhibition of colony formation at 1 μM). For comparison, ICI 198583 and CB3717 gave approx 90% and no inhibition, respectively. When tested against the same tumor in mice the N^{10}-methyl and ethyl compounds were significantly more potent than CB3717 and ICI 198583 (Table 2). These and other studies were beginning to suggest that these compounds were being very well polyglutamated and later supported by studies carried out by R. Moran who demonstrated their high first-order rate constants for mouse liver FPGS (Table 2) *(3,27)*. These discoveries were of immense importance and complementary in vitro and in vivo evaluation confirmed their high degree of cytotoxic potency in both short- and continuous-exposure assays *(27,35)*. Although cytotoxic potency *per se* was not considered a prerequisite for compound selection, it indicated a high dependence on FPGS for activity that may offer some advantage in tumors expressing high levels of FPGS. A more practical consideration was the threshold level of potency that would allow activity to be expressed in human tumor xenografts and toxicity in the host mouse. The use of the L5178Y TK-mutant mouse lymphoma in vivo had circumvented the problem of the unusually high level of salvagable thymidine present in rodent plasma but a wide range of such mutants were not available in human tumor xenografts. This meant that high compound concentrations in repeat injection schedules (typically up to 300 mg/kg daily × 14 for even the most potent cytotoxic compounds) were required to obtain therapeutic ratios. Thus the ability to progress low-potency compounds in vivo was limited simply because they could not be solubilized in volumes of aqueous injection vehicle suitable for administration to mice.

3.3.4. Selection of Candidate Compounds

Compounds were selected for further study that satisfied the following criteria: potent in vitro activity exclusively via TS inhibition with evidence of metabolism to polyglutamates; potent in vivo activity in the intramuscular L5178Y TK−/− lymphoma, typically less than 25 mg/kg (split into 2 doses 8 h apart); and TS inhibition in the L1210 tumor grown in vivo that was sustained after plasma levels declined to very low levels (typically 12–24 h). These compounds were tested in two further in vivo evaluation systems,

Table 3
In Vivo Activity of Some of the "Short-Listed" Compounds

N_{10} aryl ring	CH_3 thiophene	CH_2CH_3 thiophene	CH_3 thiazole	CH_2CH_3 thiazole	CH_2CH_3 2'F-benzoyl
L5178Y TK+/− active dose[a]	6.6	90	72	110	120
15% body-weight loss dose[b]	8.0	400	8	130	200
therapeutic ratio[c]	1.2	4.4	0.1	1.2	1.7
HX62 ovarian tumour xenograft[d]	1	approx 20	approx 20	<10	10

[a] Activity end point was dose (mg/kg/d) giving 5 d of growth delay.
[b] Dose (mg/kg/d) giving rise to 15% loss in body weight relative to the weight at the start of the dosing period.
[c] Therapeutic ratio = (weight loss dose) ÷ (antitumor dose).
[d] Dose (mg/kg/d) to give 15 d growth delay.

first the L5178Y thymidine-salvage-competent (TK+/−) tumor grown in the gastrocnemius muscle of DBA2 mice in which daily or twice daily × 5d injections were necessary to give activity, and secondly, in nontumor-bearing mice of the same strain. This allowed a therapeutic ratio to be generated using weight loss as a marker of toxicity (resulting from small intestinal damage) (Table 3). Of the compounds of interest, the N^{10}-methyl thiazole showed a very poor therapeutic ratio (approx 0.1) and was not progressed further.

Four compounds, which had already shown interesting activity in the HX62 human ovarian tumor xenograft (Table 3), were progressed to further detailed in vivo evaluation including testing against a panel of human tumor xenografts—the N^{10}-ethyl, 2'F-benzene, the N^{10}-ethyl thiazole, and the N^{10}-methyl (ZD1694) and ethyl thiophenes. ZD1694 was generally the most potent compound in both the L5178Y TK+/− tumor and the xenografts, and importantly displayed a wide spectrum of antitumor activity against the xenograft panel (two ovarian, two colon, and two small-cell lung carcinomas [SCLC]), albeit generally at high doses (because of high plasma dThd in host mouse). Effective doses (to give a 15-d growth delay) ranged from 1 mg/kg/d × 14 d (HX62 ovarian) to 100 mg/kg/d (N592 SCLC) *(37)*. More recent data has demonstrated the suspected lack of correlation between tumor sensitivity in vitro and in vivo *(3)*. The evaluation of TS inhibitors in rodents remains a major problem.

3.3.5. ZD1694, A Clinical Development Compound

Based on the above analysis, ZD1694 was chosen for clinical development. In mice, liver toxicity was only seen at doses of 1000 mg/kg (single dose) and no nephrotoxicity was observed at either 500 mg/kg or by repeat bolus injection (250 mg/kg/wk × 6wk) *(38,39)*. This compares with an effective single bolus dose of 10 mg/kg against the L5178Y TK−/− tumor *(40)*. On repeat daily × 5 bolus administration (10 mg/kg/d) toxicities observed were a reduction in neutrophils and approx 15% weight loss (DBA2 or DBA2/C57 mice) because of some damage to the small intestinal mucosa *(40,* reviewed in *3)*. These toxicities were largely prevented by coadministration of dThd. The same repeat bolus injection schedule cured approx 60% of mice bearing the L5178Y TK+/− tumor *(41)*.

ZD1694 is a compound with considerably reduced non-TS-related toxicities in mice and the improved water-solubility clearly circumvented the nephrotoxicity of CB3717. Plasma pharmacokinetics demonstrated a rapid plasma clearance of ZD1694 (β-half life of 30 min in mice with a more prolonged terminal half life) *(42)*, but rapid uptake and polyglutamation in tissues accounted for its antitumor activity by single or infrequent bolus administration (*see* below). Regulatory studies in dogs (a species with plasma dThd levels similar to man) suggested that a safe starting dose for a phase I clinical study would be 0.1 mg/m² given by 15-min infusion every three weeks. The first clinical study with Tomudex began in 1991 and Chapter 7 reports its progress from phase I and II studies, through randomized phase III studies in colorectal cancer, to registration in several countries for the palliative treatment for advanced colorectal cancer.

4. ZD1694—CELLULAR PHARMACOLOGY
4.1. Enzymology and Cytotoxicity
4.1.1. TS AND DHFR INHIBITION

ZD1694 is a mixed, noncompetitive inhibitor of both mouse and human TS with a K_i of 60–90 nM *(43,44)*. However, addition of a second glutamate increases this inhibition by an order of magnitude and further addition to give even higher-chain-length polyglutamates gives increasing smaller enhancements. The K_i for the tetraglutamate, a major intracellular metabolite (*see* below in this subheading), is approx 1 nM.

Recent X-ray structural data of the ternary enzyme complex data generated by the laboratories of R.M. Stroud (University of California, San Francisco) with ZD1694 bound to *E. coli* TS was used to confirm that, like CB3717, the quinazolinone and the pyrimidine ring of ZD1694 are held in a close stacking interaction. The quinazolinone, is also held by a series of specific hydrogen bonds to residues in the protein (Fig. 2A,B) and is partially folded with the thiophene PABA isostere inclined at an angle of 65° to the quinazolinone. The more open geometry of the thiophene forces the γ-carboxylic acid (rather than the α in CB3717) of the glutamic acid to bind through water to Lys-50. This somewhat less ordered fit probably accounts for the worse enzyme inhibition of ZD1694.

ZD1694 is a weak inhibitor (K_i for rat liver = 93 nM) of DHFR relative to the usual antifolate inhibitors of this enzyme (typically 0.01 nM). Furthermore, the ZD1694 polyglutamates bind to DHFR similarly, which is in contrast with their effects on TS *(43)*. Experimental data such as dThd protection studies suggested that the growth-rate-limiting event in cells treated with ZD1694 was TS inhibition *(43)*.

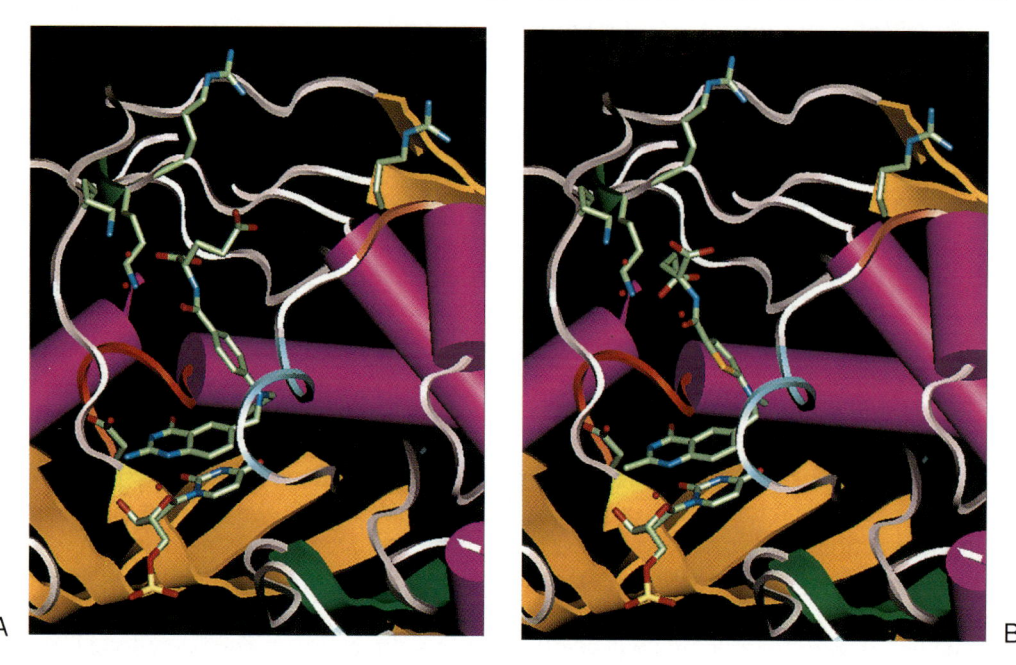

Fig. 2. Computer graphics model of CB3717 (**A**) and ZD1694 (**B**) in the active site of *E. coli* TS using ternary enzyme complex X-ray crystallography data generated by the laboratories of Prof. Stroud (University of California, San Francisco).

4.1.2. FPGS and RFC Substrate Activity and Intracellular Polyglutamation

ZD1694 is an excellent substrate for FPGS with a K_m for mouse liver FPGS of 1.3 μM (mono to diglutamate) which compares with approx 40 μM for CB3717 *(27,43)*. Furthermore the first-order rate constant (V_{max}/K_m) is approx 100 times higher than that of CB3717. Coupled with the more rapid uptake of ZD1694 via the RFC (K_m approx 2 compared with approx 40 μM) this leads to an extremely rapid rate of polyglutamation in the cell. This was confirmed by direct polyglutamate analysis using HPLC coupled with radiochemical detection *(43,45,46)*. The preferred polyglutamate forms, depending on cell lines examined, are tri-pentaglutamates, whereas the parent drug is usually found at insignificant concentrations (approx 2–10% of total drug pool).

4.1.3. Cytotoxicity and Resistance

The properties described above confer a high degree of cytotoxic potency upon ZD1694, provided FPGS is present in the cell to convert the relatively weak TS inhibition of the parent drug into the highly potent inhibition of the polyglutamate forms. Tumor cells that express reduced levels of FPGS, or possess a mutated enzyme, are resistant to ZD1694 *(47–50)*. Recently, some human tumor ovarian cells lines have been identified that intrinsically express a lower amount of FPGS RNA, which appears to confer some resistance upon these lines when compared with ovarian lines that express slightly higher amounts *(51)*. Generally the FPGS levels in ovarian cell lines are lower than those of colon cell lines which explains, in part, the lower sensitivity of ovarian cells to the drug.

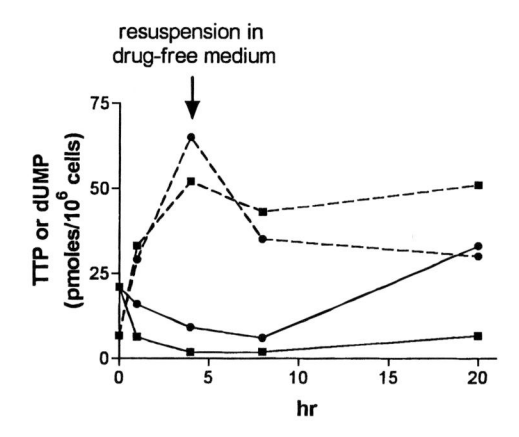

Fig. 3. Effect of dose of ZD1694 and time of exposure on TTP (—) and "dUMP" (– –) pools in L1210 mouse leukemia cells and the effect of resuspension in drug-free medium. L1210 cells were incubated with 0.1 μM (●) or 0.5 μM (■) ZD1694. TTP and dUMP were measured by immunoassay. Immunoreactive dUMP includes dUTP and dUMP.

The RFC is also essential to the potent activity of ZD1694 and cell lines with reduced or absent expression of this cell membrane carrier protein are resistant to the drug *(43,47,52)*.

Typically growth inhibition, or clonogenic IC$_{50}$ values for ZD1694 are about 1–10 nM for a 24 h exposure or longer. Smith et al. confirmed this high cytotoxicity in the human colon WiDr cell line where as little as 40 nM ZD1694 gave three decades of cell kill *(53)*. Cells do not need to be exposed continually to ZD1694 because the polyglutamates are not easily effluxed from the cells. In fact this metabolism is so rapid that L1210 cells exposed for 4 h gave an IC$_{50}$ for growth inhibition only one order of magnitude higher than for continuous exposure *(54)*. Similarly, a high degree of mouse L5178Y lymphoma cell kill was observed, with 4 h exposure to 0.1 μM ZD1694 inhibiting colony formation by 99.99% *(55)*.

4.2. Pharmacodynamics

Inhibition of TS by ZD1694 (polyglutamates) leads to a dose-dependent depletion of TTP and a concomitant elevation of dUMP (and dUTP) inside cells (Fig. 3) *(56,57)*. Similar results were seen in human W1L2 lymphoblastoid cells treated with 5–500 nM of ZD1694; dUMP/TTP ratios rose from 0.1 (pretreatment) to 150 (500 nM) *(56)*. These pool disturbances did not recover immediately after extracellular withdrawal of the drug as expected from the polyglutamate retention described above (Fig. 2). The relative contributions of TTP depletion and dUTP misincorporation into DNA to cytotoxicity are discussed in Chapter X. The concomitant elevation of deoxyuridine (dUrd) with dUMP elevation serves as a useful plasma pharmacodynamic marker for TS inhibition in vivo (*see* Chapter 20).

4.3. Cytotoxicity Reversal Studies

Thymidine reverses the cytotoxic effects of ZD1694 because thymidine kinase can activate this nucleoside to thymidylate, thereby circumventing any drug-induced TS in-

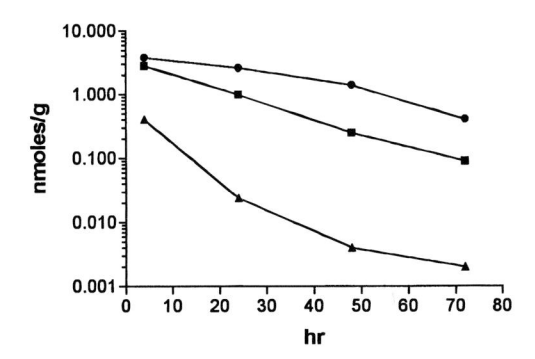

Fig. 4. Tissue drug levels after a single 10 mg/kg ip injection of ZD1694. ZD1694 levels were measured in plasma (▲), and total immunoreactive drug (parent drug + polyglutamates) was measured in liver (●), and intramuscular tumor (L5178Y TK−/−) (■).

hibition. The manner in which leucovorin (LV) reverses drug activity is both dose- and time-dependent *(43,45,54)*. This is because LV competes with ZD1694 for uptake and then for polyglutamation (probably as a result of reduced-folate pool expansion). Data suggests that LV is poorly effective at reversing ZD1694 cytotoxicity once ZD1694 polyglutamates are formed. Folic acid, because it is a weak substrate for the RFC and slow to form intracellular reduced-folate metabolites, can only partially reverse cytotoxicity when given to cells at high concentrations *(58)*.

5. IN VIVO PHARMACOLOGY

5.1. Plasma and Tissue Levels in Mice and Dogs

Two plasma elimination phases have been measured for ZD1694 (100 mg/kg ip) in mice using reversed-phase HPLC, a rapid phase of approx 0.5 h followed by a slower phase of approx 3.5 h *(42)*. Recently, a more sensitive radioimmunoassay has measured drug in the plasma 24 h after injection of 1, 10, and 100 mg/kg (5, 7, and 31 n*M*, respectively). After the highest dose, drug was still detected after 7 d (1 n*M*) *(59)*. This assay was adapted to measure total tissue ZD1694 levels including polyglutamates and relied on the cross-reactivity of the antisera to all the polyglutamate forms. Levels in the liver, kidney, and small gut epithelium exceeded those in the plasma by approx 400-, 60-, and 40-fold respectively 24 h after injection of 1 or 10 mg/kg ZD1694. Similar ratios were observed at 100 mg/kg and could still be detected in the liver and kidney 7 d later (0.15 and 0.1 nmol/g giving tissue/plasma ratios of approx 100).

The L5178Y TK-/- intramuscular tumor model was used to estimate drug accumulation relative to plasma and normal tissues. Tumor levels were 50–60 times higher than the plasma 24 and 48 h after ip bolus injection of a curative dose of 10 mg/kg ZD1694 (Fig. 4) *(60)*. These tumor levels were approx 1 and 0.25 nmol/g respectively, and similar to the normal tissue levels described above. Although not directly comparable, it is interesting that the 24 h tumor drug level is of the same order as the intracellular level found in a range of tissue-culture cells after 4- and 24-h incubation with 0.1 μ*M* tritiated ZD1694 *(61,* unpublished data). This concentration of ZD1694 is highly cytotoxic (*see* Subheading 4.1.3.).

Limited studies in dogs has confirmed a similar pattern of elimination in plasma and tissues *(59)*. Plasma levels of approx 1 nM was measured even 28 d after administration of 0.2 mg/kg. Liver and kidney levels were consistently two orders of magnitude higher than the plasma throughout the study. Levels in the gastrointestinal tissues (duodenum, jejunum, and colon) were less but still exceeded the plasma by approx 10-fold.

5.2. Polyglutamation in Mouse Tissues

The high tissue/plasma ratios described above are caused by the formation and retention of ZD1694 polyglutamates. Tritiated ZD1694 was administered to mice at a dose of 5 mg/kg and tissue levels were measured 24 h later by HPLC coupled with radiochemical detection *(61)*. Tissue/plasma total drug ratios were approx 50–100 (liver, kidney, and small intestinal epithelium) and approx 80% of the drug in the tissues was as polglutamates (di-hexaglutamates). Consistent with FPGS being expressed in liver, and tissues with a high proliferation rate, very little drug was found in the gastrocnemius muscle.

5.3. Pharmacodynamics

Pharmacodynamic markers of biological response in vivo are useful in translational research as a number of assumptions have to be made when comparing in vitro, in vivo, and clinical data. Furthermore, limitations in the usefulness of tumor models, particularly with regard to TS inhibitors (described in Subheading 3.3.3.), underscores the need for some pharmacodynamic indications of biological effect.

5.3.1. In Situ TS Assay in the Mouse L1210 Tumor

Mice bearing the ascitic L1210 tumor model were injected with an iv dose of ZD1694 *(43)*. At varying times, tumor was removed and incubated in a dThd-free medium with 5-^{3}H-deoxyuridine and hence the rate of TS activity was indirectly estimated. A dose of 1 mg/kg inhibited the flux through TS approx 90 and 75%, 2 and 12 h after injection, respectively, and 5 or 10 mg/kg inhibited it approx 80% for at least 24 h. This is a tumor capable of salvaging dThd and therefore its growth is not affected by drug administration.

5.3.2. TTP Pools in Mouse L5178Y TK-/- Tumor

The L5178Y TK-/- mouse lymphoma is thymidine-salvage incompetent and consequently when implanted into mice is highly sensitive to single injections of ZD1694. Although the *in situ* TS assay cannot be used in this model (unable to convert dUrd to dUMP) it may be used to measure TTP depletion. Preliminary measurements of tumor TTP concentrations after a curative single ip injection of 10 mg/kg ZD1694 indicated a significant reduction at 4 h (16% of control), some recovery by 24 h and complete recovery by 48 h *(60)*.

5.3.3. Plasma Deoxyuridine Levels in Mice

The pharmacodynamic markers of TS inhibition described above are not ammenable to routine measurement, particularly in humans. However, the detection of deoxyuridine (dUrd) in the plasma has been of some value. This nucleoside effluxes from cells following build up of dUMP when TS is inhibited. The main source of the dUrd is probably the normal proliferating tissues such as bone marrow and gut, so that plasma levels of this nucleoside are used as a surrogate marker of the duration of biological effect in the normal tissues which may be similar in the tumor. Plasma dUrd was first used to monitor effects following CB3717 treatment in mice and humans *(62,63)* and has recently been applied to the phase I studies with Thymitaq (AG337) *(64)*. A threefold increase in the level of plasma dUrd was found in the plasma of nontumor-bearing mice 6 and 24 h after injection of 5 mg/kg ZD1694 consistent with prolonged TS inhibition *(65, unpublished data)*. Following a course of 5 daily injections the level rose approx fivefold but returned to pretreatment levels 7 d later (intermediate time points not measured).

5.4. Protection and Reversal Studies

The selective protection or rescue of normal proliferating tissues from the cytotoxic effects of antifolates has been an intellectually exciting but challenging area, yet the original expectations from this approach have not entirely been fullfilled. However, high-dose MTX with leucovorin (LV) rescue has found a place in some clinical protocols (*see* Chapter 3). The mechanisms by which LV effects this rescue may be several including competition for MTX uptake and restoration of the reduced-folate cofactor pool. The in vitro studies described above suggested that LV may need to be administered with, or very soon after ZD1694, as once the polyglutamates were formed, LV seemed to have little effect. The most obvious reversal agent for ZD1694 was dThd, although no argument for selectivity was obvious. In vitro, dThd could be given up until the time of the induction of an irreversible cytotoxic event, e.g., DNA damage and induction of apoptosis, which could be several hours after the drug was added. However, it was recognized that in vivo: drug pharmacokinetics, distribution, and metabolism is more complex; the expression of folate-metabolizing enzymes may differ between normal and tumor tissues; and tissue proliferation kinetics is complex. Thus a number of experiments were conducted in vivo.

5.4.1. COADMINISTRATION OF LV OR DTHD WITH ZD1694

The antitumor activity of ZD1694 in L1210:ICR tumor-bearing mice (10 mg/kg daily × 5) was partly or fully prevented by coadministration of 2 and 20 mg/kg LV, respectively *(43)*. This is consistent with the prevention of drug uptake and polyglutamation observed in vitro. More recent data, using the L7178Y TK+/− tumor model, suggests that a lower dose of LV may reduce the degree of drug-induced weight loss without compromising the antitumor activity and this will be investigated further. Following the report from Smith et al. that oral folic acid selectively prevented the gastrointestinal toxicity induced by the TS inhibitor 1843U89, and to a lesser extent that induced by ZD1694 *(66)*, similar studies were conducted in our laboratories. A daily oral dose of 300 mg/kg folic acid given 1 h prior to five daily ip doses of ZD1694 (10 mg/kg) prevented both drug-induced weight loss and antitumor activity (L5178Y +/−) *(58)*. The effect of lower doses of folic acid are under investigation.

In the L1210:ICR tumor model described above, dThd (500 mg/kg 3 times a day × 8 d) prevented the antitumor activity and toxicity of ZD1694.

5.4.2. DELAYED RESCUE OF ZD1694-INDUCED TOXICITY

Balb/c mice are particularly vulnerable to ZD1694-induced gastrointestinal toxicity and were therefore used to monitor the effects of the delayed administration of either LV or dThd *(67)*. Rescue agents were commenced 24 h after completion of a 4-d course of ZD1694 (100 mg/kg/d) and were continued for several days thereafter. LV (30 or 200 mg/kg twice daily) or dThd (500 mg/kg thrice daily) generally prevented further severe weight loss and mice recovered faster (weight gain and histopathological improvement of the small gut). LV-treated mice consistently had a lower concentration of ZD1694 (polyglutamates) in the small intestinal epithelium and plasma *(68)*. The high dose and frequency of administration of ZD1694 required to induce toxicity and the rapid recovery of weight once recovery is initiated in mice not receiving rescue agents limits the direct translation of rescue protocols to the clinic. Nevertheless this work led to the recommendation that LV rescue should only be considered for the occasional patient with severe ZD1694 toxicity to avoid compromising antitumor activity.

6. SUMMARY

The process leading to the identification of ZD1694 for clinical study evolved continually as more was learned about the biochemistry and pharmacology of representative compounds. ZD1694 (Tomudex™; Raltitrexed) is the first specific, antifolate TS inhibitor to be licensed for the treatment of cancer (advanced colorectal cancer). Tomudex is a classical antifolate in that it uses carrier-mediated cellular uptake mechanism(s) (RFC) and is a substrate for FPGS. Polyglutamation is of major pharmacological importance because the polyglutamates are more potent TS inhibitors than the parent drug and are retained inside cells for prolonged periods. The latter property has lent itself to a convenient, infrequent clinical dosing regimen (15 min infusion three weekly). Preclinical research with Tomudex continues. This is aimed at increasing our understanding of the drug's action; the reasons for its selectivity in certain tumor types, its pharmacodymamic properties, its activity in combinations with other drugs, and the mechanisms involved in induction of apoptosis and the influence of the expression of certain oncogenes and tumor-suppressor genes. Many of these issues are covered in following chapters in this volume.

REFERENCES

1. Borsa J, Whitmore GF. Cell killing studies on the mode of action of methotrexate on L cells in vitro. *Cancer Res* 1969; 29:737–744.
2. Harrap KR, Taylor GA, Browman GP. Enhancement of the therapeutic effectiveness of methotrexate and protection of normal proliferating tissues with purines and pyrimidines. *Chem-Biol Interactions* 1977; 18:119–128.
3. Jackman AL, Boyle FT, Harrap KR. Tomudex (ZD1694): from concept to care, a programme in rational drug discovery. *Inv. New Drugs,* in press.
4. Harrap KR, Hill BT, Furness ME, Hart LI. Sites of action of amethopterin: intrinsic and acquired resistance. *Ann NY Acad Sci* 1971; 186:312–324.
5. Jackson RC, Niethammer D. Acquired methotrexate resistance in lymphoblasts resulting from altered kinetic properties of dihydrofolate reductase. *Eur J Cancer* 1977; 13:567.
6. Bird OD, Vaitkus JW, Clarke J, 2-amino-4-hydroxyquinazolines as inhibitors of thymidylate synthetase. *Mol Pharmacol* 1970; 6:573–575.
7. Jackman AL, Jones TR, Calvert AH. Thymidylate synthase inhibitors: experimental and clinical aspects, in *Experimental and Clinical Progress in Cancer Chemotherapy* (Muggia FM, ed.). Martinus Nijhoff, Boston, 1985, pp. 155–210.
8. Calvert AH, Jones TR, Jackman AL, Brown SJ, Harrap KR. An approach to the design of antimetabolites active against cells resistant to conventional agents illustrated by quinazoline antifolates with N^{10}-

substitutions, in. *Advances in Tumour Prevention, Detection and Characterisation* vol 5 (Davis W, Harrap KR, eds.) Excerpta Medica, Amsterdam, 1980, pp. 272–283.

9. Jones TR, Calvert AH, Jackman AL, Brown SJ, Jones M, Harrap KR, A potent antitumour quinazoline inhibitor of thymidylate synthetase: synthesis, biological properties and therapeutic results in mice. *Eur J Cancer* 1981; 17:11–19.
10. Jones TR, Calvert AH, Jackman AL, Eakin MA, Smithers MJ, Betteridge RF, Newell DR, Hayter AJ, Stocker A, Harland SJ, Davies LC, Harrap KR. Quinazoline antifolates inhibiting thymidylate synthase: variation of the N^{10} substituent. *J Med Chem* 1985; 28:1468–1476.
11. Jackson RC, Jackman AL, Calvert AH. Biochemical effects of the quinazoline inhibitor of thymidylate synthetase, CB3717, on human lymphoblastoid cells. *Biochem Pharmacol* 1983; 32:3783–3790.
12. Diddens H, Niethammer D, and Jackson RC. Patterns of cross-resistance to the antifolate drugs trimetrexate, metoprine, homofolate, and CB3717 in human lymphoma and osteosarcoma cells resistant to methotexate. *Cancer Res* 1983; 43:5286–5292.
13. Cheng Y-C, Dutschman GE, Starnes MC, Fisher MH, Nanavathi NT, Nair MG. Activity of the new antifolate N^{10}-propargyl-5,8-dideazfolate and its polyglutamates against human dihydrofolate reductase, human thymidylate synthase and KB cells containing different levels of dihydrofolate reductase. *Cancer Res* 1985; 45:598–600.
14. Jackman A. Folate-based inhibitors of thymidyate synthase as potential anticancer agents, Ph.D. thesis, University of London, 1986.
15. Clarke, SJ, Jackman AL, Judson IR. The history of the development and clinical use of CB3717 and ICI D1694. in (Rustum Y, ed.) Proc. of the International Symposium on Novel Approaches to Selective Treatments of Human Solid Tumours. *Adv. Exptl. Med. Biol.* Vol 339: Plenum, New York, 1993, pp. 277–287.
16. Jackman AL, Calvert AH. Folate-based thymidylate synthase inhibitors as anticancer drugs. *Ann Oncol* 1995; 6:871–881.
17. Moran RG, Colman PD, Rosowsky A, Forsch RA, Chan KK. Structural features of 4-amino folates required for substrate activity with mammalian folylpolyglutamate synthetase. *Mol Pharmacol* 1985; 27:156–166.
18. Sikora E, Jackman AL, Newell DR, Calvert AH. Formation and retention and biological activity of N^{10}-propargyl-5,8-dideazafolic acid (CB3717) polyglutamates in L1210 cells *in vitro*. *Biochem Pharmacol* 1988; 37:4047–4054.
19. Jones TR, Thornton TJ, Flinn A, Jackman AL, Newell DR, Calvert AH. Quinazoline antifolates inhibiting thymidylate synthase: 2-desamino derivatives with enhanced solubility and potency. *J Med Chem* 1989; 32:847–852.
20. Jackman AL, Taylor GA, O'Connor BM, Bishop JA, Moran RG, Calvert AH. Activity of the thymidylate synthase inhibitor 2-desamino-N^{10}-propargyl-5,8-dideazafolic acid and related compounds in murine (L1210) and human (W1L2) systems *in vitro* and in L1210 *in vivo*. *Cancer Res* 1990; 50:5212–5218.
21. Hughes LR, Jackman AL, Oldfield J, Smith RC, Burrows KD, Marsham PR, Bishop JAM, Jones TR, O'Connor BM, Calvert AH. Quinazoline antifolate thymidylate synthase inhibitors: alkyl, substituted alkyl, and aryl substituents in the C2 position. *J Med Chem* 1990; 33:3060–3067.
22. Marsham PR, Chambers P, Hayter AJ, Hughes CR, Jackman AL, O'Connor BM, Bishop JAM, Calvert AH. Quinazoline antifolate thymidylate synthase inhibitions: nitrogen, oxygen, sulfur and chlorine substituents in the C2 position. *J Med Chem* 1989; 32:569–575.
23. Stephens TC, Calvete JA, Janes D, Hughes LR, Jackman AL, Calvert AH. Assessment of quinazoline thymidylate synthase inhibitors using a thymidine kinase deficient cell line (L5178Y TK-/-). *Proc Am Ass Cancer Res* 1989; 30:477.
24. Taylor GA, Jackman AL, Balmanno K, Hughes LR, and Calvert AH. Estimation of the *in vitro* and *in vivo* inhibitory effects of antifolates upon thymidylate synthase in whole cells, In: (Mikanagi K, Nifhioka K, Kelley WN, eds.) *Purine Metabolism in Man* vol. 6. Plenum, New York; 1989, pp. 383–388.
25. Moran RG, Colman PD, Jones TR. Relative substrate activities of structurally related pteridine, quinazoline, and pyrimidine analogs for mouse liver folylpolyglutamate synthetase. *Mol Pharmacol* 1990; 36:736–743.
26. Jackman AL, Newell DR, Gibson W, Jodrell DI, Taylor GA, Bishop JA, Hughes LR, Calvert AH. The biochemical pharmacology of the thymidylate synthase inhibitor, 2-desamino-2-methyl-N^{10}-propargyl-5,8-dideazafolic acid (ICI 198583). *Biochem Pharmacol* 1991; 42:1885–1895.

27. Jackman AL, Marsham PR, Moran RG, Kimbell R, O'Connor BM, Hughes LR, Calvert AH. Thymidylate synthase inhibitors: the *in vitro* activity of a series of heterocyclic benzoyl ring modified 2-desamino-2-methyl-N^{10}-substituted-5,8-dideazafolates. *Adv Enz Regul* 1991; 31:13–27.
28. Harrap KR, Jackman AL, Newell DR, Taylor GA, Hughes LR, Calvert AH. Thymidylate synthase, a target for anticancer drug design, in *Advances in Enzyme Regulation* vol 29 (Weber G, ed.) Pergamon, New York, 1989, pp. 161–179.
29. Chabner BA, Allegra CJ, Curt GA, Clendenin NJ, Baram J, Koizumi S, Drake JC, Jolivet J. Polyglutamation of methotrexate. *J Clin Invest* 1985; 76:907–912.
30. Poser RG, Sirotnak FM, Chello PL. Differential synthesis of methotrexate polyglutamates in normal proliferative and neoplastic mouse tissues in vivo. *Cancer Res* 1981; 41:4441–4446.
31. Warner P, Barker AJ, Jackman AL, Burrows K, Roberts N, Bishop JAM, O'Connor BM, Hughes LR. Quinoline antifolate thymidylate synthase inhibitors: variation of the C2 and C4-substituents. *J Med Chem* 1992; 35:2761–2768.
32. Jackman AL, Marsham PR, Thornton TJ, Bishop JAM, O'Connor BM, Hughes LR, Calvert AH, Jones TR. Quinazoline antifolate thymidylate synthase inhibitors: 2'-fluoro-N^{10}-propargyl-5,8-dideazafolic acid and derivatives with modifications in the C2 position. *J Med Chem* 1990; 33:3067–3071.
33. 52. Marsham PR, Jackman AL, Oldfield J, Hughes LR, Thornton TJ, Bisset GMF, O'Connor BM, Bishop JAM, Calvert AH. Quinazoline antifolate thymidylate synthase inhibitors: benzoyl ring modifications in the C2-methyl series. *J Med Chem* 1990; 33:3072–3078.
34. Thornton TJ, Jackman AL, Marsham PR, O'Connor BM, Bishop JAM, Calvert AH. Quinazoline antifolate thymidylate synthase inhibitors: difluoro substituted benzene ring analogues. *J Med Chem* 1992; 35:2321–2327.
35. Jackman AL, Kimbell R, Brown M, Brunton L, Bisset GMF, Bavetsias V, Marsham P, Hughes LR, Boyle FT. Quinazoline-based thymidylate synthase inhibitors: relationship between structural modifications and polyglutamation. *Anticancer Drug Design* 1995; 10:573–589.
36. Marsham PR, Hughes LR, Jackman AL, Hayter AJ, Oldfield J, Wardleworth JM, Bishop JA, O'Connor BM, Calvert AH. Quinazoline antifolate thymidylate synthase inhibitors: heterocyclic benzoyl ring modifications. *J Med Chem* 1991; 34:1594–1605.
37. Stephens TC, Valaccia BE, Sheader ML, Hughes LR, Jackman AL. The thymidylate synthase inhibitor ICI D1694 is superior to CB3717, 5-fluorouracil and methotrexate against a panel of human tumour xenografts. *Proc Am Assoc Cancer Res* 1991; 32:328.
38. Jodrell DI, Newell DR, Morgan SE, Clinton S, Bensted JPM, Hughes LR, Calvert AH. The renal effects of N^{10}-propargyl-5,8-dideazafolic acid (CB3717) and a non-nephrotoxic analogue ICI D1694, in mice. *Br J Cancer* 1991; 64:833–838.
39. Jodrell D, The pharmacology and toxicology of novel thymidylate synthase inhibitors, potential new anticancer agents, MD thesis, University of Southhapton, 1990.
40. Jackman AL, Jodrell DI, Gibson W, Stephens TC. ICI D1694, an inhibitor of thymidylate synthase for clinical study. In: Harkness RA, Elion GB, Zollner N, eds. Purine and Pyrimidine Metabolism in Man VII, Plenum, New York, 1991; pp. 19–23.
41. Jackman AL, Kimbell R, Aherne GW, Brunton L, Jansen G, Stephens TC, Smith M, Wardleworth JM, Boyle FT. The cellular pharmacology and in vivo activity of a new anticancer agent, ZD9331: a water-soluble, non-polyglutamatable quinazoline-based inhibitor of thymidylate synthase. *Clin Cancer Res* 1997; 3:911–921.
42. Jodrell DI, Newell DR, Gibson W, Hughes LR, Calvert AH. The pharmacokinetics of the quinazoline antifolate ICI D1694 in mice and rats. *Cancer Chemother Pharmacol* 1991; 28:331–338.
43. Jackman AL, Taylor GA, Gibson W, Kimbell R, Brown M, Calvert AH, Judson IR, Hughes LR. ICI D1694, a quinazoline antifolate thymidylate synthase inhibitor that is a potent inhibitor of L1210 tumor cell growth *in vitro* and *in vivo*: a new agent for clinical study. *Cancer Res* 1991; 51:5579–5586.
44. Ward WHJ, Kimbell R, Jackman AL. Kinetic characteristics of ICI D1694: a quinazoline antifolate which inhibits thymidylate synthase. *Biochem Pharmacol* 1992; 43:2029–2031.
45. Jackman AL, Gibson W, Brown M, Kimbell R, Boyle FT. The role of the reduced-folate carrier and metabolism to intracellular polyglutamates for the activity of ICI D1694, in *Proc. of the International Symposium on novel approaches to selective treatments of human solid tumours: laboratory and clinical correlation. Adv. Exptl. Med. Biol.* vol. 339 (Rustum Y, ed.) Plenum, New York, 1993, pp. 265–276.
46. Gibson W, Bisset GMF, Marsham PR, Kelland LR, Judson IR, Jackman AL. The measurement of polyglutamate metabolites of the thymidylate synthase inhibitor, ICI D1694, in mouse and human cultured cells. *Biochem Pharmacol* 1993; 45:863–869.

47. Jackman AL, Kelland LR, Kimbell R, Brown M, Gibson W, Aherne GW, Hardcastle A, Boyle FT. Mechanisms of acquired resistance to the quinazoline thymidylate synthase inhibitor, ZD1694 (Tomudex) in one mouse and three human cell lines. *Br J Cancer* 1995; 71:914–924.
48. Takemura Y, Gibson W, Kimbell R, Kobayashi H, Miyachi H, Jackman AL. Cellular pharmacokinetics of ZD1694 in cultured human leukaemia cells sensitive, or made resistant to this drug. *J Cancer Res Clin Oncol,* 1996; 122:109–117.
49. Takemura Y, Kobayashi H, Gibson W, Kimbell R, Miyachi H, Jackman AL. The influence of drug-exposure conditions on the development of resistance to methotrexate or ZD1694 in cultured human leukaemia cells. *Int J Cancer,* in Press.
50. McGuire JJ, Heitzman KJ, Haile WH, Russell CA, McCloskey DE, Piper JR. Studies on the cross resistance of folylpolyglutamate synthetase-deficient, methotrexate-resistant CCRF-CEM human leukemia sublines, in *Chemistry and Biology of Pteridines and Folates, Advances in Experimental Medicine and Biology,* vol. 338 (Ayling JE, Nair MG, Baugh CM, eds.) Plenum, New York, 1993, pp. 667–670.
51. Jackman AL, Melin C, Brunton L, Kimbell R, Aherne W, Walton M. Some determinants of response to folate-based thymidylate synthase (TS) inhibitors in human colon and ovarian tumour cell lines. *Proc Amer Assoc Cancer Res* 1998; 39:434.
52. Westerhof GR, Schornagel JH, Kathmann I, Jackman AL, Rosowsky A, Forsch RA, Hynes JB, Boyle FT, Peters GJ, Pinedo HM, Jansen G. Carrier and receptor-mediated transport of folate antagonists targeting folate dependent enzymes: correlates of molecular-structure and biological activity. *Mol Pharmacol* 1995; 48:459–471.
53. Smith SG, Lehman NL, Moran RG. Cytotoxicity of antifolate inhibitors of thymidylate and purine synthesis in WiDr colonic carcinoma cells. *Cancer Res* 1993; 53:5697–5706.
54. Jackman AL, Kimbell R, Brown M, Brunton L, Boyle FT. Quinazoline thymidylate synthase inhibitors: methods for assessing the contribution of polyglutamation to their in vitro activity. *Anticancer Drug Design* 1995; 10:555–572.
55. Stephens TC, Calvete JA, Janes D, Waterman SE, Valcaccia BE, Hughes LR, Calvert AH. Antitumour activity of a new thymidylate synthase inhibitor, D1694. *Proc Am Assoc Cancer Res* 1990; 31:342.
56. Aherne W, Hardcastle A, Kelland L, Jackman A. The measurement of deoxynucleotide (dNTP) pools by radioimmunoassay, in *Purine and Pyrimidine Metabolism in Man, Adv. Exp. Med. Biol* vol. 370 (Sahota A, Taylor MW, eds.) 1995, pp. 801–804.
57. Aherne GW, Hardcastle A, Raynaud F, Jackman AL. Immunoreactive dUMP and TTP pools as an index of thymidylate synthase; effect of Tomudex (ZD1694) and non-polyglutamated quinazoline antifolate (CB30900) in L1210 mouse leukemia cells. *Biochem Pharmacol* 1996; 51:1293–1301.
58. Rees C, Kimbell R, Valenti M, Brunton L, Farrugia D, Jackman AL. Effects of leucovorin and folic acid on the cytotoxicity of the thymidylate synthase inhibitors, Tomudex (ZD1694) and ZD9331. *Proc Am Assoc Cancer Res* 1997; 38:476.
59. Aherne GW, Ward E, Lawrence N, Dobinson D, Clarke SJ, Musgrove H, Sutcliffe F, Stephens T, Jackman AL. Comparison of plasma and tissue levels of ZD1694 (Tomudex), a highly polyglutamatable quinazoline thymidylate synthase inhibitor in preclinical models. *Br J Cancer,* in press.
60. Hardcastle A, Dobinson D, Farrugia D, Jackman AL, Aherne GW. *In vivo* pharmacokinetic and pharmacodynamic studies of two specific thymidylate synthase inhibitors. *Br J Cancer* 1997; 75(Suppl. 1):25.
61. Jackman AL, Farrugia DC, Gibson W, Kimbell R, Harrap KR, Stephens TC, Azab M, Boyle FT. ZD1694 (Tomudex): a new thymidylate synthase inhibitor with activity in colorectal cancer. *Eur J Cancer* 1995; 31A:1277–1282.
62. Jackman AL, Taylor GA, Calvert AH, Harrap KR. Modulation of antimetabolite effects: effects of thymidine on the efficacy of the quinazoline-based thymidylate synthetase inhibitor, CB3717. *Biochem Pharmacol* 1984; 33:3269–3275.
63. Taylor GA, Jackman AL, Calvert AH, Harrap KR. Plasma nucleoside and base levels following treatment with the new thymidylate synthetase inhibitor, CB3717, in *Adv Exptl Med Biol* 1984, pp. 379–382.
64. Rafi I, Boddy AV, Taylor GA, Calvete JA, Bailey NB, Lind MJ, Newell DR, Calvert AH. A phase I clinical study of the novel antifolate AG337 given by 5 day oral administration. *Ann Oncol* 1996; 7(Suppl. 1):86.
65. Clarke S, Jackman AL. Plasma thymidine and deoxyuridine concentrations as pharmacodynamic indicators of thymidylate synthase inhibition following Tomudex administration to mice. *Proc Am Assoc Cancer Res* 1996; 37:385.

66. Smith GK, Amyx H, Boytos CM, Duch DS, Ferone R, Wilson HR. Enhanced antitumour activity for the thymidylate synthase inhibitor 1843U89 through decreased host toxicity with oral folic acid. *Cancer Res* 1995; 55:6117–6125.
67. Jackman AL, Farrugia DC, Clarke SJ, Aherne GW, Boyle FT, Seymour L, Azab M, Kennealey G. Delayed rescue of ZD1694 toxicity in Balb/c mice with thymidine or leucovorin. *Proc Am Assoc Cancer Res* 1995; 36:377.
68. Aherne GW, Farrugia DC, Ward E, Sutcliffe F, Jackman AL. ZD1694 (Tomudex) and polyglutamate levels in mouse plasma and tissues measured by radioimmunoassay and the effects of leucovorin. *Proc Am Assoc Cancer Res* 1995; 36:376.

7　Tomudex
Clinical Development

Philip Beale and Stephen Clarke

Contents

Introduction
Phase I Studies
Pharmacokinetic Studies
Phase II Studies
Phase III Studies
Ongoing Trials
Conclusions

1. INTRODUCTION

This chapter describes the development and clinical experience to date with Tomudex (raltitrexed, formerly ZD1694), a potent new folate-based anticancer drug that owes its cytotoxicity to inhibition of the enzyme thymidylate synthase (TS). TS catalyzes the reductive methylation of deoxyuridylate monophosphate (dUMP) to thymidylate (TMP), the rate-limiting step in the *de novo* synthesis of thymidine triphosphate (TTP), the only nucleotide specific for DNA synthesis and thus a logical target for antiproliferative agents. Specific inhibition of TS should only impact on proliferating tissues and thus avoid adverse effects on cellular metabolism as could occur with concurrent inhibition of purine synthesis (methotrexate) or incorporation of metabolites into RNA (5FU). In addition, a specific folate-based TS inhibitor, unlike 5FU, would not require the metabolism that is essential for 5FU to achieve TS-inhibitory activity. Furthermore, unlike the situation with methotrexate, in which inhibition of dihydrofolate reductase (DHFR), in the presence of ongoing *de novo* TS synthesis, could lead to an increase of reduced folate (FH2) that could compete for DHFR, a decrease in reduced folates accompanying TS inhibition should favor further TS inhibition by depleting the levels of the natural folate cofactor. Similarly drug resistance caused by elevation of dUMP, as may occur with 5FU, should promote rather than impair the action of a folate-based TS inhibitor.

From: *Anticancer Drug Development Guide: Antifolate Drugs in Cancer Therapy*
Edited by: A.L. Jackman © Humana Press Inc., Totowa, NJ

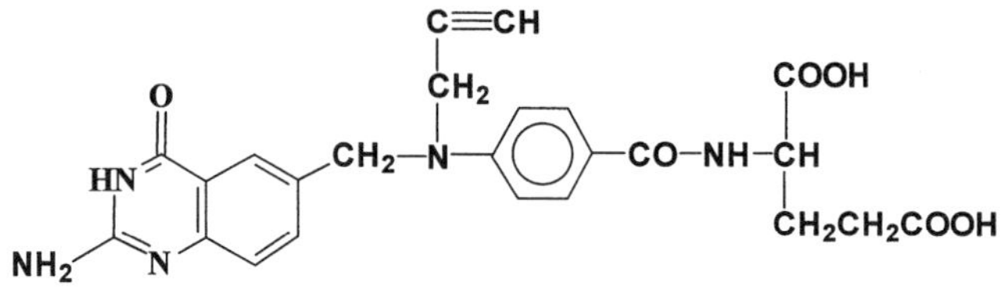

Fig. 1. Structure of CB3717.

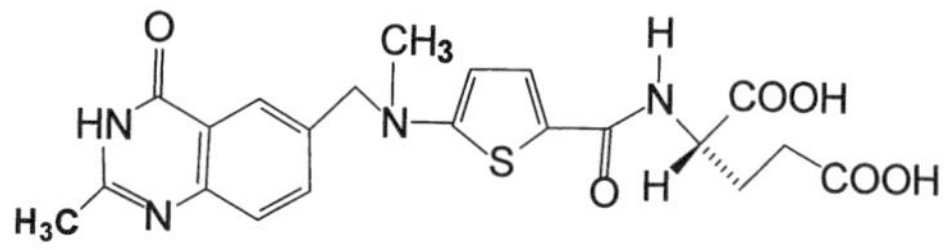

Fig. 2. Structure of Tomudex.

CB3717, (Fig. 1) the lead quinazoline folic acid analog that inhibits TS, is a substrate for folylpolyglutamate synthetase (FPGS), an enzyme that adds extra glutamic acid residues to natural and synthetic folates. In the initial phase I trial of CB3717, the dose-limiting toxicity was nephrotoxicity, which occurred in 70% of patients at doses greater than 450 mg/m^2 *(1)*. The other prominent and more prevalent toxicities were elevations in liver function tests and disabling malaise. Phase II trials of CB3717 were performed in mesothelioma, breast, colon, ovarian, and hepatocellular cancers with activity demonstrated in the latter three tumor types, but even with alkaline diuresis and more protracted infusions, the toxicities mimicked those of the phase I trials *(2–6)*. Thus, in spite of encouraging activity it was felt that the toxicities of CB3717, particularly the nephrotoxicity, precluded its further development and further trials were not undertaken.

A program of analog development was undertaken aimed at divorcing the nephrotoxicity from the antitumor effects and this proved possible. At this stage, Zeneca (previously ICI Pharmaceuticals), which had an interest and involvement in the work of the Institute of Cancer Research (ICR) on CB3717 and some of its analogs, started a joint chemical synthetic program with the ICR. The initial lead of Jones et al. *(7)* on the desamino compound quickly led to the synthesis of 2-substituted analogs as TS inhibitors of which Tomudex was the best compound to emerge (Fig. 2). Tomudex has been demonstrated to have a K_i for isolated L1210 TS of 62 nM, but in spite of this 20-fold poorer potency against isolated TS than CB3717, this compound displayed 500-fold greater cytotoxic potency than the parent compound because of its use of the reduced folate carrier and great affinity for FPGS *(8)*.

Toxicological and pharmacological studies of Tomudex were performed in mouse, rat, and dog and showed no evidence of renal or hepatic toxicity *(9)*. In dog, the toxicities seen after single iv bolus doses were gastrointestinal and bone marrow without toxicity to nonproliferating tissues, thus suggesting that the toxicities of Tomudex in man should be typical of an antimetabolite with gut and bone-marrow toxicities predominating.

2. PHASE I STUDIES

The European phase I study of Tomudex was conducted at the Royal Marsden Hospital and Rotterdam Cancer Institute and was initiated in January 1991 *(10)*. An American phase I study, conducted at the Navy Branch of the NCI, commenced in late 1991 *(11)*. The European study commenced at a dose of 0.1 mg/m^2, which was 20% of the toxic dose low in dogs. The drug was administered intravenously by 15-min infusion every 3 wk. This schedule was chosen because of concerns about possible cumulative toxicity because of the extensive polyglutamation of Tomudex and because of the experience with Lomotrexol, another folate-based agent that also undergoes extensive polyglutamation. In the European study, doses of Tomudex were escalated according to a modified Fibonacci schema with three patients being accrued per dose level until toxicities were experienced and included 0.2, 0.4, 0.6, 1.0, 1.6, 2.6, 3.0, and 3.5 mg/m^2. Sixty-one patients of median age 53 yr, 85% of whom had performance status 0 or 1, received 161 courses of Tomudex (median 2 and range 1–11). There were 33 males and 28 females and 50 patients (90%) had received prior chemotherapy. This study included patients with a wide range of tumor types. Toxicity first occurred at 1.6 mg/m^2 and involved abnormalities of liver function tests that were also seen at higher doses. These changes, which were WHO grade III or IV in 32% of patients treated at doses of 3.0 and 3.5 mg/m^2, were predominantly in the transaminases, but mild elevations of alkaline phosphatase, gamma glutamyl transferase and, to a lesser extent bilirubin, were also demonstrated. The abnormalities were self limiting, did not delay dosing, and settled on completion of therapy. The dose-limiting toxicities were myelosuppression, gastrointestinal toxicities, and fatigue/malaise. At 3.5 mg/m^2, 2 of 6 patients developed grade III/IV neutropenia, one of whom also developed grade IV thrombocytopenia complicated by pulmonary hemorrhage. At 3.0 mg/m^2, 14 of 22 patients (61%) developed myelosuppression with 5 (22%) developing grade III or IV toxicity. Fourteen patients (60%) treated with 3.0 mg/m^2 developed diarrhea, of whom 6 (26%) had grade III/IV toxicity and 5 required hospital admission for rehydration. Nausea and vomiting were common at the higher dose levels, but readily controllable with simple antiemetics. There was no evidence of renal impairment.

A fatigue syndrome manifest by lethargy and decreased performance status occurred in 4 of the 6 patients treated at 3.5 mg/m^2 and was also seen in patients treated at 3.0 mg/m^2. Skin rash occurred in 35% of patients treated with 3.0 mg/m^2 and ranged from a simple pruritic maculopapular rash to a chemical cellulitis requiring steroids. Responses were demonstrated in patients with head and neck, breast, and ovarian cancers and included patients who had progressed through 5FU-based regimens. A dose of 3.0 mg/m^2 was recommended for phase II study.

The U.S. phase I study commenced at 0.6 mg/m^2 and examined dose levels of 1.0, 1.6, 2.1, 2.8, 3.5, 4.0, and 4.5 mg/m^2. The spectrum of toxicities was identical to the European study, however a dose of 4.0 mg/m^2 was recommended for phase II trials. It remains unclear as to why the American patients were able to tolerate higher dose levels of Tomudex than their European counterparts, however it has been suggested that these patients might have had superior performance status than the European patients.

Table 1
Renal Impairment Study: Tomudex Pharmacokinetic Parameters
(Mean ± Standard Deviation)

Parameter	Normal renal function (n = 8)	Impaired renal function (n = 8)
C_{max} (ng/ml)	567.1 ± 62.7	676.1 ± 204.1
AUC_{0-tldc} (ng.h/ml)	1355.8 ± 558.5	2522.0 ± 784.9[b]
$AUC_{0-\infty}$ (ng.h/ml)	1547.9 ± 521.7	3414.5 ± 2510.5[b]
t_{max} (min)	16 (15 to 20)[a]	20 (10 to 30)[a]
$t_{1/2}$ (h)	1.82 ± 1.30	1.79 ± 0.49
$t_{1/2}$ (h)	140.0 ± 55.0	274.5 ± 127.4[b]
Clearance (mL/min)	66.7 ± 21.7	32.3 ± 12.3
Volume of distribution (L)	7.3 ± 3.0	6.2 ± 2.4
Volume of distribution at steady state (L)	492.8 ± 197.5	493.0 ± 100.3

[a] Median and range.
tldc: time to last determined concentration.
[b] Statistically significant.

3. PHARMACOKINETIC STUDIES

A study of Tomudex pharmacokinetics in patients with impaired renal function *(12)* and a [^{14}C]-labeled excretion balance study *(13)* have been performed to further define the pharmacokinetics of this compound in man.

3.1. Renal Impairment Study

In this study, the pharmacokinetics of eight patients with mild-to-moderate renal impairment (^{51}Cr-EDTA clearance between 25–65 mL/min) were compared with eight patients with normal renal function (clearance > 65 mL/min). Plasma concentrations of Tomudex declined triexponentially and could be described using a three compartment model. The AUC_{0-tldc}, $AUC_{0-\infty}$ and the terminal half life $t_{1/2}$ were significantly longer in the patients with renal impairment but there was no difference in C_{max} (Table 1, Fig. 3). There was a clear relationship between Tomudex clearance and calculated creatinine clearance using the Cockcroft equation or EDTA creatinine clearance (Fig. 4). However, whereas the patients with renal impairment tolerated the treatment less well (with more grade III/IV toxicities and hospitalizations), there was no direct relationship between AUC, $t_{1/2\gamma}$, creatinine clearance, and toxicity.

The recommendation from this study was that patients with mild-to-moderate renal impairment should receive a dose of Tomudex reduced by 50% and the dosage interval be increased to 4 wk. Patients with severe renal impairment (CrCl < 25 mL/min) should not receive Tomudex.

Analysis of patients with hepatic impairment (bilirubin 1.25–3.0 times the upper limit of normal and AST/ALT 3–10 times the upper limit of normal) from the phase I/II trials revealed no significant change in the pharmacokinetic profile or toxicities *(14)*. Therefore, no alteration in dose is recommended for patients with mild-to-moderate hepatic impairment.

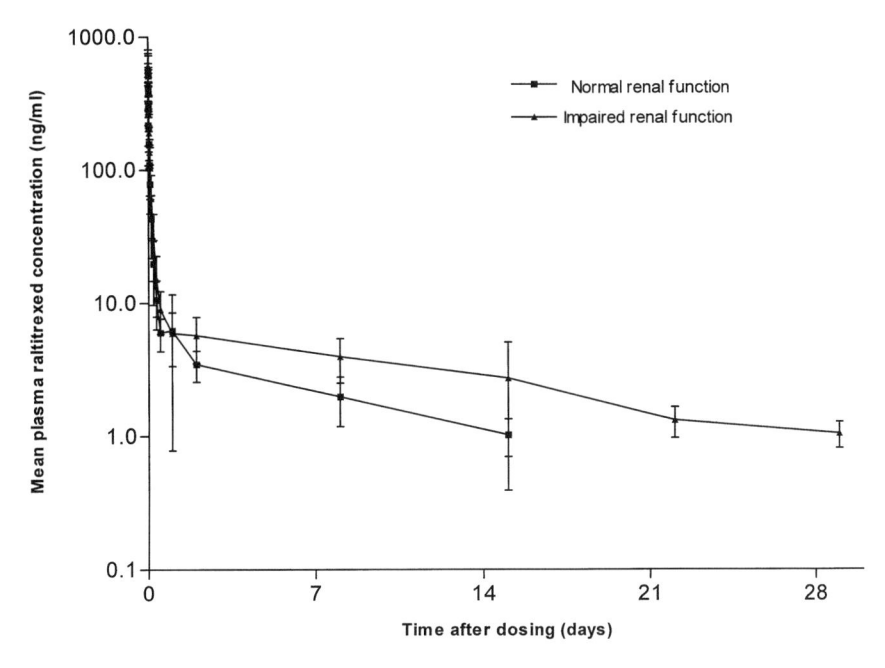

Fig. 3. Pharmacokinetic profile in patients with normal and impaired renal function.

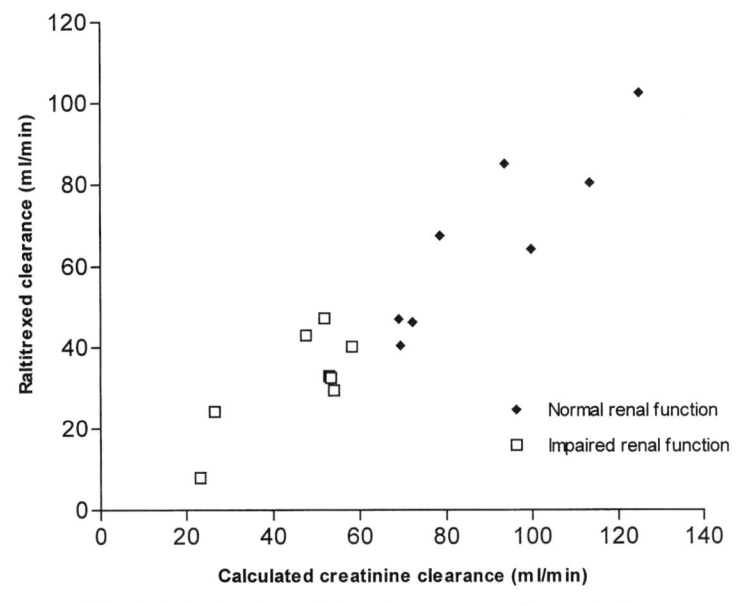

Fig. 4. Calculated creatinine clearance vs raltitrexed clearance.

3.2. [^{14}C]-Tomudex Pharmacokinetic Study

Preclinical studies have shown that the route of elimination of Tomudex varies in different species. In the rat elimination is predominantly fecal *(9),* but in the dog it is evenly divided between urine and feces (Data on Zeneca file). The excretion balance study examined the fate of a single dose of ^{14}C-labeled Tomudex in man.

Table 2
^{14}C Tomudex Plasma Pharmacokinetic Parameters

Parameter	Mean	SD	CV%
Model derived:			
C_{max} (ng/mL)	736.8	164.9	22.4
$AUC_{0-\infty}$ (ng/h/mL)	2341.7	941.1	40.2
$t_{1/2\alpha}$ (min)	12	3.0	25.8
$t_{1/2\beta}$ (min)	103	16.2	15.6
$t_{1/2\gamma}$ (h)	257	62.9	24.5
CL (mL/min)	41.3	14.0	34.0
CL_{renal} (mL/min)	21.5	5.2	24.0
Compartment model independent:			
Observed C_{max} (ng/mL)	700.6	165.3	23.6
Observed t_{max} (min)[a]	15.0	(median)	

[a] Values for 5 patients was 15.0 min: 16, 16, 17, and 20 min for the remainder. Some of the differences seen are because of the actual time samples were taken.

There was a good correlation between the measurement of total radioactivity in plasma and the RIA measurement of Tomudex. The pharmacokinetic parameters summarized in Table 2, reveals a C_{max} of 700.6 ng/mL, and a t_{max} of 15.0 min. After C_{max} was reached, the levels declined in a triexponential fashion with $t_{1/2\alpha}$, $t_{1/2\beta}$, $t_{1/2\gamma}$ being 12 min, 103 min and 257 h, respectively. However, there was a considerable range in the terminal half life (148–379 h). This value was considerably longer than calculated in the phase I trial, because of the increased length of collection of plasma samples until day 29 compared with day 4. Plasma clearance was 41.3 mL/min (range 27.3–54.3) and calculated renal clearance was 21.5 mL/min. On limited testing, there were very low plasma levels of Tomudex prior to subsequent dosing, suggesting no evidence of accumulation.

Recovery of radioactivity in the urine accounted for 21.7% of the radioactive dose in the first 24 h and this reached 28.8% by day 10 and 40.1% when extrapolated to infinity. HPLC examination of the urine showed that the drug was excreted unchanged. Fecal recovery reached 14% by day 10 in three patients for whom collections extended to this time point.

Tomudex levels fell below detection in blood and red cell pellets by 24-h postdosing, but on days 15, 22, and 29 there were low levels of radioactivity in red cell pellets and this probably represents polyglutamated metabolites of Tomudex formed in bone-marrow cells at the time of dosing. This study confirmed the very long terminal half life of Tomudex and that fecal excretion is an important route of elimination in man. However, the fate of all administered drug was not characterized and Tomudex levels in tissues at the end of the collection period represented a significant proportion of the dose.

4. PHASE II STUDIES

With the broad spectrum of activity seen in cell culture and xenograft models and the successful introduction into the clinic through the phase I trial, a number of phase II trials were commenced in centers throughout Europe, South Africa, and Australia. Completed or published results of these trials are listed in Table 3. In all studies except where otherwise indicated, the dose of Tomudex utilized was 3.0 mg/m^2 given as a 15-min in-

Table 3
Tomudex: Phase II Trial Results

Tumor type	Patient numbers	Prior therapy	Objective response rate % (95% CI)	Grade III, IV toxicity (%)		
				Leucopenia	Vomiting	Diarrhea
Colorectal	177	adjuvant only	26 (19–33)	15	11	10
Breast	46	Adjuvant therapy[b]	26 (19–42)	20	11	11
Pancreatic	42	yes	5 (1–16)	10	10	0
Ovarian	31	yes	7 (1–23)	23	NS	13
Gastric	33	yes	0 (0–13)	12	12	0
SCLC	21	yes	0 (0–19)	19	10	0
NSCLC	33	no	9[a]	N/A	N/A	N/A
Hepatoma	33	no	0 (0–13)	6	<10	9

[a] Some patients treated with 4.0 mg/m² in whom response data not known.
[b] Hormone therapy for advanced disease allowed.

fusion every 21 d. The response rates for these tumor types ranges from 0 to 26%, with the toxicities being similar across all trials.

4.1. Colorectal Cancer

5-fluorouracil has been the mainstay of treatment for advanced colorectal carcinoma (CRC) for over 30 yr and although modulation with folinic acid increases response rates, overall survival has been largely unchanged over a long period of time. Thymidylate synthase is known to be expressed in colorectal carcinomas up to 5–10-fold higher than normal mucosa and therefore represents a suitable target for Tomudex *(15)*.

A phase II trial was carried out in Europe, South Africa, and Australia in patients with advanced colorectal carcinoma who had not received prior chemotherapy except for adjuvant chemotherapy at least 1 yr prior to entry onto the study *(16)*. A total of 176 patients with advanced CRC were entered onto the study, with a mean age of 61 yr, 95% with a performance status 0 or 1, and 80% of patients with liver metastases at entry. Ten percent of patients had received adjuvant radiotherapy and 5% adjuvant chemotherapy. The mean number of cycles was 4.7 and 82% of patients received the scheduled dose.

The overall response rate was 26% including 4 complete responders and 41 partial responders with the median duration of response 170 days. The median survival of all patients was 9.6 mo. Side-effect profile was similar to other trials with Tomudex. Severe asthenia occurred in 12% of patients, 15% grade III/IV leucopenia, 10% transaminase increases, 10% grade III/IV diarrhea, and 4 patients died of possible drug-related causes. Two of these patients experienced toxicity in previous courses and did not have appropriate dose reductions. Nausea and vomiting was easily controlled with antiemetics. Following this successful trial a randomized phase III trial was initiated comparing Tomudex with 5FU and leucovorin which is discussed later in this chapter.

4.2. Breast Cancer

A phase II trial in locally advanced or metastatic breast cancer was carried out in European and Australian centers *(17)*. Forty-six patients were enrolled in the study. The mean age of the patients treated was 58 yr, the majority were of good performance status and the most frequent site of metastatic disease was liver (50%) and bone (41%). Thirty-nine percent had received prior adjuvant chemotherapy and 41% had received endocrine therapy within 3 mo of entry into the trial.

Forty-three patients were evaluable for response and the objective response rate was 26%. Two patients achieved a complete response that lasted 265 and 301 d, respectively whereas the median duration of the partial response was 209 d.

Toxicity was similar to other clinical studies with Tomudex with the most frequent grade III/IV adverse events reported being transient elevation of transaminases (22%), leucopenia (20%), diarrhea (11%), and nausea and vomiting (11%). Three patients died on study, which may have been drug related although two may not have received appropriate dose reductions.

This study showed that Tomudex has activity in advanced breast cancer as a single agent although possibly less than the taxanes and anthracyclines.

4.3. Pancreatic Carcinoma

The prognosis for unresectable pancreatic cancer is very poor with a median survival of 3–6 mo. Current therapies are aimed at palliating symptoms with no agent able to demonstrate high activity leading to prolongation of life. Forty-two patients with advanced pancreatic cancer were treated with Tomudex, of which 2 (5%) achieved a partial response, 12 (29%) had stable disease, and 21 had progressive disease *(18)*. No patient required a dose reduction but treatment was delayed in 7 patients.

Grade III, IV toxicities (>10%) seen were nausea (19%), ALT elevation (17%), AST elevation (12%), leucopenia (10%), anemia (10%), and vomiting (10%). No therapy-related deaths were recorded. One episode of allergic reaction was documented, characterized by wheezing and inspiratory stridor which responded to diphenhydramine. The conclusion of this trial was that Tomudex had minimal activity in adenocarcinoma of the pancreas.

4.4. Ovarian Carcinoma

Treatment for platinum-resistant ovarian carcinoma is currently unsatisfactory with most agents used giving a response rate of 5–30% and most responses are not durable. Patients with platinum-resistant disease, (treatment-free interval > 100 d) or who had relapsed within 12 mo of previous platinum therapy were eligible for the Tomudex phase II trial *(19)*. Thirty-one patients, median age 54 yr, receiving a median of three cycles. Twenty-eight patients were evaluable for response with 2 (7%) achieving partial responses, lasting 20 and 39 wk. Four patients had minor responses and 7 had stable disease. Toxicity was similar to other trials with grade III/IV leucopenia seen in 7 patients, diarrhea in 4 patients, and increases in AST/ALT in 3 patients. One patient developed grade IV neutropenia, thrombocytopenia, and diarrhea and subsequently died, but at the time of entry had a poor performance status and jaundice.

In summary, Tomudex displayed only moderate activity in this trial but responses were seen in patients who were truly platinum resistant.

4.5. Gastric Carcinoma

5-fluorouracil is the most active agent against gastric carcinoma with a response rate of 20%. Increased levels of TS-gene expression and protein have been shown to correlate with resistance to fluoropyrimidine treatment and therefore a more potent inhibitor of TS might have higher activity in this disease (20).

Thirty-three patients were treated in the multicenter phase II trial in advanced gastric carcinoma who may have been treated with one prior chemotherapy regimen (21). Fifteen (45%) had been treated with chemotherapy alone or in combination with surgery and/or radiotherapy. There were no objective tumor responses, 8 (24%) achieved stable disease, and 21 (64%) developed progressive disease. The toxicities were similar to other trials with grade III/IV anemia (12%), asthenia (18%), leucopenia (12%), vomiting (12%), nausea (12%), and increase in AST (9%) being the most common effects. Dyspnea, fever, mucositis, thrombocytopenia, and skin rash were seen in less than 10% of courses. There were no treatment-related deaths.

The conclusion from this trial was that Tomudex lacks activity in pretreated patients with advanced gastric carcinoma with a toxicity profile similar to other reported studies.

4.6. Lung Cancer

4.6.1. SMALL-CELL LUNG CANCER

A multicenter phase II study in 21 patients with extensive small-cell lung cancer has been reported (22). This demonstrated no activity in this group of patients, 17 of whom had received prior chemotherapy and/or surgery or radiotherapy. The patients received a median of two cycles (range 1–4) with the most common side effects reported being nausea, asthenia, bone marrow suppression, and gastrointestinal toxicity. Four patients died within 3 wk of receiving the drug in which one was a drug-related adverse event (thrombocytopenia).

No patient had a response, but 3 patients had stable disease and 16 had progressive disease. The median survival from study entry was 15 wk (range 2–126 weeks). This trial confirmed that Tomudex was not effective as second-line treatment for patients with small-cell lung cancer and that trials in patients with chemonaive disease were not indicated.

4.6.2. NON-SMALL-CELL LUNG CANCER

Data from the phase II trial in non-small-cell cancer has only been published in abstract form (23). This describes 21 patients treated at 3.0 mg/m^2 and 12 patients at 4.0 mg/m^2. Of patients treated at the lower dose level there were two partial responses lasting 7 and 5 mo and four additional minor responses. Toxicity included one episode of febrile neutropenia, 10% grade III/IV diarrhea, and 14% grade III transaminase elevation. No response data or toxicities were reported at the higher dose level.

4.7. Hepatocellular Carcinoma

Treatment for advanced hepatocellular carcinoma has yielded very disappointing results with no therapy demonstrating response rates that lead to increased survival and little in the way of palliation. CB3717 demonstrated activity against hepatocellular carcinoma (6), and given the activity of this compound, a phase II trial of Tomudex in advanced hepatocellular carcinoma was carried out in European centers (24).

Thirty-three patients were treated with 106 cycles (median 2) of Tomudex. Of 26 patients evaluable for response, none achieved a response, 12 (46%) had stable disease, and

14 developed progressive disease. Two patients however did experience minor responses with one also showing a decline in the plasma α-fetoprotein from 188 to 5 μg/L.

The most common adverse events experienced were asthenia (38%), diarrhea (38%), nausea (34%), and elevation of liver enzymes (34%). Other less-common effects were grade IV hematological toxicity in two patients, alopecia and mucositis (3–9%).

The activity of Tomudex in this disease, which is resistant to most chemotherapy agents, is modest and as a single agent is unlikely to palliate the symptoms or extend the lives of these patients.

5. PHASE III STUDIES

5.1. European Phase III Study in Colorectal Carcinoma

Following the impressive activity demonstrated by Tomudex in the phase II trial in advanced colorectal carcinoma, a randomized phase III study was commenced in November 1993 *(25,26)*. This trial which was reported in 1995 and updated in 1996, compared Tomudex 3.0 mg/m^2 every 3 wk with the Mayo Clinic schedule of 5FU (425 mg/m^2) and leucovorin (20 mg/m^2) for 5 d given every 4–5 wk in patients with previously untreated advanced colorectal carcinoma.

Four hundred and thirty-nine patients were entered and randomized into the study. Patients were well matched demographically and 97% in the Tomudex group and 94% in the 5FU/LV group had measurable disease. Responses were assessed after 12 wk of therapy and were source validated. The response rate was 19.3% in the Tomudex arm and 16.7% in the 5FU/LV arm (not significantly different) and there was no difference in the time to progression or the overall survival between the two groups. The median time to progression was 4.8 mo in the Tomudex arm and 3.6 mo in the 5FU/LV arm. There was no difference in the QOL scores or other palliative effects in both arms although both treatments resulted in improvements in performance status and weight gain. Patients however, did stay longer in hospital for dosing in the 5FU/LV arm (3.0 vs 0.7 d).

There was a significantly higher incidence of mucositis and leucopenia in the 5FU/LV arm and a higher incidence of AST/ALT rises in the Tomudex arm (Table 4). The increased rates of leucopenia however, did not result in higher infection rates and the rises in transaminases were not clinically significant. Seven patients in the Tomudex arm and 5 in the 5FU arm died from possible drug-related causes and this was not significantly different.

In a separate analysis, which included some of the patients from this trial, the mean treatment costs (excluding pharmacy costs), was similar in the two arms *(27)*. In a separate time and motion study, Tomudex was quicker and less costly to prepare, resulting in significantly less pharmacy costs for Tomudex *(28)*. In a further study, the mean total drug cost for toxicity management was 50% lower in the Tomudex group compared with 5FU/LV (Mayo regimen) *(29)*.

The conclusions from this study were that both treatment arms yielded similar response rates, time to progression, overall survival, and quality of life assessments but treatment with Tomudex once every 3 wk resulted in less hospital time and less grade III and IV mucositis and leucopenia.

Table 4
Phase III Results in Colorectal Carcinoma

	European study (Mayo)[a]		North American (Mayo)[a]		European (Machover)[b]	
	Raltitrexed (n = 223) (%)	5FU + LV (n = 216) (%)	Raltitrexed (n = 217) (%)	5FU + LV (n = 210) (%)	Raltitrexed (n = 247) (%)	5FU + LV (n = 248) (%)
Complete response	3.6	3.7	2.8	1.4	3.2	3.6
Partial response	15.7	13.0	11.5	13.8	15.4	14.5
Overall response	19.3	16.7	14.3	15.2	18.6	18.1
Median survival	10.1	10.2	9.7	12.7	10.7	11.8
Median time to progression	4.8	3.6	3.1	5.3	3.9	5.1
Weight gain	16.6	15.7	21.1	27.4	13.0	18.9
PS score improvement	36.4	29.7	39.1	40.8	38.2	31.1

[a] Tomudex 3.0 mg/m^2 5FU (425 mg/m^2) LV (20 mg/m^2).
[b] Tomudex 3.0 mg/m^2 5FU (400 mg/m^2) LV (200 mg/m^2).

5.2. Other Phase III Trials

Two other phase III trials have been published comparing Tomudex to different 5FU/LV regimens for advanced colorectal carcinoma (30,31). The first, conducted in North America was similar to the European/Australian trial except that initially there was a third study arm of Tomudex 4.0 mg/m^2 every 3 wk that was discontinued after there were three treatment-related deaths.

The response rates were similar in both arms (14.3% raltitrexed vs 15.2% 5FU/LV), but the time to progression and overall survival were significantly longer for the 5FU/LV group (Table 5). However, the time on treatment was 5.1 mo for 5FU/LV and only 2.8 mo for the Tomudex patients. Toxicity profiles were similar to the previous phase III trial.

A subsequent trial was initiated in Europe, South Africa, and Australia comparing Tomudex 3.0 mg/m^2 every 3 wk vs the Machover regimen of 5FU 400 mg/m^2 and leucovorin 200 mg/m^2 every day for 5 d given every 4 wk. This also realized similar response rates, and overall survival at the 9-mo follow up with less grade III and IV mucositis (2 vs 16%), leucopenia (6 vs 13%), and diarrhea (10 vs 19%) in the Tomudex group. However, the time to progression in the 5FU/LV arm was significantly longer (5.1 vs 3.9 mo). Dose reductions were required in 31% of patients in the 5FU/LV after the first course because of toxicity compared with 5% in the Tomudex arm, and this was reflected in an increase in QOL scores for the Tomudex-treated patients.

The conclusions from these three studies are that there are no differences in response rates between the two treatments but in two of three trials there was a significantly longer time to progression in the 5FU/LV arm. Overall survival was significantly longer in the 5FU/LV arm in one trial and comparable in the other two. There may be a better side-effect profile, a schedule advantage, and fewer hospitalizations in the Tomudex-treated patients and this may further result in quality of life differences and economic advantages. Further trials to investigate these questions are currently being conducted.

Table 5
Grade III, IV Toxicity in Phase III Trials with Tomudex

	European study (Mayo)[a]		North American (Mayo)[a]		European (Machover)[b]	
	Raltitrexed (n = 222) (%)	5FU + LV (n = 212) (%)	Raltitrexed (n = 217) (%)	5FU + LV (n = 200) (%)	Raltitrexed (n = 245) (%)	5FU + LV (n = 244) (%)
Leucopenia	14*	30	18*	41	6	13
Mucositis	2*	22	3	10	2*	16
Anemia	9	2*	9	4	5	2
Increased transaminases	10	0*	7	1	13	0*
Nausea/vomiting	13	9	13	8	9	9
Asthenia (severe)	6	2	18	10	5	2
Diarrhea	14	14	10	13	10	19
Thrombocytopenia	4	1	5	3	3	0
Constipation	3	3	2	2	2	0
Infection	5	5	6	7	4	3
Fever	3	2	2	2	0	1
Pain	5	7	14	16	5	4
Hemorrhage	2	3	3	1	0	1

[a]Tomudex 3.0 mg/m^2 5FU (425 mg/m^2) LV (20 mg/m^2).
[b]Tomudex 3.0 mg/m^2 5FU (400 mg/m^2) LV (200 mg/m^2).
*Statistically significant.

6. ONGOING TRIALS

6.1. Other Tumour Types

Several phase II trials have been initiated in other tumor types during 1996 and 1997. These include locally advanced or metastatic squamous-cell carcinoma of the head and neck, advanced hormone-resistant prostate cancer, and advanced soft-tissue sarcomas. In the pediatric population, trials have started in patients with advanced neoplastic disease (phase I) and acute leukemia.

Two trials in colorectal carcinoma are being carried out in different centers looking at the expression of thymidylate synthase, FPGS, and folypolyglutamate hydrolase (FPGH) in tumor tissue and normal mucosa and correlating these parameters with toxicity and response. Other trials in colon carcinoma are looking at those patients who have previously not responded to 5FU, comparing Tomudex and two schedules of 5FU for assessment of quality of life and survival and a comparative trial of Tomudex and 5FU/LV as adjuvant therapy.

6.2. Combination Studies

Whereas some preclinical studies in colon carcinoma cell lines have suggested synergy when Tomudex is followed by 5FU *(32)* others have only demonstrated additivity *(33)*. A dose-escalating phase I study has commenced with Tomudex (0.5–3.0 mg/m^2) followed by 5FU given over 24 h every 3 wk *(34)*. No response data are available but the combination is well tolerated and pharmacokinetic analysis has revealed a significant increase in the C_{max} and AUC of 5FU with increasing doses of Tomudex above 2.0

mg/m². The nature of this interaction is not known. A similar study has commenced using a weekly schedule of 5FU and a three weekly schedule of Tomudex.

Other combination studies ongoing include Tomudex and CPT11, and Tomudex with oxaliplatin in advanced colon carcinoma; Tomudex and doxorubicin in advanced gastric carcinoma; Tomudex and cisplatin in metastatic non small-cell carcinoma of lung; Tomudex and paclitaxel in patients with metastatic or recurrent tumours. Finally, a trial has commenced investigating the use of Tomudex in conjunction with radiotherapy for patients with rectal carcinoma.

7. CONCLUSIONS

The development of Tomudex was the result of rational drug design that has lead to a specific TS inhibitor now licensed for use in advanced colorectal carcinoma in over 10 countries. The activity is comparable to standard 5FU/LV regimens with less mucositis and leucopenia given on a more favorable schedule of once every three weeks based on its long terminal half life. Toxicities are manageable with gastrointestinal and bone-marrow toxicities being dose limiting and rises in transaminases, typical of drugs of this class not clinically significant.

The current development of Tomudex centers on drug combination with a variety of different chemotherapy agents in several different tumor types and the further evaluation of the benefit in colorectal carcinoma.

REFERENCES

1. Calvert AH, Alison DL, Harland SJ, Robinson BA, Jackman AL, Jones TR, Newell DR, Siddik ZH, Wiltshaw E, McElwain TJ, Smith IE, Harrap KR. A phase I evaluation of the quinazoline antifolate thymidylate synthase inhibitor, N^{10}-propargyl-5,8-dideazafolic acid, CB3717. *J Clin Oncol* 1986; 4:1245–1252.
2. Cantwell BMJ, Earnshaw M, Harris AL. Phase II study of a novel antifolate, N^{10}-propargyl-5,8 dideazafolic acid (CB3717), in malignant mesothelioma. *Cancer Treat Rep* 1986; 70:1335–1336.
3. Cantwell BMJ, Macaulay V, Harris AL, Kaye SB, Smith IE, Milstesad RAV, Calvert AH. Phase II study of the antifolate N^{10}-propargyl-5,8-dideazafolic acid (CB3717) in advanced breast cancer. *Eur J Cancer Clin Oncol* 1988; 24:733–736.
4. Harding MJ, Cantwell BMJ, Milstead RAV, Harris AL, Kaye SB. Phase II study of the thymidylate synthetase inhibitor CB3717 (N^{10}-propargyl-5,8-dideazafolic acid) in colorectal cancer. *Br J Cancer* 1988; 57:628–629.
5. Calvert AH, Newell DR, Jackman AL, Gumbrell LA, Sikora E, Grzelakowska-Sztabert B, Bishop J, Judson IR, Harland S and Harrap K. Recent preclinical and clinical studies with the thymidylate synthase inhibitor N^{10}-propargyl-5,8-dideazafolic acid, CB3717. *NCI Monogr* 1987; 5:213–218.
6. Bassendine MF, Curtin NJ, Loose H, Harris AL, James OFW. Induction of remission in hepatocellular carcinoma with a new thymidylate synthase inhibitor, CB3717. *J Hepatol* 1987; 4:349–356.
7. Jones TR, Thornton TJ, Flinn A, Jackman AL, Newell DR, Calvert AH. Quinazoline antifolates inhibiting thymidylate synthase: 2-desamino derivatives with enhanced solubility and potency. *J Med Chem* 1989; 32:847–852.
8. Jackman AL, Taylor GA, Gibson W, Kimbell R, Brown M, Calvert AH, Judson IR, Hughes L. ICI D1694, a quinazoline antifolate thymidylate synthase inhibitor that is a potent of L1210 tumour cell growth *in vitro* and *in vivo:* a new agent for clinical study. *Cancer Res* 1991; 51:5579–5586.
9. Jodrell D, Newell D, Gibson W, Hughes L, Calvert H. The pharmacokinetics of the quinazoline antifolate ICI d1694 in mice and rats. *Cancer Chemother Pharmacol* 1991; 28:331–338.
10. Clarke SJ, Hanwell J, de Boer M., Planting A, Verweij J, Walker M, Smith R, Jackman AL, Hughes LR, Harrap KR, Kennealey GT, Judson IR. Phase I trial of ZD1694 ("Tomudex"), a new folate based, thymidylate synthase inhibitor. *J Clin Oncol* 1996; 14:1495–1503.

11. Sorenson JM, Jordan E, Grem JL, Arbuck SG, Chen AP, Hamilton JM, Johnston P, Kohler DR, Goldspiel BR, Allegra CJ. Phase I trial of ZD1694, (Tomudex), a direct inhibitor of thymidylate synthase. *Ann Oncol* 1994; 5(suppl 5):132.
12. Judson I, Maughan T, Beale P, Primrose J, Hoskin P, Hanwell J, Berry C, Walker M, Sutcliffe F. Effects of impaired renal function on the pharmacokinetics of raltitrexed (TomudexTM ZD1694), B&J Cancer, 1998 in press.
13. Beale P, Judson I, Hanwell J, Berry C, Aherne W, Hickish T, Martin P, Walker M. Metabolism, excretion and pharmacokinetics of a single dose of [^{14}C]-raltitrexed in cancer patients. *Cancer Chemother Pharmacol*, 1998; 42:71–76
14. Judson I. Tomudex (raltitrexed) development: preclinical, phase I and II studies. *Anticancer Drugs* 1997; 8(suppl 2):S5–9.
15. Findlay MPN, Cunningham D, Morgan G, Clinton S, Hardcastle A, Aherne GW. Lack of correlation between thymidylate synthase levels in primary colorectal tumours and subsequent response to chemotherapy. *Br J Cancer* 1997; 75/6:903–909.
16. Zalcberg JR, Cunningham D, Van-Cutsem E, Francois E, Schornagel J, Adenis A, Green M, Iveson A Azab M, Seymour I. ZD1694: a novel thymidylate synthase inhibitor with substantial activity in the treatment of patients with advanced colorectal cancer. *J Clin Oncol* 1996; 14:716–721.
17. Smith I, Jones A, Spielman M, Namer M, Green MD, Bonneterre J, Wander HE, Hatscek T, Wilking N, Zalcbergn J, Spiers J, Seymour L A phase II study in advanced breast cancer: ZD1694 ("Tomudex") a novel direct and specific thymidylate synthetase inhibitor. *Br J Cancer*. 1996; 74:479–481.
18. Pazdur R, Merepol NJ, Casper ES, Fuchs C, Douglass HO, Vincent M, Abbruzzese JL. Phase II study of ZD1694 (TomudexTM) in patients with advanced pancreatic cancer. *Invest New Drugs* 1996; 13:355–358.
19. Gore ME, Earl HM, Cassidy J, Tattersall M, Mansi J, Seymour L, Azab M. A phase II study of Tomudex in relapsed epithelial ovarian cancer. *Ann Oncol* 1995; 6:724–725.
20. Johnston PG, Lenz H-J, Leichman CG, Danenberg KD, Allegra CJ, Danenberg PV, Leichman L. Thymidylate synthase gene and protein expression correlate and are associated with response to 5-fluorouracil in human colorectal and gastric tumours. *Cancer Res* 1995; 55:1407–1412.
21. Merepol N, Pazdur R, Vincent M, Willson J, Kelson D, Douglass H. Phase II study of ZD1694 in patients with advanced gastric cancer. *Am J Clin Oncol* 1996; 19:628–630.
22. Woll PJ, Basser R, Le Chevalier T, Drings P, Perez Manga G, Adenis A, Seymour L, Smith F, Thatcher N. Phase II trial of raltitrexed ('Tomudex') in advanced small-cell lung cancer. *Br J Cancer*. 1997; 76:264–265.
23. Heaven R, Bowen K, Rinaldi D, Robert F, Jenkins T, Eckardt J, Fields S, Hardy J, Patton S, Kennealey G. An open Phase II trial of ZD1694, a thymidylate synthase inhibitor, in patients with advanced non-small cell lung cancer. *Proc Amer Soc Clin Oncol* 1994; 13:A1191.
24. Rougier P, Ducreux M, Kerr D, Carr BI, Francois E, Adenis A, Seymour L. A phase II study of raltitrexed ('Tomudex') in patients with hepatocellular carcinoma. *Ann Oncol* 1997; 8:500–502.
25. Cunningham D, Zalcberg JR, Rath U, Olver I, Van Cutsem E, Svensson C, Seitz, JF, Harper P, Kerr D, Perez-Manga G, Azab M, Seymour L, Lowery K, and the Tomudex Colorectal Cancer Study Group. Tomudex (ZD1694): results of a randomised trial in advanced colorectal cancer demonstrates efficacy and reduced mucositis and leucopenia. *Eur J Cancer* 1995; 31A:1945–1954.
26. Cunningham D, Zalcberg JR, Rath U, van Cutsem, Svensson C, Seitz JF, Harper P, Kerr D, Perez-Manga G and the Tomudex Colorectal Study Group. Final results of a randomised trial comparing "Tomudex"® (raltitrexed) with 5-fluorouracil plus leucovorin in advanced colorectal cancer. *Ann Oncol* 1996; 7:961–965.
27. Ross P, Heron J, Cunningham D. Cost of treating advanced colorectal cancer: a retrospective comparison of treatment regimens. *Eur J Cancer* 1996; 32A(suppl 5):S13–17.
28. Summerhayes M, Wanklyn SJ, Shakespeare RA, Lovell J. Reduced pharmacy resource utilisation associated with raltitrexed treatment of advanced colorectal cancer. *J Oncol Pharm Practive* 1996; 3:13–19.
29. Elliot R. An analysis of drug costs for the management of chemotherapy-related side effects in advanced colorectal cancer. *J Pharm Pharmacol* 1996; 2:186–190.
30. Pazdur R, Vincent M. Raltitrexed (Tomudex) versus 5-fluorouracil and leucovorin in patients with advanced colorectal cancer (ACC): results of a randomised, multicentre trial, North American trial. *Proc Amer Soc Clin Oncol* 1997; 16:A801.

31. Harper P. Advanced colorectal cancer (ACC): results from the latest raltitrexed (Tomudex) comparative study. *Proc Amer Soc Clin Oncol* 1997; 16:A802.
32. Harstrick A, Schleucher N, Gonzales A, Schmidt C, Hoffman A, Wilke H, Rustum Y, Seeber S. Interactions and cross resistance patterns between various schedules of 5-FU and the new folate based thymidylate synthase inhibitor Tomudex (D1694). *Eur J Cancer* 1995; 31A:55p126.
33. Kimbell R, Brunton L, Jackman A. Combination studies with Tomudex and 5-fluorouracil in human colon tumour cell lines. *Br J Cancer* 1996; 73:(Suppl XXVI) p12.
34. Kragner KM, Schwartz GK, Bertino J, Kemeny N, Saltz L, Sugarman A, Kelsen DK, Tong W, Lowery C. Interim results of a phase I trial suggest that Tomudex™ (raltitrexed) may act synergistically with 5-fluorouracil (5-FU) in patients with advanced colorectal cancer. *Proc Amer Soc Clin Oncol* 1998; 17:A868.

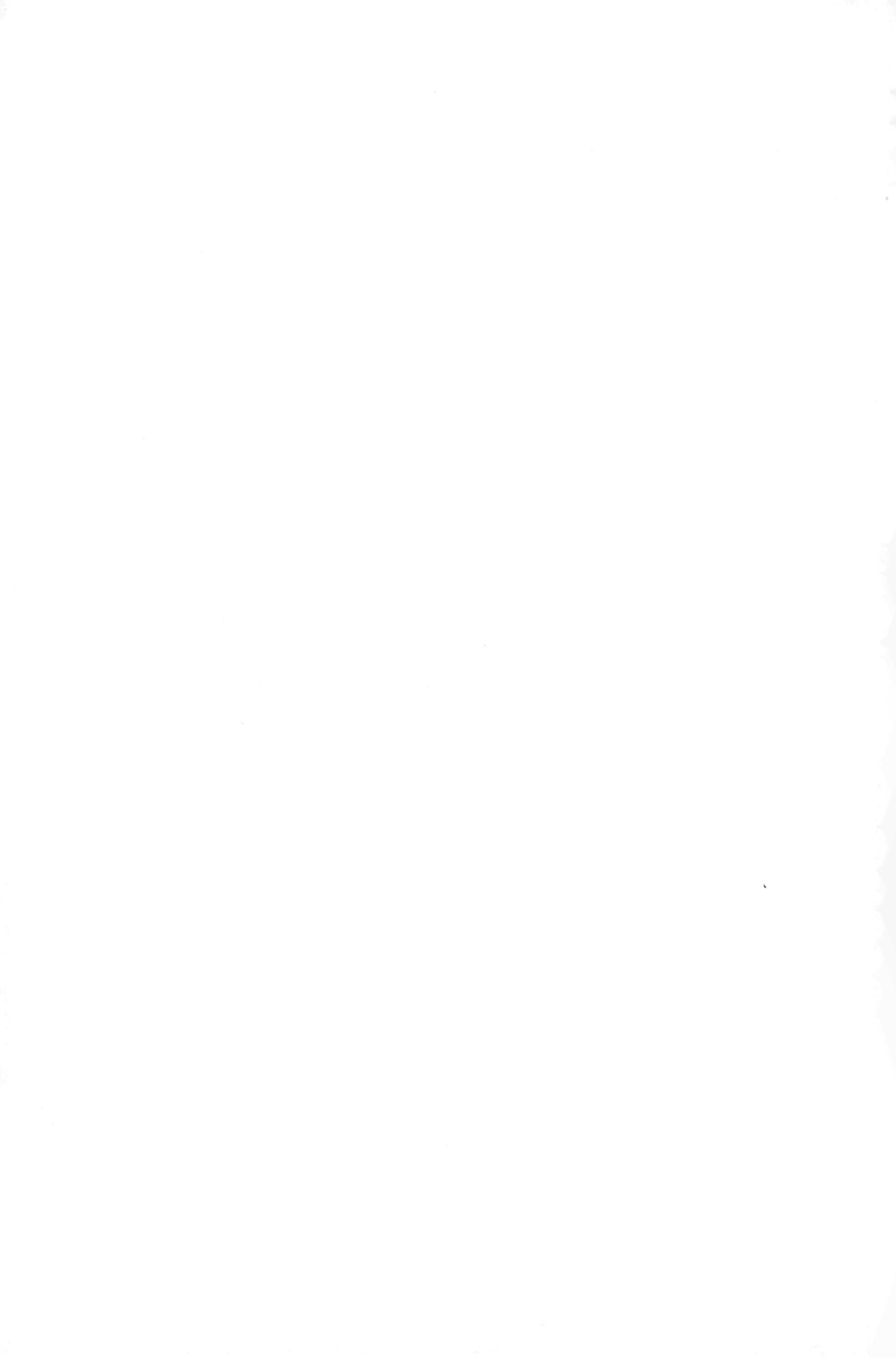

8 Preclinical Pharmacology Studies and the Clinical Development of a Novel Multitargeted Antifolate, MTA (LY231514)

Chuan Shih and Donald E. Thornton

CONTENTS

INTRODUCTION
PRECLINICAL PHARMACOLOGY STUDIES OF MTA
CLINICAL STUDIES OF MTA
CONCLUSION AND PERSPECTIVE

1. INTRODUCTION

Since the early 1950s, extensive research efforts have been devoted to the discovery and development of antifolate antimetabolites as chemotherapeutic agents for the management of neoplastic diseases. However, it was only in the last 10–15 yr, because of the rapid advances of medicinal chemistry, X-ray protein crystallography, molecular biology, pharmacology, and clinical medicine, that a significant number of new generation antifolates were brought forward for clinical development. Several folate-based antimetabolites are currently being investigated in clinical trials. These include lometrexol (6R-5,10-dideazatetrahydrofolic acid) *(1–3)*, LY309887 *(4)*, and AG2034 *(5)*, which are potent and selective inhibitors of glycinamide ribonucleotide formyltransferase (GARFT), an enzyme in the purine *de novo* biosynthetic pathway; trimetrexate *(6)*, edatrexate *(7,8)*, and PT523 *(9)* which act on dihydrofolate reductase (DHFR); raltitrexed *(10,11)*, AG337 *(12)*, BW1843U89 *(13)*, and ZD9331 *(14)* which specifically target the enzyme thymidylate synthase (TS) involved in pyrimidine biosynthesis.

N-[4-[2-(2-amino-3,4-dihydro-4-oxo-7H-pyrrolo[2,3-d]pyrimidin-5-yl)ethyl]-benzoyl]-L-glutamic acid, LY231514, is a structurally novel antifolate that possesses a unique 6-5 fused pyrrolo[2,3-d]pyrimidine nucleus instead of the more common 6-6 fused pteridine or quinazoline ring structure. LY231514 was discovered through struc-

From: *Anticancer Drug Development Guide: Antifolate Drugs in Cancer Therapy*
Edited by: A.L. Jackman © Humana Press Inc., Totowa, NJ

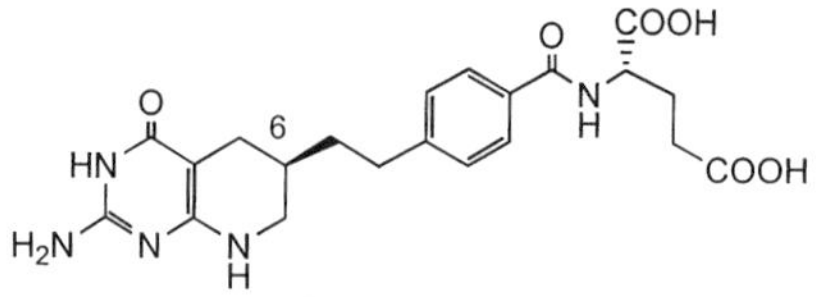

Fig. 1. The structures of lometrexol (6R-5,10-dideazatetrahydrofolic acid, DDATHF) and MTA (N-[4-[2-(2-amino-3,4-dihydro-4-oxo-7H-pyrrolo[2,3-d]pyrimidin-5-yl)ethyl]-benzoyl]-L-glutamic acid).

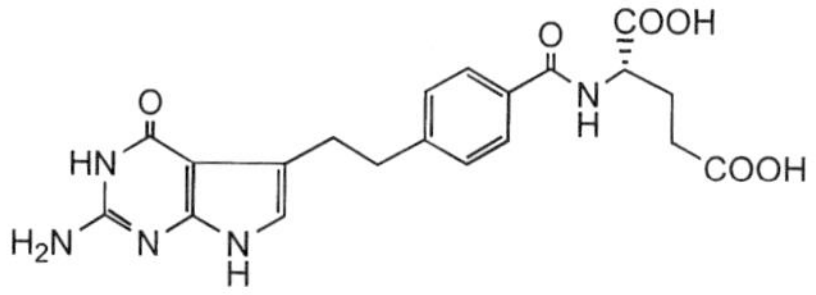

ture activity relationship (SAR) studies of the novel antipurine antifolate lometrexol series, by eliminating the C5 methylene of lometrexol and converting the sp3 center at C6 to sp2 geometry (Fig. 1) *(15,16)*. These modifications give rise to a very potent cytotoxic agent (IC_{50} = 15 nM) against human CCRF-CEM leukemia cells in culture. However, the end-product reversal pattern of this new pyrrolopyrimidine-based antifolate was completely different to the GARFT inhibitor lometrexol. The purine precursor hypoxanthine (100 μM) or aminoimidazole carboxamide (AICA) (300 μM) was incapable of protecting the cells from the cytotoxicity of LY231514. In contrast, thymidine (5 μM) was able to provide partial protection to the cells up to 10X IC_{50} concentrations of LY231514. The replacement of the tetrahydropyridine ring of lometrexol with a pyrrole moiety caused a major loss of activity in the inhibition of purine biosynthesis and shifted the major site of action of LY231514 to the inhibition of pyrimidine biosynthesis (thymidylate cycle). As a "classical" antifolate, LY231514 was found to be one of the best known substrates for mammalian folylpolyglutamate synthetase (FPGS) *(17)* and it is believed that polyglutamation and the polyglutamated metabolites of LY231514 play profound roles in determining both the selectivity and antitumor activity of this novel agent. Recent studies have shown that the polyglutamates of LY231514, (e.g., the triglutamate glu_3 and the pentaglutamate glu_5) potently inhibit several key enzymes of the folate metabolism, including TS, DHFR, GARFT, and aminoimidazole carboxamide ribonucleotide formyltransferase (AICARFT) *(18)*. As a result of this activity against several enzymes, LY231514 has become known as MTA, multitargeted antifolate.

The phase I clinical evaluation of MTA began in late 1992. Objective tumor responses were observed in patients with colorectal cancer and pancreatic cancer, some of whom had failed treatment with other TS inhibitors such as 5FU and raltitrexed *(19–21)*. Phase II studies have shown activity in a range of solid tumors, including colorectal, breast and nonsmall-cell lung cancers *(22–27)*. The purpose of this chapter is to comprehensively review the unique biochemical and pharmacological modes of action, and the recent phase I and II clinical findings of this novel multitargeted antifolate, MTA.

Table 1
Inhibitory Activity of MTA, Methotrexate and Their Polyglutamates Against rhTS,
rhDHFR, rmGARFT, and rhAICARFT (K_i [mean $\pm$ SE, nM])

Compound	rhTS	rhDHFR	rmGARFT	rhAICARFT
MTA	109 $\pm$ 9	7.0 $\pm$ 1.9	9300 $\pm$ 690	3580
MTA-glu$_3$	1.6 $\pm$ 0.1	7.1 $\pm$ 1.6	380 $\pm$ 92	480
MTA-glu$_5$	1.3 $\pm$ 0.3	7.2 $\pm$ 0.4	65 $\pm$ 16	265
MTX	13,000	0.004	80,000	143,000
MTX-glu$_5$	47	0.004	2500	56

2. PRECLINICAL PHARMACOLOGY STUDIES OF MTA

2.1. Folate Enzyme Inhibition Studies

The inhibition of recombinant human (rh)TS, rhDHFR, recombinant mouse (rm)GARFT, and rhAICARFT by MTA and its polyglutamates (glu$_3$ and glu$_5$) *(18)* is summarized in Table 1. The parent monoglutamate MTA inhibited rhTS with a K_i of 109 $\pm$ 9 nM. It has been well documented that mammalian TS shows a strong preference for polyglutamated folate substrates. The longer chain γ-glutamyl derivatives of MTA had significantly enhanced affinity toward rhTS. The addition of two extra γ-glutamyl residues (glu$_3$) to MTA resulted in 68-fold reduction of the K_i value (K_i = 1.6 nM). Further extension of the glutamate tail (MTA-glu$_5$) only slightly increased the affinity toward rhTS (K_i = 1.3 nM). MTA was also found to be a very potent inhibitor of human DHFR (K_i = 7.0 nM). In contrast to rhTS, attachment of additional γ-glutamyl residues to MTA had little effect on the inhibition of DHFR; MTA-glu$_3$ and MTA-glu$_5$ exhibited identical K_i values against rhDHFR, 7.1 nM. Tight-binding analysis showed that MTA-glu$_n$ inhibited both TS and DHFR competitively. When MTA was tested against the enzymes along the purine *de novo* biosynthetic pathway, it only demonstrated moderate inhibition toward rmGARFT (K_i = 9.3 $\mu$$M$). The triglutamate and pentaglutamate of MTA had significantly enhanced inhibitory activity against GARFT, with K_i values of 380 nM (24-fold) and 65 nM (144-fold), respectively. The pentaglutamate of MTA also inhibited human AICARFT with a K_i of 265 nM. Kinetic analysis confirmed the competitive inhibition pattern of MTA polyglutamates against both GARFT and AICARFT. Finally, MTA and its polyglutamates were competitive inhibitors of both the dehydrogenase and synthetase domains of C1 tetrahydrofolate synthase. The K_i values for the mono-, tri- and pentaglutamyl derivatives of MTA were 9.9, 3.9, and 4.7 μM, respectively, for dehydrogenase and 329, 25, 4 and 1.6 μM for synthetase. MTA was a relatively less potent inhibitor of C1 tetrahydrofolate synthase than other enzyme targets such as TS, DHFR, and GARFT. However, cell-culture experiments have suggested that the intracellular drug concentration of MTA can reach levels of 50 $\mu$$M$ (RM Schultz, unpublished observation), and at these concentrations the activity of C1 tetrahydrofolate synthase can also be greatly suppressed by MTA polyglutamates. The important role of TS in serving as a rate-limiting enzyme in folate metabolism, as well as the relative order of inhibitory potency toward TS by MTA-glu$_n$ indicate that TS is a major site of action for MTA. Inhibition of DHFR and other enzymes in the *de novo* purine biosynthetic pathway may also contribute significantly to the overall antiproliferative effect of MTA

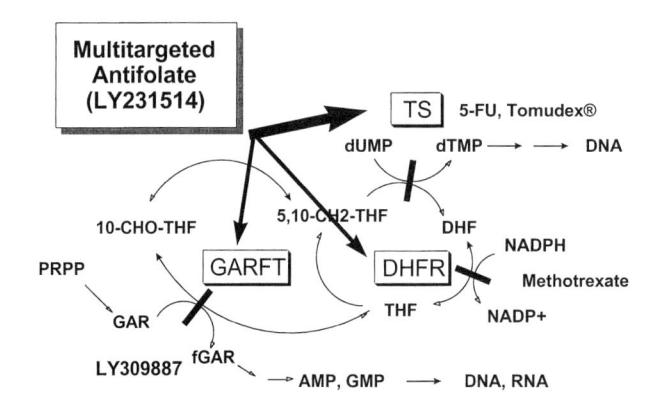

Fig. 2. Inhibition of multiple folate enzymes (TS, DHFR, and GARFT) by MTA and its polyglutamated metabolites.

(Fig. 2). This unique mode of action was further supported by additional cell-based studies (*vide infra*).

As a reference for comparison, the polyglutamates of methotrexate (MTX) also inhibit multiple folate-dependent enzymes. Chabner et al *(28)* reported that the pentaglutamate of MTX (MTX-glu$_5$) demonstrated a significant increase in affinity toward rhTS (K_i = 47 nM) and AICARFT (K_i = 56 nM) when compared with the parent monoglutamate. However, the affinity of MTX and its polyglutamates for DHFR (K_i = 4 pM) was several orders of magnitude (>12,000-fold) higher than its affinity for TS and AICARFT, suggesting that the primary intracellular target of MTX may still be DHFR.

2.2. Cell-Based End-Product Reversal Studies

MTA is very cytotoxic against CCRF-CEM leukemia cells in culture. This potent antiproliferative effect of MTA can be prevented by leucovorin, whereas only partial protection was observed with thymidine. In the presence of 5 μM thymidine, the IC$_{50}$ of MTA increased only 6–10-fold and this was significantly less than that of a pure TS inhibitor such as raltitrexed. This reversal pattern of MTA was further characterized in various human tumor cell lines such as GC3/C1 colon carcinoma and HCT-8 ileocecal carcinoma (Table 2). It was observed that 5 μM thymidine fully protected the cells from cytotoxicity with raltitrexed, whereas similar treatment with thymidine only increased the IC$_{50}$ of MTA by 18.7-fold (GC3/C1), and by 15-fold (HCT-8). Hypoxanthine (100 μM) alone did not markedly influence the cytotoxicity of MTA. Similarly, AICA (300 μM) did not modulate cytotoxicity. However, the combination of thymidine plus hypoxanthine completely reversed the cytotoxicity of MTA in all cell lines (IC$_{50}$s > 20 μM). The reversal pattern of MTA was also significantly different from that of MTX. Neither thymidine nor hypoxanthine could protect the cells from the cytotoxic actions of MTX at all drug concentrations. The unusual reversal pattern observed for MTA suggests that in addition to TS, other important inhibitory sites may exist for this agent. The higher degree of protection by thymidine at low drug concentrations indicates that TS is a major target for MTA. Addition of hypoxanthine together with thymidine fully re-

Table 2
End-Product Reversal Studies with MTA[a] (IC_{50} (nM))

Cell line	MTA alone	dThd[b] (5 μM)	Hypoxanthine[c] (100 μM)	dThd and Hypoxanthine
CCRF-CEM	25	138	32	>40,000
GC3/C1	34	637	34	>40,000
HCT	220	3104	1077	>40,000

[a]Cytotoxicity determined by MTT analysis after 72 h exposure to drug, SE of triplicate determinations did not exceed 10% of mean.
[b]With the addition of 5 μM of thymidine.
[c]With the addition of 100 μM of hypoxanthine.

Table 3
Substrate Activity of MTA and Other Antifolates for Mouse and Hog Liver FPGS

Compound	K_m (μM)[a]	rel. V_{max}[b]	rel. V_{max}/K_m[c]
Mouse Liver FPGS			
Lometrexol	9.3 ± 1.6	1.0	1.0
MTA	0.80 ± 0.11	0.63 ± 0.18	13.7
Methotrexate	166.0 ± 14	0.50 ± 0.09	0.031
Hog Liver FPGS			
Lometrexol	16.4 ± 1.0	1.0	1.0
MTA	1.9 ± 0.5	0.74 ± 0.10	6.40
Methotrexate	116.0 ± 14	0.51 ± 0.08	0.07

[a]Values listed are mean ± standard error for $n \geq 3$ or ± 1/2 range for $n = 2$ replicate experiments.
[b]The ratio of V_{max} for a substrate to the V_{max} of lometrexol with either mouse or hog liver FPGS.
[c]The V_{max} of a substrate relative to lometrexol divided by the K_m of a substrate relative to lometrexol, the kinetics of a standard compound was measured in each experiment to allow accurate comparisons among substrate.

versed the cytotoxicity of MTA, suggesting that at higher concentrations, inhibition of DHFR and/or purine *de novo* biosynthetic enzymes were responsible for other secondary cytotoxic actions of the drug, a conclusion that is consistent with results from enzymatic studies. Recent finding that H630-R10 cells *(29)* (resistant to 5FU with a 39-fold amplification of TS protein) demonstrated a significantly reduced resistance to MTA (fivefold vs 6900-fold for raltitrexed) further support the conclusion that TS is not the sole molecular target for this novel agent.

2.3. The Role of Polyglutamation and Folate Transport

Polyglutamation plays an essential role in determining the overall biochemical and pharmacological properties of the classical antifolates. The formation of polyglutamates leads to the accumulation of polyglutamated metabolites to levels that are significantly higher than could otherwise be achieved at steady state by the parent monoglutamates, and thus serves as an important cellular retention mechanism for folates and antifolates. Studies have shown that MTA is an excellent substrate for mammalian FPGS. The substrate activity of MTA and several other antifolates for mouse and hog liver FPGS *(15,17)* are listed in Table 3. Both the substrate constants (K_m) and the relative first-order

**Table 4
Antiproliferative Activity MTA Against ZR-75-1 Human Breast
Carcinoma Cell Lines with Differing Transport Characteristics**[a]

Cell Line	Transport[b]	MTA, IC_{50} (nM)
WT-AA6-FR+	RFC+, FBP+	22.7
Wild Type (WT)	RFC+, FBP−	110.2
MTX^R-BB3-FR+	RFC−, FBP+	1190.6

[a]Cytotoxicity determined after 72-h drug exposure by MTT assay. Assay medium contained 2 nM folinic acid as the sole folate source. SE of triplicate determinations did not exceed 10% of mean.
[b]Reduced folate carrier (RFC); folate binding protein-α (FBP).

rate constants (k', V_{max}/K_m) have revealed the superior propensity of MTA for polyglutamation by mouse and hog liver FPGS. Recent studies indicate that MTA is an even better substrate for recombinant human FPGS (R.G. Moran, personal communication) and this makes MTA one of most efficient substrates for the enzyme FPGS studied to date.

To evaluate the role of FPGS in the cytotoxicity of MTA in cells, the CR15 line, a lometrexol-resistant CCRF-CEM subline, was utilized. Impaired polyglutamation in CR15 cells was identified as the primary mechanism of resistance to lometrexol (30). It was estimated that CR15 cells had approx 10% of the FPGS activity of the wild-type cells and were markedly cross-resistant to MTA (>7800-fold increase in IC_{50} vs the parent CEM line), suggesting that polyglutamation is a major determinant in the cytotoxicity of MTA.

To investigate the mechanism for MTA transport, a panel of ZR-75-1 human breast carcinoma sublines, prepared by Dixon(31) and colleagues, with different transport characteristics was utilized (Table 4). The MTX-resistant cells (RFC+, FBP−), deficient in folate binding protein (FBP) activity, demonstrated only a 4.8-fold decrease in sensitivity to MTA, when compared to wild-type AA6-FR+ cells that expressed both reduced folate carrier (RFC) and FBP. Resistant cells (MTXR-BB3-FR+) deficient in RFC exhibited a much higher resistance to MTA (52-fold) than the wild-type cells. These data, plus the finding that MTA had rather poor affinity toward folate binding protein(s) in general ($K_i = 99.7$ nM vs $K_i = 0.29$ nM for lometrexol), suggest that RFC plays a predominant role in the transport and internalization of MTA.

2.4. Effects of MTA on Folate and Nucleoside Triphosphate Pools

The effects of MTA and several other antifolates (MTX, LY309887) on cellular folate and nucleotide metabolism have been examined in CCRF-CEM cells(32). Exposure of cells labeled with 100 nM 5-formylTHF to 0.1 μM MTX caused the loss of 10-formylTHF, THF, and 5-methylTHF and a concomitant accumulation of dihydrofolate (DHF), metabolic responses consistent with the blockade of DHFR by MTX. The GARFT inhibitor LY309887, on the other hand, caused accumulation of 10-formylTHF, a direct consequence of the inhibition of GARFT, which utilizes 10-formylTHF as the one-carbon donor for its enzymatic reactions. These effects are fully consistent with the known mechanisms of action of MTX and LY309887.

Because of the assay's inability to distinguish THF and methyleneTHF, the effects of MTA on cells could not be readily studied. However, exposure of cells to MTA (300 nM, also 10 times the IC$_{50}$) can trigger a slight decrease in THF and a compensatory increase in the level of 10-formylTHF. In light of the observed accumulation of 10-formylTHF by the specific GARFT inhibitor LY309887, it is tempting to attribute this small, yet significant, increase of 10-formylTHF to the inhibition of GARFT and AICARFT (antipurine effect) by MTA-glu$_n$, a hypothesis that can be verified by direct measurement of the effect of MTA on the metabolic flux from glycine to inosinic acid.

In the ribonucleotide pool studies, it was discovered that both MTX and LY309887 caused rapid depletion of both purines, ATP and GTP, and had moderate effects on the pyrimidines, UTP and CTP. However, MTA produced no significant effects on any of the ribonucleotide triphosphates at concentrations 10 times their IC$_{50}$ in CEM cells. In contrast, all three compounds demonstrated more dramatic effects on deoxyribonucleotide pools. In response to LY309887, dATP declined rapidly, followed closely by dCTP, and then later by dGTP and dTTP at a slower rate. MTX rapidly depleted all four deoxyribonucleotide levels. The effect of MTA on deoxyribonucleotide levels is consistent with reports of other TS inhibitors (33). It was found that MTA was able to induce rapid losses in dTTP, dCTP, and dGTP. However, an increase of dATP level was observed for cells treated with MTA. It will be interesting to examine the difference of the rate of accumulation of dATP induced by MTA or by other specific TS inhibitors, since Chong and Tattersall(33) reported that the combination of a GARFT inhibitor and TS inhibitor prevented the rise in the dATP pool seen with the TS inhibitor alone. The mechanism for the changes in dATP levels induced by TS inhibitors has not been well understood. However, it is noteworthy that for MTX, a drug with both antipyrimidine and antipurine effects, depletion of dTTP occurred without a concomitant increase in dATP. In summary, these studies showed that MTA exhibited unique metabolic effects that were quite distinct from those of MTX and LY309887. The folate pools (accumulation of 10-formylTHF) data suggest that in addition to the primary effect on the thymidylate synthesis, MTA may produce an antipurine effect by interfering with the enzymes along the *de novo* purine biosynthetic pathway.

2.5. Effects of MTA on Cell-Cycle Alterations and Cell Proliferation(34)

MTA affects the growth rate of CCRF-CEM leukemia cells in a concentration-dependent manner. When CEM cells were treated with concentrations of MTA greater than 100 nM, cell growth was completely inhibited and apoptosis occurred within 36 h of drug treatment. Multiple cell-cycle alterations occurred in CCRF-CEM populations when cells were treated with either a sublethal (30 nM) or a lethal (300 nM) dose of MTA. Within 8 h of drug addition, both treatments synchronized cells into G1 or G1/S population. At the sublethal dose, the cell population was distributed throughout S phase after 24 h of drug addition, and was able to complete DNA synthesis. In contrast, the population treated with 300 nM of MTA was effectively synchronized into early S phase after 24 h and was unable to complete DNA synthesis. Further studies also showed that levels of cyclin E, a G1/S-specific protein in cell-cycle control, were dramatically increased relative to control in cells treated with either sublethal or lethal dose of MTA. Dual parameter flow cytometry confirmed that cyclin E levels were 2–5-fold higher in treated vs. untreated cells. In contrast, cyclin A levels did not begin to increase until af-

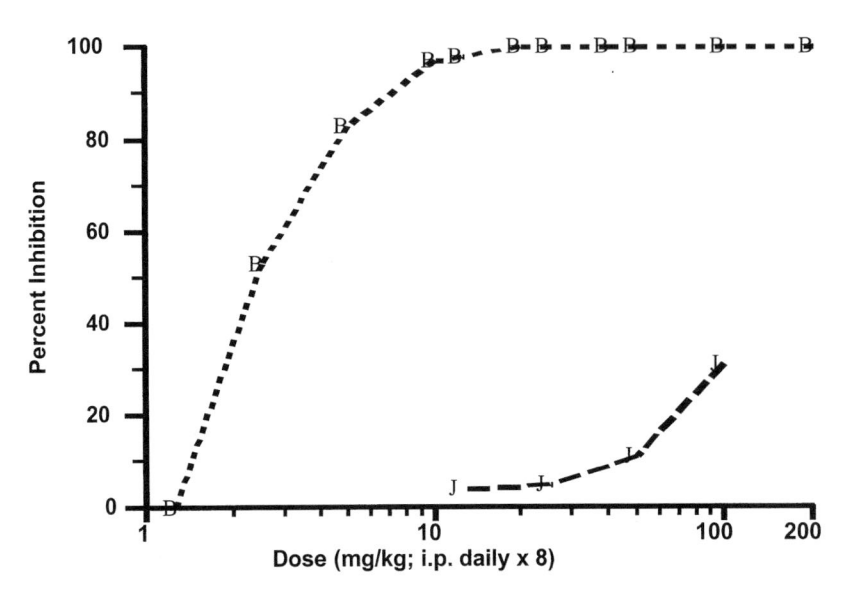

Fig. 3. Antitumor activity of MTA (LY231514, **B**) or CB3717 (**J**) against L5178Y/TK$^-$/HX$^-$, in DBA/2 mice. Both MTA and CB3717 were administered ip, daily × 10.

ter 24 h of treatment. These observations indicate that both lethal and sublethal concentrations of MTA are able to cause an initial blockade in the cell cycle prior to the G1/S checkpoint. This is followed by synchronization of the cells into the S phase under lethal concentrations. Continued exposure of the drug triggers major apoptotic events that eventually lead to cell death.

2.6. The in Vivo Antitumor Effects and the Role of Folic Acid in Modulating the Efficacy and Toxicity of MTA

MTA was found to be highly active against the L5178Y/TK-/HX-lymphoma in mice *(35)* (Fig. 3). An excellent therapeutic index was seen, along with antitumor activity in this thymidine kinase-deficient murine model, a result that is consistent with TS inhibition being the primary mode of action of MTA. Good antitumor activity was also observed for MTA in other human tumor xenografts that expressed normal level of thymidine kinase, including VRC5 (colon, 80% growth inhibition) and GC3 (colon, 94% growth inhibition), BXPC3 (pancreas), LX-1 (lung), and MX-1 (breast) xenografts (Table 5).

To evaluate the importance of dietary folate in modulating the toxicity of MTA, LD$_{50}$ values were determined in mice maintained on standard diet (SD) or on a special low-folate diet (LFD) *(35)*. MTA was administered ip daily for 10 d. It is estimated that mice on LFD consumed an average of approx 0.003 mg/kg/d of folic acid vs 0.75–1.5 mg/kg/d for mice on SD. Thus mice on SD had a daily intake of approx 250–500 times more folic acid than mice on LFD. MTA was more toxic to several different strains of mice maintained on LFD (Table 6), with the LD$_{50}$ values being 30- to 250-fold lower than mice maintained on SD. A similar effect had been observed for antipurine antifolates such as lometrexol. The MTD of lometrexol on LFD was 1000- to 5000-fold lower than in mice

Table 5
Comparison of Antitumor Activity of MTA with DDATHF and Methotrexate Against Human Tumor Xenografts

Xenograft Model	MTA[a]	DDATHF[b]	Methotrexate
GC3 colon carcinoma	+++	+++	−
VRC5 colon carcinoma	++	+++	−
BXPC3 pancreatic carcinoma	+	+	−
LX-1 lung carcinoma	+	++	[c]
MX-1 mammary carcinoma	+	+	[c]

+++: 95–100% inhibition.
++: 80–94% inhibition.
+: 60–79% inhibition.
−: <60% inhibition inactive.
[a] MTA was given ip, qd × 10 at doses up to 300 mg/kg/dose.
[b] DDATHF was given ip, q2d × 5 at doses up to 100 mg/kg/dose.
[c] NCI data.

Table 6
Effect of Dietary Folate on the Lethality of MTA

Strain of Mouse	Diet	Route, Schedule	LD_{50} (mg/kg)	Ratio of LD_{50} (SD/LFD)
DBA/2	Standard diet	ip qd × 10	approx 600	approx 60
	Low folate diet		approx 10	
CD1 nu/nu	Standard diet	ip qd × 10	approx 400	approx 250
	Low folate diet		1.56	
C3H	Standard diet	ip qd × 10	>1600	approx 30
	Low folate diet		50–100	

maintained on SD (36). DHFR inhibitors such as methotrexate had a similar effect but to a lesser extent (50- to 100-fold, J.F. Worzalla, unpublished observation). The therapeutic index of MTA against the L5178Y/TK-/HX-tumor was greatly diminished when the mice were put on a LFD (2 wk) with no folate supplementation. Good antitumor activity was observed at 0.3 mg/kg and 1.0 mg/kg (ip daily × 10) doses only, and significant toxicity was observed for MTA at higher doses (Fig. 4). However, if daily folic acid supplementation (15 mg/d/mouse, po) was given in conjunction with MTA, excellent antitumor dose-response (10 mg/kg to 1000 mg/kg, with antitumor activity ranging from 80 to 100%) and no lethality were observed. This antitumor dose response (with folate supplementation) is identical to the dose response that was observed for MTA on mice fed with SD (Fig. 3). These data suggest that folate supplementation not only modulates the toxicity but also slightly enhances the antitumor response of MTA.

2.7. Drug Disposition and Metabolism of MTA

The metabolism and disposition of MTA was studied in mice and dogs (37). Some selected pharmacokinetic parameters are summarized in Table 7. Intravenous injections of MTA gave high plasma levels of the drug, resulting in an AUC value of 30–33 μg-h/mL for mice and dogs after 20 and 7.5 mg/kg doses, respectively. In vitro protein binding of

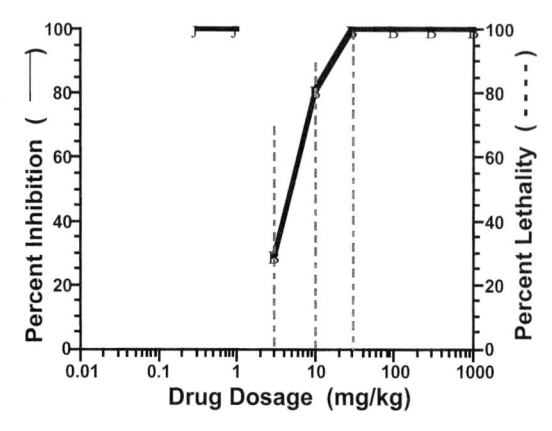

Fig. 4. Antitumor activity of MTA against L5178Y/TK⁻/HX⁻ lymphoma for mice on low folate diet (LFD) with no folate supplementation (**J**) and for mice on low folate diet that received 15 mg/kg/d daily folate supplementation (**B**); vertical dashed lines represent percent lethality in mice on low folate diet with no folate supplementation.

Table 7
Pharmacokinetic Parameters for Mouse and Dog with MTA

	Mouse		*Dog*	
Sex	M	F	M	F
Dose (mg/kg)	20	20	7.5	7.5
Route	iv	ip	iv	iv
t_{max} (h)	0.083	0.25	0.083	0.083
C_{max} (μg/mL)	41	33	38 ± 2	49 ± 9
$t_{1/2}$ (h) (interval)	7 (1–48)	7.8 (2–48)	2.8 (1–24)	1.8 (1–12)
AUC (μg/h/mL)	31	44	33 ± 1.9	30 ± 2
Cl (mL/h/kg)	645	—	230 ± 24	246 ± 29

[^{14}C]MTA in plasma was estimated at concentrations of 0.5 and 5 μg/mL using an ultracentrifugation procedure. In mouse plasma, the binding of [^{14}C]MTA was 54–58% and in dog plasma it was 46–47%. The binding was notably higher (81%) in human plasma. MTA was primarily eliminated unchanged in feces (57%) of mice after a single iv dose of [^{14}C]MTA. Urine was the major route of excretion (69%) in dogs. Half-life values were approx 7 and 2.8 h for mice and dogs, respectively.

Unchanged MTA accounted for the majority of urinary radiocarbon in mice (90%) and dogs (68%), although two minor metabolites were found in these species. The first metabolite, LY338979, was formed by oxidation of the pyrrole ring of MTA (position 6) giving the corresponding lactam (Fig. 5). This type of oxidative transformation is also seen with tryptophans and other indole-containing compounds. Further oxidation of the lactam ring of LY338979, followed by one-carbon extrusion, gave a second metabolite, LY368962, with a complete loss of the pyrrole ring structure. The structures of both metabolites were confirmed by total synthesis and NMR (long-range heteronuclear coupling) experiments. Testing of the major metabolite LY338979 showed that this agent is

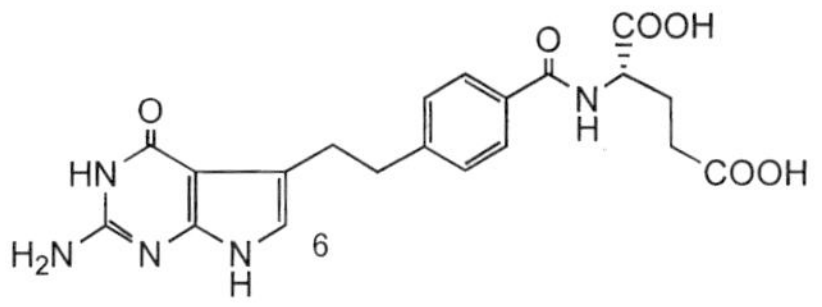

Fig. 5. Structures of the two minor metabolites of MTA isolated from the urine of mice and dogs, LY338979 and LY368962.

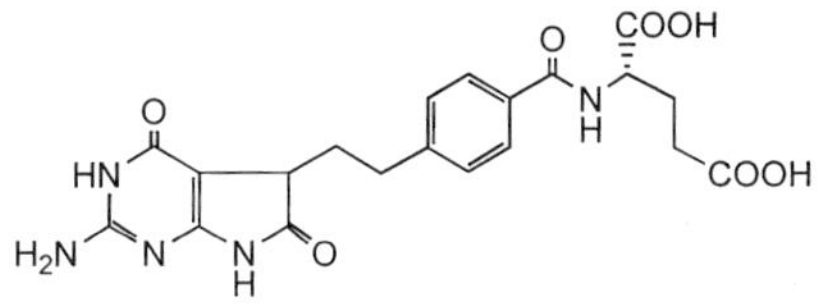

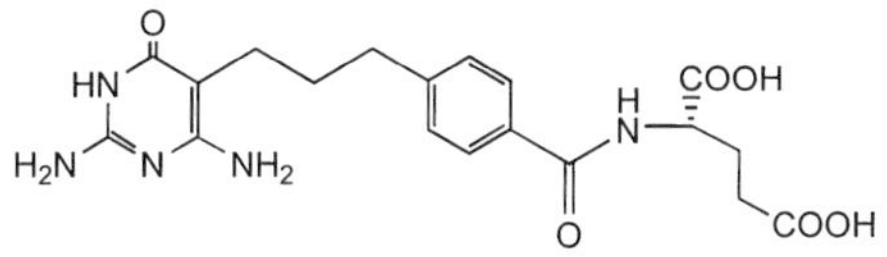

biologically inactive as a TS inhibitor (using a rhTS assay) and has no antiproliferative effects on CEM cells in culture.

2.8. Preclinical Toxicological Findings of MTA (38)

Genetic toxicology studies indicated that MTA is negative in the Ames test, in vitro chromosome aberration test, and mammalian HGPRT+ locus forward mutation assay. In acute toxicology studies, it was found that the iv median lethal dose (MLD) of MTA for female and male Fisher 344 rats was >1574 and 1322 mg/kg, respectively. In comparison, the MLD of MTX in rats is 6 to 25 mg/kg. The iv MLD for female and male CD-1 mice was >1574 mg/kg. The LD_{10} for mice could not be calculated, but was estimated to be >1574 mg/kg. The MLD of MTX for mice was 94 mg/kg.

Single and repeated dose studies of MTA were conducted in CD-1 mice and dogs. In pilot mice studies, groups of five mice of each sex per dose group were given daily ip doses of 0, 50, 100, and 150 mg/kg MTA for 2 wk. Daily doses were well tolerated by mice, all mice survived to study termination and had no clinical signs of toxicity. In longer duration studies, 10 mice/sex/dose group were dosed ip with 0, 10, and 25 mg/kg MTA daily, 105 mg/kg twice weekly, or 315 mg/kg once weekly for 6 wk. Again, all mice tolerated all doses and schedules with no compound-related mortality or clinical signs of toxicity. Intestinal necrosis was slight and was limited only to male and female mice treated daily with 10 and 25 mg/kg MTA. The higher levels of thymidine (1–5 μM) in mice is thought to reduce the impact of MTA on the proliferation and function of normal cells.

Dogs are more sensitive to MTA. Single iv slow-bolus doses of 10, 25, 50, or 100 mg/kg of MTA can be tolerated by dogs. Up to five daily doses of 5 or 10 mg/kg were given to one dog/dose and the dose of 10 mg/kg proved to be toxic. Dogs given single doses of 50 mg/kg or more had modest lymphopenia and leukopenia 6 d after dosing. The leukopenia was neither consistent nor dose related, and values returned to the reference range within 10 d of dosing. There were no important effects on erythrocyte or platelet parameters. For longer duration studies, one dog/sex/dose group was given either daily iv slow-bolus doses of 0.1, 0.5, 0.75, or 1.0 mg/kg MTA or 10 mg/kg twice weekly for up to 2 wk. Dogs treated with 0.75 or 1 mg/kg died after 7–10 daily doses. Mortality was preceded by clinical signs of decreased food consumption, hypoactivity, dehydration, emesis, abnormal stools, and increased salivation.

In summary, the toxicological profile of MTA is consistent with the known antiproliferative activities of folate antimetabolites. The major pathological effects associated with MTA occurred in the intestinal tract and lymphoid tissues; bone marrow was only minimally affected in dogs and mice given repeated doses. No hepatic or renal toxicity was observed in these preclinical toxicology studies by histopathalogic evaluation.

3. CLINICAL STUDIES OF MTA

3.1. MTA Phase I Experience

Three dosing schedules have been investigated in the phase I setting. In study JMAA, patients received MTA once every 21 d. Study JMAB looked at administering the drug once weekly for 4 wk out of every 6, and study BP-001 investigated a schedule of daily times five every 21 d.

The daily times five every 3 wk schedule resulted in a maximum tolerated dose (MTD) of 4 mg/m^2/day *(21)*. Dose-limiting toxicities on this schedule were reversible neutropenia and elevated liver enzymes. Nonhematologic toxicities were mild and included mucositis, diarrhea, rash, fatigue, and elevated transaminases. Minor responses were observed using this schedule in one patient with colorectal cancer and one patient with nonsmall-cell lung cancer (NSCLC). Phase II studies are ongoing to assess the efficacy of this schedule.

Studies JMAA and JMAB used the Modified Continual Reassessment Method for dose escalation. This involves treating a single patient at each minimally toxic dose level and adding more patients once significant toxicities are observed at a dose level. A minimum of three patients are treated at a dose level once moderate reversible toxicity is demonstrated (grade III hematologic toxicity or grade II nonhematologic toxicity excluding nausea, vomiting, and alopecia). Dose-limiting toxicity (DLT) was defined as grade IV hematologic or grade III nonhematologic toxicity, excluding nausea, vomiting, and alopecia. A minimum of six patients are treated once dose-limiting toxicities are demonstrated. In this manner, the number of patients exposed to lower, potentially less effective doses of drug is limited and more patients are treated at doses approaching the MTD *(39)*.

The DLT on the weekly times four, every 6 weeks schedule (study JMAB) was myelosuppression, particularly leukopenia and granulocytopenia *(19)*. Inability to maintain the weekly treatment schedule because of neutropenia limited dose escalation on this schedule. This schedule is not currently being pursued in phase II trials.

Table 8
Initial Phase I Experience

	BP-001	JMAA	JMAB
Schedule[a]	Daily × 5, every 21 d	Once every 21 d	Weekly × 4, every 6 wk
Number of patients treated	38	37	24
Dose range	0.2–5.2 mg/m^2	50–700 mg/m^2	10–40 mg/m^2
Recommended phase II dose	4 mg/m^2	600 mg/m^2	30 mg/m^2
DLT	neutropenia	neutropenia, mucositis, fatigue	myelosuppression, particularly granulocytopenia
Responses	Minor responses in colorectal (1) and NSCLC (1)	Partial responses in pancreas (2), and colorectal (2)	Minor responses in colorectal (2)

[a] All doses administered as a 10-min infusion.

The once every 21 d schedule has been evaluated in phase II trials (20). In the phase I trial investigating this dose (study JMAA), 37 patients were administered drug at doses ranging from 50–700 mg/m^2. Dose-limiting toxicities on this schedule were neutropenia, thrombocytopenia, and fatigue. The MTD on this schedule was determined to be 600 mg/m^2, and of the 20 patients treated at this dose, Common Toxicity Criteria (CTC) grade IV neutropenia and CTC grade IV thrombocytopenia occurred in four and one patients, respectively, in the first cycle. CTC grade II toxicities included rash, mucositis, nausea, vomiting, fatigue, anorexia, and elevations of liver transaminases. Patients experiencing rash were treated in subsequent cycles with 4 mg dexamethasone twice daily for 3 d, starting the day before MTA therapy. The severity of the rash was reduced or the rash prevented in these patients (19). The phase I experience is summarized in Table 8.

Pharmacokinetic determinations were made in 20 patients who were treated at the MTD (600 mg/m^2) in study JMAA. A mean maximum plasma concentration of 137 μg/mL was attained, with a mean half-life of 3.1 h (range 2.2–7.2 h). Mean clearance and steady-state volume of distribution values of 40 mL/min/m^2 and 7.0 l/m^2 were also measured. This mean clearance value is similar to that of creatinine clearance in the age range of the patients enrolled (approx 45–55 mL/min/m^2) and the volume of distribution reflects limited distribution outside the bloodstream (40).

Samples collected from the first dose in each course of therapy showed the disposition of MTA to be linear over the entire dose range (0.2–700 mg/m^2). The clearance of the drug is primarily renal, with 80% or more of the dose recovered unchanged in the urine during the first 24 h after dosing. No accumulation appears to occur with multiple courses, and the disposition of MTA does not change after multiple doses. Gender does not appear to affect MTA disposition. MTA clearance appears to decrease with age, although this decrease is most likely to be related to decreasing renal function (40).

Partial responses were seen in one of the phase I studies (JMAA), with two in pancreas cancer patients of duration 2 and 6 mo, and two in colorectal cancer patients of duration 7 and 11 mo. Both patients with colorectal cancer had received prior chemotherapy, one with intrahepatic FUDR and one with raltitrexed. One of the patients with pancreatic cancer had received prior therapy with 5FU.

3.2. Phase II Experience

Two phase II studies in colorectal cancer, one in pancreas cancer, two in NSCLC, and one in breast cancer began in late 1995. These studies were designed to include patients with advanced disease who were either chemonaive or had received prior chemotherapy in the metastatic setting, with a starting dose of 600 mg/m^2 once every 21 d. Results from these studies are preliminary.

Clinical activity of MTA in metastatic colorectal carcinoma has been demonstrated in two multicenter trials performed in Canada (23) and the U.S. (24). Prior adjuvant chemotherapy was allowed if completed at least 1 yr prior to study entry. In the Canadian study, the starting dose of 600 mg/m^2 was reduced to 500 mg/m^2 after dose reductions were required in five of the first eight patients. Toxicities leading to these reductions included rash, mucositis, neutropenia, and febrile neutropenia. Responses were seen at this reduced dose in six patients for an overall response rate of 21% (8–39.7%) (23). In the U.S. colorectal study, objective tumor responses were seen in 6 of 39 patients for an overall response rate of 16% (24).

Two responses, one complete and one partial, were observed in 35 evaluable patients in the pancreatic cancer phase II study for an overall response rate of 6% (25). Importantly, there were 13 additional patients with stable disease lasting for over 6 mo of treatment, suggesting a clinical benefit not immediately apparent from objective tumor measurements.

A phase II study in patients with locally advanced and/or metastatic breast cancer is ongoing and includes patients who have received prior adjuvant chemotherapy as well as one prior therapy for metastatic disease. Fourteen of 22 patients had received prior chemotherapy, 10 as adjuvant treatment, 7 for metastatic disease, and 3 patients who received both. Of the 18 patients evaluable for response, 1 complete and 5 partial responses have been documented for an overall response rate of 30%. Responses have been seen in pulmonary and hepatic metastases. Three of the six responding patients had received recent prior therapy with paclitaxel, docetaxel, or an anthracycline for metastatic disease (27).

One multi-institutional study in NSCLC has been completed in Canada (26) and an additional study is ongoing in Australia and South Africa (22). All patients were chemonaive. The majority of patients on the Canadian study used the lower starting dose of 500 mg/m^2, which was reduced from 600 mg/m^2 during the course of the study after one of the first three patients experienced CTC grade III mucositis and grade IV vomiting and myalgia. Seven partial responses have been observed in 30 evaluable patients for an overall response rate of 23.3% (95% CI 9.9–42.3%) (26). All responding patients were treated at the 500 mg/m^2 dose level.

The second NSCLC study, which is being carried out jointly between Australia and South Africa, has enrolled 21 patients to date, with 20 evaluable for response. All patients are receiving 600 mg/m^2 every 3 wk in this study. Five partial responses have been noted for an overall response rate of 25% (22). The phase II experience to date is summarized in Table 9.

Table 9
Phase II Experience

Study	JMAC	JMAD	JMAN	JMAO	JMAG	JMAL
Site	U.S.	U.S.	Canada	Canada	U.K.	Aus/S Africa
Tumor site	colorectal	pancreas	NSCLC	colorectal	breast	NSCLC
Number of evaluable patients	39	35	30	29	18	20
Median cycles	4	2	3	3	4	4
(Range)	(1–12)	(1–12)	(1–8)	(1–8)	(1–9)	(1–9)
CR	1	1	0	1	1	0
PR	5	1	7	5	5	5
Overall RR (%)	16	6	23	21	30	25
(95% CI, %)			(9.9–42.3)	(8–39.7)		

Table 10
Laboratory Toxicity ($n = 209$)

	Grade I (%)	Grade II (%)	Grade III (%)	Grade IV (%)
Alk Phos	49	13	4	
ALT	33	26	22	0
AST	42	30	10	0
Bilirubin		18	7.3	2
Creatinine	13	5	0	0
ANC	9	21	27	27
Hb	34	43	12	2.4
Platelets	31	6	7	8

A total of 209 patients have been treated on the once every 3 wk schedule in the phase II setting at 600 mg/m² and are evaluable for safety analysis. The most frequent, serious toxicity has been hematologic in nature. CTC grade III and IV hematologic toxicity included neutropenia (25 and 26%, respectively) and thrombocytopenia (7 and 10%, respectively). Although severe neutropenia is common, the frequency of serious infection has been low (grade IV infection 2%). Likewise, thrombocytopenia has been apparent, and yet serious episodes of bleeding have been rare (<1%). Whereas 8% of patients experienced grade III (4% with grade IV) skin rash, prophylactic dexamethasone is reported to ameliorate or prevent the rash in subsequent cycles. Other grade III and IV nonhematologic toxicities included stomatitis, diarrhea, vomiting, and infection. As seen in clinical studies of other antifolates, transient grade III and IV elevation of liver transaminases are common but not dose limiting. There have been no cases of persistent transaminase elevation. Tables 10 and 11 summarize the laboratory and nonlaboratory toxicity data from the phase II studies conducted at a starting dose of 600 mg/m².

4. CONCLUSION AND PERSPECTIVE

Extensive biochemical and pharmacological evidence has demonstrated that MTA is a novel antifolate that differs in its mode of action from other antifolates currently un-

Table 11
Nonlaboratory Toxicity (n = 209)

	Grade I (%)	Grade II (%)	Grade III (%)	Grade IV (%)
Cutaneous	19	39	11	5
Diarrhea	17	11	4	3
Infection	13	8	2	2
Nausea	33	30	9	0.5
Fatigue	13	11	6	0
Pulmonary	0.5	7	2	2
Stomatitis	23	16	6	1
Vomiting	13	30	2	3

dergoing investigation. MTA is transported into the cell mainly through the reduced folate carrier system and extensively metabolized to polyglutamated forms. The polyglutamates of MTA inhibit at least three key folate enzymes: TS, DHFR, and GARFT, and to a lesser extent AICARFT and C1-tetrahydrofolate synthase. The combined effects of the inhibition exerted by MTA at each target give rise to an unusual end-product reversal pattern at the cellular level that is distinct from those of other inhibitors such as methotrexate and the quinazoline antifolates. MTA is broadly active against murine solid tumors and human tumor xenografts in vivo. Many lines of evidence indicate that MTA does not behave like a pure TS inhibitor nor does it act like a conventional DHFR inhibitor, such as methotrexate, which also inhibits multiple folate enzymes. The important biochemical, pharmacological and clinical characteristics of MTA include:

- Potent inhibition of TS, DHFR, and enzymes in the *de novo* purine biosynthetic pathway including GARFT, with TS as the primary target.
- Unique end-product reversal pattern which is distinct from all other antifolates.
- Different cross-resistance pattern to cells resistant to TS inhibitors.
- Distinct metabolic effects on folate and nucleotide pools compared to other antifolates.
- Early evidence of clinical activity in NSCLC, a tumor type considered resistant to TS-based antifolate antimetabolites.
- Single-agent activity in phase II studies in patients with a broad spectrum of solid tumors including colorectal, breast, nonsmall-cell lung, and pancreatic cancers.

MTA is, therefore, a novel antifolate with unique biochemical and pharmacological properties. The efficient polyglutamation, longer cellular retention and multiple folate enzyme inhibition mechanism may contribute directly to the exciting antitumor responses now being observed in patients. Specifically, the multitargeted inhibition mechanism of MTA is intriguing. This new level of mechanistic insight evolving and around MTA prompts us to challenge the traditional approach to antifolate drug discovery and development, which has focused on developing potent and selective inhibitors of a single folate enzyme target. Given the complex nature of folate metabolism and the role of folates in maintaining the physiological functions of living systems, it is reasonable to expect that agents that can interfere with multiple enzymes in the folate pathway may trigger more biochemical imbalance of the cellular DNA and RNA synthesis of malignant cells than agents acting on a single control point.

In conclusion, MTA is a new generation antifolate with inhibitory activity against multiple folate enzymes including TS, DHFR, and GARFT. In current phase II studies, MTA is broadly active as a single agent and has shown encouraging antitumor activity in multiple solid tumors. More advanced and extensive clinical trials of MTA are currently in progress, including trials in which the effects of MTA in combination with other agents such as cisplatin and gemcitabine are under investigation. The combination of a novel mode of action, preclinical and clinical activity, manageable and tolerable side effects and a dosing schedule that is easy to administer, indicates that MTA will play an important role in the treatment of patients with solid tumors.

ACKNOWLEDGMENTS

The authors like to thank Victor Chen, Laura Mendelsohn, Bill Ehlhardt, Jeff Engelhardt, John Worzalla, Rick Schultz, Deirdre Conlon, and Jackie Walling for many helpful discussions for the preparation of this manuscript.

REFERENCES

1. Taylor EC, Harrington PJ, Fletcher SR, Beardsley GP, Moran RG. Synthesis of the antileukemic agents 5,10-dideazaaminopterin and 5,10-dideaza-5,6,7,8-tetrahydroaminopterin. *J Med Chem* 1985; 28:914–921.
2. Shih C, Grindey GB, Houghton PT, Houghton JA. The in vivo activity of 5,10-dideazatetrahydrofolic acid (DDATHF) and its diastereomers. *Proc Am Assoc Cancer Res* 1988; 29:283.
3. Beardsley GP, Moroson BA, Taylor EC, Moran RG. A new folate antimetabolite, 5,10-dideaza-5,6,7,8-tetrahydofolate is a potent inhibitor of *de novo* purine synthesis. *J Biol Chem* 1989; 264:328–333.
4. Habeck LL, Leitner TA, Shackleford KA, Gossett LS, Schultz RM, Andis SL, Shih C, Grindey GB, Mendelsohn LG. A novel class of monoglutamated antifolates exhibits tight-binding inhibition of human glycinamide ribonucleotide formyltransferase and potent activity against solid tumors. *Cancer Res* 1994; 54:1021–1026.
5. Boritzki TJ, Bartlett CA, Howland EF, Margosiak SA, Palmer CL, Romines WH, Varney MD, Webber S, Jackson RC. Biological properties of AG2034: a new inhibitor of glycinamide ribonucleotide formyltransferase. *Proc Am Assoc Cancer Res* 1996; 37:385.
6. Eisenhauser EA, Wierzbicki R, Knowling M. Phase II trials of trimetrexate in advanced adult soft tissue sarcoma. *Ann Oncol* 1991; 2:689–690.
7. Sirotnak FM, DeGraw JI, Schmid FA, Goutas LJ, Moccio DM. New folate analogs of 10-deazaaminopterin series, further evidence for markedly increased antitumor efficacy compared with methotrexate in ascitic and solid murine tumor models. *Can Chemother Pharmacol* 1984; 12:26–30.
8. Kris MG, Kinghan JJ, Gralla RJ, Fanucchi MP, Wertheim MS, O'Connel JP, Marks LD, Williams L, Farag F, Young CW, Sirotnak FM. Phase I trial and clinical pharmacological evaluation of 10-ethyl-10-deazaaminopterin in adult patients with advanced cancer. *Cancer Res* 1988; 48:5573–5579.
9. Rosowsky A, Bader H, Chen G, Mota CE, Vaidys C, Wright JE. Dihydrofolate reductase inhibition and in vivo antitumor activity of non-polyglutamatable analogs of aminopterin against human non-small cell lung carcinoma. *Proc Am Assoc Cancer Res* 1995; 36:376.
10. Jackman AL, Taylor GA, Gibson W, Kimbell R, Brown M, Calvert AH, Judson I, Hughes LR. ICI D1694, a quinazoline antifolate thymidylate synthase inhibitor that is a potent inhibitor of L1210 tumor cell growth *in vitro* and *in vivo:* a new agent for clinical study. *Cancer Res* 1991; 51:5576–5586.
11. Marsham PR, Hughes LR, Jackman AL, Hayter AJ, Oldfield J, Wardleworth JM, Bishop JA, O'Connor BM, Calvert AH. Quinazoline antifolate thymidylate synthase inhibitors: heterocyclic benzoyl ring modifications. *J Med Chem* 1991; 34:1594–1605.

12. Calvete JA, Balmanno K, Taylor GA, Rafi I, Newell DR, Lind MJ, Calvert AH, Webber S, Clendennin NJ. Preclinical and clinical studies of prolonged administration of the novel thymidylate synthase inhibitor, AG337. *Proc Am Assoc Cancer Res* 1994; 35:306.
13. Duch DS, Banks S, Dec IK, Dickerson SH, Ferone R, Heath LS, Humphreys J, Knick V, Pendergast W, Singer S, Smith G, Waters K, Wilson R. Biochemical and cellular pharmacology of 1843U89, a novel benzoquinazoline inhibitor of thymidylate synthase. *Cancer Res* 1993; 53:810–818.
14. Jackman AL, Aherne GW, Kimbell R, Brunton L, Hardcastle A, Wardleworth JW, Stephens TC, Boyle FT. ZD9331, a novel non-polyglutamatable quinazoline thymidylate synthase inhibitor. *Proc Am Assoc Cancer Res* 1994; 35:301.
15. Baldwin SW, Tse A, Taylor EC, Rosowsky A, Gossett LS, Shih C, Moran RG. Structure features of 5,10-dideazatetrahydrofolate that determine inhibition of mammalian glycinamide ribonucleotide formyltransferase. *Biochemistry* 1991; 30:1997–2006.
16. Taylor EC, Kuhnt D, Shih C, Rinzel SM, Grindey GB, Barredo J, Jannatipour M, Moran RG. A dideazatetrahydrofolate analogue lacking a chiral center at C-6; N-{4-[2-(2-Amino-1,7-dihydro-4-oxo-pyrrolo[2,3-d]pyrimidin-6-yl)ethy l]benzoyl}glutamic acid, a new and potent inhibitor of thymidylate synthase. *J Med Chem* 1992; 35:4450–4454.
17. Habeck LL, Shih C, Gossett LS, Leitner TA, Schultz RM, Andis SL, Moran RG, Mendelsohn LG. Substrate specificity of mammalian folylpolyglutamate synthetase for 5,10-dideazatetrahydrofolate analogs. *Mol Pharmacol* 1995; 48:326–333.
18. Shih C, Chen VJ, Gossett LS, Gates SB, MacKellar WC, Habeck LL, Shackelford KA, Mendelsohn LG, Soose DJ, Patel VF, Andis SL, Bewley JR, Rayl EA, Morrison BA, Beardsley GP, Kohler W, Ratnam M, Schultz RM. LY231514, a pyrrolo[2,3-d]pyrimidine based antifolate that inhibits multiple folate requiring enzymes. *Cancer Res* 1997; 57:1116–1123.
19. Rinaldi DA, Burris HA, Dorr FA, Wordworth JR, Kuhn JG, Eckardt JR, et al. Initial phase I evaluation of the novel thymidylate synthase inhibitor, LY231514, using the modified continual reassessment method for dose escalation. *J Clin Oncol* 1995; 13:2842–50.
20. Rinaldi DA, Burris HA, Dorr FA, Rodriguez G, Eckhardt SG, Fields SM, et al. A phase I evaluation of LY231514, a novel multitargeted antifolate, administered every 21 days. *Proc Am Soc Clin Oncol* 1996; 16:A489.
21. McDonald AC, Vasey PA, Walling J, Woodworth JR, Abrahams T, Bailey NP, Siddiqui N, Lind MJ, Cassidy J, Twelves CJ. Phase I and pharmacokinetic study of LY2331514, the multi-targeted antifolate, administered by daily ×5, q21 schedule. *Ann Oncol* 1996; 7(suppl 5):20.
22. Clarke S, Boyer M, Millward M, Findlay M, Ackland S, Childs A, Brew S, Walcher V, Watt D, Thornton D. Phase II study of LY231514 in patients with advanced non-small cell lung cancer (NSCLC). *Lung Cancer* 1997; 18(suppl 1), 12, A34.
23. Cripps MC, Burnell M, Jolivet J, Lofters W, Fisher B, Panasci L, Iglesias J, Eisenhauer E. Phase II study of a multi-targeted antifolate (LY231514) (MTA) as first line therapy in patients with locally advanced or metastatic colorectal cancer (MCC). *Eur J Cancer* 1997; 33(suppl 8), S172, A768.
24. John W, Clark J, Burris H, Picus J, Schulamn L, Thornton D, Lochrer P. A phase II trial of LY231514 in patients with metastatic colorectal cancer. *Proc Am Soc Clin Oncol* 1997; 16:A1038.
25. Miller KD, Loehrer PJ, Picus J, Blanke C, John J, Schulman L, Burris H, Thornton D. A phase II trial of LY231514 in patients with unresectable pancreatic cancer. *Proc Am Soc Clin Oncol* 1997; 16:A1060.
26. Rusthoven J, Eisenhauer E, Bitts C, Gregg R, Dancey J, Fisher B, Iglesias J. A phase II study of the multi-targeted antifolate in patients with advanced non-small cell lung cancer. *Proc Am Soc Clin Oncol* 1997; 16:A1728.
27. Smith IE, Miles DW, Coleman RE, Lind MJ, McCarthy S Chick J. Phase II study of LY231514 (MTA) in patients with locally recurrent or metastatic breast cancer (LR/MBC)—an interim report. *Proc Am Soc Clin Oncol* 1997; 16:A671.
28. Chabner BA, Allegra CJ, Curt GA, Clendeninn NJ, Baram J, Koizumi S, Drake JC, Jolivet J. Polyglutamation of methotrexate, Is methotrexate a prodrug? *J Clin Invest* 1985; 76:907–912.
29. $H630_{R10}$ cells were obtained from Dr. Patrick G. Johnston, Queen's University, Belfast, UK. The characterization of the $H630_{R10}$ cell line can be found in reference: *Cancer Res* 1991; 51:66–68.
30. Pizzorno G, Moroson BA, Cashmore AR, Russello O, Mayer JR, Galivan J, Bunni MA, Priest DG, Beardsley GP. Multifactorial resistance to 5,10-dideazatetrahydrofolic acid in cell lines derived from human lymphoblastic leukemia CCRF-CEM. *Cancer Res* 1995; 55:566–573.

31. Dixon KH, Mulligan T, Chung KN, Elwood PC, Cowan KH. Effects of folate receptor expression following stable transfection into wild type and methotrexate transport-deficient ZR-75-1 human breast cancer cells. *J Biol Chem* 1992; 26:24,140–24,147.
32. Chen VJ, Bewley JR, Andis SL, Schultz RM, Shih C, Mendelsohn LG, Seitz DE, Tonkinson JL. Effects of MTA (Multitargeted Antifolate, LY231514) on Intracellular Folate and Nucleoside Triphosphate Pools in CCRF-CEM cells, *Assoc Cancer Res Annual Meeting*, 1997.
33. Chong L and Tattersall MHN, 5,10-dideazatetrahydrofolic acid reduces toxicity and deoxyadenosine triphosphate pool expansion in cultured L1210 cells treated with inhibitors of thymidylate synthase. *Biochem Pharmacol* 1995; 49:819–827.
34. Tonkinson JL, Marder P, Andis SL, Schultz RM, Gossett LS, Shih C, Mendelsohn LG. Cell cycle effects of antifolate antimetabolites: implications for cytotoxicity and cytostasis. *Cancer Chemother Pharmacol* 1997; 39:521–540.
35. Worzalla JF, Self TD, Theobald KS, Schultz RM, Mendelsohn LG, Shih C. Effects of folic acid on toxicity and antitumor activity of LY231514 multitargeted antifolate (MTA). *Proc Am Assoc Cancer Res* 1997; 38:478.
36. Alati T, Worzalla JF, Shih C, Bewley JR, Lewis S, Moran RG, Grindey GB. Augmentation of the therapeutic activity of lometrexol [(6R)5,10-dideazatetrahydrofolate] by oral folic acid. *Cancer Res* 1996; 56:2331–2335.
37. Woodland JM, Barnett CJ, Dorman DE, Gruber JM, Shih C, Spangle LA, Wilson T, Ehlhardt WJ. The metabolism and disposition of the antifolate LY231514 (MTA) in mice and dogs. *Drug Metab Dispos* 1997; 25(6):693–700.
38. *Clinical Investigators' Brochure for LY231514.* Eli Lilly and Company, Indianapolis, IN.
39. Zervos PH, Faries D, Dorr FA, Rinaldi D, Storniolo AM, VonHoff DD. Practical use of the modified continual reassessment method (mCRM) for dose escalation in a phase I trial with LY231514. *Proc Am Soc Clin Oncol* 1995; 14:A473.
40. Woodworth J, Rinaldi D, Burris H, Thornton D, Reddy S, Kuhn J, VonHoff D. Assessments of hemotoxicity and relationships to pharmacokinetics from a LY231514 phase I study. *Proc Am Soc Clin Oncol* 1997; 16:A734.

9 GW1843
A Potent, Noncompetitive Thymidylate Synthase Inhibitor—Preclinical and Preliminary Clinical Studies

Gary K. Smith, Joseph W. Bigley, Inderjit K. Dev, David S. Duch, Robert Ferone, and William Pendergast

CONTENTS

INTRODUCTION
CHEMISTRY OF SOME POTENT BENZO[F]QUINAZOLINE INHIBITORS
  OF THYMIDYLATE SYNTHASE
ENZYMOLOGY
IN VITRO EFFECTS ON TUMOR CELLS
IN VIVO EFFICACY
PRECLINICAL TOXICOLOGY
CLINICAL EVALUATION OF GW1843: INITIAL PHASE I TESTING
  USING A DAILY X 5 DOSING SCHEDULE
CONCLUSIONS AND FUTURE PROSPECTIVE

1. INTRODUCTION

GW1843 is a noncompetitive inhibitor of thymidylate synthase (TS). The compound is a good substrate for folylpolyglutamate synthetase and adds glutamate moieties in vivo. However, unlike some other TS inhibitors and other antifolates, the TS inhibition constant and noncompetitive mode of inhibition is unaffected by polyglutamation. The compound is readily transported on the reduced folate carrier, and accumulates in cells. The main cellular metabolite is the diglutamate (GW1843glu$_1$). It is active in vivo against solid tumor lines. The host toxicity caused by the compound can be selectively blocked by folic acid by a mechanism that may involve blocking transport only into normal cells. Phase I clinical evaluation is promising and supports the unique preclinical

From: *Anticancer Drug Development Guide: Antifolate Drugs in Cancer Therapy*
Edited by: A.L. Jackman © Humana Press Inc., Totowa, NJ

properties. The discovery and current developmental status of the compound is the subject of this report.

2. CHEMISTRY OF SOME POTENT BENZO[F]QUINAZOLINE INHIBITORS OF THYMIDYLATE SYNTHASE: EVOLUTION OF ANTITUMOR AGENT GW1843

The thymidylate synthase (TS) program in cancer chemotherapy that led to GW1843 (compound 11g in Table 1; formerly 1843U89) grew out of a long-standing interest at Burroughs Wellcome in inhibition of enzymes of the folate pathway as a strategy for discovery of antimicrobial agents. Microbes synthesize folic acid *de novo,* possess no active folate transport mechanisms, and generally do not allow even passive diffusion of such polar molecules into their cells *(1).* Thus at the start of our antibacterial TS program, rather than seeking close analogs of folic acid containing highly polar structural elements akin to the p-aminobenzoylglutamate moiety, the emphasis was on small, relatively lipophilic folate analogs that might be capable of entering microbial cells without benefit of active folate transport. Selectivity would come from exploiting structural differences between microbial and human enzyme.

GW1843 (11g)

Among the many types of compounds examined, a series of benzo[f]quinazolin-1(2H)-ones (**1**), particularly those bearing compact lipophilic substituents in the distal benzene ring, had remarkable TS activity for such small molecules, the best of them with K_i values approx 20 nM. A considerable amount of structure-activity information was amassed on these compounds *(2,3),* and is summarized in Fig. 1. Unfortunately two overriding features common to all the compounds in this series precluded their utility as drugs, particularly as antimicrobial agents; they lacked appropriate selectivity between mammalian and bacterial TS, and they penetrated cells, bacterial or mammalian, poorly or not at all. Whereas the best TS I_{50}s were in the 20-nM range, none of the compounds had I_{50} values vs cells lower than 10 µM.

However, as we became increasingly interested in folate-based cancer chemotherapy, we came to view these molecules as offering a unique platform from which to develop TS inhibitors cytotoxic towards human tumor cells. There is little evidence that the folate enzymes, including TS, in tumor cells differ from those of normal cells; historically,

Table 1
In Vitro Activities of Benzo[f]quinazolinones

	R	X-Y	Other	TS K_i^a (nM)	Cytotoxic IC_{50}^b (nM SW-480)	Molt-4	MTX uptake K_i^c (μM)	V_m	FPGS^d K_m(uM)	V/K
6a	NH_2	8-SO_2NH	5,6-H_2	56	25,000	n.d.	0 @ 10	101	1.8	55
6b	NH_2	9-SO_2NH	5,6-H_2	2.5	7900	2400	35	n.d.^{e}	n.d.	n.d.
6c	CH_3	9-SO_2NH	5,6-H_2	18	4100	200	4.9	184	2	92
6d	CH_3	9-SO_2NMe	5,6-H_2	16.7	>5x10^4	>5x10^4	1.8	n.d.	n.d.	n.d.
6e	CH_3	9-SO_2NH		5.5	2400	118	4.9	184	2	92
6f	CH_3	7-SO_2NH		7370	>10^5	50,000	72% @ 30	55.2	7.6	7.3
6g	CH_3	8-SO_2NH	9-Br	16.4	>10^5	>10^5	45% @ 30	n.d.	n.d.	n.d.
11a	NH_2	9-CH_2NH		2.3	530	230	13	66	24.3	2.7
11b	CH_3	9-CH_2NH		1.3	365	120	1.8	126	160	0.79
11c	CH_3	9-CH_2NMe		22	1500	n.d.	0.5	117	20	5.8
11d	CH_3	8-CH_2NH		1615	>10^5	n.d.	1.5	81.3	1.96	41.5
11e	CH_3	9-CH_2NH	thiophene ^{f}	1.1	100	n.d.	3.4	113	19	5.9
11f	CH_3	9-CH_2NH	2'-F	0.09	20	6	0.85	60	45	1.33
11g	CH_3	9-CH_2NH	2',Nglu-CH_2	0.09	0.8	0.7	0.3	101	0.4	249
11h	CH_3	9-CH_2NMe	2',Nglu-CH_2	2.5	500	n.d.	0.2	131	7.3	18
11i	CH_3	9-CH_2NH	2',Nglu-S	4.0	15	n.d.	0.75	n.d	n.d.	n.d.

^{a} Inhibition constant vs. purified recombinant human TS. ^{b} Concentration for 50% reduction in the growth rate upon continuous drug exposure for 72 h (SW480) or 96 h (MCF-7). ^{c} Inhibition constant vs. the transport of [^{3}H]-MTX by MOLT-4 cells. ^{d} Substrate activity for hog liver folylpolyglutamate synthetase. V_m (rel%) is velocity compared to a control 50μM aminopterin run on each test. ^{e} Not determined. ^{f} 1,4-Phenylene ring of side chain replaced with 2,5-thiophene.

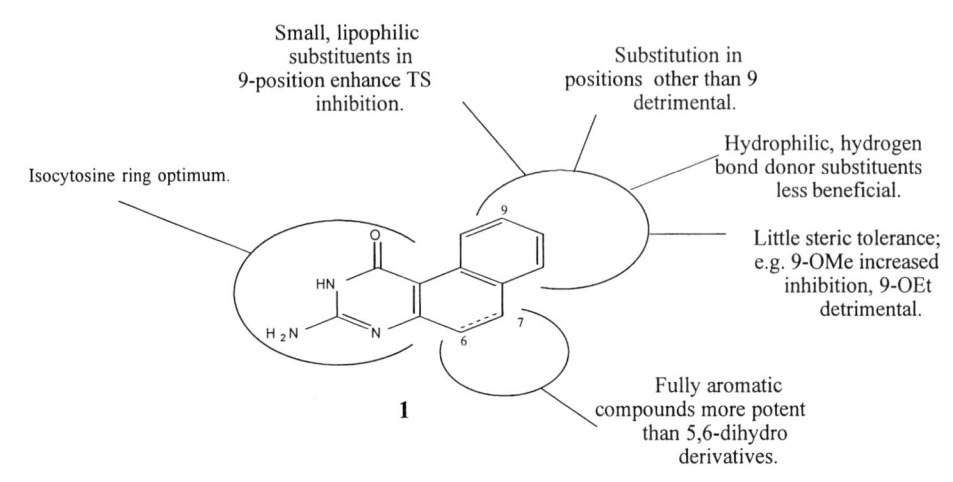

Fig. 1. Some structure/activity considerations for inhibition of thymidylate synthase (TS) by simple benzoquinazolines.

Annotations on structure **1**:
- Isocytosine ring optimum.
- Small, lipophilic substituents in 9-position enhance TS inhibition.
- Substitution in positions other than 9 detrimental.
- Hydrophilic, hydrogen bond donor substituents less beneficial.
- Little steric tolerance; e.g. 9-OMe increased inhibition, 9-OEt detrimental.
- Fully aromatic compounds more potent than 5,6-dihydro derivatives.

folate-based antitumor molecules have relied on exploiting differences in the kinetics of cell growth, or on differences in uptake, retention, and glutamation mechanisms between tumor and normal cells. Active folate transport and glutamation mechanisms are strongly dependent on the presence of the p-aminobenzoylglutamate residue, or a close analog thereof, in the natural folate or drug molecule *(4)*. Furthermore, omission of the p-aminobenzoylglutamate side chain often removes most or all of their folate-related activity. Compare, for example the low TS-inhibitory activity of the simple 2-aminoquinazolin-4(3H)-one (0% inhibition at 400 μM; Dev, unpublished) with those of potent folate analogs of the CB3717 type *(6)* (CB3717 IC$_{50}$ = 5 nM). We anticipated that with a pterin surrogate as intrinsically potent as benzo[f]quinazolinone, provided that the heterocycle continued to interact with the same region of the active site, attachment of a p-aminobenzoylglutamate residue typical of folate derivatives would result in TS-inhibitory activity that was at least additive to, or possibly synergistic with that of the heterocycle.

2.1. Sulfonamido-p-aminobenzoylglutamates

Chlorosulfonylation of the heterocycle followed by amidation with p-aminobenzoylglutamate derivatives offered a convenient synthetic entry into benzoquinazolines bearing a folate-like side chain. The sulfonamido group had received surprisingly little attention as a fraudulent linkage between the heterocycle and the aroylglutamate side chain *(7)*, despite a report of the antimalarial activity of a series of 2,4-diamino-6-quinazolinesulfonamides *(8)*, some of which were equipotent with cycloguanil or pyrimethamine; glutamate derivatives were not examined in this study, presumably because of the lack of any folate transport mechanism in the target organisms *(1)*. We had previously observed that direct sulfonylation of 3-amino-5,6-dihydrobenzo[f]quinazolin-1(2H)-one (**4a**) with chlorosulfonic acid had yielded the 8-sulfonyl chloride, whereas directivity of the electrophilic substitution was controlled by the 3-amino substituent. The acid chlorides were originally used for making simple alkylsulfonamide derivatives, which although meeting the aim of enhancing solubility, were uniformly inactive as inhibitors of TS (2). However, condensation of the acid chloride with the commercially available diethyl p-aminobenzoylglutamate and subsequent alkaline hydrolysis yielded the desired 8-sulfonamido-linked folate analog (**6a**, Scheme 2), which showed an increase of almost 200-fold in TS inhibition compared with the derivative lacking the side chain (Table 1). There was also some improvement in cytotoxicity, as measured by growth inhibitory activity against the SW480 colon tumor cell line, from inactive at 100 μM to an IC$_{50}$ of 25 μM. We found this initial result very encouraging. Whereas in the simple benzoquinazolines the addition of bulky substituents into the distal benzene ring had been uniformly detrimental to activity (2), the increase in potency observed with **6a** seemed to signify that the side chain may have been probing the area on the TS enzyme that normally binds the p-aminobenzoylglutamate residue of the natural cofactor 5,10-methylenetetrahydrofolate. Furthermore, 8-substituted benzoquinazolines had consistently been shown to be less potent than the corresponding 9-isomers in the simple series (2). In order to examine whether this effect would carry over into the benzoylglutamate derivatives, we proceeded to counteract the directivity of the 3-amino group by blocking the 8-position with a bromo substituent, whereupon chlorosulfonylation occurred exclusively at the 9-position. Condensation of the resulting 8-bromo-9-chlorosulfonyl derivative with diethyl p-aminbenzoylglutamate, removal of the bromine by hydrogenolysis over palladium, and hydrolysis as before gave the desired 9-isomer (**6b**). A further substantial gain in TS inhibitory activity was observed (20-fold) compared with the 8-isomer (Table 1). Cytotoxic activity vs SW480 cells was also improved, but the threefold gain was not as great as the TS improvement would indicate, suggesting that factors affecting cellular uptake and retention were important.

Early studies on the potent quinazoline TS inhibitor CB3717 (**3**) had shown that replacement of the 2-amino substituent by hydrogen not only had the intended effect of improving solubility, but also increased cytotoxicity 20-fold vs L1210 cells. This occurred despite a loss of TS activity of some 1.4-fold, suggesting that the desamino

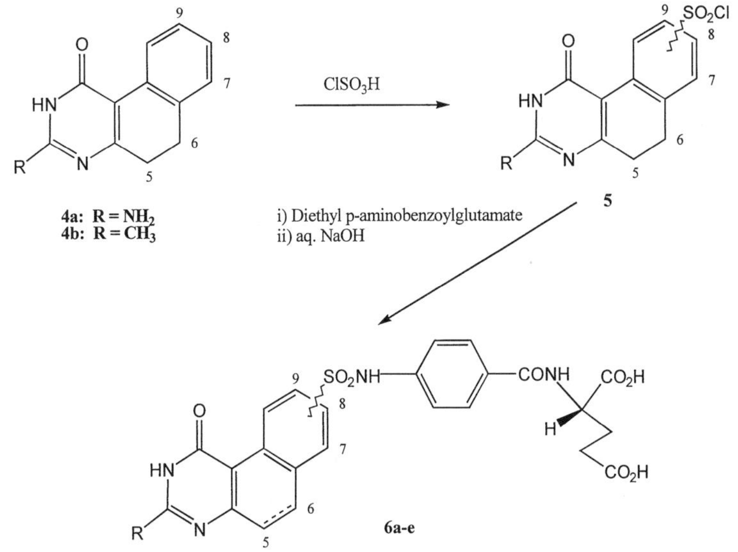

Scheme 2. Synthesis of Benzoquinazolinone Sulfonamidobenzoylglutamates.

derivative was transported and/or retained by tumor cells more effectively than was CB3717 itself *(9)*. 2-Methylquinazoline derivatives were later found to be even more effective substrates for reduced folate transport and polyglutamation *(10)*. Accordingly we targeted the analog of **6b** in which the 3-amino group was replaced by a methyl substituent. While examining chlorosulfonylation of dihydrobenzoquinazolines we fortunately found that whereas the 3-aminosubstituent in **4a** had directed the electrophile exclusively to the 8-position, only the 9-sulfonyl chloride was isolated from chlorosulfonylation of **4b**. Presumably the weaker electron-donating influence of the 3-methyl group is considerably attenuated through the pyrimidine ring, and directivity of electrophilic substitution is controlled by the bridge methylene group at the 6-position. Treatment of the acid chloride with diethyl p-aminobenzoylglutamate and hydrolysis as before gave the desired 3-methyl-9-substituted compound (**6c**, Scheme 2). The 3-methyl derivative **6c** showed a sevenfold loss of TS inhibition relative to the 3-amino derivative **6a,** rather greater than that seen in the quinazolines *(10)*. However an increased affinity to the reduced folate carrier *(11)*, which on balance, despite a slight decrease in polyglutamation *(12)*, resulted in an net gain in cytotoxicity vs SW480 (twofold) and Molt-4 (12-fold) cells.

Condensation of the acid chloride with diethyl p-(methylamino)benzoylglutamate allowed introduction of a methyl substituent onto the sulfonamide nitrogen, to yield **6d** after hydrolysis. This change was detrimental to both enzymic and cytotoxic activity, contrasting sharply with observations in the CB3717 series of quinazoline inhibitors, in which increases in TS inhibition of up to 120-fold relative to the corresponding bridge-NH derivatives were observed upon alkylation *(13)*.

We had earlier established that in the series of benzoquinazolines bearing small lipophilic substituents, "fully aromatic" derivatives, i.e., those oxidized across the 5,6-position, usually exhibited greater TS inhibitory potency than the corresponding 5,6-dihydrocompounds *(2)*. Again we predicted that this effect might also hold for the benzoylglutamate derivatives, provided that the mode of binding of the heterocyclic portion remained similar. Accordingly, **6c** was aromatized by heating the intermediate diethyl ester with palladium charcoal in diglyme and hydrolyzing as before to yield **6e**. The fully aromatic derivative showed a threefold increase in potency compared with the 5,6-dihydro-compound; increases in transport and polyglutamation were also observed, but were not particularly well reflected in the rather modest increase of less than twofold in cytotoxicity. The corresponding 7-isomer (**6f**), was prepared by chlorosulfonation of the "fully aromatic" 3-aminobenzoquinazolin-1-one. Directivity was much more ambiguous than when the 5,6-bond was saturated; amination of the mixture of sulfonyl chlorides and chromatographic separation of the resulting mixture of glutamate diester intermediates prior to hydrolysis gave the desired compound, which showed TS inhibition over 1300-fold lower than the 9-isomer. TS inhibition by the 9-bromo-8-sulfonamido analog **6g** (K_i = 16.4 μM) was 800-fold lower than that of the precursor 3-amino-9-bromoquinazolin-1-one (K_i = 20 nM) *(2)*, and 300-fold lower than that of **6a**, despite the presence in **6g** of an aromatic quinazoline nucleus and a 9-bromo substituent, both of which had proven to be advantageous in the simple benzoquinazoline series *(2)*. It may be that the presence of the bromo substituent hinders rotation of the side chain and adoption of an obligatory L-shaped conformation of the inhibitor on the enzyme suggested from recent X-ray studies *(11)*.

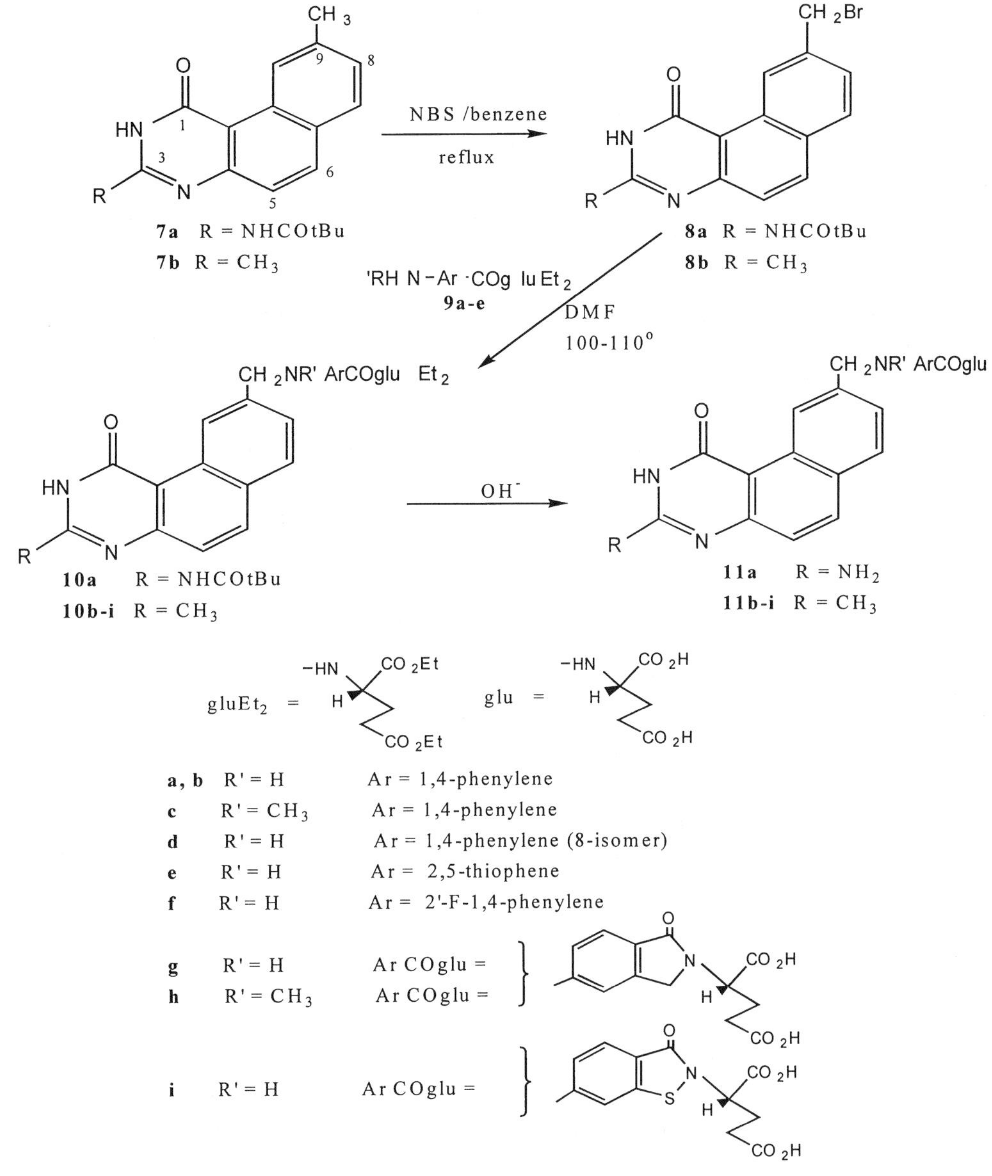

Scheme 3 Synthesis of Benzoquinazolinone Methyleneaminobenzoylglutamates

2.2. Aminomethylene-Linked Derivatives

Although a wide variety of folate-like derivatives with fraudulent linkages between the heterocycle and the side chain, including "reversed bridge" analogs *(13,15–18)* and sulfur and oxygen isosteres *(13,15,17),* had often shown significant antifolate activity, the aminomethylene link had been a feature of the most potent TS inhibitors, quinazolines such as CB3717 (**3**) *(6)* and its 2-methyl analogs *(19–25)*. Consequently, we set out to introduce this structural feature into benzoquinazolines (Scheme 3). The 3-amino substituent was protected as the pivaloyl derivative (**7a**) and the 9-methyl group brominated with n-bromosuccinimide. The bromo compound (**8a**) was condensed with diethyl p-aminobenzoylglutamate as before, and hydrolysis with sodium hydroxide removed both the protecting esters and the pivaloyl protecting groups to yield **11a**. With an I_{50} of 2.3 nM (Table 1) the compound had comparable TS inhibitory activity with the best of the sulfonamide-linked derivatives described above, but poor uptake and polyglutamation parameters explained the disappointing cytotoxic activity vs the SW480 and Molt-4 cell lines. Thus we decided to attempt the preparation of the corresponding 3-methyl derivative in anticipation of an improvement in uptake. By limiting the amount of brominating agent to slightly over one equivalent, the 9-methyl group of **7b** was brominated selectively to yield **8b**, and introduction of the p-aminobenzoylglutamate side chain effected as before. The resulting compound (**11b**) showed an increase in TS inhibition, almost twofold compared with the amino compound and fourfold compared with the corresponding sulfonamide-linked derivative **6e**. Again, however, only slight gains in cytotoxicity were observed, despite increased folate-carrier activity, perhaps because the molecule was poorly retained in the cells as evidenced by its poor FPGS substrate activity. As with the sulfonamide-linked compounds (**6c,6d**) above, replacement of the methyleneamino NH of the side chain with NMe (through condensation of the foregoing bromo compound with diethyl p-(methyl)aminobenzoylglutamate, (**9c**) resulted in a 17-fold loss in TS activity from **11b** to **11c**. Despite improvements in uptake parameters, this was reflected in a significant loss in cytotoxic activity (Table 1). Also in parallel with the sulfonamide series, the 8-substituted benzoquinazoline **11d**, prepared via bromination of the 3,8-dimethyl isomer of **7b** was 700-fold less inhibitory on TS than was the 9-isomer **11a** and showed no activity toward SW480 cells below 50 μM. Replacement of the 1,4-phenylene moiety of the p-aminobenzoylglutamate side chain with a 2,5-thiophene moiety had significantly improved cytotoxic activity in the quinazoline series, particularly with respect to cellular uptake and polyglutamation, ultimately leading to the clinical candidate Tomudex *(25)*. Attachment of the thiophene side chain to the benzoquinazoline nucleus (via condensation of the thienylglutamate diester **9e** *(25)* with the bromo derivative **8b** and hydrolysis) to yield **11e** had relatively little effect on TS activity or cytotoxicity, though the balance of methotrexate uptake inhibition (up twofold) and FPGS substrate activity (down twofold) was slightly altered (Table 1).

Introduction of a fluorine substituent into the 2'-position of the benzene ring, a strategy that had been effectively employed in the quinazoline series *(23)* gave **11f** a 14-fold greater activity against thymidylate synthase compared with **11b**, accompanied by modest increases in both transport and polyglutamation, resulting in an 18–20-fold enhancement of cytotoxic activity. The appearance of a stable hydrogen bond, observable in the NMR as a coupling between the 2'-fluorine and the glutamate NH, implied that a planar conformation in this part of the molecule was somehow significant, and suggested that an entropic advantage might be gained by rigidifying this area of the molecule in a covalent manner. Scheme 4 shows the route to such a side chain moiety, wherein a portion of the glutamate group is fixed in an isoindolinyl nucleus. 3-Nitrophthalic anhydride was condensed with diethyl glutamate to yield the phthalimido derivative that was reduced with zinc and acetic acid in THF, followed by catalytic reduction of the intermediate aminal that was not isolated. Condensation of the resulting p-aminobenzoylglutamate analog **9g** with the 9-bromomethylbenzoquinazoline **8b** as above and subsequent hydrolysis yielded the desired folate analog, GW1843, (**11g**). Whereas such a formal covalent rigidification of the side chain in this manner made little difference to the TS activity; a moderate in-

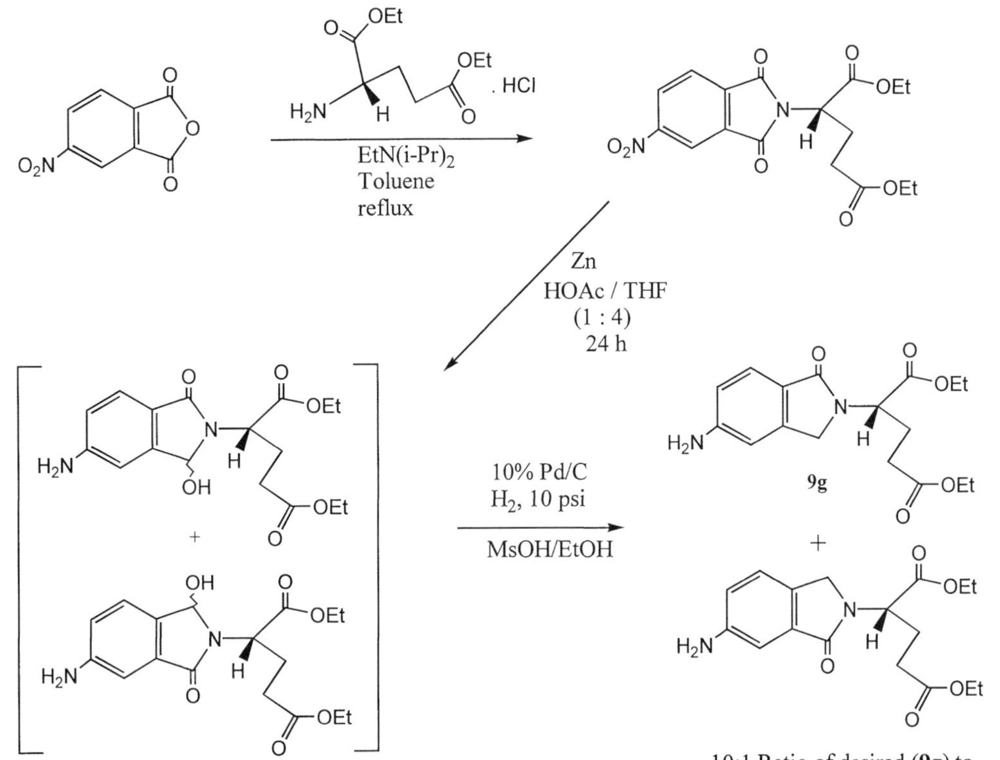

10:1 Ratio of desired (**9g**) to undesired isomer; separated by chromatography

Scheme 4. Synthesis of Conformationally Restricted Sidechain of 1843U89

crease in transportability, and an almost 200-fold increase in FPGS activity, gave significant increases in cytotoxicity, bringing the IC_{50} values into the subnanomolar range *(26)* (Table 1). Methylation of the aminomethylene bridge to yield **11h** again had a detrimental effect on TS activity (28-fold), and whereas transport was little affected, the molecule was a relatively poor substrate for FPGS. When a sulfur atom was used in place of the methylene group as the rigidifying moiety to yield **11i** *(2a),* a loss of TS activity of over 40-fold was observed, reflected in a 19-fold loss of cytotoxicity on SW480 cells.

2.3. Other Linking Groups

Several other moieties were used to link the aroylglutamate residue to the 9-position of the heterocycle, including CH_2O, CONH, CH_2CH_2 CH=CH, and the reversed-bridge sulfonamide $NHSO_2$. The compounds were all at least an order of magnitude less inhibitory toward TS than the corresponding methyleneamino compound **11b** and in no case was submicromolar cytotoxicity toward SW480 cells observed. Their syntheses and in vitro biological activities are described in ref. *2.*

2.3. Binding of GW1843 to TS

No X-ray crystal structure of thymidylate synthase was available to us during the development of GW1843. Recently Weichsel and Montfort *(14)* and Stout and Stroud *(30)* reported the crystal structure of the ternary complex of *E. coli* TS with GW1843 and dUMP bound to the active site. Whereas the heterocyclic portion of the molecule binds similarly to that of the quinazoline CB3717 and the folate cofactor, the side chain seeks out an area of hydrophobic binding that is normally not accessible. To reach this area, GW1843 distorts the wall of the active site resulting in a dislocation of active-site groups, that then bind to GW1843 in ways different from their normal binding to the cofactor. It is difficult to disagree with the authors' conclusion that GW1843 could not have been designed using current structure-based approaches.

3. ENZYMOLOGY

3.1. Inhibition of Folate-Dependent Enzymes

GW1843 is a potent and selective inhibitor of human TS with a K_i value of 0.09 nM *(27,28)*. GW1843 is an extremely poor inhibitor of other folate-dependent enzymes. Values of K_i for GW1843 against dihydrofolate reductase, AICAR transformylase, and GAR transformylase were 2000-fold (170 nM), 670,000-fold (60,000 nM), and more than 1×10^6-fold (>100,000 nM) higher than the K_i value for TS, respectively. Diglutamates of GW1843 accumulated as major species in cells treated with GW1843 *(29)*. The inhibition properties of GW1843Glu$_1$ for different folate-dependent enzymes were very similar to those of the monoglutamated form. The higher polyglutamates (Glu$_2$–Glu$_4$) of 1843U89 are approx μM K_i inhibitors of AICAR transformylase and low nM K_i inhibitors of dihydrofolate reductase (Ferone, unpublished). The observation by Duch et al. *(27)* that the cytotoxicity of GW1843 to different human tumor cell lines is completely prevented by the addition of 20 μM thymidine to the growth medium also supports the conclusion that TS is the major locus of inhibition for GW1843.

Enzyme kinetic analysis showed that the inhibition of human TS by GW1843 was noncompetitive with respect to both substrates *(28)*. Dev et al. *(28)* have presented evidence that suggests that the asymmetric binding of the folate substrates and GW1843 to the two subunits of human TS is the major factor that determines the inhibition kinetics of GW1843. Equilibrium dialysis studies showed that the folate substrate, 5,10-methylenetetrahydrofolate (5,10-CH$_2$-FH$_4$), in a ternary complex with deoxyuridylate bound to one of the subunits (site A) with a K_d of 720 nM. The binding of the substrate to the second subunit (site B) was much weaker and the K_d could not be determined by this method. In contrast, GW1843 (mono or diglutamated form) had a much higher affinity for subunit B (K_d approx 0.1 nM) compared to subunit A (K_d approx 400 nM). A crystallographic analysis of the two independent monomers provided an insight into how the two monomers, which are chemically identical before ligand binding, become asymmetric during TS activity *(30)*. A comparison of two independent active sites by a least square superimposition showed that the two molecules of GW1843 are disposed in a significantly different manner in the two monomers, showing an alignment with a 1.6-angstrom deviation *(30)*. The principal difference Stout and Stroud observed between monomer I and monomer II is a slightly less tightly held complex in the second monomer. Based on these results and the kinetic studies it appears that GW1843 exploits the intersubunit cooperativity of inhibition. Stout and Stroud *(30)* propose that in solution TS may function as a "both-the-sites active, half-the-sites catalytic" enzyme, rather than as a "half-the-sites-active" enzyme. This implies that negative cooperativity may be exhibited by TS through inhibition of the catalytic chemistry at the second site rather than through occluded binding. Weichsel and Montfort could observe no difference between the two binding sites in their crystallographic studies of GW1843 binding to *E. coli* TS *(14)*.

Human TS binds GW1843 tightly in a binary complex with a K_d of 6 nM and the binding is further stabilized by the presence of dUMP with a K_d of approx 0.1 nM *(28)*. The stabilizing effect of substrate binding to TS by GW1843 examined by thermodynamic parameters can be attributed to the extra amount of free energy released on formation of the ternary complex *(31)*. The tightness of the ternary complexes is caused by the stacking energy that results from Van der Waals contacts between the nucleotide base ring and the quinazoline ring of GW1843, which induces a conformational change in the protein *(14,30)*. This conformational change is associated with a significant positive entropy change, which suggests that water is expelled from the active site region *(31)*. The crystal structure of *Escherichia coli* TS bound to GW1843 and dUMP further revealed that the GW1843 binding surface includes a hydrophobic patch that is normally buried *(14,30)*. To reach this patch, GW1843 inserts into the wall of the TS active site, resulting in a severe local distortion of the protein. These rearrangements enable the binding of the larger dGMP and GMP molecules, overcoming the normal TS discrimination against nucleotides containing the 2′ hydroxyl *(32)*.

3.2. Polyglutamation

The polyglutamation properties of GW1843 are distinct from other "classical" antifolates—it is readily anabolized to the diglutamate, which is accumulated intracellularly. However, polyglutamation is not required for potent TS inhibition. Thus GW1843 maintains activity against tumor cell lines that contain low levels of folylpolyglutamate synthetase (FPGS) and as a result are resistant to antifols that require activation to higher polyglutamates.

GW1843 is a very efficient substrate for mammalian FPGS, with K_m values of 0.1–0.5 μM and V_{max} values equal to or higher than the best substrates *(27,29,33)*. The predominant product (70–85%) is the diglutamate with only low amounts of additional products up to the pentaglutamate. The diglutamate was also the main product found for some related benzoquinazolines *(29)*, including some with a true glutamate residue instead of the modified residue of GW1843 *(see* structure above). The di-and triglutamates of GW1843 *(29)* and three other benzoquinazolines (Ferone, unpublished) were very poor substrates for partially purified hog liver FPGS, with relative velocities ranging from 0.4–6.8% of their respective monoglutamates. Since the patterns of polyglutamation that were found intracellularly in several tumor cell lines were reproduced in overnight incubations with isolated FPGS, we conclude that the unique product distributions are inherent properties of the compounds' efficiencies as FPGS substrates. Also, the structure of GW1843 appears to be in an ideal conformation for the addition of the first glutamate by FPGS, whereas the diglutamate product is not.

Three polyglutamation factors uniquely position GW1843 among classical antifolates. Firstly, GW1843 is one of the best FPGS substrates reported for conversion to the diglutamate. Secondly, the diglutamate of GW1843 is sufficient for the intracellular accumulation and retention of the compound, based on studies on the efflux of GW1843 from HCT-8 cells in vitro *(29)*. This differentiates GW1843 from some classical antifolates that need anabolism to triglutamates or greater to be substantially retained. Finally, the high affinity of GW1843 itself for TS binding is not increased by polyglutamation. These properties enable the compound to retain its potent cytotoxicity against cell lines that are low in FPGS, and thus resistant to other classical antifolates. These include methotrexate-resistant soft-tissue sarcoma lines *(34)*, methotrexate-resistant CEM cell lines *(35)*, and a Tomudex-resistant L1210 *(36)*.

3.3. Cell Uptake and Efflux

GW1843 enters and is retained well by human tumor cells *(27,29,37)*. Inhibition of MTX transport in MOLT-4 cells was used as a screen for compounds that could bind effectively to the reduced-folate carrier (RFC). Results are shown in Table 1. That this feature measured relative affinity to the reduced-folate carrier was inferred by the ability of 5-CHO-FH4 to compete with binding and the inability of folic acid to compete. GW1843 bound with greater affinity than either MTX or 5-formyl-tetrahydrofolate (5-CHO-FH4). The K_i for GW1843 inhibition of MTX or 5-CHO-FH4 transport in these cells was 0.3 μM compared to the K_t values of 1.0 and 5.2 for MTX and 5-CHO-FH4, respectively. Using ^{14}C-labeled GW1843, the transport K_i for the compound was found to equal the K_t for GW1843 transport into these cells; thus, K_t equals 0.33 μM *(27)*. GW1843 is an excellent substrate for this transporter; V_{max}/K_t values for GW1843, MTX, and 5-CHO-FH4 are 20.3, 1.2, and 1.9 pmol/min/mg dry wt/μM, respectively. GW1843 transport was inhibited by MTX and by 5-CHO-FH4 with IC_{50} values consistent with their affinities for the reduced-folate carrier. Folic acid, however, did not inhibit GW1843 influx at folic acid concentrations below 100 μM, also consistent with RFC-dependent transport of GW1843 in this cell line *(27)*. GW1843 transport into MCF7, SW480, and WiDr cells was also found to be consistent with uptake of the compound on the RFC since transport in these lines was also inhibited by MTX and 5-CHO-FH4 but not by folic acid *(37)*.

Interestingly, the affinity of GW1843 for the RFC in rodent cells was unexpectedly poor compared to human cells *(27)*. The K_i for inhibition of MTX transport in mouse L1210 cells was 5.2 μM. The compound is poorly transported in this line as well; V_{max}/K_t for GW1843 and MTX are 0.25 and 0.9 pmol/min/mg dry wt/μM, respectively. Thus, V_{max}/K_t for GW1843 is 80-fold poorer in the rodent line, whereas that of MTX is not significantly different. Consistent with RFC-dependent uptake in the L1210 and MOLT-4 cells, accumulation of GW1843 was much greater in MOLT-4 cells than in L1210 *(27)*. Matherly and coworkers explored this phenomenon more extensively, and provided additional evidence for use of the RFC for cellular transport *(38)*. These workers cloned and expressed the human RFC, which was found to be 79 and 80% homologous to the mouse and hamster RFCs, respectively. This cDNA was transfected into an RFC-deficient mutant Chinese hamster ovary cell line. These cells were found to bind GW1843 with fourfold greater affinity than wt-CHO, consistent with the greater affinity of the human RFC for GW1843 relative to the rodent protein.

In HCT-8 cells, long-term efflux of GW1843 appears to be related to its extent of polyglutamation and is more rapid than that of the more extensively polyglutamated Tomudex (ZD1694) *(29)*. Cells were exposed to 20 nM of either GW1843 or Tomudex for 24 h. At this time, the primary GW1843 metabolite was the diglutamate (GW1843-glu$_1$) and the primary metabolite of Tomudex was the pentaglutamate. After 48 h incubation of the loaded cells with drug-free medium, 7% of the loaded GW1843 remained in the cells (as diglutatmate) and 36% of the loaded Tomudex remained (as penta- and hexaglutamates). This more rapid efflux may prevent some of the long-term toxicities associated with some extensively polyglutamated compounds.

4. IN VITRO EFFECTS ON TUMOR CELLS

4.1. Cell Growth Inhibition of Human and Rodent Cells

The relative order of potency of the benzoquinazolines observed in vitro as inhibitors of TS was also observed when the compounds were tested against human tumor cells in culture. However, relative to the differences among the benzoquinazolines as inhibitors of TS in vitro, much larger differences as inhibitors of the growth of cultured cells were seen with these compounds (Table 2). The ratio of K_i values between the least and most active compound as inhibitors of TS in vitro (1396U88 vs GW1843) was 200. In contrast, the ratio of IC_{50} values was 3000 in MCF-7, 11,000 in SW480, and 40,000 in WiDr cells in culture. These results indicated that other factors, in addition to inhibitory activity against the enzyme, were important for inhibition in intact cells.

During the development of GW1843, it was observed that the compound was considerably less effective against murine tumor cells in culture than against human cells (Table 3). This can be contrasted to the activity of Tomudex, MTX, or other antifolates, which had comparable activity against tumor cells from both species. Subsequent studies indicated that this difference in response to GW1843 between murine and human tumor cells could be explained by differences in transport between species as discussed above. Long-term accumulation studies with GW1843 in MOLT-4 and LI210 cells *(27)* illustrate the differences in the ability of human and murine cells to take up and retain GW1843. Six hours after the addition of 0.7 n*M* GW1843, intracellular levels in MOLT-4 cells were 152-fold higher than the extracellular concentration, whereas in LI210 cells, levels were only 6.6-fold higher. At an extracellular concentration of GW1843 of 17 n*M,* intracellular concentrations in MOLT-4 cells were 87-fold higher than the extracellular concentra-

Table 2
Inhibition of Cell Growth by Benzoquinazolines

	IC_{50} (nM)				
	MCF-7	*SW480*	*HCT-8*	*WiDr*	*MOLT-4*
GW1843	0.2	0.7	0.7	0.6	0.7
11f	0.7	20	48	10	6
11b	18	365	260	90	120
11a	30	530	1100	595	235
6e	100	2400	470	680	118
6b	650	7900	—	24000	2400
6c	400	3800	2300	3900	200

Table 3
Activity of GW1843 in Human
and Murine Tumor Cells in Culture

Cell Line	*GW1843* IC_{50} (nM)	*Tomudex* IC_{50} (nM)
MCF-7 (human)	0.20	0.80
SW480 (human)	0.65	0.18
LI210 (murine)	66	0.28
B16 (murine)	265	—

tion, whereas in L1210 cells, intracellular concentrations were only 4.2-fold higher. These differences were not observed with either MTX or the GAR TFase inhibitor 5-DACTHF which have similar affinities and V_{max}/K_t for the two lines.

Reversal studies in cell culture have shown that inhibition of cell growth by GW1843 in human cell lines can be reversed by the addition of thymidine alone. Concentrations of GW1843 as high as 10 μM, which are approximately 10,000-fold higher than the IC$_{50}$ value, required nothing other than thymidine to completely reverse inhibition of cell growth. In contrast, the inhibition of cell growth by GW1843 was not substantially affected by the presence of reduced folates in the medium at concentrations below 5 μM (27). 10 μM 5-CHO-FH$_4$ had no effect on the IC$_{50}$ for growth inhibition of SW480 by GW1843, and the IC$_{50}$ for growth inhibition of GC3TK$^-$ was increased only 10-fold. By contrast, the IC$_{50}$ values for growth inhibition of these cell lines by Tomudex were increased 25,000- and ≥500-fold, respectively. At extremely high concentrations (100 μM) of 5-CHO-FH$_4$, the IC$_{50}$ values for GW1843 increased only 15-fold in MCF-7 cells, 12-fold in GC3TK$^-$, and 46-fold in SW480 cells.

These observations are consistent with the noncompetitive nature of the inhibition of TS by this compound with regard to the folate cofactor since the increased cellular folate levels as a result of the 5-CHO-FH$_4$ would not be expected to compete out GW1843 binding to TS. Similarly, since both GW1843 and its singly glutamated metabolite bind well to TS, the elevated cellular folates as a result of 5-CHO-FH$_4$ treatment, would also not be expected to reverse GW1843 activity by depleting the polyglutamated forms of the compound. Rather, in the case of these 10–100 μM 5-CHO-FH$_4$ concentrations, reversal is presumably caused by competition between GW1843 and 5-CHO-FH$_4$ for transport into the cells since K_t for 5-CHO-FH$_4$ is approx 5 μM. These results can be contrasted with those obtained with Tomudex as well as MTX and 5-DACTHF, where the inhibition of cell growth is readily reversed by the addition of low concentrations of 5-CHO-FH$_4$ to the culture medium (27).

4.2. Effects of Protection and Rescue Agents: Folic Acid and Leucovorin

Reversal studies with folic acid provided additional evidence for unique features of GW1843. The activity of GW1843 was reversed 50% by folic acid concentrations of less than 100 μM in only one of eight cell lines tested. The activity against this line, the ileocecal carcinoma line HCT-8, was reversed 50% by 28 μM folic acid. In addition, the IC$_{50}$ for growth inhibition of SW480, GC3TK$^-$, and HCT-8 cells by GW1843 were increased only 1.2-, three-, and threefold, respectively, by 25 μM folic acid. In contrast, the IC$_{50}$ values for growth inhibition by Tomudex were increased 20-, 26-, and 23-fold by 25 μM folic acid. This lack of effect of folic acid on GW1843 cytotoxicity was attributed to the inability of folic acid to compete, even at these high levels, for GW1843 cell entry since IC$_{50}$ for folic acid inhibition of GW1843 transport into several cell lines is > 100 μM (see subheading 3.3.).

5. IN VIVO EFFICACY

Evaluation of the in vivo antitumor efficacy of GW1843 in rodents was difficult because of two factors—the relative insensitivity of murine cells to the cytotoxicity of benzoquinazolines (see subheading 4.1. above), and the high levels of circulating thymidine in rodents *(39)* (Ferone unpublished). To counter the first problem, we tested almost exclusively against human tumor xenografts in mice. Of course, this made it impossible to determine "therapeutic indices," since we exposed a potentially sensitive human tumor in a known insensitive host, the mouse. However, we could establish if any antitumor activity occurred in vivo and perhaps rank tumor types as to relative sensitivity.

The second problem, high plasma thymidine, was approached from several directions, two of which were widely used in our studies.

5.1. Effects on Tumors with and Without Cotreatment with Thymidine Phosphorylase

Thymidine can totally prevent the cytotoxicity of thymidylate synthase inhibitors by conversion to TMP via thymidine kinase and thus bypassing the inhibitory blockade of TS by the inhibitors *(39)*. As little as 0.1–0.5 μM thymidine can prevent TS-dependent cytotoxicity in vitro *(39,40)* (Ferone, unpublished). The plasma levels of thymidine in mice are approx 1μM, well above the <0.1 μM found in human plasma *(39)* (Ferone, unpublished). However, plasma thymidine levels in mice can be reduced to <0.05 μM by ip injection(s) of 2500 U/kg of poylethyleneglycol-adducted thymidine phosphorylase (PEG-TPase) *(41,42)*. Thymidine phosphorylase (TPase) cleaves thymidine to thymine and deoxyribose-5-phosphate, and thymine can not be converted to TMP and therefore does not bypass TS inhibition. Covalent coupling of TPase to polyethyleneglycol (PEG) reduces the antigenicity of this *E. coli* enzyme and increases circulation half life such that a single dose reduces the plasma thymidine level for 5 d, and with injections every 3–5 d, it is possible to keep thymidine levels reduced for several weeks *(43)*.

Toxicity in mice dosed ip with GW1843 at 500 mg/kg, bid for 10 d, was marginal, whereas the same dose was 100% lethal when PEG-TPase was coadministered every fourth day *(44)*.

GW1843 was active in the two systems used to evaluate human tumor xenograft sensitivity to GW1843 in PEG-TPase treated mice—tumor growth delay (in days) in tumors implanted subcutaneously, or percent tumor growth inhibition in tumors implanted under the renal capsule (subrenal capsule assay, SRCA). In the more traditional subcutaneously implanted tumor model, GW1843 caused significant tumor growth delays for colon carcinoma lines DLD-1, HT-29, and GC3C1, ovarian lines SK-OV-3 and OVCAR-3 (survival time), head and neck squamous cell carcinoma Detroit 562, lung carcinoma NCI-H460, and breast carcinoma lines MCF-7 and MX-1, but was not effective against head and neck squamous cell carcinoma A-253 or lung carcinomas NCI-H209 and A549 *(44)*. For most of these studies, the effective doses of GW1843 were in the range of 100–300 mg/kg twice daily for 7–10 d (along with PEG-TPase treatment). The typical pattern was tumor-growth suppression or cessation during dosing with outgrowth occurring after the dosing was stopped. Some of these tumor lines were insensitive in vivo to methotrexate (DLD-1, HT-29, SK-OV-3, OVCAR-3, A549) or 5-fluorouracil (HT-29, OVCAR-3, A549), even with PEG-TPase cotreatment.

The survival time of mice implanted with lung carcinoma NCI-H460 (intrathoracic implant) was increased 31% by 300 mg/kg GW1843. In another study, GW1843 at 150 mg/kg inhibited by 75% the development of liver metastases of NCI-H460 after intrasplenic injection of the tumor suspension *(45)*.

The growth rates of ileocecal adenocarcinoma HCT-8 and colon carcinoma GC3C1 were inhibited by GW1843 in the SRCA, at doses as low as 30 mg/kg dosed three times daily for five days (along with PEG-TPase treatment) *(44)*.

The conclusion from these studies is that when plasma thymidine levels are reduced to levels of < 100 n*M* (level of detection), GW1843 inhibits the growth of a diverse group of human tumor xenografts at several anatomical locations.

5.2. Effects of GW1843 on Thymidine Kinase-Deficient Tumors

Thymidine kinase-deficient (TK$^-$) tumor lines can also be used to eliminate the effects of high plasma thymidine levels on the response of tumors to GW1843. The obvious advantage of these lines for antitumor testing in rodents is their inability to activate thymidine to the nucleotide level, preventing the bypass of TS inhibition with exogenous thymidine. The disadvantages are twofold: If they are totally devoid of thymidine kinase, these cells are probably even more sensitive to TS inhibitors than thymidine kinase-positive tumors in humans, which are exposed to finite, albeit low, levels of thymidine; and very few TK$^-$ human tumor lines exist, thus limiting the range of tumors that can be tested.

GW1843 was tested extensively against two TK$^-$ human tumor lines, colon carcinoma GC3TK$^-$ *(46)* and ileocecal carcinoma HCT-8/TK$^-$ *(47)*, and most of the studies utilized the subrenal capsule assay *(37)*. Drug effects were evaluated by the amount of inhibition of growth of implanted tumor fragments and by the degree of tumor cytolysis at the lesion. GW1843 was far more potent against these TK$^-$ tumor lines than the tk$^+$ ones discussed above. On a 5 d, twice daily, ip dosing schedule (and no PEG-TPase treatment) significant growth inhibition was detected at 0.32 mg/kg for both lines and cytolysis was detected at 1.0 mg/kg *(44)*. However, GC3TK$^-$ was more sensitive than HCT-8/TK$^-$, since maximum effects occurred at lower doses for the former. At 10 mg/kg GW1843, there was continued tumor regression of GC3TK$^-$ when the tumor evaluation was extended from day 10 to day 21.

More frequent and extended dosing of GW1843 yielded stronger antitumor effects against GC3TK$^-$; twice daily was preferred to once daily, and 5>3>1 days of dosing *(44)*. These effects were more prominent with the cytolysis scores than with growth inhibition. The best result with 1 d of dosing was at 500 mg/kg; modest cytolysis and tumor stasis resulted, compared to almost complete cytolysis and tumor regression at 10 mg/kg, twice daily for five days in the same experiment. Ten-day dosing was superior to five-day in the inhibition of growth of HCT-8/TK$^-$ implanted subcutaneously. Dosed at 10 mg/kg twice daily, each group showed tumor regression while dosed and then resumption of the control growth rate 5 d after dosing was stopped.

GW1843 prevented HCT-8/TK$^-$ metastasis development in liver after intrasplenic injection of the tumor suspension *(45)*. The dosing was for 10 d, started at day 5 when metastases were first detected in controls. No hepatic tumor foci were detected on day 27 in groups dosed at 9 and 29 mg/kg, twice daily for 10 d. The survival time was doubled at 10 mg/kg and no deaths observed at 31 mg/kg in a different experiment. Also, as was observed for GC3TK$^-$ in the SRCA, 10 d of therapy was superior to 5 d in reduction of liver tumor foci, as was two 5-d cycles of therapy separated by 6 d without dosing.

The thymidine kinase-deficient cell lines were a very useful tool for assessing some of the properties of GW1843 against human tumors in vivo. In the (apparent) absence of thymidine salvage, GW1843 is very potent against these two gastrointestinal tumors—substantial cell kill, tumor regression, and complete responses were observed, in tumors growing subcutaneously, under the renal capsule and as liver metastases.

5.3. Effects of Folic Acid on Efficacy

The in vitro experiments on the effects of folic acid and leucovorin on the reversal of GW1843 cytotoxicity (Subheading 4.2., above) showed that the growth inhibition produced by GW1843 and related benzoquinazolines was poorly reversed by folates; thus the compounds were unique among polyglutamatable antifolates. This observation was then studied in mouse toxicity experiments with folic acid, and we found that high oral doses of folic acid could prevent weight loss and lethality from GW1843 *(37)*. Folic acid at 300 mg/kg dosed orally approx 0.5 h before GW1843 prevented the weight loss of 200 mg/kg GW1843 and the lethality of 400 mg/kg, twice daily for 7 d, in BALB/C mice. This mirrored the results of similar experiments in the dog (Subheading 6.2., below).

The lack of reversal against tumor lines in vitro and prevention of toxicity in vivo prompted us to determine the effects of folic acid and leucovorin on the antitumor activity of GW1843 in vivo *(37)*. Three thymidine kinase-deficient human tumor lines were used; HCT-8/TK$^-$, GC3TK$^-$, and osteosarcoma 143 B TK$^-$, in the SRCA tumor model. High oral doses of folic acid or leucovorin (300–500 mg/kg) had little to no effect on the growth inhibition or cytolysis caused by GW1843 (3.2–50 mg/kg) against GC3/TK$^-$ when evaluated 3 d after dosing stopped. The potent antitumor effects of GW1843 were maintained even with multiple dosing of folic acid around each GW1843 dose and when the tumors were evaluated 2 wk after dosing. In contrast, Tomudex and Lometrexol (a GAR TFase inhibitor) were partially reversed by folic acid in an experiment with a direct comparison to the lack of reversal against GW1843. (Low doses of folic acid are used to alleviate the toxicity of Lometrexol clinically *(48)*, but the doses used are far lower than are effective with GW1843.)

Folic acid treatment did not abate the antitumor activity of GW1843 against HCT-8/TK$^-$ or 143 B TK$^-$ when the tumors were assessed 3 d after dosing. However, there was slight reversal of activity against 143 B TK$^-$ and substantial reversal against HCT-8/TK$^-$ 2 wk later. Interestingly, HCT-8 cells have high levels of the mFBP to which GW1843 binds. If this molecule is partly responsible for GW1843 transport into HCT-8 cells, the folic acid competition in HCT-8 is consistent.

Overall, the results confirmed and extended the in vitro conclusions—that the in vivo antitumor activity of GW1843 was mostly unaffected by folic acid. Importantly, however, GW1843 toxicity in the mouse (and dog) was prevented by oral folic acid. This obviously suggested the possibility of using folic acid in the clinic to reduce the toxicity of GW1843 and/or to allow dose escalation.

6. PRECLINICAL TOXICOLOGY

6.1. Dose-Limiting Toxicology

As discussed in subheading 5., the mouse is highly resistant to GW1843-induced toxicity, which is directly attributable to the general lack of sensitivity of rodent cells to the drug and high circulating thymidine levels in the species. As such, mice can be dosed with 400 mg/kg of GW1843 bid for a week with little or no toxicity. Nonetheless, through prior treatment of mice with PEG-TPase, toxicity caused by GW1843 can be demonstrated. In BALB/C females, 200 mg/kg GW1843 bid for 7 d produces an approx 20% weight loss. Under similar thymidine-depleted conditions, 400 mg/kg of drug are lethal. Gastrointestinal toxicity is the dose-limiting toxicity under these conditions as demonstrated by bloody diarrhea and cytopathological changes consistent with maturation arrest enteritis.

The dog is far more sensitive to GW1843-induced toxicity *(37,49)*. This is presumably caused by the circulating thymidine levels of ≤ 70 nM in the dog compared to 1000 nM in the mouse *(49)* and the greater inherent sensitivity of canine cells to the drug (cells from dog bone marrow are approx 10-fold less sensitive to GW1843 than human bone marrow cells; unpublished). This sensitivity made the dog a better model for human drug toxicity, thus, toxicity was studied in this species in more detail. All experiments were performed with a 5-d, single daily dose regimen. At doses of 1 mg/kg and below, little or no toxicity was observed. At 2 mg/kg, mild reversible toxicity was observed. Toxicity at this dose included mild diarrhea, emesis, decreased activity, decreased food consumption, decreased body weight, and dehydration. Decreased lymphocyte and eosinophil levels were also observed, but neutrophil levels were seen to increase, probably because of dehydration. At 6 mg/kg GW1843, toxicity was lethal. Clinical signs, which began to appear during the last 2 d of dosing and peaked at postdose days 2 to 3, included vomiting, diarrhea, hyperthermia, labored breathing, slow or no righting reflex, prostration, and lacrimation. At this dose, the primary target of toxicity was the gastrointestinal tract, expressed clinically as severe forms of the same toxicities observed at 2 mg/kg, especially including severe bloody diarrhea and severe maturation arrest enteritis. Gross pathological changes included dark red discoloration and streaking of the lining of the intestines. Also at this dose, consistent evidence of secondary kidney toxicity (expressed as elevation of blood urea nitrogen, creatinine, globulin, and bilirubin) and liver toxicity (expressed as elevated bile acid and SGPT but not SGOT levels) was observed. However, these indicators of hepatotoxicity were not confirmed by liver histopathology, suggesting that they were secondary to stresses of dehydration and debilitation. The studies indicated that 2 mg/kg was a safe dose.

Toxicity similar to that in the dog was also observed in the cynomolgus monkey. Toxicity at 3.3 mg/kg (equivalent to 2 mg/kg in the dog on a mg/m^2 basis) was completely reversible. Sporadic clinical signs included diarrhea, emesis, and loss of appetite. These toxicities were consistent with the dose-limiting toxicity being gastrointestinal in this species as well. All toxicities resolved quickly after several days of postdose recovery.

6.2. Effect of Folic Acid Pretreatment

The effect of folic acid pretreatment was studied in the mouse and dog. In both species the toxicity of GW1843 was reversed by oral folic acid. In the mouse, weight loss associated with 200 mg/kg GW1843 was completely reversed by oral administration of 300 mg/kg folic acid 30–45 min prior to ip dosing of GW1843. Similarly, this dose of folic acid protected 8 of 10 mice treated ip with a lethal dose of 400 mg/kg GW1843.

Prevention of GW1843 toxicity was studied in more detail in the dog. At the lethal dose of 6 mg/kg of GW1843 for 5 d, 50 mg/kg folic acid dosed orally 30 min prior to the iv dose of GW1843, protected all dogs and eliminated the severe clinical signs, though mild emesis, decreased food consumption, and some weight loss persisted. Further, at twice the lethal GW1843 dose, a similar amelioration by folic acid was observed. At three times the lethal dose, however, folic acid failed to protect against the lethal toxicity of GW1843, and all animals succumbed. Thus, the lethal dose of GW1843 was elevated two- to threefold by prior oral administration of folic acid.

Alternative dosing schedules for folic acid and GW1843 were also investigated. It was found that folic acid at up to 500 mg/kg could be safely given along with a 10 mg/kg/d dose of GW1843 for 5 d. The minimal folic acid dose given once daily that was necessary to provide complete protection from the lethal 10 mg/kg dose was found to be between 10 and 50 mg/kg/d. However, if folic acid was given three times daily for 5 d, 10 mg/kg folic acid per dose was also found to protect all dogs.

The mechanism for this selective protection of normal cells by GW1843 has not been investigated in detail. Nonetheless, the results are consistent with a mechanism involving selective inhibition of drug transport into sensitive normal cells combined with noncompetitive inhibition of TS by GW1843 or its diglutamate metabolite. This mechanism assumes the presence of a folic-acid-binding transporter for GW1843 in the sensitive normal cells, and a folic-acid-insensitive transporter for GW1843 in tumor cells. The latter is consistent with the tumor transport we have described for GW1843 in MOLT-4 MCF-7, WiDr, and SW480 cells *(37)*. Systems analogous to the former, folic-acid-sensitive transport of antifolates have been described in normal gut and liver cells, and are also consistent with this mechanism *(50–59)*. An additional feature of this protection of normal cells by folic acid may be an effect of folic acid upon normal cell retention of GW1843 through competition for polyglutamation. Clearly, additional experimentation is required to sort out the mechanistic details of this very interesting feature of GW1843 selectivity.

Other reports have described the effects of folic acid on antifolate toxicity and efficacy for compounds including MTX, DDATHF, Tomudex, LY231514, and ZD9331 *(60–63)*. Low doses of folic acid have been shown to protect mice and/or humans from toxicity of MTX, DDATHF, and Tomudex. However, at doses similar to those used here, efficacy was reversed. High doses of folic acid comparable to those used above with GW1843 were not able to reverse the toxicity of the TS inhibitor ZD9331 *(62)*. Thus, GW1843 appears to be relatively unique in the selective folic acid protection feature.

7. CLINICAL EVALUATION OF GW1843: INITIAL PHASE I TESTING USING A DAILY X5 DOSING SCHEDULE

A Phase I study is being conducted under a U.S. FDA Investigational New Drug Application (IND) at the Cancer Therapy and Research Center in San Antonio, Texas. Howard Burris, *(64,65)* was the initial principal investigator, succeeded by Thomas Johnson. An important question to be addressed in this trial is the potential of high-dose oral folic acid to reduce the toxicity of iv GW1843. The object of this Phase I study is to determine the maximum tolerated dose (MTD) of GW1843 administered alone and then in combination with oral folic acid. Once the MTD of GW1843 alone was determined, that dose was used in other patient cohorts who also received 1000 mg of oral folic acid solution 45 min prior to GW1843 infusion. Daily X5 administration was chosen based on plasma drug clearance patterns observed in animals. Daily dosing was considered necessary to expose tumor cells to sustained cytotoxic levels of GW1843.

The study design included an open-label, dose-escalation study with cohorts of at least three patients per dose. All patients provided written informed consent, had to have a Karnofsky Performance Status of at least 70% and have good hematologic function. All patients had to have treatment-refractory solid tumors but were not required to have measurable disease. Hematology, clinical chemistry, and urinalysis were performed at baseline and weekly throughout the study. Blood samples for pharmacokinetic analyses were obtained periodically on days 1 through 5 during treatment courses 1 and 2. Tumor assessments (e.g., CT scans, chest X-rays, or physical examination) were performed prestudy and after each course of therapy. Cohorts of at least three patients were enrolled at sequential doses of GW1843 and doses were escalated until the MTD was reached. Maximum tolerated dose was defined as dose-limiting toxicity development in at least two of six patients at any dosage cohort.

7.1. Part 1: MTD of GW1843 Alone

GW1843 administered alone was tested at dose levels of 6, 1, 2, and 3.3 mg/m^2. The drug was administered iv over 2 min on a daily X5 schedule every 21 d. Patients were evaluated prior to the initiation of each new dosage cycle to make sure that toxicities were resolved to acceptable levels before further dosing could take place. Patients were discontinued from study participation because of withdrawal of consent, disease progression, or the development of unacceptable toxicity. Patients could continue to receive cycles of GW1843 as long as their disease status remained stable.

7.2. Part 2: MTD of GW1843 with Folic Acid

GW1843 was tested at 2, 3.3, 5, and 6 mg/m^2 coadministered with high-dose oral folic acid. Oral folic acid doses of 1000 mg were given orally 45 min prior to each 2-min iv administration of GW1843. Eligibility criteria and study discontinuation criteria were identical for parts 1 and 2.

At this time, enrollment in this trial has not reached completion. Dose-limiting toxicity has been observed in parts 1 and 2. A few additional patients are required to clarify the MTD in part 2. To date, 32 patients have been enrolled in the trial. The majority of patients have had refractory colon cancer. Most patients were male over the age of 60. Table 4 indicates the size of the dosage cohorts.

7.3. Safety and Tolerance

The first patient enrolled in this study received 6 mg/m^2 daily X5 of GW1843 without folic acid. This patient developed significant toxicity including severe anemia, neutropenia, thrombocytopenia, rash, and fever. Pharmacokinetic analyses of this patient's plasma samples postdosing indicated an 8–40 times lower clearance of the drug than predicted from preclinical studies in monkeys and dogs, respectively. The patient was hospitalized as a precaution and fully recovered from all toxicities. The protocol was subsequently amended to begin dose escalation at the lower dose of 1 mg/m^2 daily X5. The first patient chose to continue dosing at 1 mg/m^2. Dosage cohorts of 1 mg/m^2, 2 mg/m^2, and 3.3 mg/m^2 were explored in various cohorts of patients. Clinical toxicity was manifested by the development of stomatitis, skin rash, fever, and fatigue. Uncommon

Table 4
Patient Dosage Cohort Enrollment to Date (32 patients entered)

GW1843 Alone Dose	No. of Patients	GW1843 + Folic Acid Dose	No. of Patients
6 mg/m^2	1	2 mg/m^2	5
1 mg/m^2	3 (2 + 1)	3.3 mg/m^2	5
2 mg/m^2	7	5 mg/m^2	4
3.3 mg/m^2	2	6 mg/m^2	6

Dosing has ranged from 1–11 courses of treatment (median = 2).

Table 5
Toxicity Comparison of GW1843 With and Without Oral Folic Acid

Folic Acid Dose	GW1843 Dose	Number of Patients (Courses)	Stomatitis Grade 1	2	3	Rash Grade 1	2	3	Fatigue Grade 1	2	3	Fever Grade 1	2	3
0 mg	2 mg/m^2	7 (11)	3	1	1	3	4	0	4	3	1	3	4	1
1000 mg	2 mg/m^2	5 (12)	1	0	0	5	0	0	4	0	0	1	1	0
0 mg	3.3 mg/m^2	2 (3)	0	0	1	2	1	1	0	0	1	0	1	0
1000 mg	3.3 mg/m^2	5 (19)	1	0	0	0	2	0	1	0	0	1	0	0
1000 mg	5 mg/m^2	4 (9)	0	1	0	3	1	0	4	0	0	0	1	0
1000 mg	6 mg/m^2	6 (10)	1	1	0	1	2	0	4	2	1	0	2	0

adverse experiences included alopecia, anorexia, chills, diarrhea, peripheral edema, and nausea and vomiting. The MTD of GW1843 administered alone on a daily X5 regimen was determined to be 2 mg/m^2.

The initial dose of GW1843 tested in part 2 was the maximum tolerated dose observed in part 1, 2 mg/m^2. Patients pretreated with folic acid developed fewer and less severe toxicities at comparable doses of GW1843 alone. A comparison of the representative toxicities observed with GW1843 administered with or without folic acid can be seen in Table 5.

Although the initial trial is ongoing, the maximum tolerated dose of the folic acid/GW1843 drug combination appears to be 5 mg/m^2 of GW1843. A similar pattern of toxicity to GW1843 treatment alone, including stomatitis, rash, neutropenia, and malaise was observed in the patients receiving the combination, only at higher doses.

Some patients who developed significant clinical toxicities with GW1843 alone were subsequently retreated with the same dose of the drug premedicated with oral folic acid. As noted in Table 6, patients who had developed significant toxicities of stomatitis and rash with GW1843 alone had fewer and/or less-severe toxicities when oral folic acid was administered prior to drug.

7.4. Pharmacokinetics

Pharmacokinetic parameter estimates (65) indicate that the area under the curve (AUC) and the concentration of GW1843 5 min after bolus iv administration were pro-

Table 6
Toxicity in Patients Who Received GW1843 Without and Then With Oral Folic Acid

Patient Number	GW1843 Daily Dose	Stomatitis Grade		Rash Grade		Fatigue Grade		Fever Grade	
		No Folic Acid	Folic Acid	No Folic Acid	Folic Acid	No Folic Acid	Folic Acid	No Folic Acid	Folic Acid
00008	2 mg/m^2	3	0	1	0	2	0	0	0
00009	2 mg/m^2	1	0	2	1	1	1	2	0
00010	3.3 mg/m^2	3	1	3	0	1	0	2	1

portional to dose. The terminal-phase half-life of GW1843 in men is approx 7 h. Preliminary analyses indicate that the pharmacokinetic profile of GW1843 with and without folic acid is similar, but the clearance may be somewhat higher with the addition of folic acid.

7.5. Antitumor Activity

The main objective of this phase I safety and tolerance study was to determine the maximum tolerated dose of GW1843 administered either alone or in combination with oral folic acid. Determination of antitumor activity was of secondary importance in patients who were not required to have measurable disease upon entry into the study.

Evidence of antitumor activity, however, was observed in some patients *(64)*. The most striking response was seen in a patient with gastric cancer who had failed previous 5-fluorouracil therapy. The patient had evaluable disease. Evidence of major tumor shrinkage and clinical improvement was seen. The patient received two courses of GW1843 at the dose of 2 mg/m^2 without folic acid, then nine additional courses of GW1843 at the same dose along with 1000 mg of oral folic acid. Other incidences of antitumor activity were also seen in patients with colon and bladder cancer.

Administration of GW1843 following high-dose oral folic acid dosing produced fewer and less severe toxicities than observed with the drug administered by itself. In animal studies the protective effects of oral folic acid were seen in gastrointestinal toxicities, and consistent with this, stomatitis was reduced in humans. The reduction of malaise and rash in humans was somewhat surprising. The apparent maximum tolerated dose of GW1843 when given with folic acid is 5 mg/m^2, 2.5-fold higher than the drug given without the protective agent. Thus, clinical testing has indicated that oral folic acid does indeed attenuate the toxicities of this potent thymidylate synthase inhibitor in man. Additionally, some preliminary evidence of antitumor activity has been observed in patients both receiving the drug by itself and in combination with folic acid.

Because of the low clearance rate of GW1843 in humans, daily X5 administration does not appear to be the optimal dosage schedule. Additional phase I studies with other dosing regimens (e.g., weekly or once q3 weekly) are needed to determine the toxicity profile when the drug is given less frequently prior to pilot phase II efficacy testing.

8. CONCLUSIONS AND FUTURE PROSPECTIVE

This monograph on basic research and current clinical practice with antifolate drugs presents information on a number of new clinical agents and strategies. Each one provides unique properties for the clinician to exploit to aid in our continued attempts to reduce the burden of cancer. GW1843 shows promise to be one of these. It is a potent noncompetitive inhibitor of human TS. It has strong activity against human cancer cells in culture, against solid human tumors in mice, and is showing preliminary evidence of antitumor activity in humans. The potential for combination of the compound with folic acid appears to provide GW1843 with a unique mode of selectivity enhancement over other antifolates. The continued testing of GW1843 and combination with other anticancer agents will continue to be of interest toward the development of new effective therapies for a number of important cancers.

REFERENCES

1. Ferone R. *Bull WHO* 1977; 55:291–298.
2. Pendergast W, Dickerson SH, Johnson JV, Ferone R. International Patent 1991, WO 91/19700.
3. Pendergast W, Johnson JV, Dickerson SH, Dev IK, Duch DS, Ferone R, Hall WR, Humphreys J, Kelly JM, Wilson DC. *J Med Chem* 1993; 36:2279–2291.
4. Sirotnak FM, DeGraw JI, in: *Folate Antagonists as Therapeutic Agents, Vol. II, Pharmacology. Experimental and Clinical Therapeutics* Sirotnak FM, Burchall JB, Ensminger WB, Montgomery JA, eds. Academic, New York, 1984, pp. 43–95.
5. Dev IK, unpublished.
6. Jones TR, Calvert AH, Jackman AL, Brown SJ, Jones M, Harrap KR. *Eur J Cancer* 1981; 17:11–19.
7. Palmer DC, Skotnicki JS, Taylor EC. In *Progress in Medicinal Chemistry,* vol. 33, (Ellis GP, West GB, eds.). Elsevier, Amsterdam, 1988, pp. 85–231.
8. Elslager EF, Colby NL, Davoll J, Hutt MP, Johnson JL, Werbel LM. *J Med Chem* 1984; 27:1740–1743.
9. Jones TR, Thornton TJ, Flinn A, Jackman AL, Newell DR, Calvert AH. *J Med Chem* 1989; 32:847–852.
10. Hughes LR, Jackman AL, Oldfield J, Smith RC, Burrows KD, Marsham PR, Bishop JAM, Jones TR, O'Connor BM, Calvert AH. *J Med Chem* 1990; 33:3060–3067.
11. The ability of the compounds to enter tumor cells by the reduced folate transport system was assessed by measurement of their inhibition of the uptake by Molt-4 human T-cell leukemia cells of ^{3}H-methotrexate, itself a substrate for this transport system. Li SW, Nair MG, Edwards DM, Kisliuk RL, Gaumont Y, Dev IK, Duch DS, Humphreys J, Smith GK, Ferone R. *J Med Chem* 1991; 34:2746–2754.
12. The compounds were examined for their ability to function as substrates for partially purified hog liver folylpolyglutamate synthetase. Kelley JL, McLean EW, Cohn NK, Edelstein MP, Duch DS, Smith GK, Hanlon MH, Ferone R. *J Med Chem* 1990; 33:561–567.
13. Marsham PR, Jackman AL, Hayter AJ, Daw MR, Snowden JL, O'Connor BM, Bishop JAM, Calvert AH, Hughes LR. *J Med Chem* 1991; 34:2209–2218.
14. Weichsel A, Montfort WR. *Nature Structural Biol* 1995; 2:1095–1101.
15. Oatis JE, Hynes JB. *J Med Chem* 1977; 20:1393–1396.
16. Hynes JB, Garrett CM. *J Med Chem* 1975; 18:632–634.
17. Scanlon KJ, Moroson BA, Bertino JR, Hynes JB. *Mol Pharmacol* 1979; 16:261–269.
18. Fernandes DJ, Bertino JR, Hynes JB. *Cancer Res* 1983; 43:1117–1123.
19. Jones TR, Calvert AH, Jackman AL, Eakin MA, Smithers MJ, Betteridge RF, Newell DR, Hayter AJ, Stocker A, Harland SJ, Davies LC, Harrap KR. *J Med Chem* 1985; 28:1468–1476.
20. Jones TR, Smithers MJ, Taylor MA, Jackman AL, Calvert AH, Harland SJ, Harrap KR. *J Med Chem* 1986; 29:468–472.
21. Marsham PR, Chambers P, Hayter AJ, Hughes LR, Jackman AL, O'Connor BM, Bishop JAM, Calvert AH. *J Med Chem* 1989; 32:569–575.
22. Hughes LR, Jackman AL, Oldfield J, Smith RC, Burrows KD, Marsham PR, Bishop JAM, Jones TR, O'Connor BM, Calvert AH. *J Med Chem* 1990; 33:3060–3067.

23. Jackman AL, Marsham PR, Thornton TJ, Bishop JAM, O'Connor BM, Hughes LR, Calvert AH, Jones TR. *J Med Chem* 1990; 33:3067–3071.
24. Marsham PR, Jackman AL, Oldfield J, Hughes LR, Thornton TJ, Bisset GMF, O'Connor BM, Bishop JAM, Calvert AH. *J Med Chem* 1990; 33:3072–3078.
25. Marsham PR, Hughes LR, Jackman AL, Hayter AJ, Oldfield J, Wardleworth JM, Bishop JAM, O'Connor BM, Calvert AH. *J Med Chem* 1991; 34:1594–1605.
26. Similar NMR observations on 2'-fluoro derivatives were made independently in the quinazoline series, and a similarly rigidified side chain was introduced using a different synthetic route (ref. *13*). In contrast to the benzoquinazolines, however these derivatives were reported to show a two to fourfold diminution in TS activity and a 30-fold reduction in cytotoxic potency relative to the conformationally unrestricted analog.
27. Duch DS, Banks S, Dev IK, Dickerson SH, Ferone R, Health LS, Humphreys J, Knick V, Pendergast W, Singer S, Smith GK, Waters K, Wilson HR. *Cancer Res* 1993; 53:810–818.
28. Dev IK, Dallas WS, Ferone R, Hanlon M, McKee DD, Yates BB. *J Biol Chem* 1994; 269:1873–1882.
29. Hanlon MH, Ferone R. *Cancer Res* 1996; 56:3301–3306.
30. Stout TJ, Stroud RM. *Structure* 1996; 4:67–77.
31. Chen CH, Davis RA, Maley F. *Biochemistry* 1996; 35:8786–8793.
32. Weichsel A, Montfort WR, Ciesla J, Maley F. *Proc Natl Acad Sci USA* 1995; 92:3493–3497.
33. Li WW, Tong WP, Bertino JR. *Proc Am Assoc Cancer Res* 1995; 36:2274.
34. Li WW, Tong WP, Bertino JR. *Clin Cancer Res* 1995; 1:631–636.
35. Humphreys J, Smith G, Mullin R, Waters K, Duch D. *Proc Am Assoc Cancer Res* 1993; 34:272.
36. Jackman AL, Kelland LR, Kimball R, Brown M, Gibson W, Aherne GW, Hardcastle A, Boyle FT. *Br J Cancer* 1995; 71:914–924.
37. Smith GK, Amyx H, Boytos CM, Duch DS, Ferone R, Wilson HR. *Cancer Res* 1995; 55:6117–6125.
38. Wong SC, Proefke SA, Bhushan A, Matherly LH. *J Biol Chem* 1995; 270:17,468–17,475.
39. Jackman AL, Taylor GA, Calvert AH, Harrap KR. *Biochem Pharmacol* 1984; 33:3269–3275.
40. Banks SD, Waters KA, Barrett LL, Dickerson S, Pendergast W, Smith GK. *Cancer Chemother Pharmacol* 1994; 33:455–459.
41. Kozalka GW, Lobe D, Stonefield MW, Vanhooke J, Ferone R, Waters K, Ellis MN. *Antiviral Res* 1993; 20(suppl 1):143.
42. Wilson HR, Heath LS, Knick VC, Kozalka GW, Ferone R. *Proc Am Assoc Cancer Res* 1992; 33:407.
43. Wilson HR, Ferone R, Boytos CM, Heath LS, Jones JA, Knick VC, Waters K. *Proc Am Assoc Cancer Res* 1995; 36:376.
44. Wilson HR, Knick VC, Boytos CM, Dillberger J, Heath LS, Jones WA, Rudolph SK, Ferone R. manuscript in prep.
45. Boytos CM, Ferone R, Jones WA, Rudolph SK, Franklin SL, Houle CD. *Proc Am Assoc Cancer Res* 1995; 36:376.
46. Radparvar JL, Houghton PJ, Germain G, Pennington J, Rahamn A, Houghton JA. *Biochem Pharmacol* 1990; 39:1759–1765.
47. Zhang Z-G, Malmberg M, Yin M-B, Slocum HK, Rustum YM. *Biochem Pharmacol* 1993; 45:1157–1164.
48. Young CW, Currie VE, Muindi JF, Saltz LB, Pisters KMW, Esposito AJ, Dyke RW. *Proceedings of the 7th NCI-EORTC Symposium on New Drugs in Cancer Therapy* 1992, p. 136.
49. The Clinical Oncology Group, Medical Division, Burroughs Wellcome, Research Triangle Park, NC An Investigational New Drug Application for 1843U89, 1994.
50. Said HM, Ghishan FK, Redha R. *Am J Physiol* 1987; 252:229–236.
51. Sirotnak FM, Moccio DM, Yang CH. *Cancer Res* 1984; 44:5204–5211.
52. Chello PL, Sirotnak FM, Dorick DM, Donsbach RC. *Cancer Res* 1977; 37:4297–4303.
53. Zimmerman J. *Gastroenterology* 1990; 99:964–972.
54. Rosenberg IH, Zimmerman J, Selhub J. *Chemioterapia* 1985; 4:354–358.
55. Schron CM. *J Membrane Biol* 1990; 118:259–267.
56. Zimmerman J. *Biochem Pharmacol* 1992; 43:2377–2383.
57. Zimmerman J. *Biochem Pharmacol* 1992; 44:1839–1842.
58. Horne DW, Reed KA. *Arch Biochem Biophys* 1992; 298:121–128.
59. Gewirtz DA, White JC, Randolph JK, Goldman ID. *Cancer Res* 1980; 40:573–578.

60. Pavlotsky AI, Novikova LA, Svet-Moldavsky GJ, Toloknov BO, Buchman VM, Radzikhovskaya RM. *Cancer Treat Rep* 1977; 61:895–897.
61. Grindey GB, Shih C. US patent no. 5217974, 1991.
62. Rees C, Kimbell R, Valenti M, Brunton L, Farrugia D, Jackman AL. *Proc Am Assoc Cancer Res* 1997; 38:476 (abstract 3184).
63. Worzalla JF, Self TD, Theobald KS, Schultz RM, Mendelsohn LG, Shih C. *Proc Am Assoc Cancer Res* 1997; 38:478 (abstract 3198).
64. Burris HA, Smetzer LA, Eckardt JR, Rodriguez GI, Rinaldi DA, Lampkin AT, Bigley JW, Von Hoff DD. *Proc Am Soc Clin Oncol* 1996; 15:490.
65. Burris HA, Kisor DF, Smetzer LA, Eckardt JR, Rodriguez GI, Rinaldi DA, Lampkin AT, Bigley JW, Von Hoff DD. *Proc Am Soc Clin Oncol* 1996; 15:477.

10 Preclinical and Clinical Studies with the Novel Thymidylate Synthase Inhibitor Nolatrexed Dihydrochloride (Thymitaq™, AG337)

Andy Hughes and A. Hilary Calvert

Contents

Introduction
X-ray Crystallographic Design
Preclinical Studies
Clinical Studies
Summary
References

1. INTRODUCTION

Despite recent advances in chemotherapy, there remains a significant number of patients for whom no satisfactory treatment exists. It remains a high priority to evaluate drugs that may possess either greater efficacy or activity in tumors with intrinsic or acquired resistance to established treatment. Nolatrexed dihydrochloride (Thymitaq™) is a novel folate-based inhibitor of thymidylate synthase (TS). TS is the rate-limiting enzyme in the *de novo* biosynthetic pathway for thymidine nucleotides. Since thymidine is used exclusively for the synthesis of DNA, TS remains an important target for anticancer drug therapy *(1–3)*. A number of folate-based TS inhibitors have been developed and have demonstrated activity in clinical trials. It is postulated that inhibitors that utilize the folate-binding site of the TS enzyme have potential advantages over those, such as FdUMP, that act at the pyrimidine site. The folate-based cytotoxic agents are more likely, when compared with their pyrimidine-based counterparts, to have a unique locus of action, not be incorporated into nucleic acids, and not be susceptible to catabolic degradation. The first clinically evaluable folate-based TS inhibitor was CB3717. This showed antitumor activity but its development had to be abandoned because of un-

From: *Anticancer Drug Development Guide: Antifolate Drugs in Cancer Therapy*
Edited by: A.L. Jackman © Humana Press Inc., Totowa, NJ

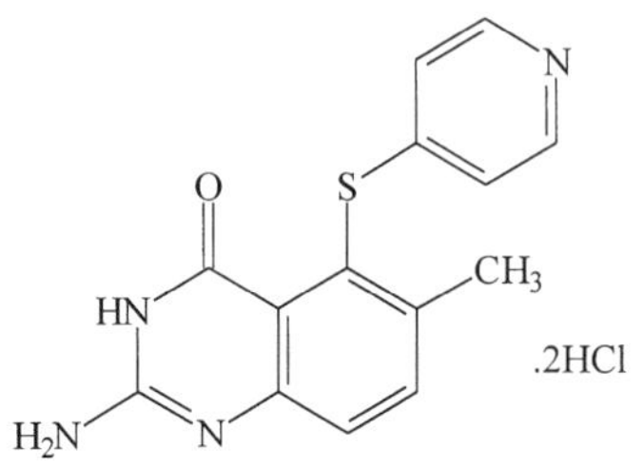

Figure 1. The structure of nolatrexed dihydrochloride.

predictable nephrotoxicity and myelosuppression *(4,5)*. A successor, raltitrexed (Tomudex), has now been extensively investigated in the clinic. Both CB3717 and raltitrexed are termed classical antifolates because they possess a terminal para-amino benzoyl glutamate moiety. Such compounds use specific carrier systems to gain entry into cells and are typically substrates for the enzyme folyl polyglutamate synthetase (FPGS). Conversion to intracellular polyglutamates by this enzyme greatly enhances the potency of classical antifolates by increasing intracellular retention and by augmenting their inhibitory potency towards TS. However, the variable toxicity of these drugs may be due to variations in the rate of formation and retention of these polyglutamates.

Nolatrexed was designed by Agouron Pharmaceuticals, San Diego, California using knowledge of the three-dimensional structure of the active site of TS (*see* Section 2). The molecular structure of nolatrexed was developed by design at the folate cofactor binding site of TS. In contrast to the classical inhibitors of TS, nolatrexed is nonclassical in that it does not possess a glutamate moiety. It therefore does not require facilitated transport for uptake into cells and is not a substrate for FPGS, and so may overcome resistance mechanisms concerned with either of these processes. The structure of nolatrexed dihydrochloride is shown in Fig. 1 and is now discussed in detail, together with its preclinical and clinical development. Attention will be given mainly to the published literature but more up-to-date information that has been presented in abstract form will also be included. Although the structure of the dihydrochloride salt is shown above, it is the free base of the drug that is the active form. All doses and plasma concentrations of nolatrexed in this chapter refer to the free base of the drug.

2. X-RAY CRYSTALLOGRAPHIC DESIGN

The molecular design of nolatrexed was guided by repetitive crystallographic analysis of protein–ligand structures *(6)*. At the time of the design, human TS was not available, so the crystal complex of *E. coli* was utilized, because the amino acid sequence of its folate binding site is nearly identical to that of the human TS enzyme. Initially, a ternary complex of *E. coli* TS, 5-FdUMP and CB3717 was examined, and then a quinazolin-4-one was substituted with a 2-methyl group in order to increase solubility. Using this new model, compounds were synthesized to fit as tightly as possible onto the folate binding site. One intermediate compound (Fig. 2) had inhibition constants of 10 μM against *E. coli* TS and 0.96 μM against human TS and was subjected to crystallization with *E. coli* and 5-FdUMP.

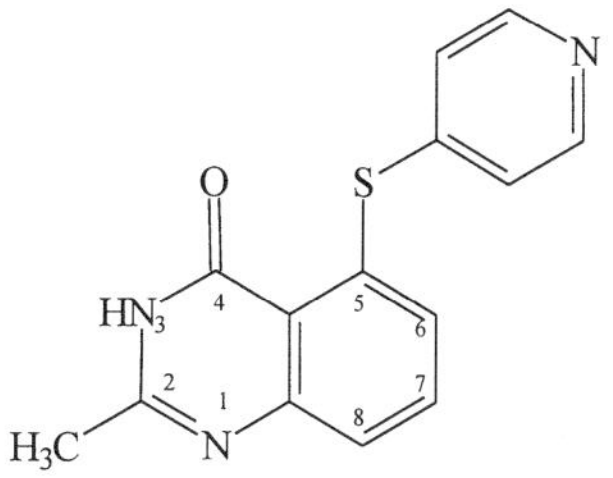

Figure 2. An intermediate compound synthesized during the design of nolatrexed.

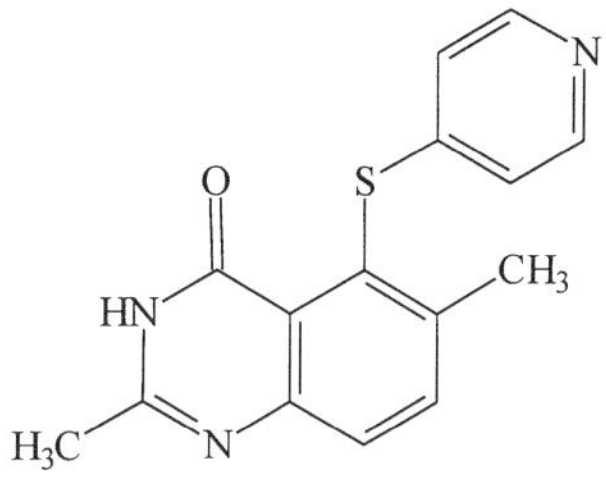

Figure 3. An intermediate compound synthesized during the design of nolatrexed.

A complex was formed and the ternary structure solved. This compound was optimized by replacing the 6-hydrogen atom with a methyl group, encouraging the thiopyridine substituent to assume an optimal configuration. This new compound (Fig. 3) was found to have a greater affinity for both *E. coli* and human TS (0.5 and 0.093 μ*M*, respectively).

This was transformed into the structure now known as nolatrexed by making a minor change to the substituents on the quinazolinone nucleus. This improved the affinity for human TS to 15 n*M*. Of several potent inhibitors designed, nolatrexed was selected for pharmaceutical formulation and clinical evaluation as a cytotoxic agent.

3. PRECLINICAL STUDIES

3.1. In Vitro

In enzyme inhibition studies, using a range of concentrations of the cofactor 5,10-methylene tetrahydrofolate, nolatrexed was found to be a potent inhibitor of purified human recombinant TS with a K_i of 11 n*M* (7). The kinetics of inhibition were found to be non-competitive with respect to the folate cofactor. In vitro experiments against a variety of murine and human cell lines demonstrated that nolatrexed inhibited cell growth. The most sensitive cell line of those studied was the L1210 (mouse leukemia) with a mean IC_{50} of 0.39 μ*M*. The least sensitive was the LoVo (human adenocarcinoma) cell line with an IC_{50} of 6.6 μ*M*. In order to determine whether TS was the intracellular locus of activity of nolatrexed, thymidine was added to the L1210 cultures treated with the drug and found to ablate significantly the antiproliferative effects of nolatrexed. The effect of nolatrexed was investigated on a thymidine-kinase deficient (TK⁻) cell line, L5178Y/TK⁻, and the wild-type parent cell line, L5178Y. Results showed a 3.5-fold enhancement in cytotoxicity in the TK⁻ cell line, which was consistent with its inability to salvage thymidine and thus bypass TS inhibition. The effect of folinic acid, hypoxanthine, and combinations of either of these with thymidine were studied. Neither folinic acid nor hypoxanthine alone altered the growth inhibitory effect of nolatrexed, suggesting that there was no effect on other folate-dependent enzyme systems. However, both folinic acid and hypoxanthine potentiated the rescue effects of thymidine in nolatrexed-treated cells. The exact mechanisms underlying these effects have not been studied further. The effect of the drug on the L1210/R6 cell line was investigated. This particular cell line overexpresses the dihydrofolate reductase (DHFR) enzyme and is extremely resistant to methotrexate. However, it was less than 2.5-fold resistant to nolatrexed compared with the parent L1210 cell line, confirming the lack of effect of this agent on DHFR. Further evidence of the link between TS inhibition and nolatrexed-induced effects was obtained. Firstly, in L1210 cells treated with nolatrexed, a significant reduction in cellular TTP pools was observed within 2 h of treatment. Secondly, flow cytometric data showed arrest in S-phase of nolatrexed-treated cells. TS activity was also measured directly, using a tritium release assay, in L1210 treated cells. This revealed that essentially complete inhibition of tritium release could be achieved, but this was not sustained after the drug was removed, suggesting that nolatrexed was rapidly removed from cells. This result was consistent with the improvement in nolatrexed cytotoxicity achieved when the duration of cell exposure to the drug was increased. These results are as would be expected from a water-soluble and lipophilic agent that has the ability to rapidly influx and efflux from cells, and does not undergo conversion to polyglutamate forms.

In vitro studies performed in Newcastle upon Tyne, U.K. using human colorectal cell lines demonstrated that 24-h exposure to nolatrexed was not sufficient to cause significant levels of cell kill *(8)*. For the HCT116 cell line, nolatrexed, at a concentration of 8 μg/mL, only killed 70% of cells. However, increasing the exposure time to 72–120 h produced concentration-dependent degrees of cytotoxicity. Exposure to nolatrexed for 120 h at the same dose of 8 μg/mL killed 99.8% of cells.

More recent in vitro data suggests a synergistic relationship between radiation and nolatrexed administration *(9)*. Studies were carried out on HT-29 human colon carcinoma cells in culture at a nontoxic concentration of nolatrexed (<10 μM). Radiation-induced cell kill was dramatically enhanced with pretreatment of the cells with nolatrexed for a time period less than 24 h. However, when the cells were exposed to nolatrexed immediately after radiation, there was no increase in cell kill. Further in vivo studies are necessary to assess the potential of the drug as a radiosensitizer. In vitro studies using a simultaneous exposure of nolatrexed and cisplatin have demonstrated a synergistic effect between these two cytotoxic agents against both ovarian (2008) and colon (HT29) cancer cells *(10)*. The synergy was observed in both 5FU and cisplatin-resistant cell lines (HT29-5FU and 2008C13, respectively). This work supports the further evaluation of this combination of drugs in the clinical setting.

Predictors of sensitivity to new thymidylate synthase inhibitors have been studied in 13 colon cancer cell lines *(11)*. The cytotoxic agents studied were raltitrexed, GW1483U89, LY231514, and nolatrexed. Nolatrexed differed from the other TS inhibitors which are all deemed classical because of their requirement for active transport and polyglutamation. Two cell lines were found to be resistant to nolatrexed, SW1116 and Colo201. The best predictors for sensitivity to the new TS inhibitors were found to be 24-h folate uptake and FPGS activity, although the latter is only applicable to the classical TS inhibitors. Nolatrexed has also been shown to enhance the growth inhibition of 5FU *(12)*. Nolatrexed facilitates binding of ^{3}H-FdUMP to purified human TS, particularly at low concentrations. More than additive growth inhibition was observed for 5FU and low dose nolatrexed in 3 of 7 colon cancer cell lines examined.

3.2. In vivo

In in vivo studies, nolatrexed showed low activity against rodent tumors with functional TK. This finding is in keeping with well-documented data on other antifolates *(13,14)* and is because rodents have high levels of circulating thymidine compared with humans and TS inhibition can be circumvented by thymidine salvage in these tumors. In order to evaluate the in vivo activity of nolatrexed, a TK$^-$ variant of the L5178Y murine lymphoma was used. Cures were achieved following intraperitoneal (ip) administration at both ip and intramuscular (im) tumor sites. The active dose levels required were nontoxic to the animals. Administering nolatrexed orally also showed activity in both ip and im tumor sites, demonstrating the ability of the drug to penetrate tissue barriers.

Further in vivo studies were undertaken and nolatrexed was administered at a dose of 60 mg/m^2 ip every 4 h to nude mice bearing the HeLa Bu25TK$^-$ human cervical cell line *(8)*. Dosing for 24 h was ineffective, but prolonging the duration of administration to 5 d resulted in significant growth retardation. Oral administration of nolatrexed was studied initially in mice *(15)* to determine bioavailability. Absorption was found to be rapid with peak plasma concentration levels achieved within 60 min. Oral bioavailability was 100%. An increase in the oral dose to 600 mg/m^2 resulted in a disproportionate increase in the area under the plasma concentration/time curve (AUC). This was accounted for by reduced clearance, implicating saturable elimination. Further studies in dogs showed an oral bioavailability greater than 80%.

3.3. Pharmacokinetics

After iv administration of nolatrexed in the rat, pharmacokinetics were best described by a two-compartment model and were dose-independent at levels from 20 to 80 mg/kg. The elimination half life was 2 h. Oral bioavailability was greater in fasted animals (53% relative to iv compared with 22% for fed animals). Absorption was more rapid, maximum plasma concentration was higher, and elimination was faster in the fasted state. In mice, the elimination half life was 2.9 h and oral bioavailability 62–90%.

3.4. Metabolites

The tissue distribution and excretion of nolatrexed were investigated in the rat utilising radiolabeled carbon *(16)*. At 48 h, 60% of the administered iv dose was excreted in the urine and 16% in the feces. Five radioactive metabolite peaks were observed in the urine and analyzed. The parent compound accounted for approx 30% of the total peak areas observed. No metabolites were observed in the rat feces. A similar urine analysis was performed on patients on a phase I study (*see* Section 4.1.2.) of nolatrexed administered as a 5-d continuous iv infusion. The parent drug accounted for approx 80% of the total peak areas. Four metabolites were found to be identical in both rat and human urine, labeled M1, M2b, M4, and M5. The major peaks in the human urine were labeled M1, M2b, and two glucuronides, M3a and M6, which were not observed in the rat.

3.4.1. TENTATIVE STRUCTURES

M1 = a benzoyl alcohol derivative of nolatrexed.
M2b = sulfoxide of M2a (M2a, AG411 = thioether hydrolysis of nolatrexed followed by S-methylation).
M3a = N-glucuronide conjugate of nolatrexed.
M4 = sulfoxide of nolatrexed.
M5 = N-oxide of nolatrexed.
M6 = N-glucuronide conjugate of M2a.

In purified forms, the above metabolites were shown to demonstrate less growth inhibition than nolatrexed itself against both the L1210 and CEM cell lines. Plasma and urinary metabolites have been further investigated in patients receiving both oral and iv nolatrexed, and similar metabolic profiles obtained *(17)*. The parent drug predominated in both urine and plasma. Among circulating metabolites, the loss of pyridine followed by S-methylation (AG411), was determined to be the most important metabolic pathway, being the precursor of two metabolites described above (M2b and M6) and of additional methylation products observed in plasma. The S-methylation of nolatrexed represented a novel biotransformation pathway. Methylation on the quinazoline ring and glucuronidation were also observed to be of importance. Further in vitro studies are now underway to examine the process by which nolatrexed is metabolized to AG411.

4. CLINICAL STUDIES
4.1. Phase I
4.1.1. 24-HIV INFUSION

This study was performed in Newcastle upon Tyne, U.K. *(18)*. It was a pharmacokinetic and pharmacodynamic study that had the following aims:

1. To investigate whether plasma concentrations of nolatrexed could be achieved in patients that were associated with antitumor activity in preclinical models.
2. To seek evidence that TS inhibition occurred in patients at clinically achievable plasma concentrations and to study the dose dependency of TS inhibition.
3. To record any toxicities or antitumor activity encountered.

Plasma nolatrexed levels were measured using a reverse-phase high performance liquid chromatography (HPLC) technique and plasma deoxyuridine (dUrd) levels were used as a surrogate marker of TS inhibition. Thirteen patients with a range of malignancies received a total of 27 courses of nolatrexed administered as a 24-h continuous iv infusion every 3 wk. The starting dose was 60 mg/m^2 which was 1/10 the LD$_{10}$ in mice. Doses were then doubled until 480 mg/m^2 at which point evidence of TS inhibition and pharmacokinetic non-linearity became evident. Doses were then escalated in 50% increments. Three or four patients were entered at each dose level although intrapatient dose escalation was permitted. The maximum dose administered was 1080 mg/m^2. Pharmacokinetic analysis revealed that plasma nolatrexed concentrations rose during the first 6 h of the infusion and were then maintained for the remaining 18 h. Once the infusion was stopped, there was a rapid monoexponential elimination of the drug and in all patients the plasma drug concentration was undetectable 48 h later. The relationship between dose and clearance suggested a reduction in clearance at higher dose levels, indicating saturable drug elimination. At doses over 240 mg/m^2, saturable elimination was confirmed by compartmental analyses *(19)*. Analysis of the urinary elimination of nolatrexed revealed that up to 28% of the administered dose was excreted unchanged in the urine within 48 h of the commencement of the infusion. Free, unbound nolatrexed constituted only 2.2–3.3% of the total drug in the plasma. This important factor was taken into consideration when determining whether plasma concentrations of nolatrexed, which corresponded to cytotoxic concentrations in vitro, were being attained. Comparisons with the in vitro data suggested that cytotoxic concentrations in the plasma were achieved. From a pharmacodynamic viewpoint, at doses of 480 mg/m^2 of nolatrexed and above, consistent elevations in plasma dUrd levels were seen at the end of the 24-h infusion. In all patients, plasma dUrd levels had returned to the pretreatment value 24 h after the end of the infusion. This suggested that TS inhibition was achieved but not maintained. There did not appear to be any increase in the magnitude of dUrd elevation at the top two doses (720 and 1080 mg/m^2) compared with 480 mg/m^2. This fact, along with the lack of maintenance of TS inhibition, led to the cessation of this study. The only significant toxicity observed was local toxicity around the infusion site. The severity of this was related to dose, but the problem was easily circumvented by administering the drug via a central venous catheter. Two explanations could account for this toxicity. Firstly, the pH of the infusate was low (pH 3.0–5.0) and secondly, buffering of the acidic drug solution within the vein may have resulted in drug precipitation. Otherwise, nolatrexed was very well tolerated with no significant myelosuppression. In summary, this study showed that cytotoxic plasma nolatrexed concentrations were readily and safely achieved, and these concentrations were associated with elevations in plasma dUrd levels. However, the lack of prolonged dUrd elevations, coupled with the lack of any biological effects such as myelosuppression, suggested that prolonged administration, either orally or via a central venous catheter, should be explored.

4.1.2. 5-D CONTINUOUS IV INFUSION

This phase I study was a multicenter, non-randomized, dose escalation trial in patients with advanced solid tumors *(20)*. Patients were treated at Newcastle upon Tyne, U.K., Metro Health, Cleveland, Ohio, and the University of California, San Diego, California. The aims of the study were to establish the maximum tolerated dose (MTD) and a recommended dose for phase II studies. The pharmacokinetics and pharmacodynamics of the drug were investigated and antitumor effects and toxicities were documented. In total, 32 patients with a range of malignancies (predominantly colorectal) were treated with nolatrexed given as a continuous 5-d iv infusion every 3 wk via a central venous catheter. The starting dose was 96 mg/m^2/d (total dose 480 mg/m^2, which corresponded to the dose in the 24-hour study at which elevations in plasma dUrd levels were consistently seen). Further dose escalations were guided by the pharmacokinetics and pharmacodynamics of nolatrexed and by any clinical toxicities encountered. Intrapatient dose escalation was permitted. The maximum dose administered was 1040 mg/m^2/d. The MTD was 904 mg/m^2/d and the recommended phase II dose was 800 mg/m^2/d. The dose-limiting toxicities were myelosuppression and mucositis. Full pharmacokinetic studies were performed on 22 patients (43 courses) *(21,22)*. At doses of 576 mg/m^2/d and below, steady-state plasma nolatrexed concentrations were achieved within 6 h of commencement of the infusion and maintained until the end of the infusion. There then followed a rapid monoexponential phase of elimination. However, at doses of 768 mg/m^2/d and above, there was evidence of saturable elimination as the plasma concentrations tended to increase throughout the infusion period, and clearance decreased at higher dose levels. Cytotoxic plasma levels were achieved at the higher dose levels. Excretion of nolatrexed in the urine was 18% (median) of the dose administered and not markedly dose-dependent.

Hematological toxicity and plasma dUrd concentrations were used to assess nolatrexed pharmacodynamics. There was a significant relationship between hematological toxicities and nolatrexed AUC. Plasma dUrd levels increased 24 h into the infusion in all cases except one and, at doses above 576 mg/m^2/d, remained elevated compared with baseline levels throughout the duration of the infusion. These levels returned quickly back to normal in all patients after cessation of the infusion. The dose-limiting toxicities of myelosuppression and mucositis were only of brief duration, possibly reflecting the short intracellular half-life of nolatrexed. Two episodes of grade IV neutropenia were encountered and one grade IV mucositis. Other toxicities seen were diarrhea, nausea and vomiting, rashes, and liver function abnormalities. One patient achieved a partial response (PR) following four courses of treatment. This patient had stage III poorly differentiated adenocarcinoma of the colon with metastatic nodal disease. The PR was maintained for 3 mo. In summary, further evaluation of nolatrexed was warranted and led to six phase II studies at the recommended dose of 800 mg/m^2/d. Preliminary results are reported later. In order to bypass the need for a central venous catheter, an oral preparation of nolatrexed has been developed.

4.1.3. PEDIATRIC STUDY

Methotrexate is an antifolate with very impressive activity in pediatric patients, particularly childhood acute lymphoblastic leukemia (ALL). It is feasible that those children resistant to methotrexate may respond to an antifolate such as nolatrexed which has different properties with respect to cellular transport and polyglutamation. For this reason, a phase I study with nolatrexed administered as a continuous 5-d infusion in pediatric patients with advanced malignancy has recently commenced in Newcastle upon Tyne, U.K. *(23)*. Patients with relapsed leukemia or solid tumors with bone marrow infiltration are eligible. Treatment courses are repeated every 28 d and the starting dose was 480 mg/m^2/d. There were no acute toxicities seen at this level so the dose was escalated to 640 mg/m^2/d. Grade II mucositis has been observed in one of the two patients so far evaluable at this dose level. This study continues to accrue patients.

4.1.4. 5-D ORAL STUDIES

Three separate studies were performed at Newcastle upon Tyne, U.K. with oral preparations of nolatrexed which were administered every 6 h for 5 d. The oral preparation was designed in order to improve patient acceptability and compliance and eliminate the problems that may be associated with an indwelling central venous catheter. Preliminary results have been published in abstract form.

4.1.4.1. Bioavailability Study. Twenty-five patients were entered on this study that investigated the bioavailability and the pharmacokinetic and pharmacodynamic properties of oral nolatrexed *(24,25)*. In addition, the dose-limiting toxicity and recommended phase II dose were determined. This was a dose-escalation study that commenced at 288 mg/m²/d. The MTD was 1000 mg/m²/d. Nolatrexed was rapidly absorbed with a median bioavailability of 89% (the majority of patients had a value above 70%). The dose-limiting toxicities were nausea and vomiting, which often precluded repeated courses of nolatrexed despite the use of combinations of standard antiemetics. At the maximum dose, peak plasma concentrations ranged from 9.6–14.4 µg/mL, exceeding the levels associated with preclinical antitumor activity in vitro and in vivo. The recommended phase II dose was 800 mg/m²/d.

4.1.4.2. Food Effect Study. Sixteen patients were studied to determine the effect of a standard meal on the absorption of orally administered nolatrexed *(26)*. On day 1, patients were randomized to receive a dose of drug either after a standard meal or an overnight fast. Day 2 was the opposite of day 1. Patients then received 200 mg/m² nolatrexed every 6 h for 5 d. On the second course of treatment 3 wk later, the order of days 1 and 2 was reversed. Plasma drug levels were measured as before. After a standard meal, the peak concentration of nolatrexed was lower (median 8.3 µg/mL compared with 15.0 µg/mL in the fasted state) and the time taken to reach the peak was longer (median 180 min compared with 45 min). AUC values were similar but the trough concentration (plasma concentration at 6 h after the dose—i.e., when the next oral dose would be scheduled) was higher (median 3.6 compared with 2.1 µg/mL) when the drug was administered after a standard meal. We know from the previous studies that inhibition of TS by nolatrexed is rapidly reversible. The slower absorption after a meal and the higher trough levels maintained may therefore result in a shorter duration of noninhibitory concentrations prior to successive doses.

In order to improve patient tolerability and compliance, higher strength capsules (200 and 50 mg) were formulated and a comparison made between these and the original formulation (80 and 20 mg). The different formulations appear to be bioequivalent.

4.1.4.3. Positron Emission Tomography (PET) Study. This study was undertaken in conjunction with the Hammersmith Hospital, London, U.K. The objectives of this study were to quantify, using PET, nolatrexed-induced changes in injected ^{11}C-thymidine uptake and retention in tumor and normal tissue following oral administration, and to investigate whether these changes can be used as a measure of TS inhibition. In addition, the aim was to determine whether PET images obtained using ^{11}C-thymidine tracer could be used as a means of optimizing dosing and scheduling of nolatrexed. Five patients with colorectal cancer were studied. Paired PET scans were performed, one before treatment and the other on the second day of treatment with oral nolatrexed. Equivalent paired studies were also performed on control subjects. Spectral analysis was used to deconvolve the plasma thymidine input function from the tissue data, yielding the fractional retention of tracer (FRT). In tumors, there was a significant ($p < 0.05$) increase in FRT post nolatrexed treatment compared with controls *(27)*. No significant change was seen in normal tissue regions or in the delivery of the tracer to the tissue. The increase in labeled tracer concentration in tumors relative to normal tissue was consistent with enhancement of the thymidine salvage pathway following TS inhibition.

4.1.5. 10-D ORAL STUDY

A phase I pharmacokinetic and pharmacodynamic study of nolatrexed administered orally every 6 h for 10 d has been performed at Edinburgh, U.K. *(28,29)*. Patient courses were repeated every 3 wk. Seventeen patients have been entered to date on the study at doses ranging from 80 to 576 mg/m^2/d. CTC grade III toxicities have been encountered and included nausea, vomiting, anorexia, fatigue, stomatitis, and liver enzyme abnormalities. Pharmacokinetic analysis revealed a 1-h postdose nolatrexed plasma concentration of 8–11.2 μg/mL and trough concentration (6 h after dose) of 1.6–2.4 μg/mL at a dose of 432 mg/m^2/d. The MTD was 576 mg/m^2/d with nausea and vomiting the dose-limiting toxicities.

4.1.6. 10-D IV STUDY

A phase I study of prolonged continuous iv administration of nolatrexed has been undertaken in Buffalo, New York *(30)*. Initially the drug was given at a dose of 288 mg/m^2/d for 7 d. This dose was then extended to 10-d duration. Preliminary results have been reported and dose-limiting toxicities were encountered at 720 mg/m^2/d for 10 d. Toxicities at doses up to 576 mg/m^2/d for 10 d had been mild with a maximum of grade II. Of interest, patients on this study were tolerating larger total doses per course than those on the 5-d continuous infusion.

4.2. Phase II Studies

Phase II studies have been undertaken in the following tumor types: advanced or metastatic head and neck cancer, non-small cell lung cancer, pancreatic cancer, prostate cancer, colorectal cancer, and hepatocellular carcinoma *(31–33)*. Nolatrexed was given as a continuous 5-d iv infusion at the recommended dose of 800 mg/m^2/d. Courses were repeated every 3 wk and doses were escalated or reduced as necessary in order to achieve grade II toxicity with each course. In order for patients to be evaluable for response, they had to have experienced grade II toxicity and then received at least one subsequent course of treatment. The studies were designed such that 14 patients were initially entered on each, with an expansion up to 25 patients in the event of an objective response. Toxicities experienced were similar to those of the phase I 5-d iv study, namely myelosuppression, mucositis, and skin rashes. In patients with hepatocellular carcinoma, preliminary results revealed one partial response (PR) out of 13 evaluable patients. In addition, two patients had minor responses such that they were able to undergo complete resection of their disease *(34)*. In the head and neck study, of 22 evaluable patients, two achieved a complete response (CR) lasting 12+ and 17+ mo *(35)*. In addition, two patients achieved a PR and two patients a minor response. Of 17 evaluable patients with adenocarcinoma of the colon, one patient achieved a PR and three patients had a decrease in their serum carcinoembryonic antigen (CEA) of 50% or greater *(36)*. Twenty-five patients with adenocarcinoma of the pancreas have been studied *(37)* and one patient had a PR and four patients a minor response. Three patients achieved stable disease for a duration ranging from 4–9 mo.

4.3. Future Studies

Due to the antitumor activity seen in the phase II studies with nolatrexed administered as a 5-d continuous iv infusion, further phase II and III studies in head and neck cancer and hepatoma have been commenced to examine this activity more closely. Also, studies involving nolatrexed in combination with other cytotoxic agents are underway. Because of the excellent bioavailability of the oral preparation of the drug, it may be feasible to develop a slow release preparation that would improve patient tolerability and maintain plasma concentrations above that needed for TS inhibition for longer periods.

5. SUMMARY

Nolatrexed is a novel, non-classical thymidylate synthase inhibitor designed by Agouron Pharmaceuticals using knowledge of the three-dimensional structure of the active site of the enzyme. It has unique properties that distinguish it from the classical antifolate cytotoxic agents. Because of the lack of a glutamate moiety, nolatrexed can diffuse passively into cells and, once there, does not require conversion to polyglutamate forms. Nolatrexed is therefore not susceptible to resistance mechanisms caused by impaired transport and decreased polyglutamation. However, work is currently underway to investigate possible mechanisms of resistance to nolatrexed *(38)*. In vitro studies showed nolatrexed to be a potent inhibitor of human TS with growth inhibitory effects against a variety of human and murine cell lines. Further tests implicated TS as the cytotoxic locus of action of the drug and suggested that prolonged exposure appeared to have the maximal effect. New data suggests that nolatrexed may have potential as a radiosensitizer.

In vivo studies confirmed that the greatest cytotoxic effects were achieved with prolonged administration of the drug. Cures could be achieved with doses that were nontoxic to the animals involved.

In the clinical setting, nolatrexed was first investigated as a continuous 24-h infusion. An increase in plasma dUrd levels during the infusion suggested that TS inhibition was being achieved, but that this was quickly reversed. Plasma concentrations that were cytotoxic in vitro were achieved in patients and the only toxicity of note was a local phlebitis. A further phase I study of a continuous 5-d iv infusion via a central venous catheter was performed. Dose-limiting toxicities were myelosuppression and mucositis and the recommended phase II dose was 800 mg/m^2/d. Saturable elimination of the drug was noted and evidence of antitumor activity was observed. TS inhibition was maintained throughout the infusion period. On the basis of these results, phase II studies were instigated in the U.S. and promising results have been achieved. Nolatrexed looks to have activity in squamous cell carcinoma of the head and neck and hepatocellular carcinoma and further studies in these tumor types are underway. In addition, antitumor effects were observed in colorectal and pancreatic cancer. This activity, and the unique properties of nolatrexed, make it a cytotoxic agent that is worth further evaluation, both as a single agent and in combination with other drugs.

REFERENCES

1. Jackman AL, Calvert AH. Folate-based thymidylate synthase inhibitors as anti-cancer agents. *Ann Oncol* 1995; 6:871–881.
2. Touroutoglou N, Pazdur R. Thymidylate synthase inhibitors. *Clin Cancer Res* 1996; 2:227–243.
3. Rustum YM, Harstrick A, Cao S, Vanhoefer U, Yin M-B, Wilke H, et al. Thymidylate synthase inhibitors in cancer therapy: direct and indirect inhibitors. *J Clin Oncol* 1997; 15:389–400.
4. Vest S, Bork E, Hansen HH: A Phase I evaluation of N^{10}-propargyl-5,8-dideazafolic acid. *Eur J Cancer & Clin Oncol* 1988; 24:201–204.
5. Cantwell BMJ, Macaulay V, Harris AL, Kaye SB, Smith IE, Milsted RA, et al. Phase II study of the antifolate N^{10}-propargyl-5,8-dideazafolic acid (CB3717) in advanced breast cancer. *Eur J Cancer & Clin Oncol* 1988; 24:733–736.

6. Webber SE, Bleckman TM, Attard J, Deal JG, Kathardekar V, Welsh KM, et al. Design of thymidylate synthase inhibitors using protein crystal structures: the synthesis and biological evaluation of a novel class of 5-substituted quinazolinones. *J Med Chem* 1993; 36:733–746.
7. Webber S, Bartlett CA, Boritzki TJ, Hilliard JA, Howland EF, Johnston AL, et al. AG337, a novel lipophilic thymidylate synthase inhibitor: *in vitro* and *in vivo* preclinical studies. *Cancer Chemother Pharmacol* 1996; 37:509–517.
8. Calvete JA, Balmanno K, Taylor GA, Rafi I, Newell DR, Lind MJ, et al. Pre-clinical and clinical studies of prolonged administration of the novel thymidylate synthase inhibitor, AG337. *Proc Am Assoc Cancer Res* 1994; 35:306 (abstract 1821).
9. Kim SH, Kim JH. Enhanced cell killing of cultured human colon carcinoma cells by a novel thymidylate synthase inhibitor and radiation. *Proc Am Assoc Cancer Res* 1996; 37:611 (abstract 4194).
10. Raymond E, Djelloul S, Buquet-Fagot C, Mester J, Gespach C. Synergy between the non-classical thymidylate synthase inhibitor AG337 (Thymitaq) and cisplatin in human colon and ovarian cancer cells. *Anti-Cancer Drugs* 1996; 7:752–757.
11. Van Triest B, Pinedo HM, Van Hensbergen Y, Telleman F, Smid K, Van der Wilt CL, et al. Polyglutamylation as a predictor for sensitivity to new thymidylate synthase (TS) inhibitors. *Proc Am Assoc Cancer Res* 1997; 38:474 (abstract 3172).
12. Van der Wilt CL, Pinedo HM, Kuiper CM, Smid K, Peters GJ. Biochemical basis for the combined antiproliferative effect of AG337 or ZD1694 and 5-Fluorouracil. *Proc Am Assoc Cancer Res* 1995; 36:379 (abstract 2260).
13. Jackman AL, Taylor GA, O'Connor BM, Bishop JA, Moran RG, Calvert AH. Activity of the thymidylate synthase inhibitor 2-desamino-N^{10}-propargyl-5,8-dideazafolic acid and related compounds in murine (L1210) and human (WIL2) systems *in vitro* and in L1210 *in vivo*. *Cancer Res* 1990; 50:5212–5218.
14. Jackman AL, Taylor GA, Gibson W, Kimbell R, Brown M, Calvert AH, et al. ICI D1694, a quinazoline antifolate thymidylate synthase inhibitor that is a potent inhibitor of L1210 tumour cell growth *in vitro* and *in vivo*: a new agent for clinical study. *Cancer Res* 1991; 51:5579–5586.
15. Calvete JA, Balmanno K, Rafi I, Newell DR, Taylor GA, Boddy AV, et al. Pre-clinical and clinical studies of the novel thymidylate synthase inhibitor AG337 given by oral administration. *Proc Am Assoc Cancer Res* 1995; 36:380 (abstract 2262).
16. Khalil DA, Real S, Zamansky I, Kosa M, Minnick S, Shetty BV. Isolation and identification of rat and human urinary metabolites of AG337 (THYMITAQ™), a potent inhibitor of thymidylate synthase. *ISSX Proc* Oct 20-24, 1996; 10:323.
17. Khalil D, Zhang K, Hee B, Shetty B. Novel S-methyl conjugates as human metabolites of AG337 (THYMITAQ™), an inhibitor of thymidylate synthase. *ISSX Proc:* Oct 26–30, 1997.
18. Rafi I, Taylor GA, Calvete JA, Boddy AV, Balmanno K, Bailey N, et al: Clinical pharmacokinetic and pharmacodynamic studies with the non-classical antifolate thymidylate synthase inhibitor 3,4-dihydro-2-amino-6-methyl-4-oxo-5-(4-pyridylthio)-quinazolone dihydrochloride (AG337) given by 24 hour continuous intravenous infusion. *Clin Cancer Res* 1995; 1:1275–1284.
19. Boddy AV, Calvete JA, Rafi I. Non-linear pharmacokinetics in cancer patients of AG337, a rationally-designed thymidylate synthase (TS) inhibitor. *Proc Am Assoc Cancer Res* 1995; 36:236 (abstract 1405).
20. Rafi I, Taylor GA, Calvete JA, Balmanno K, Boddy AV, Bailey N, et al. A Phase I clinical study of the novel antifolate AG337 given by a 5 day continuous infusion. *Proc Am Assoc Cancer Res* 1995; 36:240 (abstract 1433).
21. Rafi I, Boddy AV, Taylor GA, Calvete JA, Griffin M, Calvert AH, et al. Pharmacokinetic (PK) and pharmacodynamic (PD) studies of the non-classical thymidylate synthase inhibitor AG337 given as a 5 day i.v. infusion. *Proc Am Assoc Cancer Res* 1996; 37:177 (abstract 1216).
22. Rafi I, Boddy AV, Taylor GA, Calvete JA, Griffin M, Calvert AH, et al. Pharmacokinctic (PK) and pharmacodynamic (PD) studies of the non-classical thymidylate synthase inhibitor AG337 given as a 5 day i.v. infusion. *9th NCI-EORTC* 86, March 1996; (abstract 294).
23. Estlin E, Newell D, Pinkerton C, Taylor G, Boddy A, Pearson A, et al. Phase I study of Thymitaq (AG337) in paediatric patients with advanced malignancy. *Proc Am Assoc Cancer Res* 1997; 38:222 (abstract 1497).
24. Rafi I, Boddy AV, Taylor GA, Calvete JA, Bailey N, Lind MJ, et al. A Phase I clinical study of the novel antifolate AG337 given by 5 day oral administration. *Proc Am Assoc Cancer Res* 1996; 37:178 (abstract 1218).

25. Rafi I, Boddy AV, Taylor GA, Calvete JA, Bailey N, Lind MJ, et al. A Phase I clinical study of the novel antifolate AG337 given by 5 day oral administration. *9th NCI-EORTC* 86, March 1996 (abstract 293).
26. Hughes AN, Griffin MJ, Rafi I, Calvert AH, Johnston A, Clendeninn NJ, et al. Absorption of the TS inhibitor THYMITAQ™ when administered orally in the fed and fasted states. *Proc Am Assoc Cancer Res* 1997; 38:615 (abstract 4131).
27. Wells P, Gunn RN, Hughes A, Boddy A, Taylor GA, Rafi I, et al. Thymidine salvage as a pharmacodynamic endpoint of thymidylate synthase (TS) inhibition *in vivo*. *Proc Am Assoc Cancer Res* 1997; 38:477 (abstract 3194).
28. Jodrell D, Bowman A, Rye R, Smyth JF, Boddy A, Rafi I, et al. A Phase I pharmacokinetic/pharmacodynamic study of the lipophilic thymidylate synthase inhibitor Thymitaq™ (AG337) administered orally, 6 hourly for 10 days. *Proc Am Assoc Cancer Res* 1996; 37:184 (abstract 1256).
29. Jodrell D, Bowman A, Rye R, Smyth JF, Boddy A, Rafi I, et al. A clinical Phase I pharmacokinetic/pharmacodynamic study of the lipophilic thymidylate synthase inhibitor Thymitaq™ (AG337) administered by 10 day oral administration. *9th NCI-EORTC* 86, March 1996 (abstract 295).
30. Creaven PJ, Pendyala L, Meropol NJ, Wu EY, Clendeninn NJ, et al. Phase I and pharmacokinetic study of 3,4-dihydro-2-amino-6-methyl-4-oxo-5-(4-pyridylthio)-quinazoline dihydrochloride (THYMITAQ™, AG337). *9th NCI-EORTC* 85, March 1996 (abstract 292).
31. Loh KK, Cohn A, Kelly K, Glode LM, Stuart KE, Belani CP, et al. Phase II trials of THYMITAQ™ (AG337) in six solid tumour diseases. *Proc Am Soc Clin Oncol* 1996; 15:183 (abstract 385).
32. Clendeninn NJ, Johnston A. Phase II trials of Thymitaq™ (AG337) in six solid tumour diseases. *9th NCI-EORTC* 86, March 1996 (abstract 296).
33. Clendeninn NJ, Collier MA, Johnston AL, Loh KK, Cohn A, Kelly K, et al. Thymitaq™ (AG337): a novel thymidylate synthase inhibitor with clinical activity in solid tumours. *Proc Am Assoc Cancer Res* 1996; 37:171 (abstract 1176).
34. Stuart KE, Hajdenberg J, Cohn A, Loh KK, Miller W, White C, et al. A Phase II trial of THYMITAQ™ (AG337) in patients with hepatocellular carcinoma. *Proc Am Soc Clin Oncol* 1996; 15:202 (abstract 449).
35. Belani CP, Agarwala S, Johnson J, Cohn A, Bernstein J, Langer C, et al. A phase II trial with Thymitaq™ (AG337) in patients with squamous cell carcinoma of the head and neck. *Proc Am Soc Clin Oncol* 1997; 16:387a (abstract 1381).
36. Belani CP, Lembersky B, Ramanathan R, Cohn A, Loh K, Miller W, et al. A phase II trial of Thymitaq™ (AG337) in patients with adenocarcinoma of the colon. *Proc Am Soc Clin Oncol* 1997; 16:272a (abstract 965).
37. Loh K, Stuart K, Cohn A, White C, Hines J, Miller W, et al. A phase II trial of Thymitaq™ (AG337) in patients with adenocarcinoma of the pancreas. *Proc Am Soc Clin Oncol* 1997; 16:265a (abstract 938).
38. Tong Y, Banerjee D, Bertino JR. Mechanisms of resistance to the thymidylate synthase inhibitor AG337 in human sarcoma HT1080 cells after exposure to ethylmethanesulfonate (EMS). *Proc Am Assoc Cancer Res* 1996; 37:384 (abstract 2621).

11   ZD9331
Preclinical and Clinical Studies

F. Thomas Boyle, Trevor C. Stephens, S.D. Averbuch, and Ann L. Jackman

CONTENTS

INTRODUCTION
RATIONALE FOR DRUG DESIGN—ENZYMOLOGY AND CELLULAR PHARMACOLOGY
ZD9331: CELLULAR PHARMACOLOGY
ZD9331 PHARMACOLOGY, TOXICOLOGY, AND ANTITUMOR ACTIVITY
CLINICAL STUDIES
REFERENCES

1. INTRODUCTION

Thymidylate synthase (TS) has been the target enzyme for intensive antifolate drug development for several years and specific inhibition of TS, and hence DNA synthesis, has been achieved with a range of quinazoline analogs of folic acid, including CB3717 *(1–3)* and its non-nephrotoxic successor, Tomudex™ (ZD1694, raltitrexed) *(4–6)*. The latter compound has recently been introduced in a number of counties for the treatment of advanced colorectal cancer and is reviewed by Hughes et al. and Beale et al. (*see* Chapters 6 and 7). ZD1694 is a polyglutamatable drug that depends on cellular uptake via a carrier-mediated, saturable mechanism (the reduced-folate carrier; RFC) *(7–13)*. ZD1694 polyglutamates are significantly more potent TS inhibitors than the parent drug and retention of high-chain-length forms inside cells results in prolonged inhibition of TS in tumor cells grown in vitro and in vivo. Of more recent interest has been the development of water-soluble acidic, quinazoline-based TS inhibitors that lack FPGS substrate activity but retain high affinity for the RFC. Work from the group of F. Sirotnak *(14)* has provided evidence that compounds with favorable kinetic parameters for the RFC may offer a tumor-selective advantage, at least in murine models. Additionally, our own research demonstrated a clear potency advantage of compounds that use the RFC. Such compounds would be expected to be active against tumors expressing low FPGS

From: *Anticancer Drug Development Guide: Antifolate Drugs in Cancer Therapy*
Edited by: A.L. Jackman © Humana Press Inc., Totowa, NJ

or high folylpolyglutamyl hydrolase (FPGH) activity, both documented mechanisms of resistance in cell lines with acquired resistance to polyglutamatable antifolates *(7–13)*; and give a different, and possibly more controllable, toxicity profile than ZD1694. Whereas examples of antifolates with these biochemical attributes already existed when we started the program, e.g., the water-soluble, nonpolyglutamatable inhibitors of DHFR, none have reached the stage of clinical evaluation *(15–17)*.

In this review we outline the studies that led to the synthesis of several examples of quinazoline compounds with glutamate or dipeptide isosteres with in vitro activity *(18–22)*, and some of the in vivo evaluation of selected compounds that identified ZD9331 for clinical development *(23)*.

2. RATIONALE FOR DRUG DESIGN—ENZYMOLOGY AND CELLULAR PHARMACOLOGY

2.1. Molecular Modeling

A compound not subject to metabolic activation through polyglutamation needs to have high intrinsic potency as a TS inhibitor. For this reason, the quinazoline antifolate ICI 198583 *(24)* (the more soluble, less toxic C2-methyl analog of CB3717) was used as a starting point for synthetic modification. To support the design process, a better understanding of the inhibitor interaction with the TS enzyme was developed through molecular modeling studies based on information available on TS and its complexes with substrate and inhibitor. TS obtained from different species (from bacteria to man) show a remarkable degree of sequence homology at the primary amino acid level. Protein crystal structures had been obtained from *Lactobacillus casei* and two groups obtained structures of the ternary complex of *Escherichia coli* TS with the pyrimidine nucleotides dUMP *(25)* or F-dUMP *(26)* and CB3717. Coordinates for the ternary complex with dUMP, made available to us by R.M. Stroud (University of California, San Francisco), were used as the starting point for our studies and a model was constructed using the known primary sequence for human TS. This provided the medicinal chemistry with several valuable pieces of information for use in the design process. Firstly the benzene ring of the quinazolinone and the pyrimidine ring stack close together with the rings parallel and the two heterocyclic systems held by a series of specific hydrogen bonds to residues in the protein. Secondly it showed that CB3717 for example bound in a partially folded conformation with the PABA ring inclined at an angle of 65° to the quinazolinone and thirdly the α-carboxylic acid of the glutamate is bound through water molecules to Lys-50. A subsequent crystal structure of the ternary complex of *E. coli* TS with a tetraglutamate form of CB3717 *(27)* also showed the first glutamate residue bound in the same mode as the monoglutamate with the carboxylic acids of the subsequent glutamate residues interact electrostatically with lysine and arginine residues on the surface of the enzyme. These interactions were used as the basis of the diglutamate model (Fig. 1A) in which the α carboxyl of the second amino acid (α′) of ZM214888 could interact electrostatically with the Arg 49. A final structure obtained by the Stroud group of the ternary complex with ZD1694 *(28)*, revealed that the geometry about the PABA portion of the molecule has a profound effect on the binding of the glutamate residue. Replacement of PABA by a thiophene ring forces the γ-carboxylic acid to bind

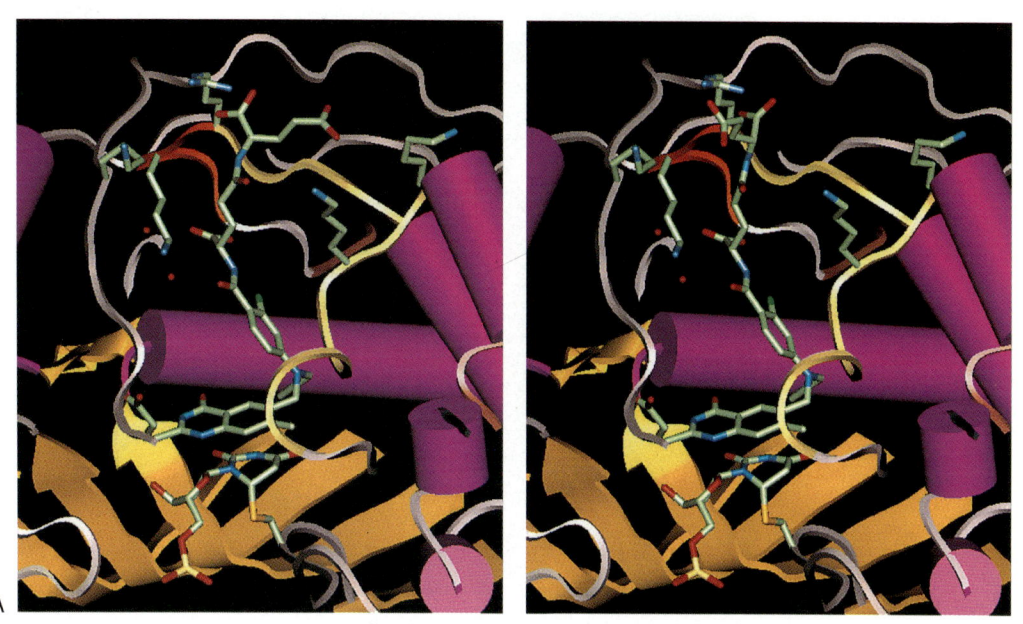

Fig. 1. (A) LL-diglutamate analog of ZM214888 and-dUMP modeled into the ternary complex of "humanized" *E. coli* thymidylate synthase. **(B)** LD-diglutamate analog of ZM214888 and-dUMP modeled into the ternary complex of "humanized" *E. coli* thymidylate synthase.

through waters to Lys-50 and this somewhat less-ordered fit probably accounts for the worse enzyme inhibition of ZD1694 monoglutamate compared with CB3717.

2.2. C7-Substitution and 2′F-Benzoyl Substitutions

These structural studies rationalized much of the activity of the early inhibitors and provided a valuable platform for the next design phase. In the first instance, the effect of substituents in various parts of the molecule to reinforce the overall binding conformation were modeled and substitution at C7 of the quinazoline looked particularly promising. Molecular mechanics (SCANOPT) and semiempirical quantum mechanical energy (AMPAC) calculations indicated that for a molecule with a substituent larger than hydrogen in the 7 position, the preferred lowest energy conformation (Fig. 2) was precisely that for optimum binding to the enzyme *(29)*. A range of C7-substituted molecules were prepared the results are presented in Table 1.

Of these analogs 7-methyl, 7-ethyl, 7-bromo, and 7-chloro derivatives gave enhanced inhibition of TS compared to the 7-H parent, but only the 7-methyl substitution gave equivalent growth inhibition. This was shown to result from the monoglutamate form alone since this compound is not a substrate for FPGS *(30)*. Strongly electron withdrawing groups at C7, exemplified by CN and CF_3 were poorer inhibitors of TS and a corresponding drop in growth inhibitory potency was seen. This probably reflects a disruption of the stacking interaction of the quinazolinone and dUMP in the ternary complex.

In these compounds a 2'-fluoro-substituent was also incorporated since earlier studies *(31)* had shown that this substituent gave a two- to threefold enhancement of TS in-

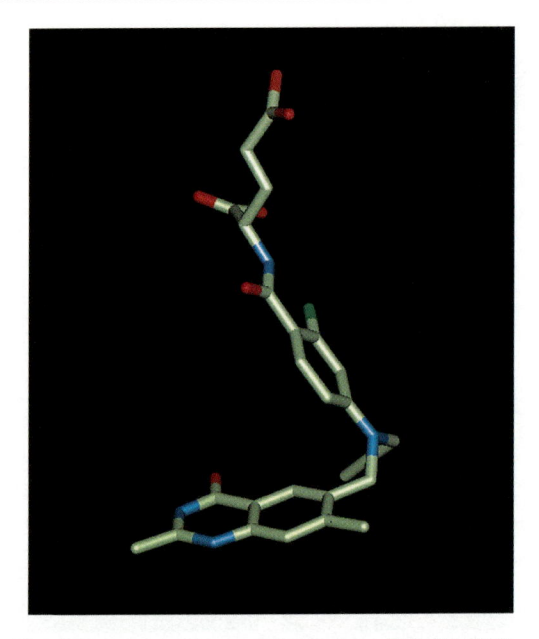

Fig. 2. Lowest energy conformation of ZM214888.

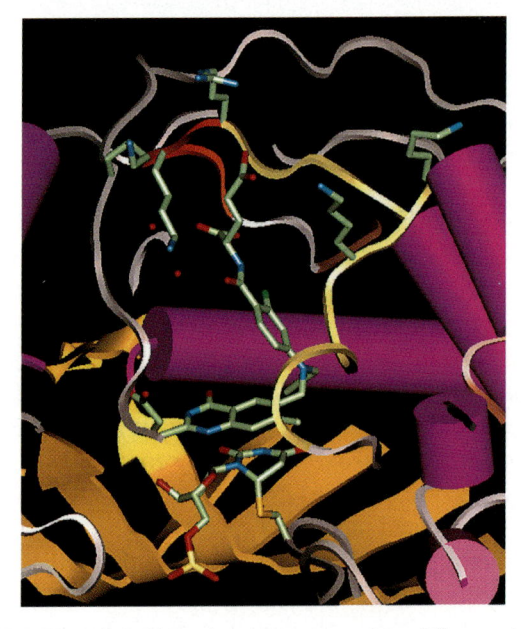

Fig. 3. ZM214888 and-dUMP modeled into the ternary complex of "humanized" *E. coli* thymidylate synthase.

hibition and growth inhibitory potency. Reinforcement of the preferred almost planar conformation in this region of the inhibitor molecule (because of the hydrogen bond between the fluorine and the glutamate NH—seen as a coupling of 7 Hz in the NMR spectrum) leading to enhanced binding through water to the C-terminal fold probably explains these results (Fig. 3). The biological data from the combined effect of 7-methyl

Table 1
Effects of C7 Substitution on TS Inhibition and L1210 Growth Inhibition

R	Inhibition of L1210 TS, IC_{50}, μM^d	Inhibition of Cell Growth, IC_{50}, μM^c		
		L1210	L1210:1565 (RFC−)	L1210:R^{D1694} (polglu−)
H (ICI198583)	0.050 (K_i = 10 nM^a)	0.15	5.8	2.7
Me	0.028 (K_i = 3 nM^a)	0.21	8	0.60
Cl	0.040	1.0		5
Br	0.017	3.0	43	8
Et	0.030	2.8	40	6.3
CF_3	0.12	>20		
CN	0.68	>20		
Me:2'F benzoyl (ZM214888)	0.010 (K_i = 7.8^b)	0.08	8	0.43
Cl:2'F	0.006	0.36	9.5	0.97

Taken from refs. 6, 22, 23.
^{a}Mixed, noncompetitive inhibition pattern.
^{b}Noncompetitive inhibition pattern.
^{c}Results are mean of at least two separate experiments.

and 2'-fluoro substituents, in ZM214888 best illustrates the consequence of this approach, with both enhancement in TS and growth inhibitory potency *(18)*. More recent data suggests that the addition of 2'F may affect the mode of inhibition, which has led to the apparent decrease in TS IC_{50}. This is concluded from the fact that the K_i for the 7-CH3,2'F compound is actually twofold higher than that of the 2'H counterpart. However, because the 2'H and 2'F compounds are mixed noncompetitive and noncompetitive respectively, the IC_{50} value (estimated at 200 μM R,S-5,10-CH_2FH_4) is misleading. The reason for the change in inhibition pattern is unclear, but may relate to unequal binding of inhibitor and substrate to the two binding sites in the dimeric enzyme *(25,26)*. Again data suggests that the cytotoxicity is entirely caused by the parent monoglutamate. The 7Cl-2'F analog shows a similar result *(22)*.

2.3. Diglutamate Mimics: Glutamate Homologs, Dipeptide Analogs and γ-Acid Mimics

Biological data obtained from the diglutamate of CB3717 and ZD1694 showed an increased potency of up to 30-fold over the monoglutamate for TS inhibition and was rationalized to be a consequence of the α' carboxyl binding to Arg 49. Applying this logic to ICI 198585 resulted in the L-Glu-γ-L-Glu—a compound some 25 times more active than the parent monoglutamate as a TS inhibitor *(32)*. Of particular importance, however, was the observation that the metabolically stabilized (to hydrolases) L-Glu-γ-D-Glu analog also showed similar enhanced enzyme activity (Table 2). The 7-methyl, 2'F analog as expected also showed the increased enzyme inhibition. Molecular modeling (Fig. 1B) suggested a common binding mode and that improved inhibitors could be made through extension of the glutamate moiety into this dipeptide-binding region.

Medicinal chemistry therefore focused on glutamate homologs (aminoadipate, pimelate, and suberate) and γ-acid mimics. Important members of these included L-glu-γ-D-amino acids (TS IC_{50} approx 1 nM), acyl sulphonamides (TS IC_{50}s 2–4 nM) and a range of sulphur-linked heterocycles of varied oxidation level and chain length (TS IC_{50} approx 2.0 nM) but the γ-tetrazole ZD9331 (Fig. 4 [2S]-2-{o-fluoro-p-[N-(2,7-dimethyl-4-oxo-3,4-dihydroquinazolin-6-ylmethyl)-N-(prop-2-ynyl)amino]benzamido}-4-(tetrazol-5-yl) butyric acid was surprisingly shown to be a potent enzyme inhibitor (L1210 TS IC_{50} approx 1 nM; K_i = 0.44 nM against isolated TS enzyme) with the highest potency against tumor cell lines *(23,33,34)*.

3. ZD9331: CELLULAR PHARMACOLOGY

3.1. Enzymology

The dissociation constants of ZD9331 for TS (mouse and/or human) are displayed in Table 3. The improvement in TS inhibition of ZD9331 over, for example, the equivalent glutamate analog (ZM214888) is believed to be caused by the interaction of the γ-tetrazole with Arg 49 within the active site. Thus ZD9331 has K_i values of approx 0.44 and 0.38 nM for isolated mouse L1210 and human W1L2 TS respectively. The mechanism of inhibition, with respect to 5,10-CH_2FH_4, is mixed noncompetitive for L1210 TS (K_{ies} approx two- to threefold higher than K_i) but noncompetitive for human TS (K_i approx K_{ies}). The K_i for ZD9331 is approx 150- and twofold lower than that of ZD1694 or its tetraglutamate metabolite, respectively.

3.2. Cell Membrane Transport

ZD9331 displayed K_is for the inhibition of ^{3}H MTX transport in the range 0.7–1.5 μM for L1210, W1L2, and CEM cells and has a K_i value that was approx twofold lower than that of ZD1694, suggesting that the RFC is likely to be an important transport route for ZD9331. This was confirmed in a cell line with a mutant RFC that was highly cross-resistant to ZD9331 (Table 4; *23*).

3.3. Cytotoxicity: Mouse and Human Cells

ZD9331 is a potent inhibitor of L1210 (mouse leukemia) and W1L2 (human lymphoblastoid) cell growth (Table 4). This pattern of cross-resistance was shared with ZD1694, but not with the nonclassical, lipophilic compound, AG337 designed by Agouron Pharmaceuticals to have activity independent of carrier-mediated transport or FPGS *(35,36)*. These comparative data clearly demonstrate that ZD9331 displays potent activity in wild-type cells, comparable with that of ZD1694, however, in contrast with ZD1694, it also has the potential to overcome antifolate resistance because of inappropriate expression of enzymes involved in folate polyglutamate homeostasis. This is il-

Table 2
Effects of Dipeptide and Glutamic γ-Acid Mimics on TS Inhibition and L1210 Growth Inhibition

R	X	Z	Inhibition of L1210 TS, IC_{50}, μM	Inhibition of Cell Growth, IC_{50}, μM[a]		
				L1210	L1210:1565 (RFC−)	L1210:R^{D1694} (polglu−)
H	H−	L-Glu——L-Glu	0.002	0.16	4.8	2.8
H	H	L-Glu——D-Glu	0.0046	0.33	16	0.68
CH_3	F	L-Glu——D-Glu	0.0009	0.2	7.8	0.4
CH_3	F	Aminoadipate	0.0032	0.25	2	0.6
CH_3	F	$(CH_2)_2$ $CONHSO_2CH_3$	0.0044	0.19	?	
CH_3	F	$(CH_2)_2$-Tetrazole (ZD9331)	0.001 $K_i = 0.0004$	0.024	1.4	0.08

Taken from refs. 22, 23.
[a] Results are mean of at least two separate experiments.

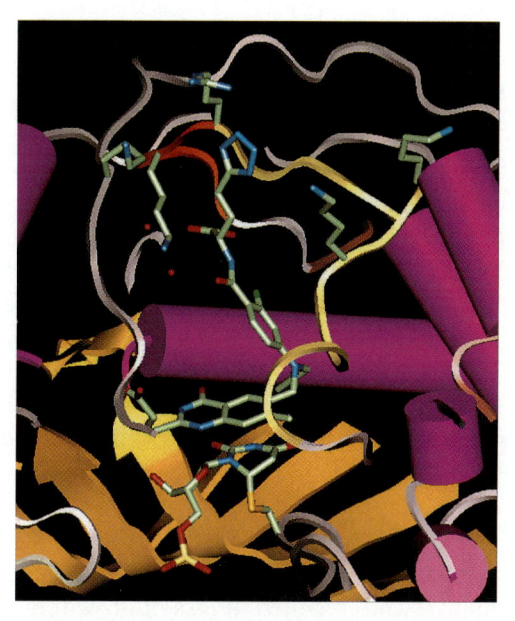

Fig. 4. ZD9331 and-dUMP modeled into the ternary complex of "humanized" *E. coli* thymidylate synthase.

Table 3
Inhibition of Partially Purified Mouse (L1210)
and Human (W1L2) TS by Quinazoline Analogs

	^aK_i, nM		$^aK_{ies}$, nM	
	L1210	W1L2	L1210	W1L2
ZM214888	7.5		K_{ies} approx K_i	
ZD9331	0.44	0.38	0.93	K_{ies} approx K_i
ZD1694	62		960	
ZD1694 glu$_4$	1.0		15	

^{a}Data taken from ref. 23.

Table 4
Inhibition of Cell Growth by ZD9331 and Other Quinazoline Analogs

	Inhibition of cell growth, IC_{50} (μM)^a						
	L1210	L1210:R7A (DHFR+++)	L1210:R^{D1694} (polyglu−)	L1210:1565 (RFC−)	W1L2	W1L2:C1 (TS+++)	W1L2 + dThd
ZM214888	0.08	0.19 (2)	0.43 (5)	7.8 (97)	0.07	>100 (>1400)	>50
ZD9331	0.024	0.08 (3)	0.076 (3)	1.4 (54)	0.0073	18 (2300)	>100
ZD1694	0.0088	0.028 (3)	>100 (>11,000)	0.76 (86)	0.0046	~100 (approx 22,000)	56
AG337	0.70	0.71 (1)	1.3 (2)	1.4 (2)	0.78	26, 24 (32)	>50

^{a}Cells were incubated with the compounds continuously for 2 or 3 d and then counted using a Coulter counter. Results are the mean of several experiments.
Numbers in parentheses are the ratios of the IC_{50} for the resistant over the parental cell lines.

lustrated by the use of the L1210 subline (L1210:R^{D1694}) which is unable to form antifolate polyglutamates (in part because of low FPGS activity). These cells, were >11,000-fold resistant to ZD1694, but were only threefold resistant to ZD9331 (Table 4). A minor transport defect (RFC) in this line (11) is thought to explain the low level of cross-resistance seen. The TS over-producing W1L2:C1 cell line was highly cross-resistant to ZD9331 as expected from a pure TS inhibitor. In contrast, and in further support of a non-DHFR locus of action, the DHFR overproducing, MTX-resistant L1210:R7A line was sensitive to ZD9331 (Table 4). Recently, it has been shown that ZD9331 may overcome intrinsic resistance to ZD1694 in a number of ovarian cell lines with low FPGS mRNA expression (37).

3.4. End-Product Reversal Studies

Consistent with TS being the locus of action of ZD9331, coincubation of drug-treated W1L2 cells with thymidine (dThd) resulted in loss of growth inhibitory activity (Table 4). Coincubation of L1210 cells with folinic acid (5 μM) under continuous exposure conditions has little effect on the growth inhibitory activity of ZD9331. At high doses

(25 μM) a threefold increase in the IC_{50} value was observed that contrasted with 5600-fold for ZD1694. A similar result was observed in human W1L2 cells. Folinic acid has been shown to markedly inhibits ZD1694 polyglutamate formation (6) and is believed to account for the large reduction in growth inhibitory activity seen in such experiments.

3.5. Cellular Pharmacodynamics

3.5.1. In Situ TS Assay

L1210 cells were incubated with equitoxic concentrations of ZD9331 and ZD1694 (0.25 and 0.1 μM, respectively) for 4 h before the addition of 5-^{3}H-deoxyuridine. The very low rate of ^{3}H release compared with controls indicated TS inhibition. However, when cells were resuspended in drug-free medium for 4 or 24 h after incubation with ZD9331 and ZD1694, only ZD1694-treated cells had TS activity below control levels at the end of the experiment and is consistent with the fact that ZD9331 is not retained in cells. Even when the initial drug incubation period with ZD9331 was extended to 24 h, cellular TS activity recovered after 4 h in drug-free medium. These data demonstrate the reversibility of TS inhibition once extracellular drug is removed and are in contrast with results obtained for ZD1694. As expected from these data, ZD9331 has low activity in short-exposure growth inhibition assays (e.g., 4 h) compared with ZD1694 (23).

3.4.2. TTP and dUMP Pools

Human W1L2 lymphoblastoid cells treated with various concentrations of ZD9331 (8–800 nM) for 4 h showed a dose-dependent increase in the dUMP/TTP ratio (23–250) which returned to control levels (0.1) after cells were incubated in drug-free medium for 4 h. In contrast, cells treated with ZD1694 (5–500 nM) had elevated ratios under these conditions (38). These data are consistent with the lack of FPGS substrate activity for ZD9331.

3.4.3. Clonogenic Assay

The low activity of ZD9331 in short-exposure assays was confirmed in a L5178Y $TK^{-/-}$ clonogenic assay in which a 4 h exposure to 10 μM ZD9331 only inhibited colony formation by approx 80% and compares with the same concentration of ZD1694 inhibiting by 99.99% (39). However, a 24-h exposure to 0.1 and 1 μM ZD9331 gave a very high level of inhibition of colony formation (Fig. 5).

4. ZD9331 PHARMACOLOGY, TOXICOLOGY, AND ANTITUMOR ACTIVITY

4.1. Mouse Tumor Models

High circulating levels of thymidine in mice have required the development of thymidine kinase deficient ($TK^{-/-}$) cell lines as model systems for the in vivo assessment of TS inhibitors (39). In a series of experiments in DBA2 mice using a dThd salvage incompetent L5178Y $TK^{-/-}$ mouse lymphoma ZD9331 was delivered by a 24-h subcutaneous infusion. A dose of 3 mg/kg cured 100% of the tumors and lower doses gave significant antitumor activity (23). Mice did not lose body weight or show other signs of toxicity up to doses of 30 mg/kg. As expected, TS-mediated toxicity was not observed for this schedule because normal tissues are still able to salvage dThd from mouse

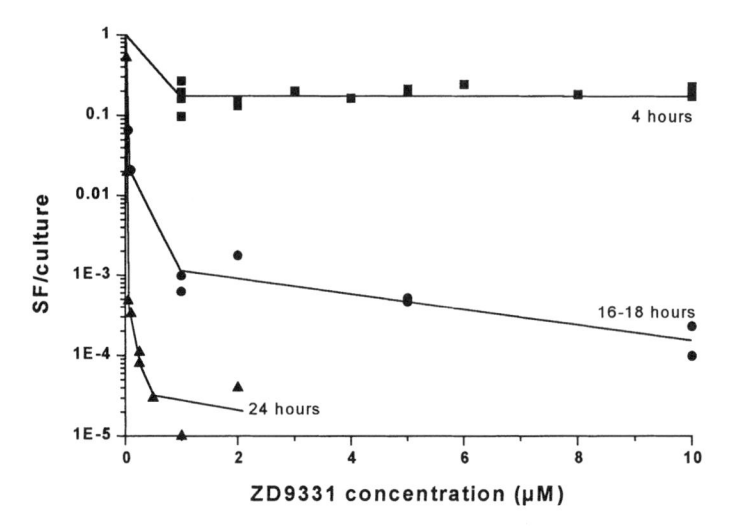

Fig. 5. Dose-response curves for L5178Y TK$^{-/-}$ cells treated in vitro with ZD9331. SF = surviving fraction in colony forming assay.

plasma. Significant L5178Y TK$^{-/-}$ antitumor activity was also seen when ZD9331 was given as a single ip injection—10mg/kg gave approx 60% cures and 25 mg/kg gave 100% cures. In the ip bolus schedule, ZD9331 and ZD1694 have approximately the same potency. This may be explained by a long terminal phase of plasma elimination ($t_{1/2}$ 5–6 h) in mice giving rise to potentially cytotoxic concentrations for at least 20 h *(40)*.

Folate-based TS inhibitors can display activity against the dThd salvage competent L5178Y TK$^{+/-}$ tumor if chronic administration protocols are used. ZD9331 was active in this model when given by continuous 7-d infusion with a mixture of cures and significant growth delays seen at doses between 25 and 75 mg/kg/d, and with 9 of 16 mice cured at 100 mg/kg/d *(23)*.

4.2. Human Tumor Xenografts

ZD9331 was tested for antitumor efficacy against a panel of nine human tumor xenografts (ovarian—HX62; colon—LoVo, Colo205, HT29; SCLC—N592, N417A; gastric—MKN45; NSCLC—A549, HX147) growing sc in nude mice. ZD9331 was administered either sc by infusion over 14 d using Alzet osmotic minipumps or by oral bolus administration using a daily ×15 schedule. Infusional ZD9331 at a dose of 80 mg/kg/d produced 9- to >15-d growth delays in eight of the nine tumors tested (Table 5). The most sensitive tumor was Colo205 and the most unresponsive tumor was A549. In earlier studies, all of these tumors also responded to daily ip treatment with ZD1694, but the doses to produce a growth delay of 15 d varied >100-fold across the tumor panel. The most sensitive tumor HX62 responded at 1 mg/kg/d, whereas the most resistant tumor N417A required >100 mg/kg/d. ZD9331 also demonstrated good activity against Colo205 when administered orally as 15 daily 200 mg/kg bolus doses (18.5- and 36-d growth delay in two separate studies). It was not active against HX62, MKN45, or HX147 by oral administration. These results may be explained by reduced bioavailabil-

Table 5
Response of Human Tumour Xenografts to ZD9331[a]

Tumor	Dose/d (mg/kg)	Median GD (d)	Errors[b] 25%	74%
HX62	25	15.7	12	19
	80	23.1	19.1	30.9
HT29	25	7.8	5.9	18.2
	80	16.9	14.1	23.8
CoLo 205	25	47.4	40.6	56.8
	80	56.2	46.9	69
LoVo	25	8.7	7	10.2
	80	20.5	17.7	25.5
MKN45	25	6.7	3.4	11.8
	80	20.1	17.3	22.1
N417A	25	14.1	9.3	16.2
	80	20.4	17	57.2
N592	25	14.4	6.7	43.6
	80	34.8	14.9	81.5
A549	25	0	0	2.1
	80	2.5	0	6.1
HX147	25	5.1	0	12
	80	9.1	4.7	14.9

[a] Treatment commenced when the tumours reached a diameter of 5–6mm
[b] Errors are 25th and 75th percentiles.

ity when ZD9331 is administered orally compared to parenterally. With the exception of A549, infusional ZD9331 has more uniform activity across a panel of human tumor xenografts than ZD1694 and if this is reflected in humans, ZD9331 could offer the prospect of broad spectrum antitumor activity in the clinic.

4.3. Toxicity

4.3.1. EFFECT OF ZD9331 ON MOUSE BODY WEIGHT AND GASTROINTESTINAL TISSUES

ZD9331, when administered by 7-d sc infusion to non-tumor-bearing DBA2 female mice, caused body weight losses that ranged from approx 5–25% after 25–200 mg/kg/d of ZD9331 with a nadir at 9–10 d. The body weight loss was considerably less in mice treated with 120 mg/kg/d if 500 mg/kg of dThd ip three times a day was given, which indicates that the drug-induced weight loss is related to inhibition of TS. Comparing the weight loss and L5178Y $TK^{+/-}$ active doses of 25–50 mg/kg/d it appears that ZD9331 is very well tolerated. In separate studies ZD1694-induced approx 15% body weight loss in male DBA2 mice at a dose of approx 10 mg/kg once daily for 5 d (nadir days 6–7) (data not shown) which is close to the active antitumor dose of 5–10 mg/kg/d. Therefore, it appears that ZD9331, compared with ZD1694, produces less body weight loss at doses closer to the active antitumor dose.

Intestinal tissues in DBA2 mice were evaluated histologically following sc infusion of ZD9331 for 7 d. ZD1694 was dosed ip twice daily for 5 d as comparator. There was no effect of ZD9331 at the 15 or 30 mg/kg/d dose level. At 60–200 mg/kg/d there were mild to moderate to marked dose-dependent changes to the villi and epithelial surfaces of the small intestine (mild—some changes in shape and nuclei of villi: moderate—some loss, blunting, and fusion of villi and some inflammation of the lamina propria mucosa; marked—extensive loss of villi, marked inflammation of the mucosa, cessation of mitosis), but there was less effect on colon. ZD1694 caused moderate epithelial changes to the small intestine at both 15 and 30 mg/kg/d. These data suggest that the onset of gastrointestinal damage with increasing dose may be more gradual with ZD9331 than with ZD1694. With ZD9331 there were mild effects on intestine at 60 mg/kg/d, which is 4 times the L5178Y TK$^{+/-}$ effective dose (dose to give approx 5-d growth delay) of 15 mg/kg/d by sc infusion, whereas for ZD1694 the effect on intestine was moderate at 15 mg/kg/d, which is only twice the antitumor dose of 6.6 mg/kg/d to give 5-d growth delay. Since body weight loss in mice is often related to the severity of gastrointestinal toxicity, this might explain the apparently higher therapeutic ratio, vs body weight loss, in mice with ZD9331. The high circulating thymidine levels in mice make it difficult to predict the relevance of these differences to man.

4.3.2. EFFECTS OF ZD9331 ON MURINE PERIPHERAL BLOOD ELEMENTS

ZD9331, when infused for 7 d into female DBA2 mice at a dose of 150 mg/kg/d, caused an approx 80% reduction in neutrophils and an approx 90% reduction in platelets at the nadir (8 d after the start of treatment) *(23)*. At the lower dose of 60 mg/kg/d it reduced neutrophils by just 50%, but still reduced platelets by approx 80%.

4.3.3. OTHER EFFECTS IN RODENTS

Plasma ALT (alanine transaminase) and liver histology were examined as indicators of possible hepatic effects of ZD9331. Although transaminemia has been observed with CB3717 and ZD1694 in clinical trials, it was asymptomatic and self-limiting. ZD9331 was administered to DBA2 mice as a 24-h sc infusion, or as single iv or po bolus doses. Plasma ALT levels were measured 4 and 24 h later and tissues samples also taken at these times for histological examination. At infusion doses of ZD9331 up to 1000 mg/kg/d, iv bolus doses up to 250 mg/kg, or po bolus doses up to 1000 mg/kg, ALT remained at control levels and liver histology was normal. For comparison, when CB3717 was infused sc over 24 h at 125–500 mg/kg/d ALT was normal, but at an infused dose of 1000 mg/kg/d and an iv bolus of 100 mg/kg both gave elevated levels of ALT. ZD9331 therefore does not demonstrate signs of acute effects on liver at doses that are substantially higher than the effective daily doses for these dose routes in the various antitumor models studied. The possibility of chronic effects on the liver were also examined. ZD9331 was infused for 7 d at 15–200 mg/kg/d and at the end of the infusion liver histology was normal except for a mild reduction in hepatocyte glycogen in some animals at doses >100 mg/kg/d. Unlike the prototype TS inhibitor CB3717, ZD9331 does not therefore appear to produce damage to the murine liver at doses well above the tumor-inhibitory range.

Plasma urea levels and kidney histology were examined as indicators of possible effects on kidney. Renal toxicity was seen in mice with CB3717, and was dose-limiting in some patients treated with this compound. No nephrotoxic effects have been seen in mice or humans with ZD1694. ZD9331 was administered to DBA2 mice either as an sc infusion over 24 h, or as an iv or po bolus and plasma urea and kidney histology were examined up to 24 h later *(41)*. No changes in plasma urea or kidney histology were observed with sc infusion dosing up to 1000 mg/kg/d, po bolus dosing up to 1000 mg/kg, or iv bolus dosing at 50 mg/kg. However, as the iv bolus dose level was raised from 100–500 mg/kg increasing levels of kidney tubular dilatation were observed, and necrosis was seen at the highest doses. Kidney function was also affected by ZD9331 at higher doses. Glomerular filtration rate (GFR) was assessed in mice by measuring ^{14}C-insulin clearance 4 and 24 h after iv or ip doses of ZD9331. At 50 mg/kg, by either dose route, no significant effects were seen at either assay time. At 150 mg/kg iv there was a minor decrease in GFR at 4 h, but this had recovered by 24 h. However, at 200 mg/kg iv, there was a major decrease in GFR at 4 h and this effect was still apparent at 24 h. The effects with ip dosing were much less. At 200 mg/kg ip there was no effect at 4 h and only a minimal effect was seen at 24 h. By comparison, CB3717, at an iv bolus dose of 100 mg/kg, increased plasma urea levels approx twofold at 4 h, with some tubular dilatation. Dose-dependent increases of kidney tubular dilatation were also observed when CB3717 was infused at 125–1000 mg/kg/d. Infusional ZD9331 does not therefore effect mouse kidney histology or function at doses that are well above the tumor-inhibitory range. The margin of safety is lower when ZD9331 is dosed by iv bolus, however because of the high tolerance of mice to TS inhibitors the doses used in these studies were much higher than are expected in humans.

From these studies it is clear that at tumor-inhibitory doses, ZD9331 does not have the liver- and kidney-damaging effects seen in rodents with CB3717. However as expected ZD9331 is toxic to rapidly proliferating hematological and intestinal tissues, but there is a suggestion that the patterns of effect on these tissues differ from those of ZD1694. These differences may be related to variations in the ability of different normal tissues to polyglutamate ZD1694, a feature not required by ZD9331.

4.3.3. STUDIES IN DOGS

Unlike rodents, dogs are not protected by high levels of circulating thymidine and are therefore much more sensitive to TS inhibitors. Single iv bolus doses of 15, 25, and 35 mg/kg ZD9331 were tolerated by beagles, but 50 mg/kg was not. There were transient reductions in body weight and food consumption at doses of 15, 25, and 35 mg/kg and total white cell count was reversibly reduced. Following 50 mg/kg the effect on body weight was more pronounced and accompanied by inappetance, emesis, and dehydration. Total white cell count was also reduced and there were cytotoxic effects on bone marrow, lymphoid tissue, thymus, and gastrointestinal tract. ZD9331 0.5–2 mg/kg was generally tolerated when administered iv daily for 5 d, but there were dose-dependent effects on proliferating tissues as expected of a cytotoxic agent. Higher dose levels (4, 6, 8 mg/kg/d) were not tolerated on the 5 daily schedule.

Toxic low dose studies performed in dogs using two ZD9331 schedules, 5 daily iv bolus doses and continuous infusion for 5 d revealed doses of 0.06 mg/kg/d and 0.04 mg/kg/d as the lowest doses which produced minimal reversible toxic effects (transient reductions in food consumption and lymphocyte count).

4.4. Preclinical Pharmacokinetics and Metabolism: Rodents and Dogs

Following iv bolus dosages of ZD9331 ranging from 0.06 through 1.5 mg/kg/d in dog, no difference in plasma concentrations between males and females was observed. Plasma concentrations declined in a bi-exponential manner, with an estimated distribution $t_{1/2}$ of approx 0.3 h and a terminal elimination $t_{1/2}$ of approx 5 h, and no accumulation after multiple dosing. After continuous infusion for 5 d at doses ranging from 0.02 to 0.5 mg/kg/d, plateau concentrations were achieved by 12 h into the infusion period. After completion of the infusion, $t_{1/2}$ (approx 5 h) and plasma clearance (approx 3–4 mL/min/kg) of ZD9331 were similar to those obtained with daily iv bolus dosing. Exposure to ZD9331 was dose proportional over the dose ranges studied by both routes.

Following iv bolus dosages of ZD9331 of 10, 25, and 100 mg/kg/d in rat, plasma concentrations were approx 30% higher in males than in females. In both sexes, plasma concentrations declined in a bi-exponential manner, with a distribution half-life (dist $t_{1/2}$) of approx 0.2 h. There was evidence of enterohepatic recirculation with increased concentrations at 12–24 h after dosing. An estimate of plasma clearance after a single dose of 10 mg/kg was consistent with a comparatively short elimination $t_{1/2}$. This was further confirmed by the absence of accumulation after multiple dosing. Exposure to ZD9331 was also dose proportional over the dose range studied in rats.

ZD9331 was eliminated mainly via the feces in both dog and rat, indicating that the major route of excretion is via biliary excretion. The majority of the administered dose was excreted as unchanged parent compound. Metabolism accounted for less than 20% of the administered dose for each species. There was no evidence of enzyme induction or of metabolism by liver hepatocytes.

ZD9331 is highly protein bound in all species. There was a 13% difference in the amount bound between human (98%) and dog (85%), giving sixfold difference in free circulating ZD9331.

5. CLINICAL STUDIES

5.1. Phase I

Based on the demonstration of marked schedule dependency, whereby prolonged exposure of ZD9331 was required for optimal TS inhibition *in situ* and antitumor activity in vivo and based on the relatively rapid clearance in dogs, two dosing schedules over 5 d were selected for initial phase I testing.

The first study, performed at the University of Chicago *(42)*, employed a 30-minute iv infusion of ZD9331 daily for 5 d, repeated every 3 wk. Doses were increased according to a two-stage escalation schema and were guided by assessment of toxicity and by pharmacokinetic data. Based on one-third of the dog low toxic dose, the initial dose was 0.4 mg/m^2/d ×5. In this ongoing study, 39 patients have been enrolled at doses up to 7.5 mg/m^2/d ×5. ZD9331 was well tolerated in these patients after multiple cycles and there was no evidence for cumulative toxicity. Similar to that observed after administration of ZD1694, ZD9331 was associated with a transient, asymptomatic elevation of serum liver transaminases that was unrelated to dose. Although the MTD had not been achieved, dose-limiting neutropenia and thrombocytopenia was observed in several patients receiving the highest doses to date. This myelosuppression generally was manifest after 10 d and was manageable and short-lived, often recovering within 1 wk. There were no significant clinical sequelae as a result of the myelosuppression and repeated cycle dose delays were rare. There were no other significant toxicities observed, including mucositis, diarrhea, or fatigue.

The second study, performed at the Institute of Cancer Research in Sutton (43), employed a 5-d continuous iv infusion, repeated every 3 wk. Doses were increased according to a two-stage escalation schema and were guided by assessment of toxicity and by pharmacokinetic data. Based on one-third of the dog low toxic dose, the initial dose was 0.125 mg/m^2/d ×5. In this ongoing study, 30 patients have been enrolled at doses up to 3.1 mg/m^2/d ×5. As with the daily 30-min infusion schedule, ZD9331 was well tolerated in these patients after multiple cycles, and there was no evidence for cumulative toxicity. Elevated transaminases were again observed as was mild myelosuppression. No patients had experienced dose-limiting toxicity up to the current dose studied.

Preliminary pharmacokinetic data obtained from 49 subjects in these phase I trials showed that the AUC and C_{max} were linear with dose and the $t_{1/2}$ and volume of distribution (approx 25 L) were independent of dose. The clearance was slow (approx 5 mL/min) and the elimination $t_{1/2}$ was long (approx 4 d with a range of 1.5 to 7.5 d). This has resulted in a 1.7- to 3.7-fold accumulation following daily 30-min iv infusions and steady-state plasma concentrations of ZD9331 were not achieved following 5 d of ZD9331 infusion.

In both phase I trials, objective responses have not been observed to date. However, evidence for antitumor activity was noted in one patient with rectal carcinoma who received 12 cycles and two patients with breast cancer who received up to six cycles of ZD9331, respectively.

5.2. Future Studies

The preliminary data from the initial phase I trials suggest that dose-limiting toxicity will be myelosuppression and that patients with advanced malignancy can readily tolerate repeated 3-wk cycles of 5-d dosing of ZD9331 by intermittent bolus infusion or continuous infusion. Surprisingly, the human pharmacokinetic data demonstrating low clearance and an elimination $t_{1/2}$ of approx 4 d were quite different from that predicted from dog and rodent pharmacokinetic studies. Because of the relatively long elimination $t_{1/2}$ in humans, it is unlikely that daily dosing over 5 d will be necessary. Thus, two additional schedules of a 30-min iv infusion once every 3 wk and a 30-min iv infusion on days 1 and 8 every 3 wk have been selected and are being studied in two ongoing phase I trials in San Antonio, London, and Newcastle, respectively. In addition, as ZD9331 demonstrated oral bioavailability in preclinical studies, oral ZD9331 phase I clinical trials have been initiated in Rotterdam. Once the toxicity profile and the MTD have been established from the phase I trials, phase II trials to determine the activity of ZD9331 against a broad range of tumors are planned.

REFERENCES

1. Jackman AL, Calvert AH. Folate-based thymidylate synthase inhibitors as anticancer drugs. *Ann Oncol.* 1995; 6:871–881.
2. Jones TR, Calvert AH, Jackman AL, Brown SJ, Jones M, Harrap KR. A potent antitumour quinazoline inhibitor of thymidylate synthetase: synthesis, biological properties and therapeutic results in mice. *Eur J Cancer* 1981; 17:11–19.
3. Jackson RC, Jackman AL, Calvert AH. Biochemical effects of a quinazoline inhibitor of thymidylate synthetase, CB3717, on human lymphoblastoid cells. *Biochem Pharmacol* 1983; 32:3783–3790.

4. Jackman AL, Judson IR. The new generation of thymidylate synthase inhibitors in clinical study. *Exp Opin Invest Drugs* 1996; 5:719–736.
5. Jackman AL, Farrugia DC, Gibson W, Kimbell R, Harrap KR, Stephens TC, Azab M, Boyle FT. ZD1694 (Tomudex): a new thymidylate synthase inhibitor with activity in colorectal cancer. *Eur J Cancer* 1995; 31A:1277–1282.
6. Jackman AL, Gibson W, Brown M, Kimbell R, Boyle FT. The role of the reduced-folate carrier and metabolism to intracellular polyglutamates for the activity of ICI D1694. *Adv Exptl Med Biol* 1993; 339:265–276.
7. Li WW, Waltham M, Tong W, Schweitzer BI, Bertino JR. Increased activity of γ-glutamyl hydrolase in human sarcoma cell lines: a novel mechanism of intrinsic resistance to methotrexate, in *Chemistry and Biology of Pteridines and Folates, Advances in Experimental Medicine and Biology* vol. 338 (Ayling JE, Nair MG, Baugh CM, eds.) Plenum, New York, 1993, 635–638.
8. Pizzorno G, Mini E, Coronnello M, McGuire JJ, Moroson BA, Cashmore AR, Dreyer RN, Lin JT, Mazzei T, Periti P, Bertino JR. Impaired polyglutamation of methotrexate as a cause of resistance in CCRF-CEM cells after short-term, high-dose treatment with this drug. *Cancer Res* 1988; 48:2149–2155.
9. McCloskey DE, McGuire JJ, Russell CA, Rowan BG, Bertino JR, Pizzorno G, Mini E. Decreased folylpolyglutamate synthetase activity as a mechanism of methotrexate resistance in CCRF-CEM human leukemia sublines. *J Biol Chem* 1991; 266:6181–6187.
10. Pavlovic M, Leffert JJ, Russello O, Bunni MA, Beardsley GP, Priest DG, Pizzorno G. Altered transport of folic acid and antifolates through the carrier-mediated reduced folate transport system in a human leukemia cell line resistant to (6R) 5,10-dideazatetrahydrofolic acid (DDATHF). In: (Ayling JE, Nair MG, Baugh CM, eds.) Chemistry and Biology of Pteridines and Folates, Advances in Experimental Medicine and Biology vol. 338 Plenum, New York, 1993, 775–778.
11. Jackman AL, Kelland LR, Kimbell R, Brown M, Gibson W, Aherne GW, Hardcastle A, Boyle FT, Mechanisms of acquired resistance to the quinazoline thymidylate synthase inhibitor, ZD1694 (Tomudex) in one mouse and three human cell lines. *Br J Cancer* 1995; 71:914–924.
12. Takemura Y, Kobayashi H, Gibson W, Kimbell R, Miyachi H, Jackman AL. The influence of drug-exposure conditions on the development of resistance to methotrexate or ZD1694 in cultured human leukaemia cells. *Int J Cancer.* 1996; 66:29–36.
13. Rhee MS, Wang Y, Nair, MG, Galivan J. Acquisition of resistance to antifolates caused by enhanced γ-glutamyl hydrolase activity. *Cancer Res* 1993; 53:2227–2230.
14. Sirotnak FM, DeGraw JI, Moccio DM, Samuels LL, Goutas L. New folate analogues of the 10-deazaaminopterin series. Basis for structural design and biochemical and pharmacologic properties. *Cancer Chemother Pharmacol* 1984; 12:18–25.
15. Galivan J, Inglese J, McGuire J, Nimec Z, Coward JK, γ-fluoromethotrexate: synthesis and biological activity of a potent inhibitor of dihydrofolate reductase with greatly diminished ability to form poly—glutamate. *Proc Natl Acad Sci USA* 1985; 82:2598–2602.
16. McGuire JJ, Russell CA, Bolanowska WE, Freitag CM, Jones CS, Kalman TI, Biochemical and growth inhibition studies of methotrexate and aminopterin analogues containing a tetrazole ring in place of the g-carboxyl group. *Cancer Res* 1990; 50:1726–1731.
17. Abraham A, Nair MG, McGuire JJ, Galivan J, Kisliuk RL, Vishnuvajjala. Antitumour efficacy of classical non-polyglutamylatable antifolates that inhibit dihydrofolate reductase, in *Chemistry and Biology of Pteridines and Folates, Advances in Experimental Medicine and Biology* vol. 338 (Ayling JE, Nair MG, Baugh CM, eds.) Plenum, New York, 1993, 663–666.
18. Marsham PR, Jackman AL, Barker AJ, Boyle FT, Pegg SJ, Wardleworth JM, Kimbell R, O'Connor BM, Calvert AH, Hughes LR. Quinazoline antifolate thymidylate synthase inhibitors: replacement of glutamic acid in the C2-methyl series. *J Med Chem* 1995; 38:994–1004.
19. Bavetsias V, Jackman AL, Kimbell R, Gibson W, Boyle FT, Bisset GMF. Quinazoline antifolate thymidylate synthase inhibitors: g-linked L-D, D-D and D-L dipeptide analogues of 2-desamino-2-methyl-N[10]-propargyl-5,8-dideazafolic acid (ICI 198583), *J Med Chem* 1995; 39:73–85.
20. Wardleworth JM, Boyle FT, Barker RJ, Hennequin LF, Pegg SJ, Stephens TC, Kimbell R, Brown M, Jackman AL. ZD9331, the design and synthesis of a novel non-polyglutamatable TS inhibitor. *Ann Oncol* 1994; (suppl 5):247.
21. Boyle FT, Wardleworth JM, Hennequin LF, Kimbell R, Marsham PR, Stephens TC, Jackman AL. ZD9331—design of a novel non-polyglutamatable quinazoline-based inhibitor of thymidylate synthase. *Proc Am Assoc Cancer Res* 1994; 35:302.

22. Jackman, AL, Kimbell R, Brown M, Bisset GMF, Bavetsias V, Marsham P, Hughes LR, Boyle FT. Quinazoline-based thymidylate synthase inhibitors: relationship between structural modifications and polyglutamation. *Anti-Cancer Drug Design* 1995; 10:573–589.
23. Jackman, AL, Kimbell R, Aherne GW, Brunton L, Jansen G Stephens TC, Smith MN, Wardleworth JM, Boyle FT. Cellular pharmacology and in vitro activity of a new anticancer agent ZD9331: a water soluble, nonpolyglutamatable quinazoline-based inhibitor of thymidylate synthase. *Clin Cancer Res* 1997; 3:911–921.
24. Hughes, LR, Jackman, AL, Oldfield, J, Smith, RC, K. Burrows, KD, Marsham, P, Bishop, JAM, Jones, TR. O'Connor BM, Calvert AH. Quinazoline antifolate thymidyate synthase inhibitors: alkyl, substituted alkyl and aryl substituents in the C2 position. *J Med Chem* 1990; 33:3060–3078.
25. Montfort WR, Perry KM, Fauman EB, Finer-Moore JS, Maley GF, Hardy L, Maley F, Stroud RM. Structure, multiple site binding and segmented accommodation in thymidylate synthase on binding dUMP and an anti-folate. *Biochemistry* 1990; 29:6964–6976.
26. Matthews DA, Appelt K, Oatley SJ, Xuong NgH. Crystal structure of Escherichia coli thymidylate synthase containing bound 5-fluoro-2'deoxyuridylate and 10-prpoargyl-5,8-dideazafolate. *J Mol Biol* 1990; 214:923–936.
27. Kamb AJ, Finer-Moore J, Calvert AH, Stroud RM. Structural basis for recognition of polyglutamated folates by thymidylate synthase *Biochemistry* 1992; 31:9883–9890.
28. Stroud RM. personal communication.
29. Boyle FT, Matusiak ZS, Hughes LR, Slater AM, Stephens TC, Smith MN, Kimbell R, Jackman AL. Substituted-2-desamino-2-methyl-quinazolinones. A series of novel antitumour agents, in *Chemistry and Biology of Pteridines and Folates, Advances in Experimental Medicine and Biology* vol. 388 (Ayling JE, Nair MG, Baugh CM, eds.) Plenum, New York, 1993; 585–588.
30. Sanghani PC, Jackman AL, Evans VR., Thornton T, Hughes L, Calvert AH, Moran RG, A strategy for the design of membrane-permeable folylpolyglutamate synthetase inhibitors: "bay region" -substituted 2-desamino-2-methyl-5,8-dideazafolate analogues. *Mol Pharmacol* 1994; 45:341–351.
31. Marsham PR. Jackman AL, Oldfield J, Hughes LR, Thornton TJ, Bisset GMF, O'Connor BM, Bishop JAM, Calvert AH. Quinazoline antifolate thymidylate synthase inhibitors: benzoyl ring modifications in the C2-methyl series. *J Med Chem* 1990; 33:3072–3078.
32. Bavetsias V, Jackman AL, Kimbell R, Gibson W, Boyle FT, Bisset GMF. Quinazoline antifolate thymidylate synthase inhibitors: γ-linked L-D, D-D and D-L dipeptide analogues of 2-desamino-2-methyl-N^{10}-propargyl-5,8-dideazofolic acid (ICI 198583). *J Med Chem* 1996; 39:73–85.
33. Wardleworth JM, Boyle FT, Barker RJ, Hennequin LF, Pegg SJ, Stephens TC, Kimbell R, Brown M, Jackman AL. ZD9331, the design and synthesis of a novel non-polyglutamatable TS inhibitor. *Ann Oncol* 1994; 5 (suppl 5):247.
34. Boyle FT, Wardleworth JM, Hennequin LF, Kimbell R, Marsham PR, Stephens TC, Jackman AL. ZD9331—design of a novel non-polyglutamatable quinazoline-based inhibitor of thymidylate synthase. *Proc Am Assoc Cancer Res* 1994; 35:302.
35. Webber SE, Bleckman TM, Attard J, Deal JD, Kalhardekar V, Welsh KM, et al. Design of thymidylate synthase inhibitors using protein crystal structures: the synthesis and biological evaluation of a novel class of 5-substituted quinazolinones. *J Med Chem* 1993; 36:733–746.
36. Webber S, Bartlett CA, Boritzki TJ, Hilliard JA, Howland EF, Johnston AL, Kosa M, Margosiak SA, Morse CA, Shetty BV. AG337, a novel lipophilic thymidylate synthase inhibitor: in vitro and in vivo preclinical studies. *Clin Chemother Pharmacol* 1996; 37:509–517.
37. Jackman AL, Melin C, Brunton L, Kimbell R, Aherne W, Walton M. Some determinants of response to folate-based thymidylate synthase inhibitors in human colon and ovarian tumour cell lines. *Proc Am Assoc Cancer Res.* 1998; 39:434.
38. Aherne W, Hardcastle A, Kelland L, Jackman AL. The measurement of deoxyuridine (dNTP) pools by radioimmunoassay. *Adv Exp Med Biol* 1995; 370:801–804.
39. Stephens TC, Smith MN, Waterman SE, McCloskey ML, Jackman AL, Boyle FT. Use of murine L5178Y lymphoma thymidine kinase mutants for *in vitro* and *in vivo* antitumour efficacy evaluation of novel thymidine synthase inhibitors. *Adv Exp Med Bio* 1993; 338:589–592.
40. Aherne GW, Ward E, Dobinson D, Hardcastle A, Jackman AL. Pharmacokinetics of abolus injection of ZD9331, a non-polyglutamated thymidylate synthase inhibitor. *Proc Am Assoc Cancer Res* 1996; 37:382.

41. Walton MI, Aherne GW, Hardcastle A, Mitchell F, Dobinson D, Boyle FT, Jackman AL. Effects of dose and route of administration of the novel, non-polyglutamatable thymidylate synthase inhibitor ZD9331 on the renal function in mice. *Br J Cancer,* in press.
42. Ratain MJ, Cooper N, Smith R, Vogelzang NJ, Mani S, Shulman K, Lowe PG, Averbuch SD. Phase I study of ZD9331: a novel thymidylate synthase (TS) inhibitor *Proc ASCO* 1997; 16:A729.
43. Rees C, Judson I, Beale P, Mitchell F, Smith R, Mayne K, Averbuch S, Jackman A. Phase I trial of ZD9331, a non-polyglutamatable thymidylate synthase (TS) inhibitor given as a five day continuous infusion. *Proc ASCO* 1997; 16:A730.

12 Preclinical and Clinical Evaluation of the Glycinamide Ribonucleotide Formyltransferase Inhibitors Lometrexol and LY309887

Laurane G. Mendelsohn, John F. Worzalla and Jackie M. Walling

CONTENTS

INTRODUCTION
INHIBITION OF GARFT AND POLYGLUTAMATION BY
  FOLYLPOLYGLUTAMATE SYNTHETASE
FOLATE-RECEPTOR SELECTIVITY OF ANTIFOLATES
CELLULAR PHARMACOLOGY
IN VIVO ANTITUMOR ACTIVITY OF LY309887
THERAPEUTIC INDEX DETERMINATIONS
THE EFFECT OF DIETARY FOLATE ON DISPOSITION OF LOMETREXOL
  AND LY309887 IN LIVER
THE EFFECT OF LFD AND DIETARY FOLATE SUPPLEMENTATION ON
  THE EFFICACY AND TOXICITY OF LOMETREXOL AND LY309887
HUMAN FOLATE STATUS
CLINICAL EVALUATION OF LOMETREXOL AND LY309887
PHASE I STUDIES WITHOUT FOLIC ACID SUPPLEMENTATION
PHASE I STUDIES WITH FOLIC ACID SUPPLEMENTATION
PHASE I STUDY OF LOMETREXOL WITH FOLINIC ACID
HOW DOES FOLIC ACID MODULATE TOXICITY?
ANTITUMOR ACTIVITY IN PHASE I
PHARMACOKINETICS
CLINICAL DEVELOPMENT OF LY309887
CONCLUSION
REFERENCES

From: *Anticancer Drug Development Guide: Antifolate Drugs in Cancer Therapy*
Edited by: A.L. Jackman © Humana Press Inc., Totowa, NJ

1. INTRODUCTION

The importance of the purine *de novo* pathway in providing DNA precursors for cancer cell growth led to the hypothesis that novel antifolate inhibitors of glycinamide ribonucleotide formyltransferase (GARFT), the first folate-dependent enzyme in this pathway, might have utility in the treatment of cancer. In 1987, clinical investigations were initiated with lometrexol (6R-dideazatetrahydrofolic acid, 6R-DDATHF), a novel "tight-binding" inhibitor of GARFT with potent antitumor activity in a number of murine and human xenograft solid tumors. Unexpected observations of delayed cumulative toxicity in phase I clinical trials prompted extensive preclinical investigations of the dynamics of folate status on the efficacy and toxicity of GARFT inhibitors and other antifolates (1). In addition, structure-activity studies have led to the identification of a second generation GARFT inhibitor, LY309887 (2′,5′-thienyl-dideazatetrahydrofolic acid), which is more potent than lometrexol and has greater antitumor efficacy in vivo (2). Biochemical and pharmacological differences between LY309887 and lometrexol with respect to potency to inhibit GARFT, differential transport and storage in liver, and polyglutamation suggest that LY309887 may have greater antitumor efficacy and more manageable toxicity in the clinic than lometrexol. A murine model of the delayed cumulative toxicity seen with lometrexol has been refined and characterized to provide greater understanding of the pharmacokinetics and pharmacodynamics of these events. In concert with recently published nutritional data on the folate status of humans and more sophisticated methods of assessing and modulating antifolate toxicities through vitamin supplementation, antifolate therapy may be poised to enter a new phase of clinical success. In this report, we describe LY309887, a GARFT inhibitor with unique biochemical and pharmacological properties that has antitumor activity against a broad panel of human xenograft tumors, and greater potency than lometrexol both as an inhibitor of GARFT and as an inhibitor of tumor growth in vivo. An overview of the phase I clinical results with lometrexol and the design of the phase I clinical trial with LY309887 will be presented.

2. INHIBITION OF GARFT AND POLYGLUTAMATION BY FOLYLPOLYGLUTAMATE SYNTHETASE

The natural forms of folic acid and "classical" inhibitors of folate-dependent enzymes are polyglutamated intracellularly by the enzyme folylpolyglutamate synthetase. Polyglutamylation enhances both intracellular retention and affinity of folates and antifolates for many of the folate-utilizing enzymes (3). Table 1 summarizes the inhibition of GARFT by lometrexol, compound LY254155 (6R,S-2′,5′-thienyl-DDATHF, a diastereoisomeric mix of LY309887 and LY309886, respectively) and their polyglutamates. Monoglutamated LY254155 was approx 30-fold more potent than lometrexol. Polyglutamation enhanced inhibition by both compounds: lometrexol-triglutamate (LY235337) was approx 4.5-fold more potent than parent compound; a 10-fold increase in inhibition was seen with the triglutamated thiophene (LY314209). These data demonstrate that the thiophene was inherently more potent as a GARFT inhibitor and that in the polyglutamated state it achieved picomolar affinity for GARFT.

The kinetic constants (K_m, V_{max}, and first-order rate constant [V_{max}/K_m]) for activa-

Table 1
Inhibition of hGARFT by Lometrexol, 254155, and Polyglutamates

Compound No.	Compound Name	hGARFT K_i (nM)
LY249543	lometrexol	59.7 ($n = 2$)
LY235540	diglu	15.4 ($n = 2$)
LY235337	triglu	13.3 ($n = 2$)
LY266978	tetraglu	7.1 ± 2.2 ($n = 4$)
LY235542	pentaglu	5.3 ($n = 2$)
LY254155	thienyl-DDATHF	2.1 ± 0.2 ($n = 5$)
LY314565	diglu	1.2 ($n = 1$)
LY314209	triglu	0.25 ($n = 2$)

The potency of antifolate analogs to inhibit monofunctional human GARFT was assessed spectrophotometrically using the Morrison equation, which is appropriate for determining the affinity of "tight-binding" compounds that produce stoichiometric inhibition (2,4).

Table 2
Kinetic Constants for Activation of GARFT Inhibitors by FPGS

Compound	K_m (μM)	Vmax (μmoles/h/mg)	k' (V_m/K_m)
lometrexol	16.4 ± 1.0	977 ± 128	60
LY309887	6.5 ± 1.1	686 ± 116	43
MTA	1.9 ± 0.5	725 ± 95	381

tion of lometrexol and LY309887, determined using hog liver FPGS are summarized in Table 2 (5). Lometrexol and LY309887 had similar K_m values as FPGS substrates. However, lometrexol had a significantly higher V_{max}. The relative efficiencies of substrate utilization by an enzyme can be determined by comparing first-order rate constants, k' (V_{max}/K_m). The data suggest that despite equal K_m values, lometrexol was a better substrate, which would be more extensively polyglutamated in vivo. For comparison, data obtained with the multitargeted antifolate inhibitor, LY231514 (MTA), is shown. With a first-order rate constant of 381, it clearly had the greatest affinity and efficacy as an FPGS substrate. In other experiments, polyglutamated products formed during a 24-h incubation of lometrexol, LY309887 or MTA with FPGS were separated by quantitative HPLC. At low substrate concentrations, i.e., below the K_m (1 μM), polyglutamation of all substrates was more extensive and a higher percentage of the total product was converted to tetra- and pentaglutamated forms than at high substrate concentrations (20 μM) in which over 70% of each antifolate was present as the triglutamate analog. These observations are consistent with the known substrate inhibition of FPGS that occurs in vivo at high intracellular folate concentrations (6).

An important inference from these data is that folate-deficient patients may accumulate and retain greater amounts of highly polyglutamated "classical antifolates," particularly in liver, a known folate depot, than patients who are folate-replete. Continuous cycling of stored antifolate through the enterohepatic pathway may explain the phenomenon of delayed and cumulative toxicity in cancer patients on lometrexol and in

Table 3
Affinity of Folic Acid and Antifolates for Isoforms of the Folate Receptor

Compound	$K_{i\,(n}M \pm SEM)$		Ratio $K_i\beta/K_i\alpha$
	Human KB cell (FRα)	Human Liver (FRβ)	
folic acid	0.07 ± 0.11	0.23 ± 0.03	3.29
methotrexate	30.0 ± 10.6	108.00 ± 4.4	3.6
lometrexol	0.29 ± 0.05	1.44 ± 0.13	4.97
S-DDATHF	0.20 ± 0.07	0.82 ± 0.01	4.10
raltitrexed	29.1 ± 7.44	285.00 ± 76.9	9.79
LY309887	1.74 ± 0.18	18.2 ± 4.4	10.5
LY309886	1.04 ± 0.31	4.48 ± 0.36	4.31
LY231514	99.7 ± 22.9	482.00 ± 141	4.83
5-CH$_3$-THF(6S)[a]	1.00	55.0	55.0

$K_i\alpha$ values were determined in equilibrium binding assays using ^{125}I-folic acid and membranes prepared from human (KB) nasopharyngeal carcinoma cells or human liver. Values are the mean from three or more determinations.

[a]FRα, KB cell; FRβ, human placenta (9).

lometrexol-treated mice on a low folate diet. Compound LY309887 may have a reduced potential for delayed toxicity in humans because it is less extensively polyglutamated. Furthermore, since it is a more potent GARFT inhibitor than lometrexol and requires less polyglutamation to achieve tight-binding inhibition, lower doses can be administered without compromising potency. Thus, in folate-replete patients having normal liver folate concentrations, accumulation, polyglutamation and retention of LY309887 in liver would be expected to be lower than observed with lometrexol. In vivo experiments to test this hypothesis were carried out in mice and results are summarized in subheading 7 (5,7).

3. FOLATE-RECEPTOR SELECTIVITY OF ANTIFOLATES

Activation of classical antifolates through formation of polyglutamates and consequent deposition in liver may only partially account for the extended bioavailability and risk of delayed cumulative toxicity of classical antifolates. Folate-transport mechanisms, including the reduced folate carrier and folate receptor (FR) isoform-selectivity are important features of antifolates that may also modulate clinical efficacy and toxicity of these compounds. It is noteworthy that FRα is highly overexpressed in many epithelial forms of cancer including ovarian and head and neck cancer (8). Dissociation constants of folic acid and several antifolates for the human FRα and FRβ isoforms are presented in Table 3. The smaller the K_i, the more tightly the compound binds to the FR. Inspection of the ratio of affinities of these antifolates for the isoforms reveals that all of the compounds have a lower affinity for the liver (FRβ) isoform relative to their FRα affinity. Such selectivity may enhance uptake of the natural folates, e.g., 5-CH$_3$-THF into normal tissues or tumors over uptake into liver, particularly at physiological serum folate concentrations (10–40 nM). The affinity of lometrexol for both FR isoforms was very high, and the poor selectivity ratio of 4.97 suggests that lometrexol would readily accumulate in human liver as well as tumors expressing FR. The affinity of LY309887 for the liver receptor was 12.6-fold lower than lometrexol's affinity and the selectivity of LY309887 for the α over the β isoform was 10.5, suggesting that this new compound will not accumulate in liver as much as lometrexol. In addition to transport by FR, both lometrexol and LY309887 are taken up by the reduced folate carrier. This carrier, however, has a high capacity but a low affinity (>micromolar) for reduced folates. In vivo experiments in mice using radiolabeled lometrexol or LY309887 have confirmed these suggestions and these data are presented in Subheading 7.

The clinical significance of these observations is relevant to the risk of delayed, cumulative toxicity. Murine studies have demonstrated that lometrexol is taken up and stored in the liver *(10)*. It is thought that the clinical observations of delayed and cumulative toxicity may result from gradual release of stored lometrexol over time resulting in an extended γ-phase plasma half life *(11)*. The affinity of LY309887 for liver folate receptors suggest that it is less likely to be transported into the liver, and, because it is less efficiently polyglutamated than lometrexol, it should not be retained in the liver as well. The greater potency of LY309887 to inhibit GARFT suggests that lower doses of this compound may be used. Collectively, these properties suggest that LY309887 may have a reduced risk of delayed toxicity in humans.

4. CELLULAR PHARMACOLOGY

LY309887 showed potent in vitro cytotoxicity (IC_{50} of 2.9 n*M*) against CCRF-CEM leukemia cells and was approx fivefold more cytotoxic than lometrexol (IC_{50} of 15.2 n*M*) *(2)*. The cytotoxicity of both compounds was reversed by hypoxanthine, but not by thymidine. The cell cycle effects of LY309887 were evaluated using the human leukemia cell line CCRF-CEM. Exposure of cells to 29 n*M* of this inhibitor for 24–96 h resulted in a slowed progression of cells through S-phase and an increase in the number of S-phase cells *(12)*. Measurement of deoxynucleotide pools demonstrated marked decreases in dATP pools in these cells within 6 h of exposure *(13)*.

5. IN VIVO ANTITUMOR ACTIVITY OF LY309887

The dose-response curves of LY309887 and lometrexol against the murine C3H mammary tumor are shown in Fig. 1. LY309887 demonstrated antitumor activity over a broad dose range in this model with 94% tumor inhibition seen at 1 mg/kg/dose and up to 99% inhibition seen at 100 mg/kg/dose. LY309887 was a more potent antitumor agent especially since lometrexol was dosed more frequently (q2d × 5) compared to LY309887 (dosed q3d × 4). Thus LY309887 showed 99% inhibition of tumor growth from 3 to 100 mg/kg/dose with acceptable toxicity (lethality <20% at all efficacious doses), whereas lometrexol showed 97% inhibition of tumor growth at 400 mg/kg/dose. No lethality was noted at any of the doses of lometrexol including the 400 mg/kg dose, the highest dose tested for lometrexol in this study.

The antitumor activity of LY309887 (or LY254155, the mixture of its "6-R" and "6-S" stereoisomers) and lometrexol (or the mixture of its "6-R" and "6-S" stereoisomers, LY237147) in a number of preclinical models is summarized in Table 4. Maximum inhibition was obtained at doses producing 25% or less lethality. There were no significant differences in the maximum inhibition between the LY254155 isomers and lometrexol

Table 4
Antitumor Activity of GARFT Inhibitors

Tumor	Thiophene[b]		DDATHF[c]	
	6 R diastereomer LY309887	6 R,S diastereomers LY254155	6 R diastereomer LY249543 (lometrexol)	6 R,S diastereomers LY237147
CX-1 colon		64% (40)		73% (100)
GC3 colon	95% (30)	96% (40)	94% (200)	98% (100)
HC1 colon	97% (30)	98% (40)	99% (50)	94% (200)
VRC5 colon	86% (30)	96% (5)		99% (100)
LX-1 lung		98% (10)	81% (100)	
MX-1 mammary	52% (10)	61% (40)		76% (100)
BXPC3 pancreatic		87% (40)		59% (50)
PANC1 pancreatic	92% (30)	85% (40)	67% (300)[b]	

[a]Compound dosed ip at the indicated dose (mg/kg) and schedule; e.g., for the CX-1 colon xenograft, 6R,S-diastereomer was dosed ip q3d × 4 at 40 mg/kg.
[b]Dose schedule: q3d × 4.
[c]Dose schedule: q2d × 5.

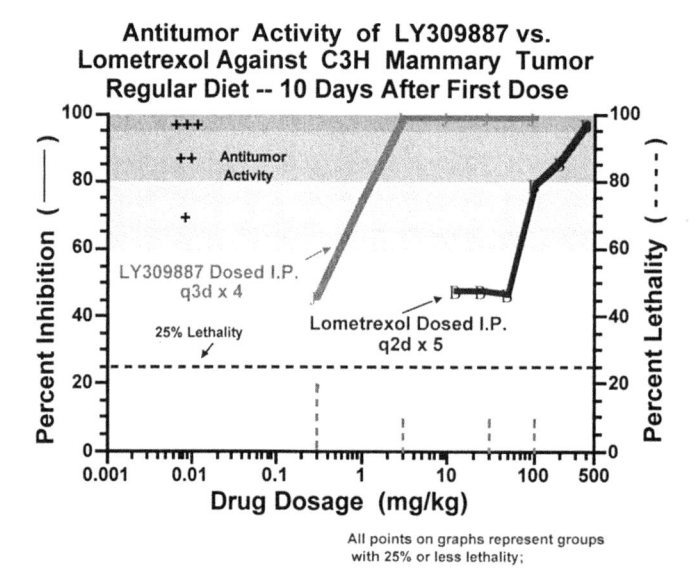

Fig. 1. Antitumor Activity of LY309887 vs. Lometrexol Against C3H Mammary Tumor.

isomers. Against the LX-1 lung, VRC5, HC1, and GC3 colon xenografts, both the LY309887 and lometrexol produced over 80% tumor inhibition. Against the MX-1 mammary and CX-1 colon, both the thiophene isomers and lometrexol produced between 60% and 80% inhibition. In these studies, the thiophene analogs were dosed q3d × 4 while lometrexol was dosed q2d × 5.

The ability of LY254155 to prevent tumor regrowth of the human colon xenograft

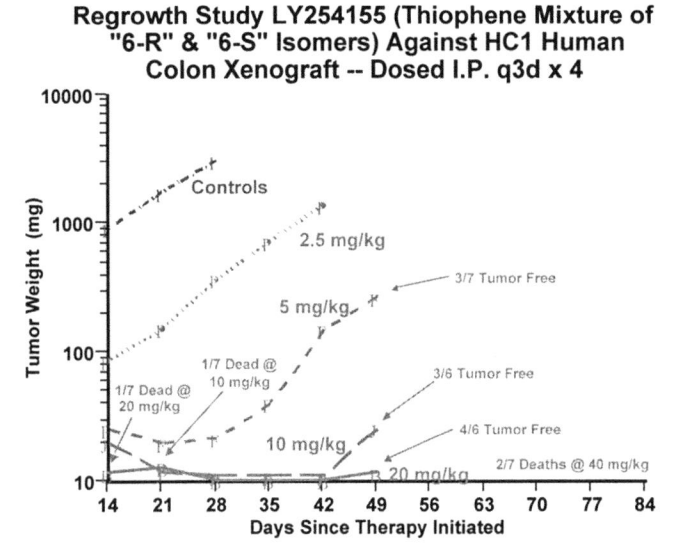

Fig. 2. Regrowth Study LY254155 (Thiophene Mixture of "6-R" & "6-S" Isomers) Against HC1 Human Colon Xenograft.

was investigated (Fig. 2). A single course of LY254155 (mixture of "6-R" and "6-S" isomers of the thiophene) was given starting 14 d after inoculation with the HC1 human colon xenograft. At the lowest doses, tumor growth was slowed; at higher doses tumor regrowth was prevented for at least 42 d. The highest dose of 40 mg/kg in this study was also very effective, but two of the seven mice died (>25% lethality), and thus this data was not included. At the 10 mg/kg dose, three of six mice were tumor free, and at the 20 mg/kg dose, four of six mice were tumor free 39 d after completion of a single course of therapy.

Similar results were obtained using GC3 xenograft tumors. Thus for two colon xenograft models, the LY254155 prevented growth of tumor for periods of 4–7 wk, and in one of these tumor models, the HC1 colon tumor, a single course of the thiophene resulted in a majority of mice being tumor free more than 5 wk after the therapy had been completed.

6. THERAPEUTIC INDEX DETERMINATIONS

The activities of LY309887 and lometrexol were compared using calculations of therapeutic index ranges for the two drugs. For this comparison, both drugs were tested in human xenograft tumor models (dosing schedule: q3d × 4). Ideally these comparisons should be made using tumor models in which both drugs were highly active. The ratio of LD_{10} divided by the ED_{90} would give therapeutic indices relevant to clinical safety. However, in some tumor models, a maximal tumor growth inhibition of 70% was obtained. Therefore, calculations of therapeutic index were based on the ratio of LD_{10} to ED_{70} (2). Calculations of therapeutic indices using ED_{90} values would give slightly lower values. The LD_{10} for these studies was assessed in nontumor-bearing mice to eliminate uncertainty regarding cause of death, i.e., from tumor burden vs drug toxicity, especially since lethality resulting from antifolate toxicity was delayed for many days.

Table 5
Estimates of Therapeutic Index^a Ranges for LY309887
and Lometrexol Based on Ratio of LD_{10}/ED_{70}

	LY309887	Lometrexol (LY249543)
PANC-1 pancreatic	10–30	3–10
LX-1 lung	3–10	1–3
MX-1 mammary	1–3	1–3
HC1 colon	3–10	1–3
VRC5 colon	3–10	3

^{a}Therapeutic index range:
(e.g., for LY309887 against PANC-1) = LD_{10}/ED_{70} = (30–100 mg/kg)/(3 mg/kg) = 10–30
All values for LD_{10} and ED_{70} based on q3d × 4 ip dosing with regular diet.
LD_{10} values determined in C3H female mice.
ED_{70} values determined in CD1 Nu/Nu mice.

Lethality was determined in C3H mice which were used for testing murine tumor models. However, the human xenograft models utilized CD1 Nu/Nu mice. Thus the therapeutic index calculations use efficacy data from this strain of mouse.

Compound LY309887 was more potent than lometrexol in producing antitumor activity in several models, and it also was more potent in producing lethality in mice. In the PANC-1 pancreatic tumor and the LX-1 human lung xenografts, LY309887 was about 100 times more potent in its antitumor activity compared to lometrexol when both were dosed q3d × 4. The LD_{10} for LY309887 was between 30 and 100 mg/kg, whereas for lometrexol, an LD_{10} between 1000 and 3000 mg/kg was obtained. Thus, LY309887 was approx 30 times more potent for producing lethality in mice compared to lometrexol. Estimates of therapeutic indices were calculated as shown in Table 5. In PANC-1 pancreatic, LX-1 lung, HC1 colon, and VRC5 colon xenograft tumor models, preliminary estimates of therapeutic index showed an approx threefold greater therapeutic index for LY309887 compared to lometrexol. In MX-1 mammary tumors, both compounds were less active, and there was no difference in therapeutic index in this tumor model.

7. THE EFFECT OF DIETARY FOLATE ON DISPOSITION OF LOMETREXOL AND LY309887 IN LIVER

In phase I clinical trials with lometrexol, unexpected delayed and cumulative toxicity in patients was encountered (1). The observed toxicities, mucositis and myelosupression, are classically associated with antifolate therapy. However, the duration of toxicity following a single-drug dose and the cumulative nature of the toxicity were novel observations of antifolate toxicity. It was hypothesized that cancer patients may be marginal in their folic acid stores. To this end, a folate-deficient murine model was established to characterize biochemical and pharmacological effects of low dietary folate (LFD) on the efficacy and delayed toxicity of antifolate inhibitors.

In mice receiving a LFD for 2 wk, Schmitz et al. showed that folate pools were reduced in plasma, liver, intestine, and tumors (14). In addition, significant changes were noted in the density of FR in tumors and liver and in the isoforms expressed in tumors

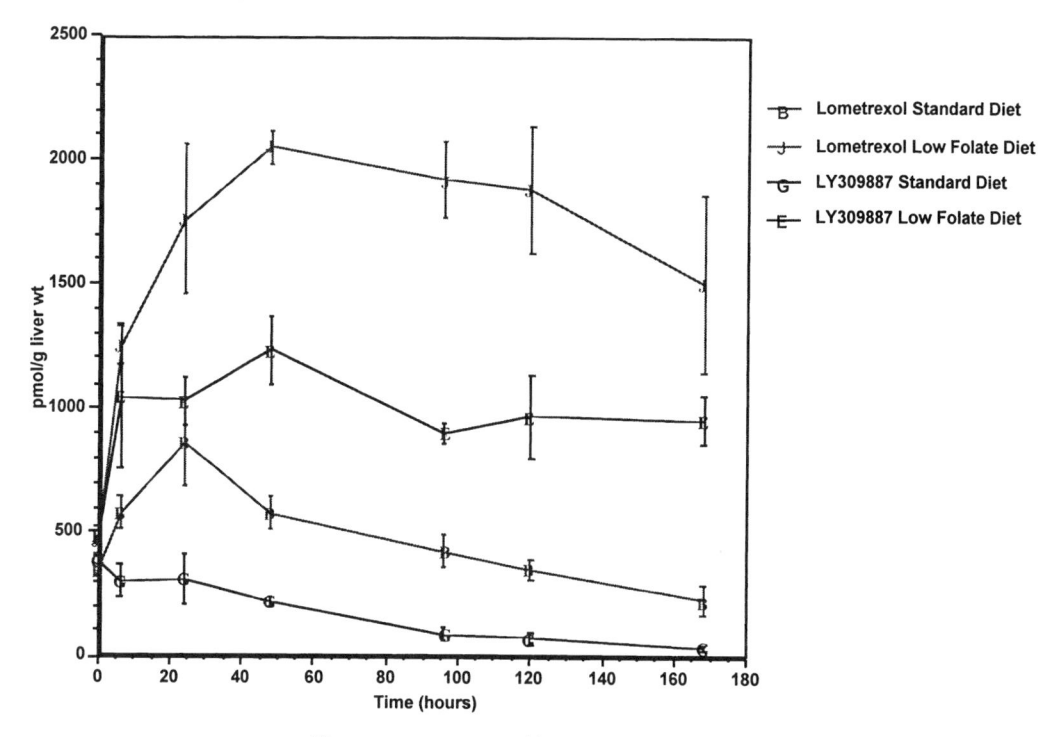

Fig. 3. Total Disposition of [^{14}C]-lometrexol and [^{14}C]-LY309887 in Murine Liver.

(15). Increases in tumor and liver FPGS activity were also noted *(16)*. Whole-body autoradiography studies in mice on standard diet or LFD receiving either [^{14}C]-lometrexol or [^{14}C]-LY309887 demonstrated significantly higher accumulation of drug in livers of mice on LFD *(10,7)*. The accumulation and polyglutamation state of lometrexol and LY309887 in livers of mice on SD and LFD were compared by dosing mice iv with equitoxic doses (LD$_{50}$ doses in LFD mice) of radiolabeled parent compound. The total accumulation of each drug in liver was determined over a 7-d period (Fig. 3). Polyglutamates were also determined by reversed-phase HPLC *(7)*.

Regardless of diet, more lometrexol accumulated in murine liver than LY309887. Furthermore, animals on LFD accumulated roughly 6–10-fold more drug than animals on SD and clearance of drug from livers of LFD mice was slower than clearance from SD mice. Polyglutamation profiles showed that on SD, the most common metabolite after 24-h for both drugs was pentaglutamate (80–90%). In mice on LFD receiving LY309887, penta- and hexa-glutamyl-metabolites were still the predominant forms; 70 and 30%, respectively. In contrast, lometrexol was polyglutamated more extensively: an additional percentage, approx 15%, was recovered as the septa- and octa-glutamyl forms *(17)*.

8. THE EFFECT OF LFD AND DIETARY FOLATE SUPPLEMENTATION ON THE EFFICACY AND TOXICITY OF LOMETREXOL AND LY309887

In mice on a LFD for 2 wk, the toxicity of lometrexol and LY309887 increased 300–1000-fold. Antitumor activity cannot be assessed because of the lethality of these agents. Oral supplementation with folic acid (0.6–600 mg/kg) restores sensitivity to the antitumor activity of both GARFT inhibitors. High doses of folic acid (>600 mg/kg) eliminated both toxicity and antitumor activity.

The therapeutic indexes (LD_{10}/ED_{90}) of LY309887 and lometrexol were determined over a range of supplemental folic acid doses in two antitumor models, the human xenograft GC3 colon and the murine mammary tumor C3H (Table 6). The data show that increasing folic acid supplementation doses from 0.0 to 6–15 mg/kg/d resulted in an enhanced therapeutic index ranging from 6 to 60 for LY309887 in both models. Furthermore, the ability to delay regrowth of the GC3 tumors over a broad dose range was only seen at the higher doses of folate supplementation. A small but modest increase in lometrexol's therapeutic index to 2–5 was also observed. Higher doses of folic acid supplementation resulted in less robust increases in the therapeutic index.

9. HUMAN FOLATE STATUS

The folate status of cancer patients has not been systematically evaluated. However, early studies reported decreased serum folic acid activity in patients with metastatic cancer [18–20]. Other investigators have demonstrated decreased urinary clearance of a folic-acid load [21,22]. Saleh et al. demonstrated that patients with metastatic disease incorporated more folic acid into their reduced folate pools, had decreased catabolism of folate and more rapid clearance of serum folate than controls even in the presence of maintained serum $5-CH_3$-THF concentrations [22]. They concluded that patients were folate deficient and that there was an increased demand for folate in patients with malignant disease. In these patients, variability in the metabolism, pharmacokinetics, and toxicity of classical antifolates compared to humans with normal folate status would not be unexpected. Furthermore, dietary supplementation with folic acid may "normalize" the dose response for achieving antitumor activity and reduce toxicity to normal tissues by restoring folate pools in tissues having low folate requirements, without meeting the high folate demands of rapidly dividing tumor cells.

The biochemical pathways that utilize folate cofactors also require adequate amounts of vitamins B_{12} and B_6. Thus, the status of all three vitamins in patients may significantly influence the severity of toxicity observed during chemotherapy. R. Allen and his colleagues have established that measuring specific amino acid metabolites, especially homocysteine, N-methyl glycine and others, from these metabolic pathways provides a more sensitive and reliable assessment of patient vitamin status [23]. These surrogate indicators of functional folate status are more indicative of deficiencies and more responsive to dietary supplementation.

10. CLINICAL EVALUATION OF LOMETREXOL AND LY309887

Cancer chemotherapy was born in 1948 with the discovery that the antifolate antimetabolite aminopterin, an inhibitor of dihydrofolate reductase (DHFR), induced remissions in patients with acute lymphoblastic leukemia [24]. Over the last 50 yr, intensive structure-activity studies directed at the folate pathway led initially to the identification of methotrexate [25], also an inhibitor of DHFR, and 5 fluorouracil (5FU) an inhibitor of the enzyme thymidylate synthase (TS) [26]. More recently a number of pure

Table 6
Effect of Increasing Folic Acid Supplementation on the Therapeutic Index

Tumor	Folate Supplement mg/kg/d	Therapeutic Index LY309887	LD_{10}/ED_{90} lometrexol
GC3 colon	none	0	0
	0.6	3 (2,4)	0.6
	6.0	25 (25,25)	1.5
	15.0	60	n.d.
	60.0	n.d.	2
C3H mammary	none	0	0
	0.6	1.4 (1.3,1.5)	2
	6	9 (6, 12)	5
	15	6	n.d.
	60	n.d.	1

n.d.: not determined.

TS inhibitors have been studied, the lead compound being CB3717. Despite initial evidence of activity (27,28), this compound failed in the clinic largely because of unpredictable renal toxicity, which was thought to result from crystallization of the compound within the kidney (27). The replacement of the 1'-amino and 10 propargyl groups to a methyl group and the replacement of the 1',4'-phenylene to 2',5'-thienyl bioisostere on CB3717 gave a more potent and soluble TS inhibitor, raltitrexed (ZD1694). Raltitrexed has recently been shown in randomized comparative trials to be active in the treatment of colorectal cancer. These studies have led to the granting of a product license in several countries including the U.K. Other antifolate antimetabolites are currently under development including the 5FU prodrugs, capecitabine (29) and UFT (30), and the multitargeted antifolate (MTA, LY231514) (31–33). However, no specific inhibitors of purine biosynthesis are yet utilized in routine clinical practice. The first molecule to enter clinical trials that was directed at inhibition of an enzyme essential for *de novo* purine biosynthesis, glycinamide ribonucleotide transformylase (GARFT), was the 6R diastereomer of dideazatetrahydrofolic acid (DDATHF), an analog of tetrahydrofolate, known as lometrexol (34,35). Lometrexol was selected for clinical development on the basis of its preclinical activity in vitro and in vivo (36,37). Hematologic and gastrointestinal toxicity was dose limiting in both mice and dogs. The dog was the most sensitive of the animal species tested, with 100 mg/m^2/wk being tolerated in chronic dosing schedules. In contrast, mice tolerated 600 mg/m^2/wk in chronic studies (38). The first phase I study was initiated in 1989/1990. It was not until a number of phase I studies had been started that the preclinical data showing an effect of dietary folic acid on modulation of therapeutic index become available. Hence the initial phase I studies were conducted without folic acid supplementation. A number of dosing schedules, of both lometrexol, and of folic acid were examined in the phase I program, and these are described in Table 7 below.

A number of key clinical questions have been addressed in these studies as follows.

1. What is a suitable dosing schedule of lometrexol that can be given repeatedly?
2. What is the maximum tolerated dose (MTD), and the projected phase II dose?
3. What is the nature of the toxicity and pharmacokinetic profiles?
4. Do the preclinical observations on the effect of folic acid on toxicity translate into a clinical setting, i.e., does coadministration of folic acid ameliorate or prevent toxicity, and hence allow a higher MTD of lometrexol (and hence projected phase II dose) to be established.
5. What is the effect of different doses and schedules of folic acid?
6. Does folic acid influence the pharmacokinetics of lometrexol?
7. Can folinic acid (leucovorin) be used as an alternative to folic acid to ameliorate toxicity or as a potential rescue strategy?

11. PHASE I STUDIES WITHOUT FOLIC ACID SUPPLEMENTATION

In summary, without folic acid coadministration, regardless of the schedule utilized, lometrexol caused cumulative toxicity, with myelosuppression and mucositis being dose limiting. Other toxicities included neutropenia and anemia. A number of different schedules were evaluated in an attempt to identify one in which the drug could be used repeatedly. The initial studies included a trial of a once every two week dosing schedule (q2 weeks), which was then extended to a maximum of 6 wk when observations of cumulative toxicity were made *(36)*. A total of 16 patients were treated at 15, 30, and 60 mg/m^2, although with repeat dosing, it became clear that at least the two higher doses were above the maximum tolerated dose and were associated with severe toxicity, i.e., prolonged myelosuppression (anemia, thrombocytopenia, and neutropenia) and mucositis. In some cases, empiric treatment of patients with leucovorin for 4 to 8 d appeared to be helpful. Toxicity was correlated with prolonged retention of lometrexol in plasma. An alternative w × 3 q5 dosing schedule was evaluated by Muggia and colleagues, in a targeted phase I study of patients with colorectal cancer, using a starting dose of 3 mg/m^2 *(40)*. Three patients were treated at this dose level, 4 at 4.5 mg/m^2 and 17 at 6 mg/m^2. Again toxicity became limiting in second and subsequent cycles, and led to the recommendation that 6 mg/m^2 was safe in the initial course, but that dose intensity should be reduced in subsequent cycles by a change in schedule to w × 2 in subsequent cycles. Seven patients who developed hematologic toxicity were given leucovorin, and recovery of counts occurred within a week, although the nadir of myelosuppression is not quoted. Three patients who developed mild toxicity were given folic acid but this appeared to be ineffective, since platelet counts continued to decline. There was no correlation of toxicity of lometrexol with baseline red blood cell folate levels. A further trial of a twice weekly × 4, every 28–35 d schedule studied 34 patients, and defined an MTD of 2.7 mg/m^2, but again severe cumulative toxicity was observed *(41)*.

12. PHASE I STUDIES WITH FOLIC ACID SUPPLEMENTATION

During the course of this twice weekly × 4 q28–35 d study *(41)*, Gerry Grindey published data demonstrating that dietary folic acid status had a profound effect on the tox-

Table 7
Phase I Studies of Lometrexol

Without folic acid modulation

Investigator/References	Schedule	Dose Levels Studied mg/m²	Comments
Nelson et al. (39)	Q2–6 wks	15, 30, 60	Cumulative toxicity at 15 mg/m²
Muggia et al. (40)	w × 3 Q5 w × 3 Q5 w × 2 Q4	3.0, 4.5, 6.0 6.0	GIII/IV tox seen at all dose levels 6 mg/m² safe in the initial course then change to w × 2Q4
Young et al. (41)	Twice weekly × 2 Q4 wk	2.7, 3.6, 4.8	MTD = 2.7 mg/m²

With modulation: folic acid

Investigator/References	Schedule	Dose Levels Studied mg/m²	Folic Acid Dose	Folic Acid Schedule	Comments
Young et al. (41)	Twice weekly ×2 Q4	4.8, 5.0, 6.4	1 mg	daily continuously	MTD = 4–5 mg/m²
Cole et al. (42)	w × 3	4	1 mg	d 1 continuously	significant tox; anemia, neuropenia, thrombocytopenia, and stomatitis less tox
Laohavinij et al. (43)	Q3 or 4 wk	12–170	5 mg	d 7 to d + 6	Schedule tolerable and suitable for phase II evaluation.
Roberts et al. (44)	w × 8	5 initially, (max 4 escalations)	3 mg/m²	continuous	Initial dose level tolerated. Folate to be dose reduced only if MTD not reached.
Muggia et al. (45)	Q3 w	15, 20, 25, 30	25 mg/m²	3 h before lometrexol	iv folic acid does not improve tolerance. Study closed early.

With modulation: folinic acid

Investigator/References	Schedule	Dose Levels Studied mg/m²	Folinic Acid Dose	Folinic Acid Schedule	Comments
Sessa et al. (46) Part (1)	d × 3 Q4 wks	1.5–4	—	—	thrombocytopenia and mucositis dose limiting
Part (2)	Q4 wk	12–21	15 mg 4 × daily	days 3–5	
Part (3)	Q4 wk	21	15 mg 4 × daily	interval between lometrexol and folinic acid extended d5–7	
Part (4)	Q4 wk	30, 45, 60	15 mg 4 × daily	day 7 to day 9	Anemia dose limiting

icity of lometrexol *(47,48)*. Hence subsequent patients in the study were treated with 1 mg folic acid/d given continuously. This level of supplementation permitted an escalated MTD of 4 to 5 mg/m^2 twice weekly × 4 dose to be defined, and appeared to reduce the cumulative aspects of the toxicity profile.

A key question that remained was how much folic acid was required to achieve optimal amelioration of toxicity, accepting that any effects on efficacy could only be evaluated in a phase II setting. Accordingly, a study of a weekly × 3 schedule was conducted *(42)*, in which folic acid was given orally each day, beginning 24 h prior to the first dose of lometrexol. At the first (4 mg/m^2) and second dose level (5 mg/m^2) of lometrexol, patients were treated with 1 mg/d folic acid, and in the third cohort, 2 mg of folic acid was given to patients treated with 5 mg/m^2 lometrexol. An initial report suggested less toxicity at the 2 mg folic acid dose, but data from only two patients was reported, compared to six and four patients treated at the first two dose levels. Again, anemia was the most prevalent toxicity, and neutropenia, thrombocytopenia, and stomatitis were also common. These observations led to a further look at the single dose every 4 wk schedule, using a higher dose of folic acid, 5 mg/d for 14 d, given for 7 d before and for 7 d after the dose of lometrexol. This dose of folic acid was chosen from extrapolation from the preclinical studies. Additional objectives for this study were to study the effect of lometrexol on pharmacodynamics, in order to determine whether folic acid improves tolerance of lometrexol, to determine the toxicity of lometrexol in patients receiving multiple courses of the drug with folic acid supplementation, and to describe the pharmacokinetics. This study recruited 43 patients from 1991 to December, 1995. Dose levels between 12 and 45 mg/m^2 were studied using a once every 4 wk schedule. This interval was then reduced to 3 wk since recovery of the platelet count after dosing was achieved by day 21. Dose escalation proceeded with patients being studied at the 45, 60, 78, 100, 130, and 170 mg/m^2 dose levels. The MTD was not formally defined in this study, and the investigators felt that there was capacity for further dose escalation. Thirty-five patients received two courses of therapy and a total of 99 courses was given to the 43 patients. The major toxicity observed was thrombocytopenia; WHO grade III or IV toxicity was observed in 9/99 courses, but a downward trend in platelet counts was observed across successive courses in all patients even if the criteria for grading toxicity was not reached (i.e., a platelet count of less than 100). Similarly anemia became more marked in those patients receiving more than two courses, although there was only a 4% incidence of WHO grade III and IV toxicity. Four patients developed WHO grade III/IV neutropenia, and in one case this was associated with fever requiring iv antibiotics. Two patients developed WHO grade III mucositis, and three patients had decreases in GFR, but this was not in the setting of raised serum creatinine. These toxicities were observed at various dose levels during dose escalation. The investigators treated two of the patients who developed grade IV thrombocytopenia with leucovorin at 30 mg every 6 h for 12 and 14 d, respectively, and although platelet recovery was achieved it was not clear that leucovorin had played a role in this, hence no further patients were treated with leucovorin. Given the previous experience with this schedule in the absence of folic acid, discussed in Subheading 11 *(39)*, this study clearly demonstrated that folic acid supplementation at 5 mg/d for 14 d reduced clinical toxicity permitting a dose of greater than 10 times that in the absence of supplementation, and in particular the cumulative nature of the toxicity was reduced. More recently, two other studies have addressed the question of how much folic acid is required to ameliorate toxicity. In a weekly lometrexol schedule in which folic acid 5 mg/d was given continuously, the initial dose of 5 mg/m² lometrexol for 12 wk was tolerated *(44)*. Data from the completed study is awaited with interest. In contrast 25 mg/m² folic acid given iv 3 h before lometrexol failed to ameliorate toxicity *(45)*. Taken together this data would suggest that 2 mg folic acid per day is not adequate but that 5 mg folic acid given orally does ameliorate toxicity. The duration of folic acid required is not clear, but the Laohavinij study would suggest that 14 d when given 7 d before and 7 d after the dose of lometrexol in a 3-wk cycle affords protection. In contrast iv folic acid, at least when given at 25 mg/m², 3 h before lometrexol, is inadequate.

13. PHASE I STUDY OF LOMETREXOL WITH FOLINIC ACID

The early observations of being able to rescue some patients with leucovorin prompted an additional study to look at the most appropriate rescue regime. The study was conducted in four parts. In the first part, lometrexol was given once daily for 3 d, to be repeated every 4 wk. The highest dose that could be administered was 4 mg/m²/d i.e., a total dose of 12 mg/m² every 3 wk. As with other studies, thrombocytopenia and mucositis were dose limiting, so in the second part of the study, lometrexol was given as a single dose on d 1 and oral folinic acid, 15 mg four times a day, was given on d 3–5. The time interval between lometrexol and folinic acid was then extended in part III and in the last part of the study, folinic acid was given from d 7–9. An MTD of 60 mg/m² was reached, with cumulative delayed and persistent anemia being dose limiting. When folinic acid was given on d 5–7 rather than d 7–9, this appeared to reduce anemia, hence this would be the recommended timing of folinic acid for a phase II study. Since leucovorin (5 formyltetrahydrofolate) is converted intracellularly to 5,10-methylene tetrahydrofolate, one would expect that it would reduce the antitumor activity of lometrexol. This has been confirmed in end-product reversal experiments, and hence in the clinic a folic acid-supplemented regime may be preferable. Not withstanding these considerations, it should be noted that a patient with clear cell carcinoma of the ovary had a partial response on this study (*see* Subheading 15).

14. HOW DOES FOLIC ACID MODULATE TOXICITY?

There are a number of possible explanations for the preclinical and clinical observation that dietary folate levels modulate toxicity. As reviewed by Laohavinij and colleagues *(43),* these include:

1. A pharmacokinetic interaction.
2. Modulation of lometrexol transport.
3. An effect on lometrexol polyglutamation
4. An increase in intracellular folate pools in sensitive normal tissues.

There is no evidence to support a pharmacokinetic interaction in humans, although this may be species dependent (*see* Subheading 16). The only evidence to support a transport-mediated mechanism comes from studies in which mice were administered radiolabeled lometrexol and the disposition followed by whole-body autoradiography, *(10).* Under conditions of low folate status, there was an increase in hepatic retention of between 2.5- and 4.2-fold. Further studies are clearly needed to study both transport, polyglutamation, and folate pools in normal tissues.

15. ANTITUMOR ACTIVITY IN PHASE I

Although determination of activity is not an objective of phase I studies in oncology, a number of responses were noted in the phase I studies of lometrexol, in the presence or absence of folic acid supplementation, and at varying dose levels during dose escalation. In the weekly ×3 q5 study without folic acid, a PR was obtained in a patient with NSCLC, who was treated initially at the 4.5 mg/m^2 dose level and then dose reduced to 3 mg/m^2. This patient had a complete response in a node in the supraclavicular fossa, a decrease in nonmeasurable disease on CT scanning, and symptomatic benefit. The response duration was not reported. Young and coworkers *(41,49)* reported a complete response of 18+ mo duration in a patient with oropharyngeal cancer and a PR of 4 mo in a patient with a malignant fibrous histiocytoma. These patients were treated on the twice weekly ×4 q 28–35 d study. In this study the last 19 patients to be accrued of 53 total were supplemented with oral folic acid at 1 mg/d continuously. Whether the responders were among the supplemented cohort of patients is not reported. In the study of lometrexol given q3 wk with 14 d of 5 mg oral folic acid given orally around the dose of lometrexol, the authors *(43)* reported a partial response at the 30 mg/m^2 dose level in a patient with advanced breast cancer with soft-tissue disease. This was sustained for 48 d. In the same study at the 45 mg/m^2 dose level, a further patient with advanced breast cancer had a minor response with improvement in skin lesions. This patient also reported reduced dyspnea sustained for 10 wk. In the d × 3 study q28 d study supplemented with leucovorin *(46)*, a patient with a clear-cell carcinoma of the ovary with a retroperitoneal recurrence who had received prior therapy with cisplatin, alkylating agents, and radiotherapy had a partial response lasting 8 mo.

16. PHARMACOKINETICS

Plasma lometrexol concentrations were measured in both the studies using an HPLC method involving derivatization and fluorescence detection *(43,46)*. Pharmacokinetic parameters derived from patients treated up to 45 mg/m^2 in the Laohavinj folic acid study are described in the Wedge et al. study *(50)*. Of particular note is the long terminal half life, 2593 ± 1671 min, which could result either from enterohepatic recirculation, or from release of the compound from hepatic stores. The relationship between dose and area under the lometrexol plasma concentration vs time curve (AUC) is linear. Samples from seven patients treated at 45 or 60 mg/m^2 in the study in which folinic acid was given after lometrexol *(46)* were also studied. There was no difference in plasma half life, clearance, (30.1 ± 8.1 mL/min/m^2) or extent of protein binding (78%). This result, which suggests a lack of interaction between lometrexol and folic acid in humans, is in contrast to a finding of a sustained plasma concentrations of lometrexol in mice fed a folate-free diet compared to those fed a regular diet *(10)*.

17. CLINICAL DEVELOPMENT OF LY309887

The observations of severe cumulative toxicity in the absence of folic acid supplementation and the need to repeat studies with folic acid, meant that the phase I clinical development of lometrexol was very protracted. During the course of this clinical development, Eli Lilly and Company developed the second-generation compound

LY309887. As has been reviewed earlier in this chapter, LY309887 has a different ratio of binding the different isoforms of the folate receptor, such that one would predict a greater distribution of the molecule into target tumor compared with the liver, and consequently, an improved therapeutic index. In preclinical models of efficacy, LY309887 appears to be more active than lometrexol in two pancreatic xenografts and the LX1 lung model (Table 4). Therefore, on completion of the preclinical toxicology for the compound, Eli Lilly decided to discontinue development of lometrexol in favor of developing LY309887. Hence, no phase II studies were conducted with lometrexol to assess efficacy.

However, a number of questions remained from the phase I studies of lometrexol that needed to be investigated clinically, including the appropriate schedule of lometrexol and the length of folic acid supplementation and the appropriate dose. The phase 1 clinical trials of LY309887 have therefore set out to address the questions of a suitable schedule for LY309887 and the appropriate duration of oral folic acid supplementation using a 5 mg daily dose. The end points of these studies include determination of the MTD, characterization of toxicity and pharmacokinetics, and a determination of functional folate status assessed by measuring amino acid metabolites identified by Allen et al. *(23)*. Two studies use an every 3 wk schedule and LY309887 is given weekly in the remaining study. Folic acid is given for 5 d in one of the q3 wk studies, and for 14 d around the dose of LY309887 in the other. The latter schedule is therefore identical to that used in the lometrexol study performed by Laohavinij et al. *(43)*. In the weekly LY309887 study folic acid is given daily at 5 mg. Data on the patients' functional folate status is being collected, since it may provide valuable clues as to potentially useful predictors of toxicity. These studies are ongoing.

During the course of the phase I development, additional preclinical studies have been performed showing that unlike lometrexol, if the dose of folic acid is increased above 6 mg/kg/d, then there is an increasing effect on the therapeutic index, with both amelioration of toxicity and improvement in efficacy. These experiments are described in detail (*see* Subheading 8). Given these observations, we felt that it was important to evaluate them in a clinical setting and once the MTD on the q3 week study with 14 d of folic acid has been established, the dose of folic acid will be increased to 25 mg daily in subsequent cohorts of patients in an attempt to further escalate LY309887 and define a new MTD. This dose of folic has been chosen from extrapolation from the animal studies.

18. CONCLUSION

In the absence of folic acid supplementation, patients treated with lometrexol in phase I clinical trials developed severe and cumulative myelosuppression and mucositis. The preclinical observations of the role of folic acid in preventing toxicity but preserving activity has been partially investigated in a clinical setting. We know that a 5 mg dose of folic acid given for 14 d around the dose of lometrexol allows at least 10 times more drug to be administered. Any effect on efficacy can of course not be evaluated except in the context of a phase II study. However it is encouraging to note that a number of partial responses were observed in the phase I clinical development in those patients who received folic acid supplementation. Similarly leucovorin given after dosing with lometrexol increases tolerance. Exactly how much folic acid needs to be given and for how long remains to be elucidated. We do know that an iv dose given 3 h before lometrexol is inadequate. These questions are being addressed in the clinical development of LY309887. The preclinical observations of an increasing therapeutic index at increased doses of folic acid are intriguing. It remains to be seen whether this translates into an effect clinically. However the preclinical profile of lometrexol and LY309887 are different and it would appear that the two molecules are also different clinically. The continued clinical development of inhibitors of purine biosynthesis is therefore important and has contributed greatly to our knowledge of preclinical and clinical correlates with antifolates.

REFERENCES

1. Ray MS, Muggia FM, Leichman GC, Nelson RL, Dyke RW, Moran RG. Phase I study of 6 (R)-5,10-dideazatetrahydrofolate: a folate antimetabolite inhibitory to *de novo* purine synthesis. *J Natl Cancer Inst* 1993; 85:1154–1159.
2. Habeck LL, Leitner TA, Shackelford KA, Gossett LS, Schultz RM, Andis SL, Shih C, Grindey GB, Mendelsohn LG. A novel class of monoglutamated antifolates exhibits tight-binding inhibition of human glycinamide ribonucleotide formyltransferase and potent activity against solid tumors. *Cancer Res* 1994; 54:1021–1026.
3. McGuire JJ, Bertino JR. Enzymatic synthesis and function of folylpolyglutamates. *Mol Cell Biochem* 1981; 39:19–48.
4. Morrison JF. Kinetics of reversible inhibition of enzyme catalyzed reactions by tight-binding inhibitors. *Biochem Biophys Acta* 1969; 185:269–286.
5. Habeck LL, Moran RG, Shih C, Gossett LS, Leitner TA, Schultz RM, Andis S, Mendelsohn LG. Substrate specificity of mammalian folylpolyglutamate synthetase for 5,10-Dideazatetrahydrofolate and related analogues. *Mol Pharmacol* 1995; 48:326–333.
6. McGuire JJ, Hsieh P, Coward JK, Bertino JR. Enzymatic synthesis of folylpolyglutamates. *J Biol Chem* 1980; 255:5776–5788.
7. Habeck LL, Chay SH, Pohland RC, Worzalla JF, Shih C, Mendelsohn LG. Whole-body disposition and polyglutamate distribution of the GAR formyltransferase inhibitors LY309887 and lometrexol in mice: effect of low folate diet. *Cancer Chemotherapy Pharmacol* 1998; 41:201–209.
8. Ross JF, Chaudhuri PK, Ratnam M. Differential regulation of folate receptor isoforms in normal and malignant tissues *in vivo* and in established cell lines. *Cancer Res* 1994; 73:2432–2434.
9. Wang X, Shen F, Freisheim JH, Gentry LE, Ratnam M. Differential stereospecificities and affinities of folate receptor isoforms for folate compounds and antifolates. *Biochem Pharmacol* 1992; 44:188–1901.
10. Pohland RC, Alati T, Lantz RJ, Grindey GB. Whole body autoradiographic disposition and plasma pharmacokinetics of 5, 10 dideazatetrahydrofolic acid in mice fed folic acid deficient or regular diets. *J Pharm Sci* 1994; 83:1396.
11. Taber LD, O'Brien P, Bowsher RR, Sportsman JR. Competitive particle concentration fluorescence immunoassay for measuring 5,10-dideazatetrahydrofolic acid (lometrexol) in serum. *Clin Chem* 1991; 37:254–260.
12. Tonkinson JL, Marder P, Andis SL, Schultz RM, Gossett LS, Shih C, Mendelsohn LG. Cell cycle effects of antifolate antimetabolites: implications for cytotoxicity and cytostasis. *Cancer Chemotherapy Pharmacol* 1997; 39:521–530.
13. Chen VJ, Bewley JR, Andis SL, Schultz RM, Iversen PW, Shih C, Mendelsohn LG, Seitz DE, Tonkinson JL. Preclinical cellular pharmacology of LY231514: a comparison with methotrexate, LY309887 and raltitrexed for their effects on intracellular folate and nucleoside triphosphate pools in CCRF-CEM cells. *Br J Cancer* 1988; 77,S53:27–34.
14. Schmitz JC, Grindey GB, Schultz RM, Priest DG. Impact of dietary folic acid on reduced folates in mouse plasma and tissues. Relationship to dideazatetrahydrofolate sensitivity. *Biochem Pharmacol* 1994; 48:319–325.
15. Gates SB, Mendelsohn LG, Shackelford KA, Habeck LL, Kursar JD, Rutherford PG, et al. Characterization of folate receptor from normal and neoplastic tissue: influence of dietary folate on folate receptor expression. *Clin Cancer Res* 1996; 2:1135–1141.

16. Gates SB, Worzalla JF, Shih C, Grindey GB, Mendelsohn LG. Dietary folate and folypolyglutamate synthetase activity in normal and neoplastic murine tissues and human tumor xenografts. *Biochem Pharmacol* 1996; 52:1477–1479.
17. Mendelsohn LG, Gates SB, Habeck LL, Shackelford KA, Worzalla J, Shih C, Grindey GB. The role of dietary folate in modulation of folate receptor expression, folylpolyglutamate synthetase expression and the efficacy and toxicity of lometrexol. *Advances Enzyme Regul* 1996; 36:365–381.
18. Magnus E. Folate activity in serum and red cells of patients with cancer. *Cancer Res* 1967; 27:490–497.
19. Hoogstraten B, Baker H, Gilbert HS. Serum folate and serum vitamin B_{12} in patients with malignant hematologic diseases. *Cancer Res* 1965; 25:1933–1938.
20. Einhorn J, Reizenstein P. Metabolic studies on folic acid in malignancy. *Cancer Res* 1966; 26:310–313.
21. Rao PBR, Lagerlof BJ, Einhorn J, Reizenstein PG. Folic acid activity in leukemia and cancer. *Cancer Res* 1965; 25:221–224.
22. Saleh AM, Pheasant AE, Blair JA, Allan RN, Walters J. Folate metabolism in man: the effect of malignant disease. *Br J Cancer* 1982; 46:346–353.
23. Allen RH, Stabler SP, Savage DG, et al. Metabolic abnormalities in cobalamin (vitamin B-12) and folate deficiency. *FASEB J* 1994; 71:344–353.
24. Farber S, Diamond LK, Mercer RD, Sylvester RF, Wolff JA. Temporary remissions in acute leukemia in children produced by folic acid antagonist, 4-aminopteroylglutamic acid (aminopterin). *N Engl J Med* 1948; 238:787–793.
25. Venditti JM, Kline I, Tyrer DD, Goldin A. 1,3 bis (22-chloroethyl)-1-nitrosourea (NSC-400009962) and methotrexate (NSC-740) as combination therapy for advanced mouse leukemia L1210. *Cancer Chem Reports* 1965; 48:5–9.
26. Cornell GN, Cahow CE, Frey C, McScherry C, Beal JM. Clinical experience with 5-fluorouracil (NSC-19893) in the treatment of malignant disease. *Cancer Chem Biol Response Modif* 1960; 9:23–30.
27. Calvert AH, Alison DL, Harland SJ, Robinson BA, Jackman AL, Jones TR, et al. A phase I evaluation of the quinazoline antifolate thymidylate synthase inhibitor, N10-propargyl-5,8-dideazafolic acid, CB3717. *J Clin Onc* 1986; 4:1245–1252.
28. Bassendine MF, Curtin NJ, Loose H, Harris AL, James OFW. Induction of remission in hepatocellular carcinoma with a new thymidylate synthase inhibitor, CB3717. *J Hepatology* 1987; 4:349–356.
29. Bajetta E, Carnaghi C, Somma L, Stampino CG. A new oral fluoropyrimidine in patients with advanced neoplastic disease. *Tumori* 1996; 82:450–452.
30. Kimura K, Suga S, Shimaji T, Kitamura M, Kubo K, Suyuski Y, Isobe K. Clinical basis of chemotherapy for gastric cancer with uracil and 1-2'-tetra hydrofuryl)-5-fluoro uracil. *Gastroeuterologia Japonica* 1980; 15:324–329.
31. Shih C, Chen VJ, Gossett LS, Gatess SB, MacKellar WC, Habeck LL, Shackelford KA, Mendelsohn LG, Soose DJ, Patel VF, Andis SL, Bewley JR, Rayl EA, Moroson BA, Beardsley GP, Kohler W, Ratnam M, Schultz R. LY231514, a pyrrolo {2,3-d} pyrimidine-based antifolate that inhibits multiple folate-requiring enzymes. *Cancer Res* 1997; 57:1116–1123.
32. Rinaldi D, Burris H, Dorr F, Eckardt J, Fields S, Langley C, et al. A phase I evaluation of LY231514 administered every 21 days, utilizing the modified continual reassessment method for dose escalation (Meeting abstract). *Proc Am Soc Clin Oncol* 1995; 14(31 Meet):474–A1539.
33. Cripps MD, Burnell M, Jolivet J, Lofters W, Fisher B, Panasci, L, et al. Phase II study of a multi-targeted antifolate (LY231514) (MTA) as first-line therapy in patients with locally advanced or metastatic colorectal cancer (MCC). *Proc Am Soc Clin Oncol* 1997; 16(33 Meet.):267a.
34. Taylor EC, Harrington PJ, Fletcher SR, Beardsley GP, Moran RG. Synthesis of the antileukaemic agents 5,10-dideazaaminopterin and 5,10-dideaza-5,6,7,8-tetrahydroaminopterin. *J Med Chem* 1985; 28:914–921.
35. Beardsley GP, Moroson GA, Taylor EC, Moran RG. A new folate antimetabolite, 5,10 dideaza-5,6,7,8-tetrahydrofolate is a potent inhibitor of de novo purine synthesis. *J Biol Chem* 1989; 264:328–333.
36. Jansen G, Westerhof GR, Kathmann I, Rijksen G, Schornagel JH. Growth inhibitory effects of 5,10 dideazatetrahydrofolic acid on murine variant L1210 and human CCRF-CEM leukemia cells with different membrane transport characteristics for (anti) folate compounds. *Cancer Chemother Pharmacol* 1991; 28:115–117.
37. Shih C, Grindey GB, Houghton PJ, Houghton JA. *In vivo* antitumor activity of 5,10 Dideazatetrahydrofolic acid (DDATHF) and its diastereomeric isomers. *Proc Amer Assoc Cancer Res* 1988; 29:293.
38. Alati T, Worzalla J, Shih J, Bewley JR, Lewis SL, Moran R, Grindey G. Augmentation of the therapeutic activity of lometrexol [(6-R) 5,10-dideazatetrahydrofolic acid by oral folic acid. *Cancer Res* 1996; 56:2331–2335.

39. Nelson R, Butler F, Dugan W, et al. Phase I clinical trial of LY264618 (Dideazatetrahydrofolic acid: DDATHF). *Proc ASCO* 1990; 9:76.
40. Muggia F, Martin T, Ray M, Leichman CG, Grunberg S, Gill I, Moran R, Dyke R, Grindey G. Phase I study of 5, 10 dideazatetrahydrofolate (LY264618, DDATHF-B). *Proc ASCO* 1990; 9:285.
41. Young CW, Currie VE, Muindi JF, Saltz LB, Pisters KMW, Esposito AJ, Dyke RW. Phase I study of lometrexol (LY264618 or LTX) improved clinical tolerance with oral folic acid. *Proc NCI EORTC* 1992.
42. Cole JT, Gralla RJ, Kardinal CG, NP Rivera. Lometrexol (DDATHF): phase I weekly trial of a weekly schedule of this new antifolate. *Proc Am Assoc Cancer Res* 1992; 33:2468.
43. Laohavinij S, Wedge SR, Lind MJ, Bailey N, Humphreys, Proctor M, Chapman F, Simmons D, Oakley A, Robson L, Gumbrell, Taylor GA, Thomas HD, Boddy A, Newell DR, Calvert AH. A phase I study of the antipurine antifolate lometrexol (DDATHF). *Invest New Drugs* 1996; 14:325–335.
44. Roberts JD, Poplin EA, Mitchell RB, Tombes MB, Kyle B, Moran R. Phase I study of weekly IV lometrexol with continuous folic acid supplementation. *Proc ASCO* 1996; 15:488.
45. Muggia FM, Synold TW, Newman EM, Jeffers S, Lichman LP, Doroshow JH, et al. Failure of pretreatment with intravenous folic acid to alter the comulative hematologic toxicology of lometrexol. *J Natl Cancer Inst* 1996; 88:495–496.
46. Sessa C, de Jong M, D'Incalci M, Hatty S, Pagani O, Cavalli F. Phase I study of the antipurine antifolate lometrexol (DDATHF) with folinic acid rescue. *Clin Cancer Res* 1996; 2:1123.
47. Grindey GB, Alati T, Shih C. Reversal of the toxicity but not the antitumor activity of lometrexol by folic acid. *Proc Am Assoc Cancer Res* 1991; 32:1921.
48. Grindey GB, Alati T, Lantz R, Pohland R, Shih C. Role of dietary folic acid in blocking the toxicity but not the antitumor activity of lometrexol (DDATHF). *Proc NCI EORTC* 1992.
49. Young CW, Currie V, Balter L, Trochanowski B, Eton O, Dyke R. Phase I and clinical pharmacologic study of LY264618, 5,10-dideazatetrahydrofolate. *Proc Am Assoc Cancer Res* 1990; 31:177.
50. Wedge SR, Laohavinij S, Taylor GA, Boddy A, Calvert AH, Newell DR. Clinical pharmacokinetics of the antipurine antifolate (6R) -5,10-dideazatetrahydrofolic acid (lometrexol) administered with an oral folic acid supplement. *Clin Cancer Res* 1995; 1:1479–1486.

13 AG2034

A GARFT Inhibitor with Selective Cytotoxicity to Cells that Lack a G1 Checkpoint

Theodore J. Boritzki, Cathy Zhang, Charlotte A. Bartlett, and Robert C. Jackson

CONTENTS

INTRODUCTION: THE COMPLEX PHARMACOLOGY OF LOMETREXOL
THE BIOCHEMICAL PHARMACOLOGY OF AG2034
THE ANTITUMOR ACTIVITY OF AG2034 IN VIVO
TOXICITY TO FOLATE-DEPLETED MICE
THE KISLIUK EFFECT
CYTOTOXICITY IN RELATION TO FOLATE AND P53 STATUS
CELL-CYCLE EFFECTS OF AG2034
CONCLUSIONS
ACKNOWLEDGMENTS
REFERENCES

1. INTRODUCTION: THE COMPLEX PHARMACOLOGY OF LOMETREXOL

Lometrexol (6*R*-DDATHF) was synthesized by E.C. Taylor and colleagues *(1)*, and shown by Beardsley, Grindey, and Moran *(2)* to be a selective inhibitor of glycinamide ribonucleotide formyltransferase (GARFT). Lometrexol was a landmark anticancer compound for a number of reasons: it was the first potent and selective GARFT inhibitor, it had in vivo antitumor activity in models in which earlier classes of antifolate drugs were inactive *(3)*, and it was, arguably, the first anticancer drug whose activity could be unequivocally attributed to depletion of cellular purine nucleotides. In clinical trials, lometrexol gave responses in a number of hard-to-treat solid tumors, but it was unexpectedly toxic, in particular giving severe and prolonged delayed thrombocytopoenia *(4)*. This toxicity was particularly serious in patients who may have been folate deficient. Grindey and his colleagues then reported the surprising observation that a brief period of dietary folate depletion made mice several hundred-fold more susceptible to lome-

From: *Anticancer Drug Development Guide: Antifolate Drugs in Cancer Therapy*
Edited by: A.L. Jackman © Humana Press Inc., Totowa, NJ

trexol toxicity *(5)*. It was observed that lometrexol bound tightly to the membrane folate-binding protein (mFBP), and one hypothesis advanced to account for its greatly increased toxicity in conditions of folate depletion was that under conditions of low extracellular folate concentration, mFBP was upregulated, which could be responsible for greater cellular uptake, and hence greater toxicity, of circulating lometrexol *(6)*. Alati et al. reported preclinical studies showing that folic acid protected mice from lometrexol toxicity without compromising its antitumor activity *(7)*. As a result, clinical trials of lometrexol are now being conducted in conjunction with folic acid supplementation *(8)*. Whereas this approach makes lometrexol much safer, as we shall show later, folic acid supplementation may cause major changes in the effects of GARFT inhibitors on the cell cycle.

An alternative explanation for the delayed toxicity of lometrexol was suggested by Alati et al. *(7)* who noted that in folate-depleted mice the plasma pharmacokinetics of lometrexol showed a long gamma elimination phase that was not observed in folate-replete mice. Two possible approaches to developing novel GARFT inhibitors with less delayed toxicity would be to make compounds that bind less tightly to the mFBP and rely on the reduced folate carrier (RFC) for entry into cells and secondly to make compounds that are more rapidly cleared under the conditions of normal human plasma folate concentration.

There has been a debate as to whether the antiproliferative effect of GARFT inhibitors is primarily a cytotoxic effect or a cytostatic effect. An important early contribution to this topic was the work of Smith et al. *(9)* who showed unequivocally that lometrexol was cytotoxic to a human colon carcinoma cell line, but that the degree of cell kill was less than that given by an equally growth-inhibitory concentration of a thymidylate synthase (TS) inhibitor, and the onset of cytotoxicity was much slower. We shall return to the subject of cytostatic and cytotoxic effects of GARFT inhibitors later, in the discussion of AG2034.

2. THE BIOCHEMICAL PHARMACOLOGY OF AG2034

The design of novel GARFT inhibitors at Agouron used the X-ray crystal structure of *E. coli* GARFT as a starting point, which was solved with a bound inhibitor *(10)*. In mammalian cells, GARFT forms one domain of a trifunctional enzyme, and the mammalian GARFT domain has extensive homology with *E. coli* GARFT (which is a monofunctional enzyme). Initially the bacterial structure was used for inhibitor design, but the human GARFT structure has now been solved (R. Almassy, personal communication). A number of novel GARFT inhibitors were designed using structure-based drug-design approaches, and structures of two of them, AG2032 and AG2034, are shown in Fig. 1 *(11,12)*. Both AG2034 and AG2032 were potent GARFT inhibitors, and they were competitive with the folate cofactor substrate *(12)*. Kinetic parameters are shown in Table 1; both AG2032 and AG2034 were good substrates for folylpolyglutamate synthetase (FPGS). CCRF-CEM and HeLa cells do not form detectable amounts of AG2034 polyglutamates when grown under cytostatic or cytotoxic conditions. However, HeLa cells, cultured in the presence of hypoxanthine, extensively polyglutamylate AG2034. The major polyglutamate species are the AG2034-glutamate conjugates after addition of four or five additional glutamic acids (K. Zhang, personal communication). Therefore, AG2034 is a substrate for human FPGS and each intermediate compound, after addition

Lometrexol

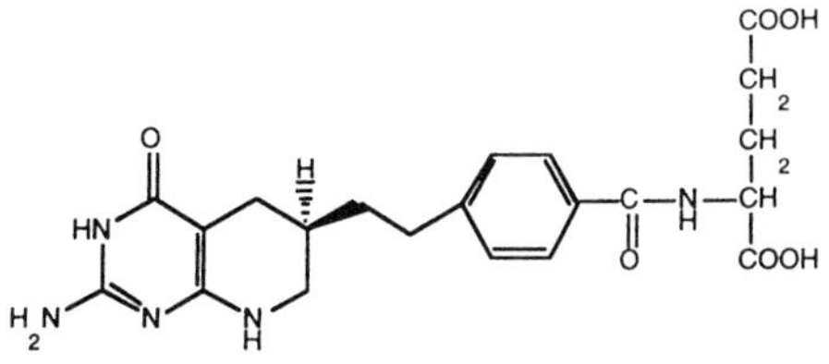

AG2032

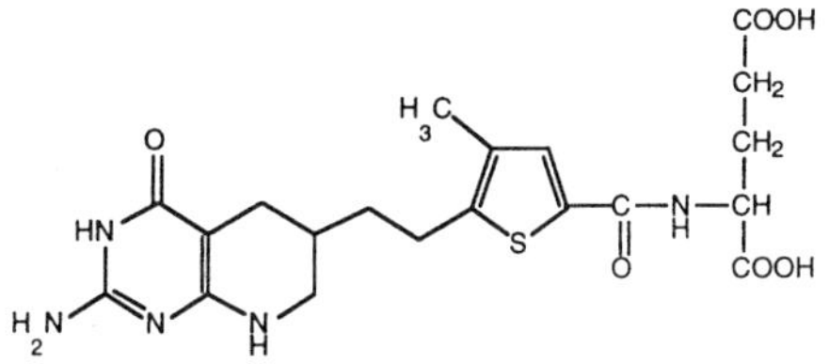

AG2034

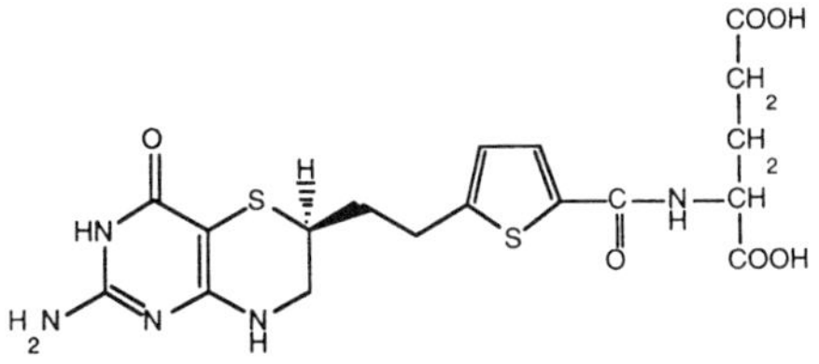

Fig. 1. Chemical structures of lometrexol, AG2032 and AG2034.

Table 1
Kinetic Parameters for Inhibitors of Glycinamide Ribonucleotide Formyltransferase

Compound	GARFT K_i (nM)	mFBP K_d (nM)	FPGS K_m (μM)	V_{max} (nmol/h/mg)
AG2032	1	28	nd	nd
AG2034	28	0.004	6.4	0.48
Lometrexol	25	0.016	4.5	0.71
Folic acid	—	0.060	108	0.56

K_i for GARFT was calculated using a K_m for 10-formy-5,8-dideazafolate of 0.6 μM.

K_d for mFBP was determined using the competitive binding method and assuming a K_d for ^{3}H-folic acid of 0.06 nM. nd = not determined.

Table 2
In Vitro Activity Summary for GARFT Inhibitors

Compound	IC_{50} for L1210 (nM)	Hx reversal (fold)	IC_{50} for CCRF-CEM (nM)	AICA reversal (fold)	IC_{50} for L1210/CI-920 (nM)
AG2032	11	20,000	7	20,000	6900
AG2034	4	68,000	4	820	1400
Lometrexol	17	131,000	11	21,000	3400

IC_{50} values were estimated over a 72-h continuous exposure, after which cells were stained with MTT and measured colorimetrically. The concentrations of hypoxanthine (Hx) and AICA in the reversal experiments were 100 and 175 μM, respectively.

Table 3
Ribonucleotide Contents of HeLa/S3 Cells after 168-h Exposure to AG2034

Treatment	UTP	CTP	ATP	GTP
Control	729	130	1643	561
AG2034, 168 h	708	113	569	479

HeLa/S3 cells in folate-free minimal essential medium containing 2 nM leucovorin were treated with 10 nM AG2034, and nucleotide levels were determined in 0.7 N perchloric acid extracts by strong anion-exchange HPLC.

Values are expressed as nanomoles/10^9 cells.

of 1, 2, 3, or 4 glutamic acids is also a substrate. Based on K_i, AG2034-glu$_5$ binds GARFT approx 28 times more tightly than AG2034. Therefore, polyglutamylation of AG2034 results in more potent GARFT inhibition.

AG2034 was 3.8-fold more potent than lometrexol as a ligand to mFBP, but AG2032 was 1750-fold weaker. When tested as inhibitors of cell growth, all three GARFT inhibitors gave inhibition at low nanomolar concentrations against both murine (L1210) and human (CCRF-CEM) leukemia cells (Table 2). In all cases, extensive protection was given by both hypoxanthine and by 5-aminoimidazole-4-carboxamide (AICA), confirming the site of action as upstream of AICAR formyltransferase. Against the L1210/CI-920 subline, which lacks a functional reduced-folate carrier (RFC), all three compounds were much less active, suggesting that all three compounds are extensively transported by the RFC.

Under conditions in which AG2034 caused cell-cycle arrest of HeLa/S3 cells in G2 phase (see below) the ribonucleotide pools showed a specifically antipurine effect (Table 3). After a week of continuous exposure to 10 nM AG2034, pools of the pyrimidine nucleotides UTP and CTP were almost identical to control values. GTP was decreased 15% and ATP was depleted by 65%. Table 4 shows the short-term (4 h) effect of three concentrations of AG2034 on L1210 cells. Again, the pyrimidine ribonucleotides were not much changed (except for an increase in UTP at the highest concentration). A modest, dose-dependent decrease in GTP was seen (up to 45% depletion), and a somewhat greater decline in ATP (up to 61%). These decreases in purine ribonucleotide levels were sufficient to cause a marked decline in rates of nucleic acid synthesis. Fig. 2 shows DNA and RNA synthesis in L1210 cells treated with 1 μM AG2034 for up to 4 h. By 4 h, both DNA and RNA synthesis rates had decreased by more than 60%,

Table 4
Ribonucleotide Contents of L1210 Cells after a 4-h Exposure to AG2034

Treatment	UTP	CTP	ATP	GTP
Control	330	199	2210	552
AG2034, 10 nM, 4 h	379	225	2190	535
AG2034, 100 nM, 4 h	393	229	1370	353
AG2034, 1 μM, 4 h	558	239	882	304

Early log-phase cells were treated with AG2034 for 4 h, and nucleotide levels were determined in 0.7 N perchloric acid extracts by strong anion-exchange HPLC.

Values are expressed as nanomoles/10^9 cells.

DNA and RNA Synthesis in L1210 Cells Treated with AG2034

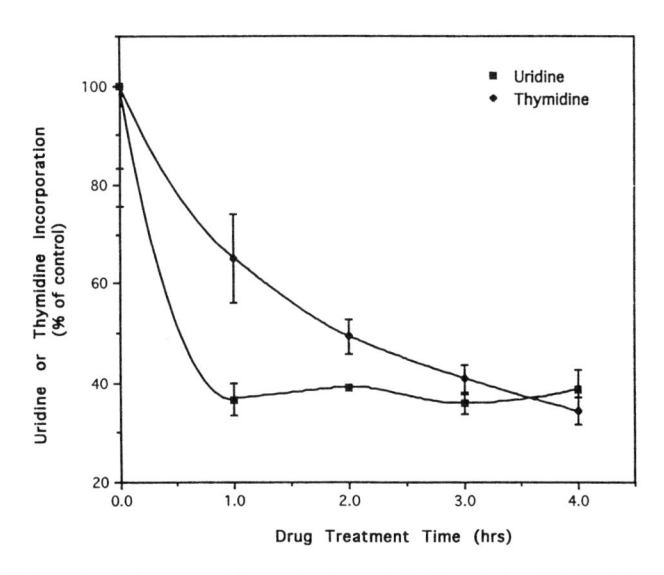

Fig. 2. Inhibition of DNA and RNA synthesis in L1210 cells by AG2034 (1 μM) based upon incorporation of radiolabeled thymidine and uridine, respectively, into material insoluble in 10% trichloroacetic acid.

with the most rapid decline being in RNA synthesis. These results are consistent with purine nucleotide depletion, resulting from GARFT inhibition, being the primary site of action of AG2034.

3. THE ANTITUMOR ACTIVITY OF AG2034 IN VIVO

The antitumor activity of AG2034 against three transplanted murine tumors and four human tumor xenografts (all as sc implants) was reported by Boritzki et al. *(12)*. In these studies, drugs were administered by ip injection, daily for 9 d, beginning 1 d after tumor

Table 5
Comparative in Vivo Toxicities of AG2032 and AG2034 in Mice Fed Normal and Low Folate Diets

Compound	Diet	Treatment schedule	Maximum tolerated dose (mg/kg)	
			per injection	cumulative
Lometrexol	normal	qd 1–9	40	360
Lometrexol	normal	qd 1–5	100	500
Lometrexol	low folate	qd 1–5	0.5	2.5
AG2032	normal	qd 1–9	150	1350
AG2032	normal	qd 1–5	200	1000
AG2032	low folate	qd 1–9	5	25
AG2034	normal	qd 1–9	12.5	112.5
AG2034	normal	qd 1–5	40	200
AG2034	low folate	qd 1–5	0.2	1

The treatment route was intraperitoneal

implantation. Based upon maximum tolerated doses on this protocol, AG2034 was approximately fourfold more dose-potent than lometrexol. AG2034 showed activity similar to or greater than that of lometrexol against the murine tumours, 6C3HED lymphosarcoma, C3H/BA mammary carcinoma, and B16 melanoma (these studies compared the two compounds head-to-head). Lometrexol was not tested against the xenograft lines. AG2034 gave growth delays ranging from 6.5 d against the KM20L2 human colon carcinoma to 21 d against the H460 human nonsmall-cell lung carcinoma (the other lines in which activity was seen were the LX-1 lung carcinoma and the HxGC3 colon carcinoma

The schedule dependence of AG2034 in vivo activity was assessed against the C3H/BA mouse mammary carcinoma *(12)*. Treatment once daily for 3 d gave a moderate growth delay (9 d), and daily treatment for 9 d was slightly more active (10.9 d growth delay). Surprisingly, daily treatment (or twice daily treatment) for 5 d was less active than the 3-d regimen. The most active protocol was treatment twice weekly for 2 wk (i.e. 1, 4, 7, and 10) which gave a growth delay of 14.9 d. Much higher doses of AG2034 could be given on the intermittent regimen than with daily dosing: The maximum tolerated dose on the twice-weekly regimen was 200 mg/kg/injection, compared with 10 mg/kg/injection on the daily ×9 protocol.

4. TOXICITY TO FOLATE-DEPLETED MICE

Because of the observation of Grindey and his colleagues that lometrexol was much more toxic to folate-depleted mice *(5–7)* it was of interest to determine whether the same effect was seen with AG2032, whose binding to mFBP is almost 2000-fold weaker than that of lometrexol. Results are shown in Table 5. With lometrexol we approximately reproduced the results of Grindey et al. *(5)*, obtaining a 200-fold decrease in maximum tolerated dose (MTD) in the folate-depleted mice, relative to mice fed standard laboratory diet. AG2034 was also 200-fold more toxic to the folate-depleted mice. With AG2032 the difference was 40-fold, suggesting that mFBP binding may contribute to the potentiation of toxicity under low-folate conditions, but that it cannot be the only contributory

Table 6
In Vivo Activity of Combinations of AG2034 and Trimetrexate Against the C3H/BA Murine Mammary Tumor

Dose of AG2034 (mg/kg)	Dose of trimetrexate (mg/kg)	Growth delay (days)
0	1.5	1.8
2.5	0	4.5
5.0	0	4.9
10.0	0	5.0
2.5	1.5	5.3
5.0	1.5	7.8
10.0	1.5	toxic

Groups of six mice were inoculated with trochar fragments subcutaneously in the flank, and treatment was initiated 1 d later. Treatment was intraperitoneal, daily for 5 d. Tumors were measured in two orthogonal dimensions with calipers, and tumor mass calculated by the ellipsoid formula. Results are expressed as the median growth delay in days (days for treated tumour to reach evaluation size of 750 mg minus days for control tumour to reach 750 mg).

factor. Perhaps for both AG2032 and AG2034 greater amounts of inhibitor polyglutamates accumulate under low-folate conditions.

5. THE KISLIUK EFFECT

In 1985, Kisliuk et al. *(13)* reported that the antibacterial activities of CB3717 (a TS inhibitor) and of lometrexol were strongly potentiated by the lipophilic dihydrofolate reductase (DHFR) inhibitor, trimethoprim. This observation was extended to mammalian cells by Galivan et al. *(14–16)* who reported that trimetrexate, metoprine, or methotrexate potentiated CB3717 and lometrexol in H35 rat hepatoma cells, that the effect was related to depletion of tetrahydrofolate polyglutamates in presence of a DHFR inhibitor, and that this enhanced the polyglutamylation of lometrexol. We shall refer to this synergistic interaction between a DHFR inhibitor and a polyglutamylatable inhibitor of TS or GARFT as "the Kisliuk effect." Ferguson et al. *(17)* showed that therapeutic synergism between methotrexate and lometrexol could be obtained in mice bearing the L1210 leukemia, though the combination was less efficacious than the maximum tolerated dose of methotrexate used as a single agent. Kisliuk et al. extended the observation to human lymphoma cells in vitro, and reported that the degree of synergy was enhanced by high folic acid concentration in the medium *(18)*. Gaumont et al. quantified the drug interaction using the response-surface method *(19)*. This technique calculates an interaction parameter, α; for an additive interaction, α is zero, for antagonism α is negative, and a positive α indicates synergism. In standard tissue-culture medium (which contains 2.2 μM folic acid), Gaumont et al. found α of 4.7 (marked synergism) and in medium containing 40 μM folic acid, α was 53.6 (extremely strong synergism). Finally, Faessel et al. *(20)* showed that the combination of trimetrexate and AG2034 gave α as high as 480 in HCT-8 cells.

Table 6 presents the first in vivo data showing that a combination of trimetrexate plus a GARFT inhibitor may be more active than either single agent at its MTD. In the C3H/BA mouse mammary tumor, the optimal dose of AG2034, used as a single agent, gave a 5-d growth delay. A low dose of trimetrexate (1.5 mg/kg) gave a growth delay of under 2 d. When this dose of trimetrexate was combined with 10 mg/kg of AG2034 (or if higher doses of trimetrexate were used) the combination was extremely toxic. However, the combination of AG2034 at 5 mg/kg with trimetrexate at 1.5 mg/kg was well tolerated, and gave a longer growth delay than either single agent at its optimal dose.

6. CYTOTOXICITY IN RELATION TO FOLATE AND P53 STATUS

Clonogenic assay studies with HeLa/S3 human cervical carcinoma cells showed that the cytotoxicity of AG2034 was highly dependent upon the composition of the cell-culture medium: in standard minimal essential medium (MEM), which contained 2.2 μM folic acid, AG2034 gave complete cytostasis at concentrations above 10 nM, but no cell kill, even at a concentration of 100 μM for 14 d. When the cells were cloned in MEM containing 50 nM folic acid (closer to physiological conditions), AG2034 was highly cytotoxic, giving approx 90% cell kill at 10 nM, and 100% cell kill at 100 nM *(21)*. In contrast, growth in low-folate conditions only slightly increased the cytotoxicity of AG2034 to A549 human lung carcinoma cells: after a 21-d exposure, 100 μM AG2034 gave approx 40% cell kill in normal MEM, and approx 50% kill in low-folate medium. Because of the marked effect of the folate concentration in the culture medium on the response of the cells to AG2034, all the subsequent experiments described below were carried out in medium containing 50 nM folic acid. The observation that 0.1 μM AG2034 was completely lethal to HeLa/S3 cells, but that a concentration 1000-fold higher gave only 50% kill (at physiological folate concentration) indicated an unusual degree of cell selectivity for an antimetabolite, and prompted an extension of this study to further cell types *(21)*. The SW480 human colon carcinoma cell line responded similarly to HeLa/S3, in this case 10 nM AG2034 giving complete cell kill. The human breast carcinoma line, MCF-7, like A549, only suffered approx 50% cell kill after prolonged exposure to 100 μM AG2034. These results suggested a sharp dichotomy between the response to AG2034 of cells with normal p53 and a functional G1 checkpoint (A549, MCF-7), in which only a minor degree of cytotoxicity was seen, even at extremely high concentrations, and cells lacking a functional G1 checkpoint, probably because they do not have normal p53 function (HeLa/S3, SW480) which were highly sensitive to AG2034-induced cytotoxicity. Measurements of purine ribonucleotide pools by anion-exchange high pressure liquid chromatography in HeLa/S3, MCF-7, and A549 cells showed marked decreases in all these cell lines *(21)*. Thus the inability of AG2034 to kill A549 and MCF-7 cells was not a result of lack of effect on *de novo* purine biosynthesis.

7. CELL-CYCLE EFFECTS OF AG2034

Many studies have shown that p53 mediates a G1 arrest in cells following treatment with DNA-damaging agents, and it is generally believed that DNA damage is the upstream signal that triggers p53-mediated cell cycle arrest *(22–24)*. Our results showed that 24-h exposure of L1210 cells to a known TS inhibitor, Thymitaq (AG337), gave a dose-dependent incidence of DNA strand breaks, as measured by alkaline elution *(21)*. When HeLa/S3 cells were cultured in the presence of 10 μM AG2034 in folate-free

MEM supplemented with 50 nM folic acid, and DNA was extracted and subjected to agarose gel electrophoresis, even after 1 wk of treatment, DNA from the attached cells showed no indication of strand breaks. If DNA was extracted from the dying floating cells, it streaked on the gel, indicating a continuum of lower molecular weights, but showed no sign of the DNA ladder pattern characteristic of apoptosis. However, DNA extracted from L1210 cells that had been treated for 48 h at 10 nM, 100 nM, 1 μM, 10 μM, or 100 μM showed classical DNA ladder patterns, indicating that L1210 cells treated with AG2034 undergo apoptosis. Another approach to measuring DNA damage, the TUNEL assay, measures DNA nicks by end-labeling the DNA strands with deoxyuridine, which is then visualized with a fluorescent antibody. This assay showed that AG2034 at 100 μM gave no DNA breaks after 48 h, but that by 72 h 20% of A549 cells (which has a functional p53) and over 90% of SW480 (which lacks functional p53) were labeled, presumably indicating that the treated cells were undergoing apoptosis.

Flow cytometric studies of cell-cycle distribution *(21)* indicated that in two cell lines with a G1 checkpoint, A549 and H460, treatment with AG2034 at 10 μM gave an increased fraction of cells in G1, and decreased the fraction in S + G2 + M. Conversely, in two lines that lacked a G1 checkpoint, HeLa/S3 and SW480, the fraction of cells in S-phase was sharply increased. Another experiment followed HeLa/S3 cells that were treated with 10 nM AG2034; by 24 h the fraction of cells in S-phase was increased, relative to control. The cells moved slowly through S-phase, and by 168 h (1 wk) the surviving cells were mainly in G2-phase. In L1210 cells, also, accumulation in S-phase was seen following treatment with AG2034: A control population had 30% G1:56% S:14% G2 + M. By 48 h after treatment with either 10 nM or 1 μM AG2034, over 90% of cells were in S, and the G2 + M compartment was totally depleted. By 72 h, cells were starting to accumulate in G2 + M, especially at the higher concentrations of AG2034; e.g., after 72 h in 1 μM the distribution of L1210 cells was 15%:G1:62% S:23% G2 + M. These results suggest that under conditions of purine stress, cells continue to move through S-phase, but more slowly than usual.

8. CONCLUSIONS

The starting point for the development of these novel GARFT inhibitors was the desire to design a compound that had the broad-spectrum antitumor activity of lometrexol without its potentially dangerous delayed toxicity. The availability of an X-ray crystal structure, first of the *E. coli* GARFT enzyme with an antifolate inhibitor bound in the active site, and later, the GARFT domain of the human trifunctional enzyme made it possible to adopt a structure-based design approach *(25)*. Two of the compounds resulting from this work were AG2032 and AG2034, compounds that differ only in the presence or absence of a methyl substituent on the thiazole side chain and the substitution of sulphur for carbon at the 5 position (Fig. 1), but whose pharmacological differences have been quite revealing. The methyl substituent resulted in AG2032 being 7000-fold weaker than AG2034 as an mFBP ligand, though it was a better GARFT inhibitor (Table 1), and the two compounds were similar as in vitro growth inhibitors, when measured in standard culture medium (Table 2). In terms of in vivo antitumor activity, AG2032 differed from AG2034 in two respects: it was approx 10-fold less dose-potent, and it had a narrower antitumor spectrum. AG2032 had good activity against the 6C3HED murine lymphosarcoma and the H460 xenograft, but was inactive against the B16 melanoma and the C3H/BA mammary carcinoma (data not shown). Thus removal of mFBP binding made AG2032 less toxic (to mice fed a standard laboratory diet), but resulted in it having the narrow spectrum of activity characteristic of methotrexate, rather than the broad spectrum of lometrexol or AG2034.

In animals fed a low folate diet, AG2032 was 40-fold more toxic than to animals fed a standard laboratory diet. This compares with a 200-fold difference for lometrexol and for AG2034 (Table 5). Perhaps, as suggested by Grindey et al. *(5)* upregulation of mFBP in low folate conditions may explain part of the difference in toxicity of these compounds in low-folate conditions, but the greater part of the effect must be caused by other factors. It seems likely that in low folate conditions, more polyglutamate derivatives of the GARFT inhibitors are formed than under high-folate conditions, and perhaps the polyglutamates turn over more slowly. The effect may be the result of less competition for folylpolyglutamate synthetase (FPGS) from natural folates, or less feedback inhibition of FPGS by natural folylpolyglutamates, or both.

It seems likely that the Kisliuk effect—the remarkable potentiation of polyglutamylatable antifolates by DHFR inhibitors—is related to the greatly enhanced toxicity of GARFT inhibitors under low-folate conditions. DHFR inhibitors cause depletion of tetrahydrofolates, and their polyglutamates, and thus result in greater levels of the other antifolates being polyglutamylated. The degree of potentiation seen with AG2034 and trimetrexate in vitro is one of the strongest synergistic drug interactions ever reported *(20)*. Since the interaction increases toxicity as well as therapeutic activity, it is not yet clear whether this effect will be clinically useful, but the encouraging preliminary combination data shown in Table 6 suggest that it may be.

The other surprising observation to emerge from these studies was that using low, physiological concentrations of folate in vitro did not simply increase the inhibitory potency of AG2034, but (in some cell lines) actually altered the qualitative effect of the inhibitor. The studies with HeLa/S3 and SW480 cells *(21)* showed that in standard cell-culture media, which have an unnaturally high folate concentration, AG2034 was only cytostatic, but that when lower levels of folate (or leucovorin), closer to physiological plasma levels, were used, AG2034 was highly cytotoxic. It is not yet known whether this difference will be seen with other GARFT inhibitors. An implication of this observation is that literature data on in vitro effects of GARFT inhibitors obtained in standard culture medium or medium supplemented with undialyzed serum (such as the NCI in vitro tumor panel, or the human tumour cloning assay) must be interpreted with caution. The second important implication is for clinical trial design: It has been shown *(8)* that folic acid supplementation makes lometrexol a better-tolerated drug, but this work raises the possibility that folic acid supplementation converts the antitumor response from a cytotoxic effect to a cytostatic effect.

Finally, our series of studies with AG2034 showed that cells that lack functional p53, and thus have no G1 checkpoint, respond very differently to treatment with AG2034 at physiological folate concentrations: HeLa/S3 cells and SW480 cells, which lack a functional p53, were killed by 10 nM AG2034, whereas MCF-7 and A549 cells, with normal p53, had only a cytostatic response at a drug concentration 10,000-fold higher, an unprecedented degree of selectivity for an antimetabolite. The explanation for this selectivity became clear from the cell-cycle studies *(21)*. In cells with a G1 checkpoint, purine depletion triggers this checkpoint, and cells accumulate at the G1:S boundary. This observation supports the previous report of Linke et al. *(26)* that ribonucleotide depletion can trigger p53-dependent cell-cycle arrest in the absence of DNA strand breaks. In cells that lack a functional G1 checkpoint (as do about half of advanced human carcinomas), the AG2034-treated cells progress out of G1, and move slowly through S-phase into G2, and at some point undergo apoptotic death. This cell cycle effect of GARFT inhibitors differs markedly from the effect of inhibitors of DHFR or TS, which cause accumulation of cells at the G1/S boundary or in very early S-phase regardless of the p53 status of the cells. Whereas there is still a paucity of data, studies with 5-fluorouracil *(23)* and Tomudex *(27)* suggest that p53-defective cells may be less sensitive to these TS inhibitors. Tonkinson et al. *(28)* reported that human leukemia cells treated with a TS inhibitor were arrested at the G1/S boundary, but that the GARFT inhibitor LY309887 caused an increased number of cells in S-phase (this study was done in standard, high-folate, culture medium).

In summary, the complex cellular pharmacology of the GARFT inhibitors, their multiple modes of cellular uptake, the slow turnover of their polyglutamates, with the potential that this poses for delayed toxicity, and their dependence upon nutritional status, will make the design of optimal clinical trials for this class of drugs quite challenging. However, since most anticancer drugs are less active against the 50% of human cancers that lack a G1 checkpoint, the availability of a new class of antimetabolites, exemplified by AG2034, that have a high degree of selectivity against such cells, should be of great utility.

ACKNOWLEDGMENTS

The authors thank Steve Margosiak and Eleanor Dagostino for providing enzyme kinetic data.

REFERENCES

1. Taylor EC. New pathways from pteridines. Design and synthesis of a new class of potent and selective antitumor agents. *J Heterocyclic Chem* 1990;27:1–12.
2. Beardsley GP, Taylor EC, Grindey GB, Moran RG. Deaza derivatives of tetrahydrofolic acid. A new class of folate antimetabolite. In: Cooper BA, Whitehead VM, eds. Chemistry and Biology of Pteridines. DeGruyter, Berlin, 1986, pp. 953–957.
3. Shih C, Grindey GB, Houghton PJ, Houghton JA. In vivo antitumor activity of 5,10-dideazatetrahydrofolic acid (DDATHF) and its diastereomeric isomers. *Proc Am Assoc Cancer Res* 1991; 32:324.
4. Muggia F, Martin T, Ray M, Leichman CG, Grunberg S, Gill I, Moran R, Dyke R, Grindey G. Phase I clinical trial of weekly 5,10-dideazatetrahydrofolate (LY 26418, DDATHF-B). *Proc Amer Assoc Clin Oncol* 1990; 9:74.
5. Grindey GB, Alati T, Shih C. Reversal of the toxicity but not the antitumor activity of lometrexol by folic acid. *Proc Am Assoc Cancer Res* 1991; 32:324.
6. Schmitz JC, Grindey GB, Schultz RM, Priest DG. Impact of dietary folic acid on reduced folates in mouse plasma and tissues. Relationship to dideazatetrahydrofolate sensitivity. *Biochem Pharmacol* 1994; 48:319–325.
7. Alati T, Worzalla JF, Shih C, Bewley JR, Lewis S, Moran RG, Grindey GB. Augmentation of the therapeutic activity of lometrexol [(6-*R*)5,10-dideazatetrahydrofolate] by oral folic acid. *Cancer Res* 1996; 56:2331–2335.
8. Bailey N, Lind M, Laohavinij S, Robson L, Walling J, McCarthy S, Smith C, Newell D, Calvert AH. A phase I study of 3 weekly lometrexol (DDATHF) with folic acid supplementation. Abstracts, 9th NCI-EORTC Symposium on New Drugs in Cancer Therapy, 1996, p. 90.

9. Smith SG, Lehman NL, Moran RG. Cytotoxicity of antifolate inhibitors of thymidylate and purine synthesis to WiDr colonic carcinoma cells. *Cancer Res* 1993; 53:5697–5706.
10. Almassy RJ, Janson CA, Kan CC, Hostomska Z. Structures of apo and complexed *Escherichia coli* glycinamide ribonucleotide transformylase. *Proc Natl Acad Sci USA* 1992; 89:6114–6118.
11. Varney MD, Palmer CL, Romines WH, Boritzki TJ, Margosiak SA, Almassy R, Janson CA, Bartlett C, Howland EJ, Ferre R. Protein structure-based design, synthesis and biological evaluation of 5-thia-2,6-diamino-4-(3H)-oxopyrimidines: inhibitors of glycinamide bibonucleotide transformylase with potent cell growth inhibition. *J Med Chem* 1997; 40:2502–24.
12. Boritzki TJ, Bartlett CA, Zhang C, Howland EF, Margosiak SA, Palmer CL, Romines WH, Jackson RC. AG2034: a novel inhibitor of glycinamide ribonucleotide formyltransferase. *Invest New Drugs* 1996; 14:295–303.
13. Kisliuk RL, Gaumont Y, Kumar M, Coutts M, Nanavate NT, Kalman TI. The effect of polyglutamylation on the inhibitory activity of folate analogs. In: Goldman ID, ed. Proceedings of the Second Workshop on Folyl and Antifolyl Polyglutamates. Praeger, New York, 1985, pp. 319–328.
14. Galivan J, Nimec Z, Rhee M. Synergistic growth inhibition of hepatoma cells exposed in vitro to propargyl-5,8-dideazafolate with methotrexate or the lipophilic antifolates trimetrexate and metoprine. *Cancer Res* 1987; 47:5256–5260.
15. Galivan J, Nimec Z, Rhee M, Boschelli DH, Oronsky AL, Kerwar SS. Antifolate drug interactions. Enhancement of growth inhibition due to the antipurine 5,10-dideazatetrahydrofolic acid by the lipophilic dihydrofolate reductase inhibitors metoprine and trimetrexate. *Cancer Res* 1988; 48:2421–2425.
16. Galivan J, Rhee MS, Johnson TB, Dilwith R, Nair MG, Bunni M, Priest DG. The role of cellular folates in the enhancement of activity of the thymidylate synthase inhibitor 10-propargyl-5,8-dideazafolate against hepatoma cells *in vitro* by inhibitors of dihydrofolate reductase. *J Biol Chem.* 1989; 264:10,685–10,692.
17. Ferguson K, Boschelli D, Hoffman P, Oronsky A, Whiteley J, Webber S, Galivan J, Freisheim J, Hynes J, Kerwar SS. Synergy between 5,10-dideaza-5,6,7,8-tetrahydrofolic acid and methotrexate in mice bearing L1210 tumors. *Cancer Chemother Pharmacol* 1989; 25:173–176.
18. Kisliuk RL, Gaumont Y, Powers JF, Thorndike J, Nair MG, Piper JR. Synergistic growth inhibition by combinations of antifolates. In: MF Picciano, ELR Stokstad, JF Gregory, eds. Evaluation of Folate Metabolism in Health and Disease. Liss, New York, 1990, pp. 79–89.
19. Gaumont Y, Kisliuk RL, Parsons JC, Greco WR. Quantitation of folic acid enhancement of antifolate synergism. *Cancer Res* 1992; 52:2228–2235.
20. Faessel H, Slocum HK, Jackson RC, Boritzki T, Rustum YM, Greco WR. Super in vitro synergy between trimetrexate and the polyglutamatable antifolates AG2034, AG2032, AG2009 and Tomudex against human HCT-8 colon cells. *Proc Am Assoc Cancer Res* 1986; 37:385.
21. Zhang CC, Boritzki TJ, Jackson RC. An inhibitor of glycinamide ribonucleotide formyltransferase is selectively cytotoxic to cells that lack a functional G1 checkpoint. *Cancer Chemother Pharmacol* 1998; 41:223–8.
22. Yin Y, Tainsky MA, Bischoff FZ, Strong LC, Wahl GM. Wild-type p53 is required for radiation-induced cell cycle control and inhibits gene amplification in cells with mutant p53 alleles. *Cell* 1992; 70:937–48.
23. Lowe SW, Ruley HE, Jacks T, Housman DE. p53-Dependent apoptosis modulates the cytotoxicity of anticancer agents. *Cell* 1993; 74:957–967.
24. White E. p53, guardian of Rb. *Nature* 1994; 371:21–2.
25. Jackson RC. Contributions of protein structure-based drug design to cancer chemotherapy. *Semin Oncol* 1997; 24:164–172.
26. Linke SP, Clarkin KC, DiLeonardo A, Tsou A, Wahl GM. A reversible, p53-dependent G0/G1 cell cycle arrest induced by ribonucleotide depletion in the absence of detectable DNA damage. *Genes Dev* 1996; 10:934–7.
27. Arredondo MA, Yin MB, Lu K, Schüber C, Slocum HK, Rustum YM. Decreased c-myc protein accompanied by increased p53 and Rb is associated with thymidylate synthase inhibition and cell cycle retardation induced by D1694. *Proc Am Assoc Cancer Res* 1994; 35:304.
28. Tonkinson JL, Marder P, Andis SL, Schultz RL, Gossett LS, Shih C, Mendelsohn LG. Cell cycle effects of antifolate antimetabolites: implications for cytotoxicity and cytostasis. *Cancer Chemother Pharmacol* 1997; 39:521–31.

14 Receptor- and Carrier-Mediated Transport Systems for Folates and Antifolates

Exploitation for Folate-Based Chemotherapy and Immunotherapy

G. Jansen

CONTENTS

INTRODUCTION
FOLATE INFLUX AND EFFLUX SYSTEMS
REDUCED FOLATE CARRIER (RFC)
MEMBRANE FOLATE RECEPTOR (MFR)/MEMBRANE-ASSOCIATED FOLATE BINDING PROTEIN (mFBP)
LOW pH TRANSPORT ROUTE
HIGH CAPACITY/LOW AFFINITY ROUTE
PASSIVE/FACILITATED DIFFUSION
RFC AND MFR TRANSPORT OF ANTIFOLATE DRUGS; STRUCTURE-ACTIVITY RELATIONSHIPS
MFR AS A TARGET FOR MOV18-GUIDED IMMUNOTHERAPY AND MACROMOLECULE TRANSPORT
CONCLUSIONS
ACKNOWLEDGEMENTS
REFERENCES

1. INTRODUCTION

Eukaryotic cells lack the possibility of *de novo* biosynthesis of reduced folate cofactors that are required as one-carbon donors in the biosynthesis of thymidylate, purines, and amino acids *(1)*. For this reason, cellular folate homeostasis depends on the delivery of reduced folate cofactors from extracellular fluids. At a physiological pH, the negatively charged α- and γ-carboxyl groups of the glutamate side chain of reduced folate cofactors change these molecules into divalent anions that cannot simply pass the plasma membrane but require (a) specific transport system(s) for their cellular entry. The importance of folate metabolism in tumor cells has been recognized for a long time as a potential target for chemotherapy *(2–6)*. Historically, classical folate analogs such as aminopterin (AMT) and methotrexate (MTX) were recognized to disrupt folate metabolism through inhibition of dihydrofolate reductase (DHFR) *(7)*. More recently, folate analogs were synthesized that could target other key enzymes in folate metabolism, including thymidylate synthase (TS) *(8,9)*, glycinamide ribonucleotide transformylase (GARTFase) *(10,11)*, and folylpolyglutamate synthetase (FPGS) *(12)*. A number of these novel antifolates have demonstrated potential clinical activity *(3,13–18)*. The majority of these folate analogs share the common feature that efficient membrane transport is the first determining factor in exerting their biological activity. This chapter will mainly focus on the role of two folate transport systems that are considered to be of the greatest relevance from the perspective of mediating folate homeostasis and the delivery of folate-based chemotherapeutic drugs into tumor cells. These transporters include the reduced folate carrier (RFC) *(19–22)* and a membrane-associated folate receptor (MFR) *(22–25)*, also referred to as membrane-associated folate-binding protein (mFBP). A summary of some molecular, biochemical, and functional properties of these transporters will be given (*see*, e.g., Table 1) along with a few examples how these properties (see Fig. 2A, B, below) may be translated into an improved biological/cytotoxic activity of antifolate drugs (*see* Table 2).

2. FOLATE INFLUX AND EFFLUX SYSTEMS

The net cellular uptake of (anti)folates is largely determined by the dynamic interaction of (multiple) unidirectional or bidirectional transport routes that control their influx and efflux rates. Whereas over the past three decades a large number of studies have been dedicated to delineate the molecular and biochemical events of (anti)folate influx into malignant cells, the role of (anti)folate efflux transporter(s) has remained relatively disregarded. For MTX, multiple efflux transporters have been identified, including multispecific organic anion transporters (MOAT) and the RFC itself *(26–29)*. Although the efflux issue will not be addressed further in this chapter, a number of recent studies have underlined that the (in)activity of efflux routes can contribute significantly to the biological activity of antifolates. Schlemmer and Sirotnak *(30)* demonstrated a large differential in efflux efficiency between folic acid and antifolates in L1210 cells. Antifolates such as AMT and the TS inhibitor ZD1694 *(13,14)* were markedly more efficient substrates for efflux than MTX, which itself was more efficiently effluxed than folic acid. In Chinese hamster ovary cells, a defective efflux of folic acid *(31)* resulted in an increased intracellular level of folates which, consequently, abolished the biological activity of a number of (lipophilic) antifolates *(32)*.

Since differential transport may contribute to antifolate drug selectivity, characterization of folate transporter(s) in normal cells is of great relevance. Unfortunately, this type of information is not largely available, perhaps with the exception of the tissue distribution of membrane folate receptors *(33–36,* see also subheading 4.3), and intestinal folate transporters which are involved in the dietary uptake of folates. These 'nutritional' transporters (reviewed in refs. *25,37–39*) are structurally and functionally different from folate transporters in malignant cells. For example, intestinal transport of folates is a carrier-mediated process that is driven by a transmembrane pH gradient and proceeds

Table 1
Characteristic Features of RFC and MFR-isoforms

	RFC	MFR-α	MFR-β	MFR-γ	Refs
Encoding gene(s)	RFC1	MFR-α	MFR-β	MFR-γ	(59–66,100–104)
Molecular weight	46–48 kDa (rodents) 70–120 kDa (human)	28–40 kDa	28–38 kDa	25–32 kDa	(23–25,51,54,57)
Membrane orientation	transmembrane	GPI-anchored	GPI-anchored	secretory protein	(20–22,95,96)
Mechanism of transport	anion-exchange mechanism driven by anion gradients	(a) endocytosis (b) potocytosis	(a) endocytosis (?) (b) potocytosis (?)		(44,45,111–115)
K_m RFC transport/ Ki [^{3}H] Folic acid binding to MFR	Folic acid: 200–400 μM (6S)5-CH$_3$THF: 1–5 μM (6R)5-CH$_3$THF: 3–10 μM MTX: 2–10 μM	Folic acid: 0.35 nM (6S)5-CH$_3$THF: 1 nM (6R)5-CH$_3$THF: 4 nM MTX: 114 nM	Folic acid: 1.5 nM (6S) 5-CH$_3$THF: 55 nM (6R)5-CH$_3$THF: 7.5 nM MTX: 1900 nM	Folic acid: 0.4 nM (6S) 5-CH$_3$THF: 2.2 nM (6R)5-CH$_3$THF: 2.4 nM	(20–22,108,109,122)
Molecular specific activity (molecules MTX/binding site/hr)[a]	116	1.2	2.7		(125,141)

[a]For L1210 cells with defective RFC transport at V_{max} conditions (125,141).

Table 2
Growth Inhibitory Effects of Antifolates as a Function of RFC- and/or MFR-Mediated Transport in Murine and Human Leukemia Cells (IC$_{50}$ [nM], 72 h drug exposure)

	CCRF-CEM (RFC+/MFR−) (2 μM FA)	CEM/MTX (RFC−/MFR−) (2 μM FA)	CEM-7A (RFC+++/MFR−) (1 nM LV)	L1210 (RFC+/MFR−) (2 μM FA)	L1210-B73 (RFC+/MFR+++) (1 nM LV)	L1210-B73 (RFC+/MFR+++) (20 nM FA)	L1210-MFR (RFC−/MFR+++) (1 nM LV)	L1210-MFR (RFC−/MFR+++) (20 nM FA)
MTX	8.1	1950	1.2	2.2	3.4	10	19	1400
EDX	1.3	533	0.3	1.6	2.9	4.3	24	703
PT523	1.1	33	0.7	0.7	2.7	3	54	2504
CB3717	705	7750	36	395	2.8	29	1.1	24
IAHQ	1090	17075	71	705	2.1	30	0.9	39
ICI-198583	17	605	3.2	9.1	0.2	57	0.3	74
ZD1694	3.5	444	0.7	3	0.5	23	0.2	117
GW1843	2.4	520	1.1	23	1.9	12	0.8	12
LY231514	23	470	5.2	14	4.1	16	1.6	162
ICI-198583-D-Glu	500	6680	46	460	2.1	84	4	970
ZD9331	16	286	6.7	16	1.2	12	0.8	73
DDATHF	11	80	2.2	9.2	4.1	88	1.6	93
AG2034	27	122	4.3	30	22	n.d.	18	225

Data in this table were taken, in part, from ref. *122*. This reference provides additional background information regarding characteristics of the cell lines and growth inhibition conditions.

FA: folic acid, LV: leucovorin, IC50: drug concentration providing 50% growth inhibition.

with relatively similar affinities for folic acid, reduced folate cofactors, and antifolates such as MTX *(40,41)*.

Collectively, detailed information regarding differences in molecular, biochemical, and functional properties of folate transporters in normal cells and malignant cells will be helpful for a rational design of strategies that improve the chemotherapeutic efficacy of antifolate drugs by increasing drug uptake in malignant cells and protecting normal cells from toxic effects. Subheadings 3. and 4. will give an overview of the current status of experimental and clinically directed research regarding RFC and MFR. The potential relevance of other transporters will be discussed just briefly (subheadings 5., 6., and 7.).

3. REDUCED FOLATE CARRIER (RFC)

3.1. Kinetic Properties, Mechanism of Uptake, Regulation of Transport Activity

Since the original reports of Kessel *(42)* and Goldman *(43)* on the kinetics of MTX uptake in murine leukemia cells, a carrier-mediated transport process was characterized for the uptake of reduced folate cofactors in a variety of other mammalian cells *(20–22)*. This reduced folate carrier (RFC) displays saturable and high-affinity transport for reduced folate cofactors 5-formyltetrahydrofolate (5-CHO-THF, leucovorin) and 5-methyltetrahydrofolate (5-CH$_3$-THF) (K_m 1–3 µM), and the antifolate MTX (K_m 3–26 µM). In contrast, folic acid is transported with a poor affinity (K_m 200–400 µM) by the RFC. Furthermore, RFC transport is pH-, energy-, and temperature-dependent (Q_{10} 27–37°C 6–8). A characteristic feature of RFC-mediated transport is the inhibitory effect of structurally (un)related organic and inorganic anions, e.g., 5-CHO-THF, phosphate, bicarbonate, NADP, and AMP/ADP *(44,45)*. On the other hand, preloading of intact cells with 5-CHO-THF, or loading of plasma membrane vesicles with 5-CHO-THF or phosphate, (trans)stimulated the uptake of MTX *(46,47)*. These and other results have supported the currently accepted concept of RFC-mediated MTX transport being a bidirectional carrier process that requires anion gradients to drive uphill transport of MTX. However, since direct evidence for the exchange of an intracellular anion for an extracellular MTX anion has not been clearly demonstrated, it is possible that anions can have other (regulatory) effects on RFC transport that may facilitate transport, e.g., by altering of the carrier mobility in the membrane or altering the ionization status of MTX *(47)*.

The cellular expression and functional activity of the RFC can vary significantly as a result of up- or downregulation of synthesis of the transport protein and/or efficiency of carrier functioning. In addition to changes in the anionic status of the extracellular medium, several other conditions can have an impact on RFC transport: in cell-culture experiments, RFC expression is optimal in the logarithmic phase of growth and up to threefold lower in the stationary phase of growth *(48)*; differentiation/maturation of HL60 leukemia cells decreased RFC-mediated influx of MTX and the amount of RFC protein by at least fivefold *(49)*; and prolonged cell culture in medium containing low concentrations of folates (<1 nM) can upregulate the expression of RFC protein and transport activity *(50–53)*. In this regard, our laboratory has isolated a variant (CEM-7A) of human CCRF-CEM leukemia cells that displayed a 30-fold increased expression of

RFC protein along with a 95-fold increased V_{max} for MTX influx *(52)*. In this cell line, transport activity (but not transport protein) could be downregulated 7–9-fold in a rapid (<1 h) response to changes in the cellular folate pool and purine (nucleotide) status *(52,54,55)*. Subsequently, several cell lines with different histological phenotypes were isolated that displayed a 3–10-fold increased RFC activity upon adaptation in low-folate medium *(56)*. So, this phenomenon seems to be a universal characteristic.

Finally, one other potential site of regulation of RFC transport activity has been indicated from studies by Price *(57)*, Freisheim *(54)*, and Jansen et al. *(55,56)* who showed that RFC-mediated transport of a radiolabeled photoaffinity of MTX proceeded via a specific pathway: following membrane translocation via the RFC, the photoprobe is initially transferred to a 38-kDa protein prior to its final target DHFR. It has been postulated that this 38-kDa protein, which is either a cytosolic protein or loosely associated with the plasma membrane or cytosolic, serves as an intracellular shuttle protein for (anti)folates. Additional elucidation of the underlying biochemical and metabolic mechanism(s) of RFC transport regulation will be of importance as it may be a determining factor in establishing folate homeostasis and intracellular levels of antifolate uptake.

3.2. Biochemistry and Genetics

Affinity-labeling experiments identified the RFC in rodent cells as being a membrane protein with a molecular weight of 46–48 kDa *(51,57)*. In human cells, extensive N-linked and O-linked glycosylation yields a much higher apparent molecular weight of the RFC (80–120 kD) *(54,55,58,59)*.

Recently, several research groups have reported the isolation of cDNA clones from rodent and mammalian cells that encode for a protein *(RFC1)* that is involved in (anti)folate transport *(59–66)*. These studies revealed a number of features of the human *RFC1* gene/protein. The gene is localized on chromosome 21 (21q22.2-q22.3) *(64,67)*, there is 65–80% amino acid sequence homology between human and rodent *RFC1* *(59,62–64)*, and, on the basis of hydropathy plots, the *RFC1* appears to be a glycoprotein which has 12 transmembrane spanning domains *(60,64)*. Furthermore, several lines of evidence support a correlation between *RFC1* and RFC-mediated transport of (anti)folates: bidirectional MTX transport as well as MTX sensitivity is restored in MTX-transport defective cells upon transfection with *RFC1* cDNA *(29,59,60,62,64,68)*; *RFC1* mRNA transcript levels were differentially expressed in MTX-transport upregulated and downregulated cells *(56,59,69)*; *RFC1* gene amplication has been noted in RFC upregulated cells *(56,69)*; and mutations in the *RFC1* gene have been associated with transport-related resistance to MTX *(70–73)*. It is noteworthy that elevated RFC transport following *RFC1* cDNA transfection *(29)* has a different effect on cellular (anti)folate accumulation than elevated RFC transport that can be observed in cells selected in folate-restricted medium *(50,52)*. *RFC1* cDNA transfections in transport-defective murine L1210 cells established only a minor (twofold) increase in the intracellular exchangeable pool of MTX *(29)* since the bidirectionality of transport also increased the rate of MTX efflux through the RFC route. In contrast, efflux rates were largely unaltered in cell lines with upregulated RFC transport after selection in folate-restricted medium *(50,52)*. In another study, Wong et al. *(68)* showed that upon *RFC1* cDNA transfection in human leukemia cells the large increase in the expression of RFC protein was not accompanied by a concomitant increase in RFC transport capacity. Altogether, these studies indicate that additional factor(s) may play a role in regulating influx/efflux rates of (anti)folates *(54,55)* and/or sequestration into intracellular compartments from which efflux is impaired *(74)*.

Besides the above-mentioned correlates between RFC and *RFC1*, there are still a number of unresolved issues that remain to be addressed in the near future, e.g., rodent and human *RFC1* cDNAs encode for a protein with a predicted molecular weight of 58 and 64–66 kDa, respectively *(59–64)*, whereas affinity-labeling techniques have identified a different apparent molecular weight for rodent RFC (46–48 kDa) and human RFC (80–120 kDa); antibodies raised against *RFC1* synthetic peptides *(64)* do not seem to recognize the glycosylated human RFC protein; human *RFC1* cDNA contains only one site of N-linked glycosylation *(59–64)* which seems inconsistent with the extensive degree of glycosylation of RFC; and *RFC1* displays homology with a 58-kDa folate transporter in mouse small intestine *(75,76)*.

3.3. Biodistribution RFC

Prior to the application of RT-PCR technology to detect RFC levels *(77)*, differences in the cellular expression of RFC have been documented on the basis of functional activity *(20)*. Original reports on the immunohistochemical staining of RFC *(22,78,79)* were revisited because of the lack of full specificity of the antibody that was directed against the glycosylated human RFC *(59)*. Recently, Chiao et al. *(80)* reported the generation of a specific antibody against murine RFC, but this antibody has not yet been employed for immunohistochemical purposes. Constitutive functional RFC activity has been demonstrated in a variety of tumor cell lines of different origin *(20,22)*. In general, RFC activity is relatively high in undifferentiated neoplastic and fetal tissues, whereas its activity declines significantly upon cellular maturation/differentiation *(48,49)*. Detailed studies on clinical specimens have been limited predominantly to (childhood) leukemia cells and soft-tissue sarcoma cells that display a wide variation in molecular and functional RFC(1) expression *(72,81–83)*. Moscow et al. *(77)* reported on the RT-PCR analysis of *RFC1* mRNA expression in 40 of the 60 cell lines in the NCI drug screen panel. *RFC1* mRNA levels varied over a range of 15-fold and correlated (rho: 0.294) positively with MTX cytotoxicity. *RFC1* mRNA expression was relatively the highest in breast-cancer cell lines and leukemias, and the lowest in CNS and lung tumor cell lines. Intermediate values were observed for melanomas, colon, and renal cancer cell lines.

3.4. (RFC) Transport-Related Antifolate Resistance

Defective transport via the RFC as a result of qualitative (increased K_m or decreased V_{max} for uptake) or quantitative defects (decreased RFC expression) has been recognized as a common mechanism of antifolate resistance in cell lines and clinical specimens, including leukemias *(3,46,72,79,84–91)*. Delineation of the molecular and biochemical basis for RFC transport defects showed that either a single amino acid substitution in a putative transmembrane domain of the *RFC1* cDNA, or single/double mutations in the *RFC1* gene resulting in premature stop codons, were responsible for the expression of functionally inactive transport protein *(70–73)*. Recently, a novel mechanism of transport-related resistance to antifolates was reported to be associated with the expression of an altered RFC protein that exhibited a decreased K_m for transport of folic acid and reduced folate cofactors. As a result of the increased efficiency of folate uptake, the cellular folate pool can rise to such a high level that it abolishes polyglutamylation of antifolates along with their cytotoxic activity *(55,92,93)*.

4. MEMBRANE FOLATE RECEPTOR (MFR)/MEMBRANE-ASSOCIATED FOLATE BINDING PROTEIN (mFBP)

Folate-binding protein is a generic term for proteins including enzymes utilizing folate as a cofactor, serum protein such as albumin, and specific binding proteins that bind folates with receptor-like high affinities *(21,23–25)*. High-affinity folate binding proteins/folate receptors may exist in a particulate, cell-membrane-associated form, or in a soluble form. Soluble FBPs may have a function in folate transfer in serum and/or may act as facilitators in folate absorption *(21,94)*. The following sections will focus on the role of membrane-associated FBPs/folate receptors (MFR) in (anti)folate transport.

4.1. MFR Biochemistry and Genetics

MFRs reside in the outer layer of the plasma membrane by means of a linkage via glycosylphosphatidylinositol (GPI) anchor attached to the C-terminus of the protein *(95–97)*. Soluble forms of MFR may arise from proteolytic cleavage (metalloproteases) or by cleavage via GPI-specific phospholipase C *(95–98)*. MFRs are membrane proteins with a high affinity for folic acid (K_d 0.1–1 nM); the affinity of the receptor for reduced folate cofactors and MTX is approx threefold and 100-fold lower, respectively, compared to folic acid *(21,23–25,99)*. Currently, at least three MFR isoforms have been identified which are encoded by MFR genes localized on chromosome 11 (q13.3–q13.5) *(100)*. The cDNA of the MFR-α isoform was isolated from human nasopharyngeal KB cells, human placenta, and CaCo-2 cells *(95,101)*. The cDNA for MFR-β from human placenta *(102)*, and the cDNA for the MFR-γ isoform was recently cloned from malignant human hematopoietic cells *(103)*. The MFR isoforms share approx 70% amino acid sequence homology. MFR-α and -β are GPI-linked to the membrane, MFR-γ is a secretory protein since it lacks a signal for GPI attachment *(104)*. The cDNAs for MFR-α and MFR-β encode for proteins consisting of 257 and 255 amino acids, respectively, leading to a mature protein with an MW of 28–30 kDa *(101,102)*. This protein undergoes posttranslational modifications including processing of the polypeptide at the N- and C-terminus, glycosylation, and phosphorylation. One of the posttranslational modifications is the cleavage of the signal sequence before attachment to the GPI anchor *(105)*. Glycosylation enlarges the MW of the 26–30 kDa MFR core protein to a 38–44 kDa mature protein *(106)*. Glycosylation appears to be important for ligand binding since various stages of deglycosylated MFR did not bind folic acid. Although MFR-α and MFR-β isoforms from human and murine sources are functionally homologous, they exhibit a markedly different substrate-affinity-binding profile. Recent studies by Shen et al. *(107)* demonstrated that one single amino acid substitution (Leu 49 in MFR-α vs Ala 49 in MFR-β) is responsible for a relatively higher binding affinity of MFR-α for (anti)folates compared to MFR-β, and opposite stereospecificities for binding reduced folate cofactors and several antifolate compounds. In particular, MFR-α displays preferential binding of the natural physiological 6S-stereoisomers of 5-CH$_3$THF and leucovorin, whereas MFR-β demonstrates a higher binding affinity for the unnatural 6R stereoisomers of these reduced folate cofactors *(108,109)*. MFR-α displayed a 3- to 16-

fold greater affinity than MFR-β for a small series of antifolate compounds, including MTX, aminopterin, CB3717, and DDATHF *(109,110)*. Binding affinities of MFR-α for a larger group of antifolates will be discussed in greater detail in subheading 8.

4.2. Mechanism/Regulation of MFR-Mediated (Anti)Folate Uptake

The exact mechanism of MFR-mediated uptake of (anti)folate compounds is still an unresolved and controversial issue. At least two different pathways have been described by which MFR-mediated transport of (anti)folates can proceed. The first pathway is the classical receptor-mediated endocytosis route via clathrin-coated pits. This pathway appeared to be the major route for MFR-mediated folate uptake in human kidney cells *(111)* and in a number of tumor cell lines *(112)*. A second transport route that has received considerable attention over the past years, is via potocytosis *(113)*. The characterization of this pathway of MFR-mediated (anti)folate transport is largely based on extensive studies using monkey kidney MA104 cells as an experimental model system *(114–116)*. In this model system MFR molecules are entirely clustered in so-called caveolae, plasma membrane-attached vesicular organelles that have caveolin (rather than clathrin) as the major structural coat protein *(117,118)*. Caveolae can temporarily close from the external environment after which rapid acidification of the caveolar lumen causes dissociation of (anti)folates from MFR. Subsequently, a putative carrier protein translocates the (anti)folates across the plasma membrane into the cytosol. During this process the caveolae remain attached to the plasma membrane. The cycle is completed when the caveolae open and expose MFR to the extracellular space again. In this respect, caveolae differ from clathrin-coated pits that pinch off from the plasma membrane to fuse with the endosomal system. An important conceptional assumption in the potocytosis model is that GPI-anchored MFR molecules *per se* lack the possibility of translocating bound (anti)folate compounds across the plasma membrane but require a (specific) carrier protein for this process. The RFC or a H^+-driven pump have been postulated to serve as potential carrier molecules *(119,120)*. However, several lines of evidence suggest that a role for RFC in potocytosis is unlikely: MFR-mediated folate uptake can be fully operative in RFC-defective cell lines *(121–125)*; functional activity of RFC is almost completely abolished under the acidified conditions of closed caveolae *(125,126)*; and finally RFC/MFR affinity-labeling studies showed no evidence for colocalization of MFR and RFC in caveolae of human KB nasopharyngeal carcinoma cells or CEM leukemia cells *(112)*.

Although several aspects of potocytosis as a route for MFR-mediated (anti)folate transport need to be clarified, it is of particular interest to speculate whether MFRs residing in caveolae can have function(s) in addition to folate transport that are associated with the expression of caveolin. The evidence is accumulating that caveolin functions as a scaffolding protein to organize and concentrate specific lipids (cholesterol and glycosphingolipids) and lipid-modified signaling molecules (e.g., Src-like kinases, an IP_3-sensitive Ca^{2+} channel, an ATP-sensitive Ca^{2+} pump, endothelial nitric-oxide synthase, and G proteins) within caveolae membranes *(127–131)*. Caveolae as well as caveolin are most abundantly expressed in terminally differentiated cells: adipocytes, endothelial cells, and muscle cells *(131)*. For instance, caveolin was highly expressed in normal mammary epithelium, but upon mammary tumorogenesis its expression was lost in several transformed cell lines from human mammary carcinomas (e.g. MCF-7 and ZR-75-

1 cells). Engelman et al. *(131)* also demonstrated that cell transformation by activated oncogenes (e.g. v-*abl* and H-*ras*) led to a marked reduction or loss of caveolin expression. Interestingly, induction of caveolin in these oncogenically transformed cells abrogated anchorage-independent growth, suggesting that downregulation of caveolin expression and caveolae organelles may be critical for maintaining the transformed phenotype in certain cell types. Additional studies will be necessary to address whether MFR present in caveolae has multiple functions as compared to MFR expressed in cells that do not contain caveolae *(123)*.

In vitro studies using cell lines with a high expression of MFR demonstrated that functional MFR transport activity can be regulated at several levels:

1. The expression of MFR itself can be subject to up- or downregulation as a function of the extracellular folate concentrations *(33,99,123,132,133)*. Although some cell lines constitutively express high levels of MFR (e.g., KB cells), a high extracellular folate concentrations may downregulate MFR synthesis (e.g., because of hypermethylation of the MFR gene) *(134)*, whereas low extracellular concentrations of folate frequently enhance the MFR expression (e.g., because of increased MFR mRNA stability) *(135)*.
2. Folate homeostasis may be another factor that can determine the functional activity of MFRs. A comparative analysis of the intracellular folate content in KB cells (approx 20 pmol/10^6 cells) *(132)* with the high level of MFR expression in KB cells (30–50 pmol/10^6 cells) suggests that either these cells use a portion of the total MFR folate-binding capacity for the delivery of folates into the cytosol, or that the recycling rates of MFRs in KB cells are very slow. In this regard, studies by Kamen et al. *(114,136)* proposed that recycling of apo-MFR to the membrane could be subject to metabolic feedback regulation as a result of preferential binding of intracellular folylpolyglutamates to apo-MFR compared to extracellular folylmonoglutamates.
3. MFR-mediated folate uptake via potocytosis in MA104 cells can be influenced by conditions that either disrupt the integrity of caveolae (e.g., cholesterol-binding agents) or inhibit molecules in caveolae in control of MFR recycling (e.g., inhibitors of PKC-α) *(137)*.
4. It is important to note that many MFR-expressing tumor cells simultaneously express functional activity of other folate transporter(s), including the RFC *(126,138–142)*. Under these conditions, folate uptake via the RFC establishes a folate status that can control MFR recycling as described in item 1, above. In fact, several studies *(125,126,139,140)* indicated that whenever RFC is expressed in tumor cells simultaneously with MFR (e.g., in KB, MA-104, IGROV-I ovarian carcinoma cells), the major contribution of (anti)folate transport comes from the RFC and not from MFR. The role of MFR becomes more prominent under conditions of low extracellular concentrations of (anti)folates where K_ds for MFR-binding predominate over K_ms for RFC transport *(121,124–126,139,143,144)*. Impairment of RFC activity can further increase the relative role of MFR in (anti)folate transport *(121–123,139)*.
5. Modifications in the GPI-anchoring of MFR can have implications for the efficacy of MFR transport. Recently, Wang et al. *(145)* showed that one MFR-expressing subline of murine L1210 cells, from which MFR was insensitive to PI-PLC, exhibited an enhanced (anti)folate binding capacity and increased 5-CH_3THF/folic acid transport capacity compared to another L1210 subline from which MFR could be released by PI-PLC. The authors concluded that variant GPI structures may modulate the function of MFR by influencing its conformation/topography in the membrane.

6. Finally, there is evidence that a high binding affinity of MFR for antifolates does not necessarily imply a better transport efficiency. One reason for this can be that tight binding also hampers the dissociation of the ligand from the receptor in an acidic environment compared to a ligand for which the MFR has a lower affinity. Second, it has been noted that antifolates for which MFR has a lower binding affinity but that are good substrates for folylpolyglutamate synthetase (FPGS) are more efficiently transported than antifolates for which MFR has a high binding affinity and a low substrate affinity for FPGS *(142,146)*. These results indicate that efficiency of polyglutamylation may be a rate-limiting factor in MFR-mediated (anti)folate uptake.

4.3. Biodistribution of MFR

The availability of immunological and molecular probes has allowed a detailed investigation of the biodistribution of MFR-isoforms. MFRs are expressed in many tissues of both normal and neoplastic origin, in primary cell cultures of normal cells, and in a variety of established tumor cell lines *(33,34,36)*. The expression of MFR isoforms appeared to be tissue-specific and can often be upregulated in neoplastic tissues. RT-PCR analysis of differential MFR-α and MFR-β expression *(33)* showed that normal tissues expressed low-to-moderate levels of MFR-β. Likewise, malignant tissues of nonepithelial origin appeared to express elevated levels of MFR-β. MFR-α alone was expressed in normal epithelial cells and was markedly elevated in a variety of carcinomas (in particular ovarian carcinomas), with the exception of head and neck squamous cell carcinomas. Unlike fresh tumor samples, established tumor cell lines constitutively expressed MFR-α as the main isoform. This may be caused by in vitro selection of cells expressing MFR-α given its more favorable kinetics of reduced folate cofactor transport compared to MFR-β (*see* also Table 1). Of particular interest is the observation of MFR expression in hematopoietic progenitor cells *(103,147,148)*. It is still unclear whether MFR in these cells plays a role in folate uptake and folate homeostasis or that MFRs are involved in (caveolae-related) signal transduction pathways.

The distribution of MFR-γ is restricted to a limited number of established cell lines (ovarian and cervical carcinoma), normal tissues (spleen, thymus), and malignant tissues (ovarian carcinoma, uterine carcinoma) *(103)*. These authors also showed that the expression of MFR-γ was elevated in spleen and bone marrow samples of patients with chronic and acute myeloid leukemias and acute lymphocytic leukemias. Altogether, a complete picture of the quantitative and functional levels of MFR-isoforms in malignant cells may facilitate their targeting by antifolates for which MFRs have an appreciable binding affinity.

5. LOW PH TRANSPORT ROUTE

Wild-type murine L1210 leukemia cells as well as L1210 cells with defective RFC transport were found to express a folate transporter that displays optimal activity at a pH below 7.4. *(149,150)*. MTX transport via this route is energy dependent, shows saturation kinetics, and has similar relative affinities for folic acid and reduced folate cofactors. Transport of MTX via this route is optimal at pH 6.2 and more than 10-fold higher than at pH 7.4. The V_{max} for MTX by the low pH route (at pH 6.2) is twofold lower than for the RFC (at pH 7.4) *(150)*. Under conditions in which RFC is defective, transport activity via the low pH route may still be sufficient to compensate for the loss of RFC activity and to accumulate sufficient folates required for cell growth. A detailed understanding of a possible physiological or pharmacological role of this low pH route in (anti)folate transport awaits an additional biochemical and molecular characterization of this transporter along with the analysis of its expression in other tumor cell types.

6. HIGH CAPACITY/LOW AFFINITY ROUTE

Sirotnak et al. *(151)* demonstrated both in wild-type and RFC-transport-defective murine L1210 cells a folate transporter that had a low affinity for folic acid (K_m 550 μM) but a V_{max} that was 20-fold higher than the RFC. It seems likely that this transport system has no physiological relevance but at high extracellular concentrations it may contribute to antifolate transport. Similar for the low pH route, the possible importance of this transporter needs to be addressed in additional studies.

7. PASSIVE/FACILITATED DIFFUSION

Passive diffusion may contribute to the uptake of MTX in high dose regimens (> 1 g MTX/m^2). This may be important in cases of tumor cells with defective MTX transport *(152)*. Yang et al. *(153)* showed that the contribution of passive diffusion of 1 μM MTX in L1210 cells was 0.0018 nmol/min/g dry wt compared to a V_{max} of 2.9 nmol/min/g dry wt for RFC-mediated transport of MTX in intact L1210 cells. Passive diffusion was linearly increased with the extracellular MTX concentration *(153)*.

8. RFC AND MFR TRANSPORT OF ANTIFOLATE DRUGS; STRUCTURE-ACTIVITY RELATIONSHIPS

For almost 50 yr, MTX has had an established role in cancer chemotherapy, both as a single agent and in combination chemotherapy *(3,4,6)*. A detailed understanding of the factors that contribute to the preclinical and clinical activity of MTX (e.g., membrane transport, polyglutamylation, target enzyme inhibition) has provided a solid basis for the design of novel antifolates that are either transported more efficiently, have a prolonged intracellular retention as a result of improved polyglutamylation, or are more potent (multitargeted) inhibitors of critical enzymes in folate metabolism. Traditionally, screening programs to assess the biological activity of novel antifolates consisted of in vitro model systems (usually leukemia cells) which express the RFC as the sole transport system for reduced folate cofactors and antifolate compounds. Recently, Westerhof et al. *(122)* reported a structure-activity analysis with respect to the transport properties and growth-inhibitory potential of a series of 37 classic and novel antifolate inhibitors of DHFR, TS, GARTFase, and FPGS against murine L1210 leukemia cells and human CEM leukemia cells with different expression levels of either the RFC and/or MFR. A selection of these antifolates (*see* Fig. 1) was made on the basis of their clinical application or a specific rational design. MTX is used as a reference compound for the class of DHFR inhibitors and as a reference compound to assess the efficiency for RFC-mediated transport. Two other DHFR inhibitors, one of which is efficiently polyglutamated: edatrexate (EDX) *(154)*, and a nonpolyglutamatable compound; PT523 *(155)*, displayed an improved transport efficiency via the RFC. CB3717 *(8,13,156)* and IAHQ *(157)* were among the first folate-based antifolate inhibitors of TS from which rationally designed

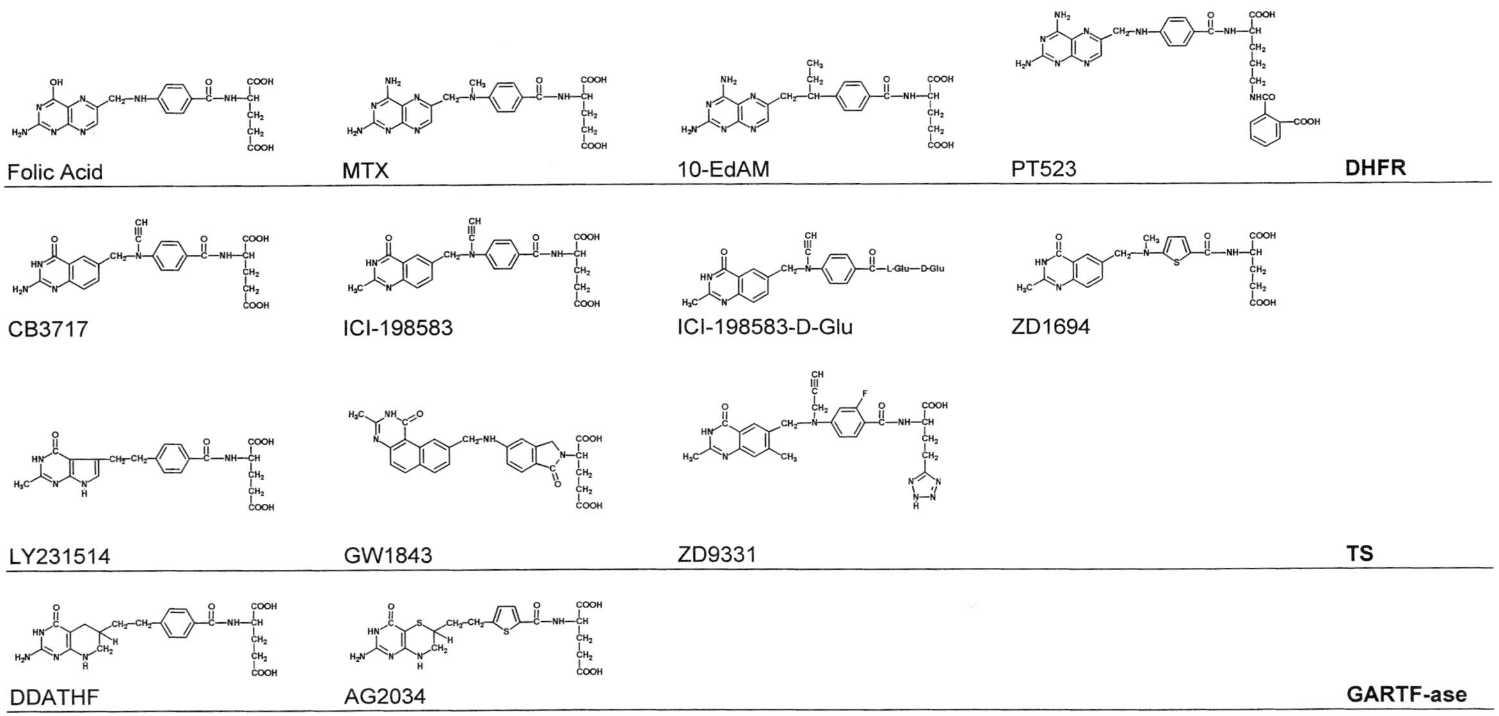

Fig. 1. Chemical structures: folic acid, the DHFR inhibitors: MTX, EDX, and PT523, the TS inhibitors CB3717, ICI-198583, ICI-198583-L-Glu-D-Glu, ZD1694, LY231514 (MTA), GW1843, ZD9331, IAHQ, and the GARTFase inhibitors DDATHF and AG2034.

analogs were synthesized that nowadays demonstrate substantial activity in preclinical model systems and in a clinical setting *(3,13,15,16,18, see* also Chapters 6–11). CB3717 served as the leading compound for the synthesis of two TS inhibitors: ICI-198583 *(158)* and ZD1694 *(159),* which were more efficiently transported via the RFC than CB3717. In addition, ZD1694 is a better substrates for FPGS than CB3717 *(159).* Two other compounds that meet this profile are GW1843 *(9,160)* and LY231514 *(161).* In addition to TS, polyglutamates of LY231514 can also inhibit DHFR and GARTFase, therefore this compound is referred to as a multitargeted antifolate (MTA) *(161).* ZD9331 belongs to the class of TS inhibitors that requires RFC transport but cannot be polyglutamated *(162).* One last group of TS inhibitors includes ICI-198583-γ-D-Glu, an antifolate with a dipeptide side chain that reduces RFC transport and polyglutamylation by FPGS *(163,164).* Two reference compounds from the class of antifolate GARTFase inhibitors are DDATHF *(10)* and AG2034 *(11).* Both compounds exhibit improved RFC transport and polyglutamylation by FPGS compared to MTX.

Figure 2A, B shows a side-by-side comparison of the affinity of RFC and MFR, respectively, for the antifolates depicted in Fig. 1. Human RFC substrate affinity is 6–17-fold lower than MTX for CB3717, IAHQ, and ICI-198583-D-Glu. All other antifolates demonstrate an improved RFC substrate affinity over MTX (Fig. 2A). Several structural features were identified which can determine (in)efficient utilization of the RFC: 2-NH_2/4-oxo oxidized structures (e.g., folic acid, CB3717, and IAHQ) are poor substrates for the RFC; replacement of the 2-NH_2-group for a 2-CH_3 group (e.g., in CB317) markedly improved the RFC substrate affinity; modifications of the glutamate side chain do not necessarily diminish RFC substrate affinity, except in the case of dipeptide side chains or with di/trivalent negatively charged residues; and modifications/substitutions in the pteridine/quinazoline ring, the C^9-N^{10} bridge or the p-aminobenzoyl ring do not cause a significant loss or improval of the RFC substrate affinity.

MFR-binding affinity for the selected group of antifolates shows a different profile (Fig. 2B). Based on the competition for [^{3}H]folic acid binding to L1210-MFR cells, expressing the murine MFR-α isoform which is functionally identical to the human MFR-α isoform expressed in KB cells *(101,107),* a characteristic picture is observed. Relative to folic acid, MFR exhibits a low binding affinity for the group of DHFR inhibitors MTX, EDX, and PT523, whereas a relatively high binding affinity is noted for the group of antifolate TS and GARTFase inhibitors. Structural features that determine a high or low MFR binding affinity are as follows: a high binding affinity is noted for 2-NH_2/4-oxo oxidized structures, whereas a low binding affinity is observed for 2,4-NH_2 structures (MTX, EDX, PT523). Other modifications/substitutions at pteridine/quinazoline ring, the C^9-N^{10} bridge, the p-aminobenzoyl ring, and the glutamate side chain are well tolerated with respect to MFR binding affinity *(122).*

A panel of human and murine leukemia cell lines with different expression levels of either the RFC *(52,165)* and/or MFR *(121,122,138)* has been helpful as a model system for assessing the differential role of the RFC and MFR in the growth inhibitory potential of the antifolate inhibitors of DHFR, TS and GARTFase. Table 2 (taken from ref. *122)* shows the growth inhibitory effects of the antifolate inhibitors of DHFR, TS, and GARTFase against the panel RFC and/or MFR expressing cell lines. Table 2 indicates that the potency of growth inhibition by the antifolate drugs was correlated with the RFC substrate affinity (Fig. 2A) and MFR binding affinity (Fig. 2B). Furthermore, antifolate

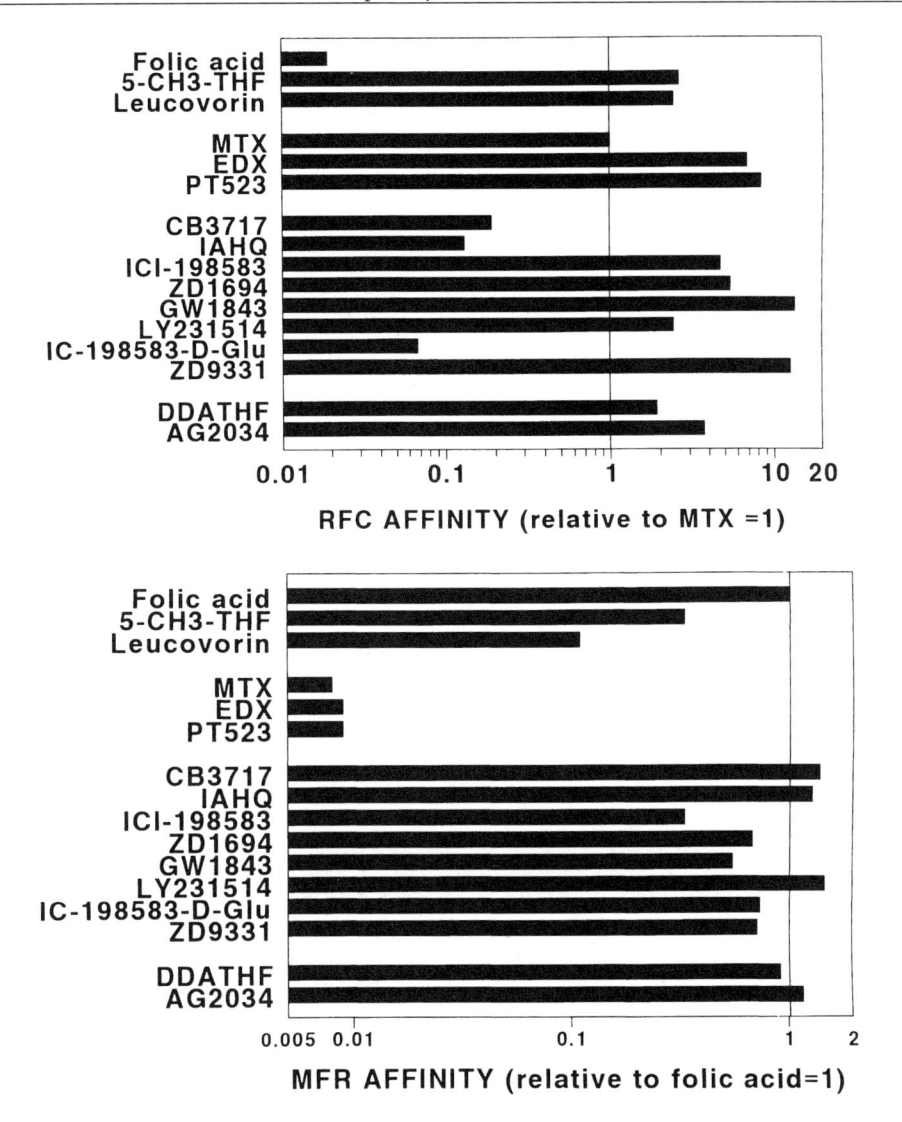

Fig. 2. (A) RFC substrate affinity for FA, reduced folate cofactors, MTX vs novel antifolates. Values represent the concentrations of compound necessary to inhibit RFC-mediated [^{3}H]MTX influx in RFC-overproducing CEM-7A cells *(51)* by 50% at an extracellular concentration of 5 μM [^{3}H]MTX (from ref. *122*). (B) Relative MFR binding affinity for FA, reduced folate cofactors, MTX vs novel antifolates. Values represent the reciprocal molar ratio required to displace/complete 50% of [^{3}H]folic acid binding to intact L1210-MFR. Relative MFR binding affinity for folic acid is set at 1 (from ref. *122*).

growth inhibition of MFR-expressing cells is influenced by the extracellular concentration of folic acid. Competition with folic acid at the level of MFR binding markedly reduced the growth inhibition by the 3 DHFR inhibitors (IC$_{50}$ 700–2500 nM). For the group of TS and GARTFase inhibitors, the growth inhibitory effects were also reduced, but to a lower extent than for the DHFR inhibitors. This can be explained by the fact that the high MFR-binding affinity for the TS/GARTFase inhibitors restrains competition for FA binding and internalization. Dual expression of RFC and MFR in L1210-B73 cells grown at 1 nM leucovorin displayed full sensitivity to all antifolate drugs tested in Table 2, suggesting that both transporters are active in internalizing compounds for which they display a high affinity. Since RFC activity is not influenced by the presence of 20 nM folic acid, RFC-mediated internalization and growth inhibition by MTX, EDX, and PT523 is not compromised in L1210-B73 cells. Collectively, Table 2 identifies antifolate compounds that are preferentially transported via either the RFC (MTX, EDX, and PT523) or MFR (CB3717, IAHQ, ICI-198583-D-Glu), or can utilize both RFC and MFR (ICI-198583, ZD1694, GW1843, LY231514, ZD9331, DDATHF, and AG2034) *(122)*.

Whereas in vitro model systems with RFC and/or high MFR expression clearly demonstrate a role for these transporters in the cellular uptake of (novel) antifolates, for clinical specimens, despite a qualitative assessment of expression levels (see subheadings 3.3. and 4.3; biodistribution of RFC/MFR), the critical functional level of RFC/MFR that can accumulate antifolates to a cytotoxic level remains to be determined. Again on the basis of in vitro studies, Pinard et al *(123)* showed that in RFC-defective breast cancer cells, MFR expression levels ≥ 2 pmol/10^7 cells were sufficient to internalize cytotoxic concentrations of antifolates for which MFR has a high affinity (e.g., CB3717 and DDATHF). Higher MFR levels may be required for antifolates that exhibit a lower MFR binding affinity (e.g., MTX, EDX). With respect to *ex vivo* RFC activity in clinical specimens, studies with childhood leukemia cells *(82,83,166)* and human soft-tissue carcinoma cells *(81,167)* showed that novel antifolates such as GW1843, LY231514, DDATHF, ZD1694, AMT, EDX, and PT523 were taken up more efficiently than MTX, which is consistent with their better substrate affinity for the RFC.

Another issue of potential clinical interest is to improve the therapeutic index of antifolates by a transport-related protection strategy against antifolate toxicity to normal tissues. Recent studies showed that the functional folate status is a prognostic indicator of hematological toxicity in clinical trials with the multitargeted antifolate LY231514 *(168)*. Based on differences in binding affinity, it can be rationalized that folic acid will be more effective than leucovorin in protecting MFR-expressing normal tissues from toxic effects of antifolates for which MFR has a high affinity. Animal and clinical studies showed that oral folic acid could enhance antitumor activity by reducing GW1843 induced intestinal toxicity *(169)* or DDATHF-induced myelosuppression *(170)*. Mechanistically, the protective effect by folic acid could be mediated at the level of competition for drug entry via the MFR, which is expressed in normal colon tissue and hematopoietic cells *(33,171)*, as well as by enhanced (MFR-mediated) folic acid uptake. Elevated intracellular folate pools can subsequently block the polyglutamylation of antifolates *(92,93,172)*. Leucovorin rescue has a longstanding tradition in high-dose MTX-containing chemotherapeutic regimens *(152,173–175)*. It is evident that the differential efficiency of RFC/MFR-mediated entry in normal vs malignant cells is one of the factors contributing to the efficacy of leucovorin rescue *(176)*. An increasing knowledge of the (functional) levels of MFR and/or RFC in normal and malignant cells along with the differential substrate affinity of RFC/MFR can therefore make an important contribution to the rational design of optimal strategies for either folic acid or leucovorin-based rescue protocols.

9. MFR AS A TARGET FOR MOV18-GUIDED IMMUNOTHERAPY AND MACROMOLECULE TRANSPORT

Besides exploitation of MFR as a target for folate-based chemotherapeutic drugs (Fig. 2B, Table 2), MFR has received considerable attention as a target for radioimmunotherapy of ovarian cancer and as a possible internalizing route for (macro)molecules.

9.1. MFR as a Target for MOv18-Guided Immunotherapy

The constitutive overexpression of MFR in ovarian cancer *(33,34,177–179)* has initiated preclinical and clinical research for therapeutic exploitation. Miotti et al. *(180)* isolated a series of antibodies against different epitopes of MFR. Two of these antibodies, MOv18 and MOv19, are currently applied in experimental *(181)* and clinical medicine *(182–184)*. Chimeric radiolabeled MOv18 appeared to be a suitable antibody for immunoscintigraphic purposes demonstrating an uptake ratio of 3.8 and 6.7 for ovarian tumor to normal tissues at 2 and 6d, respectively, after injection of the antibody *(183)*. Grippa et al. *(185)* showed promising results for the treatment of minimal residual disease of ovarian cancer by radioimmunotherapy with [^{131}I]-labeled MOv18. After one single dose of murine [^{131}I] MOv18 (100 mCi) and 90-d follow-up period, 5 out 16 patients showed a complete response, 6 patients had stable disease, and 5 patients showed progressive disease. In vitro studies indicate that MOv-18-guided immunotherapy may be improved further by conjugating MOv18 with folic acid or antifolates for which MFR has a high affinity *(186)*. (Anti)folate conjugation of MOv18 enhanced the retention as well as the internalization of the antibody in cell lines with different levels of MFR expression *(187)*.

Another potential therapeutic exploitation of antibodies against MFR was reported by Coney et al. *(188)* who showed that chimeric murine-human MOv18 and MOv19 antibodies, in combination with human peripheral blood mononuclear cells as effector cells, could induce antibody-dependent cellular cytotoxicity (ADCC) against human IGROV-I ovarian carcinoma cells. In a clinical setting, Canevari et al. *(189)* reported that specific lysis of ovarian carcinoma cells by in vitro activated peripheral blood T lymphocytes using a bispecific monoclonal antibody directed against MFR on ovarian cancer cells and the CD3 molecule on T lymphocytes *(190,191)*. An overall response rate of 27% was observed in this study (26 patients) with only mild-to-moderate toxicity. The three complete responses lasted from 18 to 26 mo.

9.2. MFR as a Vehicle for Macromolecule Transport

An original report by Leamon and Low *(192)* demonstrating that folate conjugation could induce MFR-mediated endocytosis of macromolecules in human KB carcinoma cells, has initiated further (pre)clinical research to achieve selective targeting of MFR expressing cells. Folate conjugated to cytotoxins (e.g., momordin) was selectively cytotoxic against MFR-overexpressing KB cells but not to MFR-negative cells *(193,194)*. Other conjugates with selective potential were doxorubicin and antisense oligodeoxyribonucleotides containing liposomes with folic acid linked to phospholipids via a polyethylene glycol spacer *(195–197)*. MFR-mediated endocytosis could also serve as a mechanism of selective delivering of radiopharmaceuticals (e.g., [^{67}Ga]-deferoxamine) for diagnostic imaging and/or radiation therapy of KB carcinoma xenografts in nude mice *(198,199)*. Finally, folate conjugation to anti T-cell receptor antibodies appeared to be very efficient in mediating lysis of tumor cells that express either the α- and β isoform of MFR *(200,201)*. Lysis of MFR-positive cells could be detected at antibody-conjugate concentrations as low as 1 pM, which was three orders of magnitude below the antibody concentration required to detect binding to MFR-positive cells.

The critical determinants in the above-mentioned applications of exploiting MFR as a target molecule are the cellular level of MFR expression and the extracellular folate status that can compete for MFR binding. The proof of principle is usually demonstrated for KB cells, which express high levels of MFR (up to 30×10^6 molecules per cell), or IGROV-I ovarian carcinoma cells, which express moderately high levels of MFR (up to 1×10^6 molecules per cell). Kranz et al. *(200)* showed that 4×10^3 molecules per cell was the treshold level of MFR to achieve an ADCC response with folate conjugated anti-T-cell receptor antibodies. Critical MFR expression levels for the delivery of cytotoxic concentrations of chemotherapeutic drugs via folate-conjugated macromolecules or liposomes remain to be determined before this therapeutic approach can be applied in a clinical setting.

10. CONCLUSIONS

The RFC, MFR, and folate efflux systems play a critical physiological role in controlling the reduced folate cofactor status in normal and malignant cells and thereby the effectiveness of antifolate inhibitors of DHFR, TS, and GARTFase. Furthermore, RFC and MFR display a differential transport capacity for antifolate drugs that will also contribute to their effectiveness (Fig. 3). It is anticipated that the increasing knowledge of the expression levels of RFC and MFR (isoforms) in normal and malignant cells, the molecular, biochemical, and functional properties of these transporters, and the cellular folate status, will be advantageous to improve currently active antifolate-based chemotherapy regimens for leukemias *(3,82,85)* and solid tumors *(13,15,16)* and MFR-targeted radioimmunotherapy of ovarian cancer *(184,185)*. In addition, it will be beneficial to pursue selective protection of normal cells by leucovorin or folic acid. In order to achieve this goal, clinically directed laboratory studies will be necessary to elucidate a number of unresolved issues in antifolate transport, such as: determination of functional levels of RFC and MFR (isoforms) in clinical specimens; regulatory aspects of antifolate influx and efflux; the physiological/pharmacological relevance of the cellular coexpression of multiple folate transport systems; a tumor-type delineation of potocytosis or receptor-mediated endocytosis as a mechanism of MFR-mediated antifolate uptake; and the molecular basis of RFC and MFR-defective antifolate resistance.

ACKNOWLEDGMENTS

This study was supported by a grant from the Dutch Cancer Society (NKB-VU 96-1260). G. J. Peters is acknowledged for critical reading of the manuscript. I. Kathmann is acknowledged for technical assistance and K. Smid for preparing the illustrations.

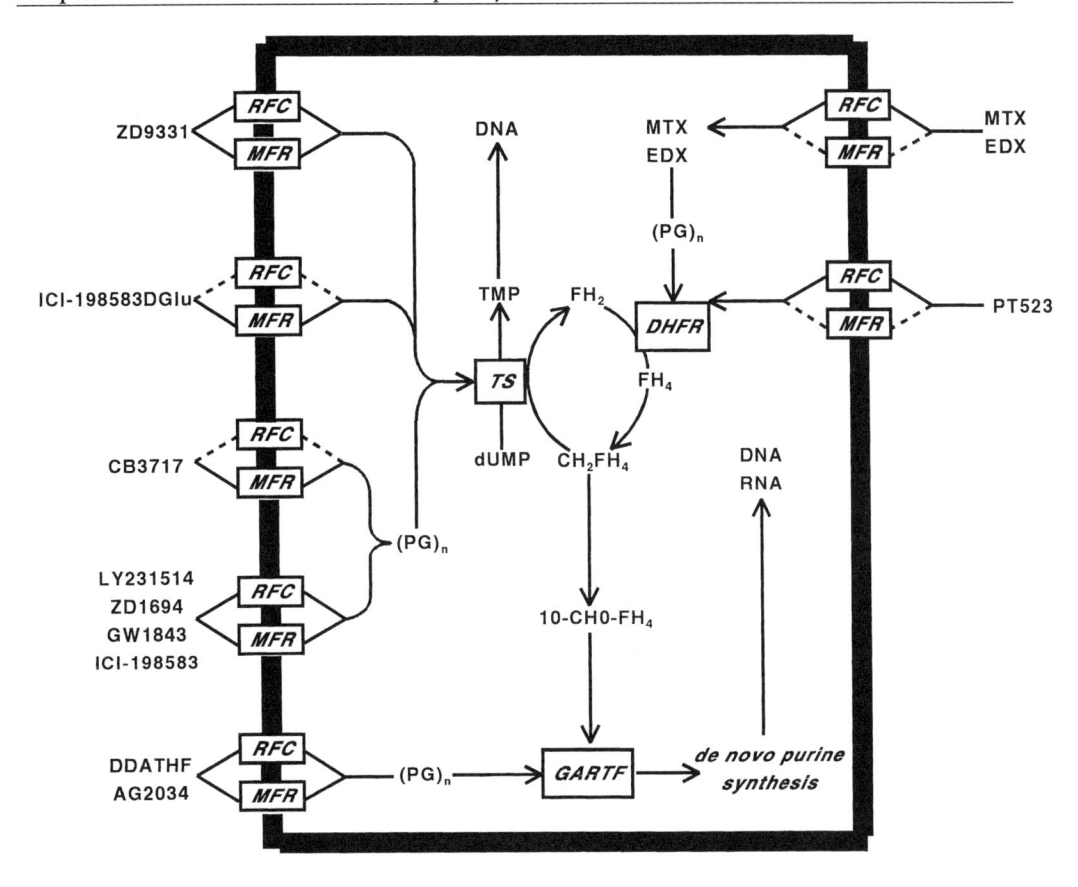

Fig. 3. Schematic representation of RFC- and MFR-mediated of transport of antifolates, metabolism of antifolates, and intracellular targeting of DHFR, TS, and GARTFase. The efficiency of RFC and MFR transport of antifolates is depicted by a continued line (representing the major transport route) or a broken line (representing a minor transport route).

REFERENCES

1. Stockstad ELR. Historical perspective on key advances in the biochemistry and physiology of folates. In: (Picciano, MF, Stokstad, ELR, Greogory, JF eds.) Folic Acid Metabolism in Health and Disease. Wiley-Liss, New York, 1990, pp. 1–21.
2. Hitchings GH. Nobel lecture in physiology or medicine 1988: selective inhibitors of dihydrofolate reductase. *In Vitro Cell Dev Biol* 1989; 25:303–310.
3. Bertino JR. Ode to methotrexate. *J Clin Oncol* 1993; 11:5–14.
4. Schornagel JH, McVie JG. The clinical pharmacology of methotrexate, a review. *Cancer Treat Rev* 1983; 10:53–75.
5. Jukes TJ. Searching for the magic bullets: early approaches to chemotherapy-antifolates, methotrexate. *Cancer Res* 1987; 47:5528–5536.
6. Goldman ID, Matherly LH. The cellular pharmacology of methotrexate. *Pharmacol Ther* 1985; 28:77–102.
7. Huennekens FM, Duffy TH, Vitols KS. Folic acid metabolism and disruption by pharmacologic agents. *NCI Monographs* 1987; 5:1–7.

8. Harrap KH, Jackman AL, Newell DR, Taylor GA, Hughes LR, Calvert AH. Thymidylate synthase: a target for anticancer drug design. *Adv Enzyme Regul* 1989; 29:161–179.
9. Duch DS, Banks S, Dev IK, Dickerson SH, Ferone R, Health LS, Humphreys J, Knick V, Pendergast W, Singer S, Smith GK, Waters K, Wilson HR. Biochemical and cellular pharmacology of 1843U89, a novel benzoquinazoline inhibitor of thymidylate synthase. *Cancer Res* 1993; 53:810–818.
10. Beardsley GP, Moroson BA, Taylor EC, Moran RG. A new folate antimetabolite 5;10-dideaza-5,6,7,8,-tetrahydrofolate is a potent inhibitor of the *de novo* purine synthesis. *J Biol Chem* 1989; 264:328–333.
11. Boritzki TJ, Bartlett CA, Zhang C, Howland EF, Margosiak SA, Palmer CL, Romines WH, Jackson RC, AG2034: a novel inhibitor of glycinamide ribonucleotide formyltransferase. *Invest New Drugs* 1996; 14:295–303.
12. Rosowsky A, Forsch RA, Reich VE, Freisheim JH, Moran RG. Side chain modified 5-deazafolate and 5-deazatetrahydrofolate analogues as mammalian folylpolyglutamate synthetase and glycinamide ribonucleotide formyltransferase inhibitors: Synthesis and in vitro biological evaluation. *J Med Chem* 1992; 35:1578–1588.
13. Jackman AL, Calvert AH. Folate-based thymidylate synthase inhibitors as anticancer drugs. *Ann Oncol* 1995; 6:871–881.
14. Jackman AL, Boyle FT, Harrap KR. Tomudex$_{TM}$ (ZD1694): from concept to care, a programme in rational drug discovery. *Invest New Drugs* 1996; 14:305–316.
15. Rustum YM, Harstick A, Cao S, Vanhoefer U, Yin MB, Wilke H, Seeber S. Thymidylate synthase inhibitors in cancer therapy: direct and indirect inhibitors. *J Clin Oncol* 1997; 15:389–400.
16. Peters GJ, Ackland SP. New antimetabolites in preclinical and clinical development. *Exp Opin Invest Drugs* 1996; 5:637–679.
17. Berman EM, Werbel LM. The renewed potential for folate antagonists in contemporary cancer chemotherapy. *J Med Chem* 1991; 34:479–485.
18. Zalcberg JR, Cunningham D, Van Cutsem E, Francois E, Schornagel J, Adenis A, Green M, Iveson A, Azab M, Seymour I. ZD1694: a novel thymidylate synthase inhibitor with substantial activity in the treatment of patients with advanced colorectal cancer. *J Clin Oncol* 1996; 14:716–721.
19. Sirotnak FM. Correlates of folate analog transport, pharmacokinetics and selective antitumor action. *Pharmac Ther* 1980; 8:71–104.
20. Sirotnak FM. Obligate genetic expression in tumor cells of a fetal membrane property mediating "folate" transport: biological significance and implications for improved therapy of human cancer. *Cancer Res* 1985; 45:3992–4000.
21. Ratnam M, Freisheim JH. Proteins involved in the transport of folates and antifolates by normal and neoplastic cells. In: (Picciano, MF, Stokstad, ELR, Greogory, JF) Folic Acid Metabolism in Health and Disease. Wiley-Liss, New York, 1990, pp. 91–120.
22. Matherly LH. Mechanisms of receptor-mediated folate and antifolate membrane transport in cancer chemotherapy. In: (Georgopapadakou NH, ed) Drug Transport in Antimicrobial and Anticancer Chemotherapy. Marcel Dekker, New York, 1995, pp. 453–524.
23. Henderson GB. Folate-binding proteins. *Ann Rev Nutr* 1990; 10:319–335.
24. Antony AC. The biological chemistry of folate receptors. *Blood* 1992; 79:2807–2820.
25. Antony AC. Folate receptors. *Ann Rev Nutr* 1996; 16:501–521.
26. Dembo M, Sirotnak FM, Moccio DM. Effects of metabolic deprivation on methotrexate transport in L1210 leukemia cells: further evidence for separate influx and efflux systems with different energetic requirements. *J Membr Biol* 1984; 78:9–17.
27. Henderson GB, Tsjui JM, Kumar HP. Characterization of the individual transport routes that mediate the influx and efflux of methotrexate in CCRF-CEM human lymphoblastic cells. *Cancer Res* 1986; 46:1633–1638.
28. Saxena M, Henderson GB. Identification of efflux systems for large anions and anionic conjugates as the mediators of methotrexate efflux in L1210 cells. *Biochem Pharmacol* 1996; 51:975–982.
29. Zhao R, Seither R, Brigle KE, Sharina IG, Wang PJ, Goldman ID. Impact of overexpression of the reduced folate carrier (RFC1), an anion exchanger, on concentrative transport in murine L1210 leukemia cells. *J Biol Chem* 1997; 272:21,207–21,212.
30. Schlemmer SR, Sirotnak FM. Structural preferences among folate compounds and their analogues for ATPase-mediated efflux by inside-out plasma membrane vesicles derived from L1210 cells. *Biochem Pharmacol* 1995; 49:1427–1433.

31. Assaraf YG, Goldman ID. Loss of folic acid exporter function with markedly augmented folate accumulation in lipophilic antifolate-resistant mammalian cells. *J Biol Chem* 1997; 272:17,460–17,466.
32. Jansen G, Barr HM, Kathmann I, Peters GJ, Bunni M, Priest DG, Assaraf YG. Altered metabolism of (anti)folates in pyrimethamine resistant Chinese hamster ovary cells. In: (Pfleiderer W, Rokos H, eds) Chemistry and Biology of Pteridines and Folates 1997. Blackwell Science Press, Berlin, 1997, pp. 253–256.
33. Ross JF, Chaudhuri PK, Ratnam M. Differential regulation of folate receptor isoforms in normal and malignant tissues in vivo and in established cell lines. *Cancer* 1994; 73:2432–2343.
34. Weitman SD, Lark RH, Coney LR, Fort DW, Frasca V, Zurawsky VR, Kamen BA. Distribution of the folate receptor GP38 in normal and malignant cell lines and tissues. *Cancer Res* 1992; 52:3396–3401.
35. Weitman SD, Weinberg AG, Coney LR, Zurawski VR, Jennings DS, Kamen BA. Cellular localization of the folate receptor: potential role in drug toxicity and folate homeostasis. *Cancer Res* 1992; 52:6708–6711.
36. Garin-Chesa P, Campbell I, Saigo PE, Lewis JL, Old LJ, Rettig WJ. Trophoblast and ovarian cancer antigen LK26. Sensitivity and specificity in immunopathology and molecular identification as a folate-binding protein. *Am J Pathol* 1993; 142:557–567.
37. Selhub J, Dhar GJ, Rosenberg IH. Gastrointestinal absorption of folates and antifolates. *Pharmac Ther* 1987; 20:397–418.
38. Halstad CH. Intestinal absorption of dietary folates. In: (Picciano MF, Stokstad ELR, Greogory JF, eds). Folic Acid Metabolism in Health and Disease. Wiley-Liss, New York, 1990, pp. 23–45.
39. Mason JD. Intestinal transport of monoglutamyl folates in mammalian systems. In: (Picciano MF, Stokstad ELR, Greogory JF, eds.) Folic Acid Metabolism in Health and Disease. Wiley-Liss, New York, 1990, pp. 47–63.
40. Said HM, Ghishan FK, Redha R. Folate transport by human intestinal brush-border membrane vesicles. *Am J Physiol* 1987; 252:G229–G236.
41. Zimmerman J. Folic acid transport in organ-cultured mucosa of human intestine. *Gastroenterology* 1990; 99:964–972.
42. Kessel D, Hall TC, Roberts D, Wodinsky I. Uptake as a determinant of methotrexate response in mouse leukemia. *Science* 1965; 150:752.
43. Goldman ID, Lichtenstein NS, Oliverio VT. Carrier-mediated transport of the folic acid analogue, methotrexate, in the L1210 leukemia cell. *J Biol Chem* 1968; 243:5007–5017.
44. Goldman ID. A model system for the study of heteroexchange diffusion: methotrexate-folate interactions in L1210 and Ehrlich ascites tumor cells. *Biochim Biophys Acta* 1971; 223:624–633.
45. Henderson GB, Zevely EM. Anion exchange mechanism for transport of methotrexate in L1210 cells. *Biochem Biophys Res Commun* 1981; 99:163–169.
46. Schuetz JD, Westin EH, Matherly LH, Pincus R, Swerdlow PS, Goldman ID. Membrane protein changes in an L1210 leukemia cell line with a translocation defect in the methotrexate-tetrahydrofolate cofactor transport carrier. *J Biol Chem* 1989; 264:16,261–16,267.
47. Yang CH, Sirotnak FM. Interaction between anions and the reduced folate/methotrexate transport system in L1210 plasma membrane vesicles: directional symmetry and anion specificity for differential mobility of loaded and unloaded carrier. *J Membr Biol* 1984; 79:285–292.
48. Henderson GB, Zevely EM. Affinity labeling of the 5-methyltetrahydrofolate/methotrexate transport protein in L1210 leukemia cells by treatment with an N-hydroxysuccinimide ester of [^{3}H]methotrexate. *J Biol Chem* 1984; 259:4558–4562.
49. Yang CH, Pain J, Sirotnak FM. Alteration of folate analogue transport inward after induced maturation of HL-60 leukemia cells. *J Biol Chem* 1992; 267:6628–6634.
50. Sirotnak FM, Moccio DM, Yang CH. A novel class of genetic variants of the L1210 cell up-regulated for folate analogue transport inward. *J Biol Chem* 1984; 259:13,139–13,144.
51. Yang CH, Sirotnak FM, Mines LS. Further studies on a novel class of genetic variants of the L1210 cell with increased folate analogue transport inward. *J Biol Chem* 1988; 263:9703–9709.
52. Jansen G, Westerhof GR, Jarmuszewski MJA, Kathmann I, Rijksen G, Schornagel JH. Methotrexate transport in variant human CCRF-CEM cells with elevated levels of the reduced folate carrier: selective effect on carrier-mediated transport of physiological concentrations of reduced folates. *J Biol Chem* 1990; 265:18,272–18,277.
53. Matherly LH, Czajkowski CA, Angeles SM. Identification of a highly glycosylated methotrexate

membrane carrier in K562 human erythroleukemia cells up-regulated for tetrahydrofolate cofactor and methotrexate transport. *Cancer Res* 1991; 51:3420–3426.
54. Freisheim JH, Ratnam M, McAlinden TP, Prasad KMR, Williams FE, Westerhof GR, Schornagel JH, Jansen G. Molecular events in the membrane transport of methotrexate in human CCRF-CEM leukemia cells. *Adv Enzyme Regul* 1992; 32:17–31.
55. Jansen G, Mauritz R, Assaraf YG, Sprecher H, Drori S, Kathmann I, Weterhof GR, Priest DG, Bunni M, Pinedo HM, Schornagel JH, Peters GJ. Regulation of carrier-mediated transport of folates and antifolates in methotrexate sensitive and resistant leukemia cells. *Adv Enzyme Regul* 1997; 35:59–76.
56. Jansen G, Kathmann I, Westerhof GR, Smid K, Noordhuis P, Peters GJ, Schornagel JH, Ratnam M, McAlinden TP, Freisheim JH, Bunni M, Priest DG, Sprecher H, Assaraf YG. Regulation of carrier-mediated transport of folates and antifolates in methotrexate-sensitive and resistant cells. In: (Pfleiderer W, Rokos H, eds) Chemistry and Biology of Pteridines and Folates 1997. Blackwell Science Press, Berlin, 1997, pp. 111–122.
57. Price EM, Ratnam M, Rodeman KM, Freisheim JH. Characterization of the methotrexate transport pathway in murine L1210 leukemia cells: Involvement of a membrane receptor and a cytosolic protein. *Biochemistry* 1988; 27:7853–7858.
58. Matherly LH, Angeles SM. Role of N-glycosylation in the structure and function of the methotrexate membrane transporter from CCRF-CEM human lymphoblastic cells. *Biochem Pharmacol* 1994; 47:1094–1098.
59. Wong S, Proefke SA, Bhushan A, Matherly LH. Isolation of human cDNAs that restore methotrexate sensitivity and reduced folate carrier activity in methotrexate-transport defective Chinese hamster ovary cells. *J Biol Chem* 1995; 270:17,468–17,475.
60. Dixon KH, Lanpher BC, Chiu J, Kelley K, Cowan KH. A novel cDNA restores reduced folate carrier activity and methotrexate sensitivity to transport deficient cells. *J Biol Chem* 1994; 269:17–20.
61. Williams FMR, Murray RC, Underhill TM, Flintoff WF. Isolation of a hamster cDNA clone encoding for a function involved in methotrexate uptake. *J Biol Chem* 1994; 269:5810–5816.
62. Williams FMR, Flintoff WF. Isolation of a human cDNA that complements a mutant hamster cell defective in methotrexate uptake. *J Biol Chem* 1995; 17:2987–2992.
63. Prasad PD, Ramamoorthy S, Leibach FH, Ganapathy V. Molecular cloning of the human placental folate transporter. *Biochem Biophys Res Commun* 1995; 206:681–687.
64. Moscow JA, Gong M, He R, Sgagias MK, Dixon KH, Anzick L, Melzer PS, Cowan KH. Isolation of a gene encoding a human reduced folate carrier (RFC1) and analysis of its expression in transport-deficient, methotrexate-resistant human breast cancer cells. *Cancer Res* 1995; 55:3790–3794.
65. Murray RC, Williams FMR, Williams WF. Structural organization of the reduced folate carrier gene in Chinese hamster ovary cells. *J Biol Chem* 1996; 271:19,174–19,179.
66. Tolner B, Roy K, Sirotnak FM. Organization, structure and alternate splicing of the murine RFC-1 gene encoding a folate transporter. *Gene* 1997; 189:1–7.
67. Yang-Feng TL, Ma YY, Liang R, Prasad PD, Leibach FH, Ganapathy V. Assignment of the human folate transporter gene to chromosome 21q22.3 by somatic cell hybrid analyses and in situ hybridization. *Biochem Biophys Res Commun* 1995; 210:874–879.
68. Wong SC, McQuade R, Proefke SA, Bhushan A, Matherly LH. Human K562 transfectants expressing high levels of reduced folate carrier but exhibiting low transporter activity. *Biochem Pharmacol* 1997; 53:199–206.
69. Sprecher H, Jansen G, Drori S, Schornagel JH, Peters GJ, Assaraf YG. Reduced folate carrier gene amplification and overexpression of altered transcripts in human leukemia CEM-7A cells. *Proc Am Assoc Cancer Res* 1996; 37:381.
70. Brigle KE, Spinella MJ, Sierra EE, Goldman ID. Characterization of a mutation in the reduced folate carrier in a transport defective L1210 murine leukemia cell line. *J Biol Chem* 1995; 270:22,974–22,979.
71. Gong M, Yess J, Connolly T, Ivy Sp, Ohnuma T, Cowan KH, Moscow JA. Molecular mechanism of antifolate transport-deficiency in a methotrexate-resistant MOLT-3 human leukemia cell line. *Blood* 1997; 89:2494–2499.
72. Gorlick R, Goker E, Trippett T, Steinherz P, Elisseyeff Y, Mazumdar M, Flintoff WF, Bertino JR. Defective transport is a common mechanism of acquired resistance in acute lymphocytic leukemia and is associated with decreased reduced folate carrier expression. *Blood* 1997; 89:1013–1018.

73. Wong SC, Proefke SA, Bushan A, Matherly LH. Mutations of the reduced folate carrier in transport impaired CCRF-CEM cells. *Proc Am Assoc Cancer Res* 1997; 38:162.
74. Schlemmer SR, Sirotnak FM. Retentiveness of methotrexate polyglutamates in cultured L1210 cells. *Biochem Pharmacol* 1993; 45:1261–1266.
75. Said HM, Nguyen TT, Dyer DL, Cowan KH, Rubin SA. Intestinal folate transport: identification of a cDNA involved in folate transport and the functional expression and distribution of its mRNA. *Biochim Biophys Acta* 1996; 1281:164–172.
76. Chiao JH, Roy K, Tolner B, Yang CH, Sirotnak FM. *RFC-1* gene expression regulates folate absorption in mouse small intestine. *J Biol Chem* 1997; 272:11,165–11,170.
77. Moscow JA, Connolly T, Myers TG, Cheng CC, Paull K, Cowan KH. Reduced folate carrier (RFC1) expression and anti-folate resistance in transfected and non-selected cell lines. *Int J Cancer* 1997; 72:184–190.
78. Matherly LH, Angeles SM, Czajkowski CA. Characterization of transport-mediated methotrexate resistance in human tumor cells with antibodies to the membrane carrier for methotrexate and tetrahydrofolate cofactors. *J Biol Chem* 1992; 267:23,253–23,260.
79. Matherly LH, Taub JW, Ravindranath Y, Proefke SA, Wong SC, Gimotty P, Buck S, Wright JE, Rosowsky A. Elevated dihydrofolate reductase and impaired methotrexate transport as elements in methotrexate resistance in childhood acute lymphoblastic leukemia. *Blood* 1995; 85:500–509.
80. Chiao JH, Yang CH, Roy K, Pain J, Sirotnak FM. Ligand-directed immunoaffinity purification and properties of the one-carbon, reduced folate carrier. *J Biol Chem* 1995; 270:29,698–29,704.
81. Li WW, Tong WP, Bertino JR. Antitumor activity of antifolate inhibitors of thymidylate and purine synthesis in human soft tissue carcinoma cell lines with intrinsic resistance to methotrexate. *Clin Cancer Res* 1995; 1:631–636.
82. Smith A, Hum M, Winick NJ, Kamen BA. A case for the use of aminopterin in treatment of patients with leukemia based on metabolic studies of blasts *in vitro*. *Clin Cancer Res* 1996; 2:69–73.
83. Rots MG, Pieters R, Veerman AJP, Van Zantwijk CH, Noorhuis P, Peters GJ, Jansen G. Mechanisms of methotrexate resistance and its circumvention by novel antifolates in childhood leukemia. In: (Pfleiderer W, Rokos, H, eds.) Chemistry and Biology of Pteridines and Folates 1997. Blackwell Science Press, Berlin, 1997, pp. 175–180.
84. Peters GJ, Jansen G. Resistance to antimetabolites. In: (Schilsky RL, Milano GA, Retain M, eds.) Principles of Antineoplastic Drug Development and Pharmacology. Marcel Dekker, New York, 1996, pp. 543–585.
85. Gorlick R, Goker E, Trippett T, Waltham M, Banerjee D, Bertino JR. Intrinsic and acquired resistance to methotrexate in acute leukemia. *N Engl J Med* 1996; 335:1041–1048.
86. Trippett T, Schlemmer S, Elisseyeff Y, Goker E, Wachter M, Steinherz P, Tan C, Berman E, Wright JE, Rosowsky A, Schweitzer B, Bertino JR. Defective transport as a mechanism of acquired resistance to methotrexate in patients with acute lymphocytic leukemia. *Blood* 1992; 80:1158–1162.
87. Kathmann I, Mauritz R, Noordhuis P, Voorn D, Aardewijn P, Schornagel JH, Pinedo HM, Peters GJ, Jansen G. Mechanisms of resistance against methotrexate and novel antifolates in human CCRF-CEM leukemia cells. In: (Pfleiderer W, Rokos H, eds.) Chemistry and Biology of Pteridines and Folates 1997. Blackwell Science Press, Berlin, 1997, pp. 257–261.
88. Assaraf YG, Schimke RT. Identification of methotrexate transport deficiency in mammalian cells using fluoresceinated methotrexate and flow cytometry. *Proc Natl Acad Sci USA* 1987; 84:7154–7158.
89. Schuetz JD, Matherly LH, Westin EH, Goldman ID. Evidence for a functional defect in the translocation of the methotrexate transport carrier in a methotrexate-resistant murine L1210 leukemia cell line. *J Biol Chem* 1988; 263:9840–9847.
90. Jackman AL, Kelland LR, Kimbell R, Gibson W, Aherne GW, Hardcastle A, Boyle FT. Mechanism of acquired resistance to the quinazoline thymidylate synthase inhibitor ZD1694 (Tomudex) in one mouse and three human cell lines. *Br J Cancer* 1995; 71:914–924.
91. Takemura Y, Kobayashi H, Gibson W, Kimbell R, Miyachi H, Jackman AL. The influence of drug-exposure conditions on the development of resistance to methotrexate or ZD1694 in cultured human leukemia cells. *Int J Cancer* 1996; 66:29–36.
92. Mauritz R, Kathmann I, Assaraf YG, Drori S, Schornagel JH, Priest DG, Bunni MA, Pinedo HM, Peters GJ, Jansen G. A novel mechanism of resistance to polyglutamatable antifolates in human CEM leukemia cells. In: (Pfleiderer W, Rokos H, eds.) Chemistry and Biology of Pteridines and Folates 1997. Blackwell Science Press, Berlin, 1997, pp. 157–162.

93. Tse A, Brigle KE, Moran RG. Dominant mutations in the reduced folate carrier confer resistance to 5,10-dideazatetrahydrofolate (DDATHF) by causing efficient transport of folic acid. *Proc Am Assoc Cancer Res* 1997; 38:162.
94. Kane MA, Waxman S. Role of folate binding proteins in folate metabolism. *Lab Invest* 1989; 60:737–736.
95. Lacey SW, Sanders JM, Rothberg KG, Anderson RGW, Kamen BA. Complementary DNA for the folate binding protein correctly predicts anchoring to the membrane by phosphatidylinositol. *J Clin Invest* 1989; 84:715–720.
96. Luhrs CA, Slomiany BL. A human membrane-associated folate binding protein is anchored by a glycosylphosphatidylinositol tail. *J Biol Chem* 1989; 264:21,466–21,449.
97. Elwood PC, Deutsch JC, Kolhouse JF. The conversion of the human membrane-associated folate binding protein (folate receptor) to the soluble folate binding protein by a metalloprotease. *J Biol Chem* 1990; 266:2346–2353.
98. Antony AC, Verma RS, Unune AR, LaRosa JA. Identification of a Mg^{2+}-dependent protease in human placenta which cleaves hydrophobic folate binding protein to hydrophilic forms. *J Biol Chem* 1989; 264:1911–1914.
99. Jansen G, Kathmann I, Rademaker BC, Braakhuis BJM, Westerhof GR, Rijksen G, Schornagel JH. Expression of a folate binding protein in L1210 cells grown in low folate medium. *Cancer Res* 49:1959–1963.
100. Ragoussis J, Senger G, Trowsdale J, Campbell IG. Genomic organization of the human folate receptor genes on chromosome 11q13. *Genomics* 1992; 14:423–430.
101. Elwood PC. Molecular cloning and characterization of the human folate-binding protein cDNA from placenta and malignant tissue culture (KB) cells. *J Biol Chem* 1989; 264:14,893–14,901.
102. Ratnam M, Marquardt H, Duhring JL, Freisheim JH. Homologous membrane folate binding proteins in human placenta: cloning and sequence of a cDNA. *Biochemistry* 1989; 28:8249–8254.
103. Shen F, Ross JF, Wang X, Ratnam M. Identification of a novel folate receptor, a truncated receptor, and receptor type β in hematopoeitic cells: cDNA cloning, expression, immunoreactivity, and tissue specificity. *Biochemistry* 1994; 33:1209–1215.
104. Shen F, Wu M, Ross JF, Miller D, Ratnam M. Folate receptor type γ is primarily a secretory protein due to lack of an efficient signal for glycosylphosphatidylinositol modification: protein characterization and cell type specificity. *Biochemistry* 1995; 34:5660–5665.
105. Yan W, Ratnam M. Preferred sites of glycosylphosphatidylinositol modification in folate receptors and constraints in the primary structure of the hydrophobic portion of the signal. *Biochemistry* 1995; 34:14,594–14,600.
106. Luhrs CA. The role of glycosylation in the biosynthesis of and acquisition of ligand-binding activity of the folate binding protein in cultured KB cells. *Blood* 1991; 77:1171–1180.
107. Shen F, Zheng X, Wang J, Ratnam M. Identification of amino acid residues that determine the differential ligand specificities of folate receptors α and β. *Biochemistry* 1997; 36:6157–6163.
108. Wang X, Shen F, Freisheim JH, Gentry LE, Ratnam M. Differential stereospecificities and affinities of folate receptor isoforms for folate compounds and antifolates. *Biochem Pharmacol* 1992; 44:1898–1902.
109. Brigle KE, Spinella MJ, Westin EH, Goldman ID. Increased expression and characterization of two distinct folate binding proteins in murine erythroleukemia cells. *Biochem Pharmacol* 1994; 47:337–345.
110. Brigle KE, Westin EH, Houghton MT, Goldman ID. Characterization of two cDNAs encoding folate binding proteins from L1210 murine leukemia cells. *J Biol Chem* 1991; 266:17,243–17,249.
111. Hjelle JT, Christensen EI, Carone FA, Selhub J. Cell fractionation and electron microscope studies of kidney folate-binding protein. *Am J Physiol* 1991; 260:C338–C346.
112. Rijnboutt S, Jansen G, Posthuma G, Hynes JB, Schornagel JH, Strous GJAM. Endocytosis of GPI-linked membrane folate receptor-α. *J Cell Biol* 1996; 132:35–47.
113. Anderson RGW, Kamen BA, Rothberg KG, Lacey SW. Potocytosis; sequestration and transport of small molecules by caveolae. *Science* 1992; 225:410–411.
114. Kamen BA, Wang MT, Streckfuss AJ, Peryea X, Anderson RGW. Delivery of folates to the cytoplasm of MA104 cells is mediated by the surface membrane receptor that recycles. *J Biol Chem* 1988; 263:13,602–13,609.

115. Rothberg KG, Ying Y, Kamen BA, Anderson RGW. The glycophospholipid-linked folate receptor internalizes folate without entering the clathrin-coated pit endocytic pathway. *J Cell Biol* 1990; 110:637–649.
116. Smart EJ, Mineo C, Anderson RGW. Clustered folate receptors deliver 5-methyltetrahydrofolate to cytoplasm of MA104 cells. *J Cell Biol* 1996; 134:1169–1177.
117. Rothberg KG, Heuser JE, Donzell WC, Ying YS, Glenney JR, Anderson RGW. Caveolin, a protein component of caveolae membrane coats. *Cell* 1992; 68:673–682.
118. Glenney JR, Soppet D. Sequence and expression of caveolin, a protein component of caveolae plasmamembrane domains phosphorylated on tyrosine in RSV-transformed fibroblasts. *Proc Natl Acad Sci USA* 1992; 89:10,517–10,521.
119. Kamen BA, Smith AK, Anderson RGW. The folate receptor works in tandem with a probenecid sensitive carrier in MA104 cells in vitro. *J Clin Invest* 1991; 87:1442–1449.
120. Prasad PD, Mahesh VB, Leibach FH, Ganapathy V. Functional coupling between a bafilomycin A_1-sensitive proton pump and a probenecid-sensitive folate transporter in human placental choriocarcinoma cells. *Biochim Biophys Acta* 1994; 1222:309–314.
121. Jansen G, Schornagel JH, Westerhof GR, Rijksen G, Newell DR, Jackman AL. Multiple transport systems for the uptake of folate-based thymidylate synthase inhibitors. *Cancer Res* 1990; 50:7544–7548.
122. Westerhof GR, Schornagel JH, Kathmann I., Jackman AL, Rosowsky A, Forsch RA, Hynes JB, Boyle FT, Peters GJ, Pinedo HM, Jansen G. Carrier- and receptor-mediated transport of folate antagonists targeting folate-dependent enzymes: correlates of molecular structure and biological activity. *Mol Pharmacol* 1995; 48:459–471.
123. Pinard MF, Jolivet J, Ratnam M, Kathmann I, Molthoff CFM, Westerhof GR, Schornagel JH, Jansen G. Functional aspects of membrane folate receptors in human breast cancer cells with transport-related resistance to methotrexate. *Cancer Chemother Pharmacol* 1996; 38:281–288.
124. Dixon KH, Mulligan T, Chung KN, Elwood PC, Cowan KH. Effects of folate receptor expression following stable transfection into wild type and methotrexate transport-deficient ZR-75-1 human breast cancer cells. *J Biol Chem* 1992; 267:24,140–24,147.
125. Spinella MJ, Brigle KE, Sierra EE, Goldman ID. Distinguishing between folate receptor-—mediated transport and reduced folate carrier-mediated transport in L1210 leukemia cells. *J Biol Chem* 1995; 270:7842–7849.
126. Westerhof GR, Rijnboutt S, Schornagel JH, Pinedo HM, Peters GJ, Jansen G. Functional activity of the reduced folate carrier in KB, MA104 and IGROV-I cells expressing folate binding protein. *Cancer Res* 1995; 55:3795–3802.
127. Anderson RGW. Caveolae: where incoming and outgoing messages meet. *Proc Natl Acad Sci USA* 1993; 90:10,909–10,913.
128. Sargiocomo M, Sudol M, Tang Z, Lisanti MP. Signal transducing molecules and glycosyl-phosphatidylinositol-linked proteins form a caveolin-rich insoluble complex in MDCK cells. *J Cell Biol* 1993; 122:798–809.
129. Parton RG, Simons K. Digging into caveolae. *Science* 1995; 269:1398–1999.
130. Ju H, Zou R, Venema VJ, Venema RC. Direct interaction of endothelial nitric-oxide synthase and caveolin-1 inhibits synthase activity. *J Biol Chem* 1997; 272:18,522–18,525.
131. Engelman JA, Wykoff CC, Yasuhara S, Song KS, Okamoto T, Lisanti MP. Recombinant expression of caveolin-1 in oncogenically transformed cells abrogates anchorage-independent growth. *J Biol Chem* 1997; 272:16,374–16,381.
132. Kane MA, Portillo RM, Elwood PC, Antony AC, Kolhouse JF. The influence of extracellular folate concentration on methotrexate uptake by human KB cells. *J Biol Chem* 1986; 261:44–49.
133. Miotti S, Facheris P, Tomassetti A, Bottero F, Bottini C, Ottone F, Colnaghi MI, Bunni MA, Priest DG, Canevari S. Growth of ovarian-carcinoma cell lines at physiological folate concentration: effect of folate-binding protein expression *in vitro* and *in vivo*. *Int J Cancer* 1995; 63:395–401.
134. Hsueh CT, Dolnick BJ. Regulation of folate-binding protein gene expression by DNA methylation in methotrexate-resistant KB cells. *Biochem Pharmacol* 1994; 47:1019–1027.
135. Hsueh CT, Dolnick BJ. Altered folate-binding protein mRNA stability in KB cells grown in folate-deficient medium. *Biochem Pharmacol* 1993; 45:2537–2545.
136. Kamen BA, Capdevilla A. Receptor-mediated folate accumulation is regulated by the folate content. *Proc Natl Acad Sci USA* 1986; 83:5983–5987.

137. Smart EJ, Ying YS, Anderson RGW. Hormonal regulation of caveolae internalization. *J Cell Biol* 1995; 131:929–938.
138. Westerhof GR, Jansen G, van Emmerik N, Kathmann I, Rijksen G, Jackman AL, Schornagel JH. Membrane transport of antifolate compounds in L1210 cells: the role of carrier- and receptor-mediated transport systems. *Cancer Res* 1991; 51:5507–5513.
139. Schultz RM, Andis SL, Schakelford KA, Gates SB, Ratnam M, Mendelsohn LG, Shih C, Grindey GB. Role of membrane-associated folate binding protein in the cytotoxicity of antifolates in KB, IGROV1, and L1210A cells. *Oncology Res* 1995; 7:97–102.
140. Miotti S, Bagnoli M, Ottone F, Tomassetti A, Colnaghi MI, Canevari S. Simultaneous activity of two different mechanism of folate transport in ovarian carcinoma cell lines. *J Cell Biochem* 1997; 65:479–491.
141. Sierra EE, Brigle KE, Spinella MJ, Goldman ID. Comparison of transport properties of the reduced folate carrier and folate receptor in murine L1210 leukemia cells. *Biochem Pharmacol* 1995; 50:1287–1294.
142. Spinella MJ, Brigle KE, Freemantle SJ, Sierra EE, Goldman ID. Comparison of methotrexate polyglutamylation in L1210 leukemia cells when influx is mediated by the reduced folate carrier or the folate receptor. *Biochem Pharmacol* 1996; 52:703–712.
143. Luhrs CA, Raskin CA, Durbin R, Wu S, Sadasivan E, McAllister W, Rothenberg SP. Transfection of a glycosylated phosphatidylinositol-anchored folate-binding protein complementary DNA provides cells with the ability to survive in low folate medium. *J Clin Invest* 1992; 90:840–847.
144. Matsue H, Rothberg KG, Takashima A, Kamen BA, Anderson RGW, Lacey SW. Folate receptor allows cells to grow in low concentrations of 5-methyltetrahydrofolate. *Proc Natl Acad Sci USA* 1992; 89:6006–6009.
145. Wang X, Jansen G, Fan J, Kohler WJ, Ross JF, Schornagel JH, Ratnam M. Variant GPI structure in relation to membrane-associated functions of murine folate receptor. *Biochemistry* 1996; 35:16,305–16,312.
146. Schornagel JH, Mauritz R, Kathmann I, Pinedo HM, Peters GJ, Jansen G. Kinetics of carrier- and receptor-mediated transport of antifolates. *Proc Am Assoc Cancer Res* 1996; 37:386.
147. Antony AC, Bruno E, Briddell RA, Brandt JE, Verma R, Hoffman R. Effect of perturbation of specific folate receptors during in vitro erythropoiesis. *J Clin Invest* 1987; 80:1618–1623.
148. Antony AC, Briddell RA, Brandt JE, Stravena JE, Verma RS, Miller ME, Kalasinski LA, Hoffman R. Megaloblastic hematopoieses in vitro. Interaction of anti-folate receptor antibodies with hematopoietic progenitor cells leads to a proliferative response independent of megaloblastic changes. *J Clin Invest* 1991; 87:313–325.
149. Henderson GB, Strauss BP. Characteristics of a novel transport system for folate compounds in wild-type and methotrexate-resistant L1210 cells. *Cancer Res* 1990; 50:1709–1714.
150. Sierra EE, Brigle KE, Spinella MJ, Goldman ID. pH dependence of methotrexate transport by the reduced folate carrier and the folate receptor in L1210 cells. *Biochem Pharmacol* 1997; 53:223–231.
151. Sirotnak FM, Goutas LJ, Jacobsen DM, Mines LS, Barrueco JR, Gaumont Y, Kisliuk RL. Carrier-mediated transport of folate compounds in L1210 cells. *Biochem Pharmacol* 1987; 36:1569–1667.
152. Ackland SP, Schilsky RL. High dose methotrexate: a critical reappraisal. *J Clin Oncol* 1987; 5:2017–2031.
153. Yang CH, Peterson RHF, Sirotnak FM, Chello PI. Folate analog transport by plasma membrane vesicles isolated from L1210 leukemia cells. *J Biol Chem* 1979; 254:1402–1407.
154. Schmid FA, Sirotnak FM, Otter GM, DeGraw JI. New antifolates of 10-deazaaminopterin series: markedly increased antitumor activity of the 10-ethyl analogue compared to the parent compound and methotrexate against some human tumor xenografts in nude mice. *Cancer Treat Rep* 1985; 69:551–553.
155. Rhee MS, Galivan J, Wright JE, Rosowsky A. Biochemical studies on PT523, a potent nonpolyglutamatable antifolate, in cultured cells. *Mol Pharmacol* 1994; 45:783–791.
156. Jones TJ, Calvert AH, Jackman AL, Brown SJ, Jones M, Harrap KH. A potent antitumor quinazoline inhibitor of thymidylate synthase: synthesis, biological properties and therapeutic results in mice. *Eur J Cancer* 1981; 17:11–19.
157. Fernandes DJ, Bertino JR, Hynes JB. Biochemical and antitumor effects of 5,8-dideazaisopteroylglutamate, a unique quinazoline inhibitor of thymidylate synthase. *Cancer Res* 1983; 43:1117–1123.

158. Jackman AL, Newell DR, Gibson W, Jodrell DI, Taylor GA, Bishop JA, Hughes LR, Calvert AH. The biochemical pharmacology of the thymidyulate synthase inhibitor 2-desamino-2-methyl-N^{10}-propargyl-5,8-dideazafolic acid (ICI 198,583). *Biochem Pharmacol* 1991; 42:1885–1895.
159. Jackman AL, Taylor GA, Gibson W, Kimbell R, Brown M, Calvert AH, Judson IR, Hughes LR. ICI D1694, a quinazoline antifolate thymidylate synthase inhibitor that is a potent inhibitor of L1210 tumor cell growth in vitro and in vivo: a new agent for clinical studies. *Cancer Res* 1991; 51:5579–5586.
160. Hanlon MH, Ferone R. *In vitro* uptake, anabolism, and cellular retention of 1843U89 and other benzoquinazoline inhibitors of thymidylate synthase. *Cancer Res* 1996; 56:3301–3306.
161. Shih C, Chen VJ, Gossett LS, Gates SB, MacKellar WC, Habeck LL, Schackelford KA, Mendelsohn LG, Soose DJ, Patel VF, Andis SL, Bewley JR, Rayl EA, Moroson BA, Beardsley GP, Kohler W, Ratnam M, Schultz RM. LY213514, a pyrrolo[2,3-d]pyrimidine-based antifolate that inhibits multiple folate-requiring enzymes. *Cancer Res* 1997; 57:1116–1123.
162. Jackman AL, Kimbell R, Aherne GW, Brunton L, Jansen G, Stephens TC, Smith M, Wardleworth M, Ward W, Boyle FT. The cellular pharmacology and *in vivo* activity of a new anticancer agent, ZD9331; a water soluble, non-polyglutamatable quinazoline-based inhibitor of thymidylate synthase. *Clin Cancer Res* 1997; 3:911–921.
163. Bavetsias V, Jackman AL, Marriot JH, Kimbell R, Gibson W, Boyle FT, Bisset GMF. Folate-based inhibitors of thymidylate synthase: synthesis and antitumor activity of γ-linked sterically hindered dipeptide analogues of 2-desamino-2-methyl-N^{10}-propargyl-5,8-dideazafolic acid (ICI 198583). *J Med Chem* 1997; 40:1495–1510.
164. Jansen G, Schornagel JH, Wardleworth M, Boyle FT, Bavetsias V, Marriot J, Jackman AL. Glutamate side chain modified quinazoline antifolate thymidylate synthase inhibitors: transport characteristics and biological evaluation. *Ann Oncol* 1996; 7(suppl. 1):90.
165. Rosowsky A, Lazarus H, Yuan GC, Beltz WR, Magnini L, Abelson HT, Modest EJ, Frei III E. Effects of methotrexate esters and other lipophilic antifolates on methotrexate-resistant human leukemic lymphoblsts. *Biochem Pharmacol* 1980; 29:648–652.
166. Bekkenk M, Mauritz R, Pieters R, Rots M, van Zantwijk CH, Veerman AJP, Peters GJP, Jansen G. Sensitivity for novel antifolates in childhood leukemia cells with resistance to methotrexate. In: (Pieters, R, Kaspers, GJL, Veerman AJP, eds.) Drug Resistance in Leukemia and Lymphoma II. Harwood Academic Publishers, Amsterdam, The Netherlands, 1997, pp. 173–181.
167. Li WW, Cordon-Cardo C, Chen Q, Jhanwar SC, Bertino JR. Establishment, characterization and drug sensitivity of four new human soft tissue sarcoma cell lines. *Int J Cancer* 1996; 68:514–519.
168. Zervos PH, Allen RH, Thornton DE, Thiem PA. Functional folate status as a prognostic indicator of toxicity in clinical trials of the multitargeted antifolate LY231514. *Eur J Cancer* 1997; 33:(suppl)S18.
169. Smith GK, Amyx H, Boytos CM, Duch D, Ferone R, Wilson HR. Enhanced activity for the thymidylate synthase inhibitor 1843U89 through decreased host toxicity with oral folic acid. *Cancer Res* 1995; 55:6117–6125.
170. Alati T, Worzalla JF, Shih C, Bewley JR, Lewis S, Moran RG, Grindey GB. Augmentation of the therapeutic activity of lometrexol [(6-R)5,10-dideazatetrahydrofolate] by oral folic acid. *Cancer Res* 1996; 56:2331–2335.
171. Holm J, Hansen SI, Hoier-Madsen M, Sondergaard K, Bzorek M. The high affinity folate receptor of normal and malignant human colonic mucosa. *APMIS* 1994; 10:828–836.
172. Schmitz JC, Grindey GB, Schultz RM, Priest DG. Impact of dietary folic acid on reduced folates in mouse plasma and tissues. Relationship to dideazatetrahydrofolate sensitivity. *Biochem Pharmacol* 1994; 48:319–325.
173. Matherly LH, Barlowe CK, Phillips VM, Goldman ID. The effects of 4-aminoantifolates on 5-formyltetrahydrofolate metabolism in L1210 cells. A biochemical basis of the selectivity of leucovorin rescue. *J Biol Chem* 1987; 262:710–717.
174. Jolivet J, Jansen G, Peters GJ, Pinard MF, Schornagel JH. Leucovorin rescue of human cancer and bone marrow cells following edatrexate or methotrexate. *Biochem Pharmacol* 1994; 47:659–665.
175. Sirotnak FM, Otter GM, Schmid FA. Markedly improved efficacy of edatrexate compared to methotrexate in a high-dose regimen with leucovorin rescue against metastatic murine solid tumors. *Cancer Res* 1993; 53:587–591.
176. Van der Veer LJ, Westerhof GR, Rijksen G, Schornagel JH, Jansen G. Cytotoxicity of methotrexate and trimetrexate and its reversal by folinic acid in human leukemic CCRF-CEM cells with carrier-mediated and receptor-mediated folate uptake. *Leukemia Res* 1989; 13:981–987.

177. Campbell IG, Jones TA, Foulkes WD, Trowsdale J. Folate binding protein is a narker for ovarian cancer. *Cancer Res* 1991; 51:5329–5338.
178. Coney LR, Tomassetti A, Carayannopoulos L, Frasca V, Kamen BA, Colnaghi MI, Zurawski VR. Cloning of a tumor-associated antigen: MOv18 and MOv19 antibodies recognize a folate binding protein. *Cancer Res* 1991; 51:6125–6132.
179. Toffoli G, Cernigoi C, Russo A, Gallo A, Bagnoli M, Boicchi M. Overexpression of folate binding protein in ovarian cancers. *Int J Cancer* 1997; 74:193–198.
180. Miotti S, Canevari S, Menard S, Mezzanzanica D, Porro G, Pupa SM, Regazzoni M, Tagliabue E, Colnaghi MI. Characterization of human ovarian-associated antigens defined by novel monoclonal antibodies with tumor-restricted specificity. *Int J Cancer* 1987; 39:297–303.
181. Molthoff CFM, Buist MR, Kenemans P, Pinedo HM, Boven E. Experimental and clinical analysis of the characteristics of a chimeric monoclonal antibody, MOv18, reactive with an ovarian cancer-associated antigen. *J Nucl Med* 1992; 33:2000–2005.
182. Grippa F, Buraggi GL, Re ED, Gasparini M, Seregini E, Canevari S, Gadina M, Presti M, Marini A, Seccamani E. Radioimmunoscintigraphy of ovarian cancer with the MOv18 monoclonal antibody. *Eur J Cancer* 1991; 27:724–729.
183. Buist MR, Kenemans P, Den Hollander W, Vermorken JB, Molthoff CJM, Burger CW, Helmerhorst TJM, Baak JPA, Roos JC. Kinetics and tissue distribution of the radiolabeled chimeric monoclonal antibody MOv18 IgG and F(ab')$_2$ fragments in ovarian carcinoma patients. *Cancer Res* 1993; 53:5413–5418.
184. Molthoff CFM, Prinssen HM, Kenemans P, van Hof AC, den Hollander W, Verheijen RHM. Escalating protein doses for chimeric monoclonal antibody MOv18 IgG in ovarian carcinoma patients: a phase I study. *Cancer* 1997; 80:2712–2720.
185. Crippa F, Bolis G, Seregni E, Gavoni N, Scarfone G, Ferraris C, Buraggi GL, Bombardieri E. Single-dose intraperitoneal radioimmunotherapy with the murine monoclonal antibody I-131 MOv18: clinical results with minimal residual disease of ovarian cancer. *Eur J Cancer* 1995; 31A:686–690.
186. Molthoff C, Klein-Gebbinck J, Verheijen R, Kenemans P, Jansen G. Membrane folate receptor mediated binding and internalization of (anti)folate-MOv18 immunoconjugates. *Tumor Targeting* 1996; 2:140–141.
187. Molthoff C, Gebbinck J, Verheijen R, Kenemans P, Jansen G. Membrane folate receptor-mediated binding and internalization of (anti)folate-MOv18 immunoconjugates. *Pteridines* 1997; 8:163–164.
188. Coney LR, Mezzanzanica D, Sanborn D, Casalini P, Colnaghi MI, Zurawski VR. Chimeric murine-human antibodies directed against folate binding receptor are efficient mediators of ovarian carcinoma cell killing. *Cancer Res* 1994; 54:2448–2455.
189. Canevari S, Stoter G, Arienti F, Bolis G, Colnaghi MI, Re EMD, Eggermont AMM, Goey SH, Gratema JW, Lamers CHJ, Nooy MA, Parmiani G, Raspagliesi F, Ravagnani F, Scarfone G, Trimbos JB, Warnaar SO, Bolhuis RLH. Regression of advanced ovarian carcinoma by intraperioneal treatment with autologous T lymphocytes retargeted by a bispecific monoclonal antibody. *J Natl Cancer Inst* 1995; 87:1463–1469.
190. Bolhuis RLH, Lamers CHJ, Goey SH, Eggermont AMM, Trimbos JBMZ, Stoter G, Lanzavecchia A, Re E, Miotti S, Raspagliesi F, Rivoltini L, Colnaghi MI. Adoptive immunotherapy of ovarian carcinoma with BS-MAb-targeted lymphocytes: a multicenter study. *Int J Cancer* 1992; 7:78–81.
191. Boerman O, Tibben JG, Massuger LFAG, Claessens RAMJ, Corstens FHM. Tumor targeting of the anti-ovarian carcinoma X anti-CD3/TCR bispecific monoclonal antibody OC/TR and its parental MOv18 antibody in experimental ovarian cancer. *Anticancer Res* 1995; 15:2169–2174.
192. Leamon CP, Low PS. Delivery of macromolecules into living cells: a methods that exploits folate receptor endocytosis. *Proc Natl Acad Sci USA* 1991; 88:5572–5576.
193. Leamon CP, Low PS. Cytotoxicity of momordin-folate conjugates in cultured human cells. *J Biol Chem* 1992; 267:24,966–24,971.
194. Leamon CP, Low PS. Selective targeting of malignant cells with cytotoxin-folate conjugates. *J Drug Targeting* 1994; 2:101–112.
195. Lee RJ, Low PS. Delivery of liposomes into cultured KB cells via folate receptor-mediated endocytosis. *J Biol Chem* 1994; 269:3198–3204.
196. Lee RJ, Low PS. Folate-mediated tumor cell targeting of liposome-entrapped doxorubicin in vitro. *Biochim Biophys Acta* 1995; 1233:134–144.

197. Wang S, Lee RJ, Cauchon G, Gorenstein DG, Low PS. Delivery of antisense oligodeoxyribonucleotides against the human epidermal growth factor receptor into cultured KB cells with liposomes conjugated to folate via polyethylene glycol. *Proc Natl Acad Sci USA* 1995; 92:3318–3322.
198. Mathias CJ, Wang S, Lee RJ, Waters DJ, Low PS, Green MA. Tumor-selective radiopharmaceutical targeting via receptor-mediated endocytosis of Gallium-67-deferoxamine-folate. *J Nucl Med* 1996; 37:1003–1008.
199. Wang S, Lee RJ, Mathias CJ, Green MA, Low PS. Synthesis, purification, and tumor cell uptake of ^{67}Ga-deferoxamine-folate, a potential radiopharmaceutical for tumor imaging. *Bioconjugate Chem* 1996; 7:56–62.
200. Kranz DM, Patrick TA, Brigle KE, Spinella MJ, Roy EJ. Conjugates of folate and anti-T-cell-receptor antibodies specifically target folate-receptor-positive tumor cells for lysis. *Proc Natl Acad Sci USA* 1995; 92:9057–9061.
201. Cho BK, Roy EJ, Patrick TA, Kranz DM. Single-chain Fv/folate conjugates mediate efficient lysis of folate-receptor positive tumor cells. *Bioconjugate Chem* 1997; 8:338–346.

15 Folates as Chemotherapeutic Modulators

Julio Barredo, Marlene A. Bunni, Raghunathan Kamasamudram, and David G. Priest

CONTENTS

INTRODUCTION
METABOLIC INTERCONVERSION OF FOLATES
MODULATION OF ANTIFOLATE TOXICITY
MODULATION OF FU ANTITUMOR ACTIVITY
PHARMACOKINETICS
SUMMARY
REFERENCES

1. INTRODUCTION

Antifolates are effective chemotherapeutic agents used to treat a wide range of malignancies *(1–3)*. At pharmacological doses, limiting toxicity occurs in hematopoietic cells and intestinal mucosa, with lesser effects on kidney, liver, and the central nervous system *(4)*. An accepted strategy to overcome these toxicities is the supplementation of folates as rescue agents *(5–7)*. In this context, the use of high doses of methotrexate (MTX) with leucovorin (LV) or 5-formyltetrahydrofolate (5-CHOFH$_4$) rescue is widely used in the clinical setting *(8,9)*. A second modulatory application of folates is potentiation of drug cytotoxicity when used in conjunction with certain inhibitors of folate-related enzymes. The prime example of this type of modulation is the combination of 5-fluorouracil (5FU) and LV leading to a more potent inhibition of thymidylate synthase (TS) and to improved therapeutic activity in several epithelial malignancies *(10–13)*. The rational use of folates as modulators of toxicity or antitumor activity requires an integral understanding of their biochemistry, pharmacokinetics, and pharmacodynamics.

From: *Anticancer Drug Development Guide: Antifolate Drugs in Cancer Therapy*
Edited by: A.L. Jackman © Humana Press Inc., Totowa, NJ

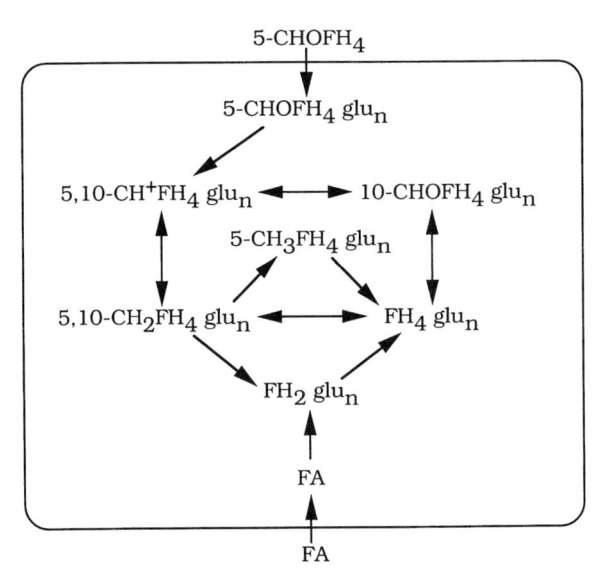

```
                    5-CHOFH$_4$
                        ↓
                 5-CHOFH$_4$ glu$_n$
                   ↙
  5,10-CH$^+$FH$_4$ glu$_n$ ⟷  10-CHOFH$_4$ glu$_n$
           ↕        5-CH$_3$FH$_4$ glu$_n$        ↕
                       ↗
  5,10-CH$_2$FH$_4$ glu$_n$ ⟷  FH$_4$ glu$_n$
                   ↘       ↗
                  FH$_2$ glu$_n$
                        ↑
                        FA
                        ↑
                        FA
```

Fig. 1. Cellular interconversions of LV (5-CHOFH$_4$) and FA.

This chapter will review the biochemistry and metabolism of folates associated with modulation, with emphasis on the pharmacokinetic aspects of these compounds.

2. METABOLIC INTERCONVERSION OF FOLATES

The two folates that have been used clinically to ameliorate toxicity are LV and folic acid (FA) *(7–14)*. LV has been used extensively both to reverse toxic side effects of antifolates and as a potentiator of 5FU cytotoxicity, whereas FA has been used on a more experimental basis. Both of these folate forms require metabolic transformation to other species in order to act as modulators. As shown in Fig. 1, following cellular uptake via an active transport process *(15)*, folates below the tetrahydrofolate (FH$_4$) oxidation level undergo reduction catalyzed by the enzyme dihydrofolate reductase (DHFR), metabolic interconversion to at least five different one-carbon forms, and polyglutamylation through the addition of γ-linked glutamyl residues catalyzed by folylpolyglutamate synthetase (FPGS) *(16,17)*. In the case of LV, it is rapidly converted by enzymatic and nonenzymatic processes to 10-formyltetrahydrofolate (10-CHOFH$_4$) *(18)*. Subsequently, this form establishes a dynamic steady state with other folate species through a series of enzymatic interconversions *(19)*. Hence, supplementation of FA or LV initiates a complex metabolic process that results in elevation of an array of reduced folates. Because folate pathways are integrally connected, all folate species tend to become elevated although some are more sensitive to extracellular changes than others *(20)*.

3. MODULATION OF ANTIFOLATE TOXICITY

Antifolates very often target TS either directly or indirectly *(1,14,21–23)*. Consequently, this enzyme lies at the core of attempts to prevent or reverse toxicity. At moderate doses, MTX and other DHFR inhibitors such as edatrexate (EDX), are thought to cause depletion of the TS substrate 5,10-methylenetetrahydrofolate (CH_2FH_4), resulting in the indirect inhibition of TS *(1,24,25)*. At higher doses, these compounds and several other novel antifolates such as Tomudex (ZD1694), ZD9331, Thymitaq (AG337), GW1843, and LY231514 act directly upon TS to inhibit generation of thymidylate *(14,22,26–29)*. Based on rescue studies with hypoxanthine, higher doses of almost all antifolates also result in disruption of purine metabolism *(1,3)*.

Most in vitro studies of LV modulation of MTX toxicity have been conducted using tumor cell lines *(30,31)*. In these systems, for LV to prevent toxicity it is generally required that MTX or polyglutamates thereof (MTX-PG), be displaced from the cell or prevented from accumulating. There are several modes by which this could occur, including competition for the uptake carrier or for FPGS sites preventing either cellular uptake or MTX-PG synthesis *(1,3,30,32)*. An additional mechanism of rescue is intracellular elevation of CH_2FH_4, resulting in accumulation of FH_2 via the TS reaction. This concept also involves displacement of MTX from DHFR by FH_2 and hence generation of "free" intracellular MTX that can be more readily displaced from the cell.

A disadvantage of in vitro studies of toxicity reversal is the difficulty in establishing selectivity of the folate modulation process for normal vs tumor cells. Jolivet et al. *(6)* and Stromhaug et al. *(33)* have investigated the role of LV in reversing MTX toxicity in human hematopoietic stem cells in culture. Their results indicate preferential rescue of normal progenitors compared to tumor cells, but more studies are needed. In vivo studies have examined the role of LV as a rescue agent using mice implanted intraperitoneally with the L1210 murine leukemia cell line *(34)*. A moderate time- and dose-dependent selectivity for the retention of MTX in tumor vs intestinal epithelial cells was observed. Additionally, LV rescue given after high dose MTX (HDMTX) extended survival in this model *(35)* and resulted in greater elevation of FH_2 pools in tumor vs intestinal epithelium *(34)*.

The clinical rationale for HDMTX with LV rescue includes the potential to overcome drug resistance as a result of dose-dependent formation of MTX-PG, and accumulation of high plasma concentrations of MTX leading to cytotoxic concentrations in cerebrospinal fluid and other sanctuary sites. In general, doses of MTX over 100 mg/m^2 require LV rescue, and doses as high as 33 gm/m^2 have been reported to be well tolerated when given with LV rescue *(36)*. More recently the use of LV rescue with EDX has also been shown to ameliorate toxicity and increase the therapeutic index in patients with lung cancer *(37)*.

Folic acid has recently received renewed attention as a means by which toxicity can be averted. The studies by Grindey and coworkers indicated a substantial increase in the toxicity of Lometrexol (DDATHF) in mice fed a FA-restricted diet *(38)*. Likewise, graded supplementation of FA demonstrated a significant reduction in toxicity without impacting negatively on antitumor activity, suggesting that FA might be used to enhance the therapeutic index. This model has been recently extended to studies using the novel multitargeted antifolate LY231514 and the TS-targeted compound GW1843 *(14,29)*.

Taken together, these data suggest that FA may also be suitable as a folate source for modulation of drug toxicity. Even though some initial clinical trials failed to demonstrate this effect in humans *(7)*, additional studies testing various doses and schedules will be needed to definitively address the clinical role of these laboratory observations.

4. MODULATION OF FU ANTITUMOR ACTIVITY

The ability to form and maintain a stable ternary complex is a critical determinant of sensitivity to fluorouracil's DNA-directed antitumor activity which has been discussed more extensively in Chapter 5. In summary, LV enhances 5FU inhibition of TS via stabilization of the covalent ternary complex formed between TS, fluorodeoxyuridine monophosphate, and CH_2FH_4 *(39,40)*. Exogenous LV administration results in elevated ternary complex formation and increased cytotoxicity *(10)*. Clinically, the combination of 5FU and LV results in improved tumor response as well as augmented toxicity (lower MTD compared to 5FU alone) *(11–13)*.

5. PHARMACOKINETICS

5.1. Methods of Folate Estimation

The use of folates both as agents to reduce the toxicity of antifolates and to potentiate 5FU antitumor activity has become accepted therapy for many human malignancies *(7–14)*. However, the dose, administration route, and time interval between administration of drug and folate vary considerably between treatment regimens. Hence, a precise and thorough examination of the pharmacokinetics of these folates and their metabolites could aid substantially in optimal clinical trial design. However, attempts to conduct such studies have been limited by analytical difficulties associated with the unstable nature of reduced folates and the number of potential metabolites. Historically estimates of plasma folates have relied on microbiological assessment through the use of a panel of three microbes *(41,42)*. Whereas this approach is very sensitive, it is tedious and limited in the number of reduced folates that can be evaluated. Methods based on chromatographic separation prior to evaluation can potentially be applied to most, if not all, reduced folates after enzymatic removal of polyglutamates *(43,44)*. However, instability of more labile folates generally limits this approach to the most abundant species present in plasma after LV administration (5-$CHOFH_4$ and 5-CH_3FH_4). A radioenzymatic method has been developed that is based on entrapment of the metabolite, CH_2FH_4, and other folates after enzymatic conversion to this form, into the covalent ternary complex formed between bacterial TS and tritiated fluorodeoxyuridine monophosphate. This approach has recently been used to determine the pharmacokinetics of LV and its less stable metabolites in human and mouse plasma *(45,46)*. Some of the results obtained will be discussed in the remaining portion of this chapter.

5.2. General Considerations

There are at least four folate metabolites that can potentially arise through known enzymatic steps following the administration of LV to humans. Although this metabolism is thought to occur predominately in hepatic tissue, other sites can participate to a lesser

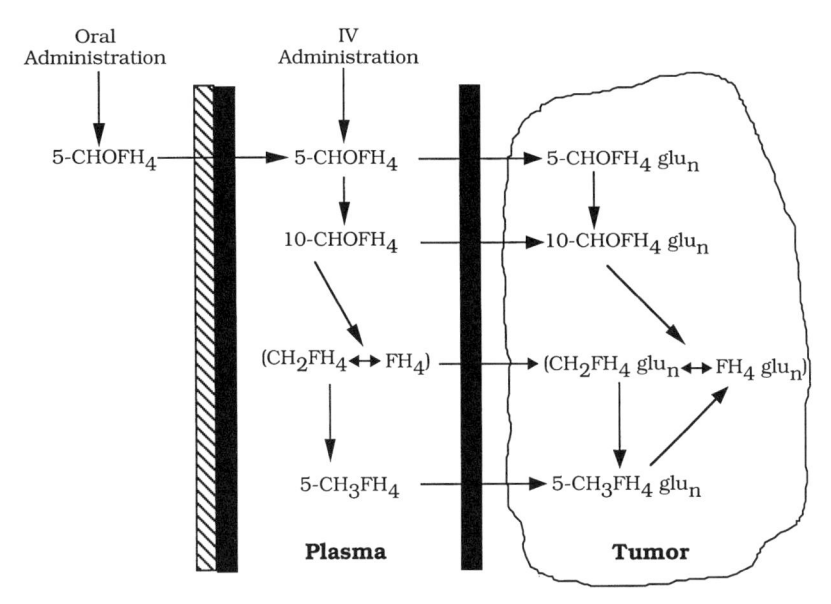

Fig. 2. A proposed model for metabolite accumulation in tumor following iv and oral administration of LV.

extent so that the kinetic behavior of these circulating metabolites following a pharmacologic dose of LV is exceptionally complex. In addition, the uptake of metabolites from plasma by the target tissue can vary depending upon the folate type and level. Whereas reversal of toxicity focuses on metabolism within normal tissues. 5FU potentiation studies require that tumor tissue as well be examined. Studies of circulating folates can provide insight into the potential for elevation of folates in tissues, but direct assessment is much more desirable. Emerging results from very limited studies provide a preliminary indication that human tumor responsiveness to 5FU depends on elevated CH_2FH_4 *(47)*, but limited availability of human tissue samples have made such studies difficult. Hence, animal models have been the only practical alternative and they will be discussed subsequently.

5.3. Pharmacokinetics of Leucovorin in Humans

The complex array of folates that can arise in plasma after administration of LV to humans is shown in Fig. 2. According to this model, it is presumed that metabolism of 5-$CHOFH_4$ or LV can occur at many sites resulting in elevation of essentially all metabolites in plasma. Hence, both circulating parent compound and metabolites would be available for uptake and utilization by tumor tissue. Administration of LV by the oral route requires uptake across the intestinal mucosa, a potentially saturable barrier. Thus, prediction of plasma accumulation and depletion of individual folates using classical algorithms becomes exceptionally difficult. Hence, detailed evaluation of each folate in

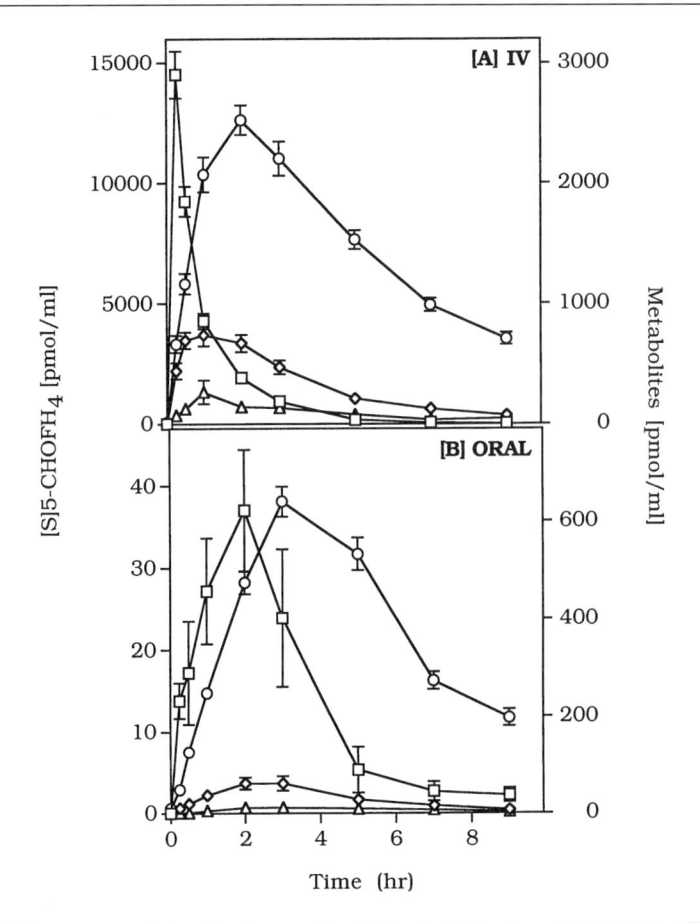

Fig. 3. Reduced folate accumulation in plasma after LV administration. 5-CHOFH$_4$ (□), CH$_2$FH$_4$ + FH$_4$ (◇), 5-CH$_3$FH$_4$ (○), and 10-CHOFH$_4$ (△) were estimated by the ternary complex assay after iv (**A**) and 2 wk later oral (**B**) administration of 125 mg/m^2 LV to healthy volunteers. Values are the mean ± SEM of duplicate analyses of samples from five volunteers.

plasma as a function of time has been necessary to assess metabolite availability to target tissues.

Figure 3A shows the time and dose dependence of [S]5-CHOFH$_4$, the active LV diastereomer, and metabolites thereof monitored in plasma by the ternary complex method following iv administration *(45)*. The parent compound, 5-CHOFH$_4$, declines in an apparent first-order process as a result of metabolism, tissue uptake, and renal elimination. The dose-dependent half life of LV is approx 30 min. 5-CH$_3$FH$_4$ is the predominant circulating metabolite, but other folates are also present at significant levels. In fact, the maximal accumulation of the CH$_2$FH$_4$ + FH$_4$ pool is only approx threefold less than the 5-CH$_3$FH$_4$ pool. Whereas the specific metabolic pathways or tissue sites of metabolism are complex, it is likely that 10-CHOFH$_4$ is the major initial stable metabolite and liver is the primary metabolic site. Additionally, CH_2FH_4 and FH_4 are probably formed next and accumulate transiently with 5-CH_3FH_4 being the terminal metabolite.

It is currently unclear to what extent 5-CH_3FH_4 can itself reverse toxicity or potentiate 5FU. Even so, clinical administration of 5FU following LV has typically targeted the time when 5-CH_3FH_4 is maximally elevated. However, the observation that CH_2FH_4 (likely to be the most important metabolite for modulation) is also present in plasma and that it achieves a peak concentration earlier than 5-CH_3FH_4 (Fig. 3A), suggests a shorter interval between 5FU and LV administration may lead to superior tumor response. This postulate assumes that tumor elevation of the active metabolite corresponds to plasma elevation. This assumption receives support from animal studies to be discussed later.

As pointed out earlier, following oral administration of LV, intestinal absorption must also be considered as an important determinant of plasma metabolite elevation (*see* Fig. 2). It can be seen in Fig. 3B that only a relatively small fraction of the parent compound accumulates after administration of an oral dose of LV, compared to an equivalent dose administered iv (Fig. 3A). Whitehead et al. *(48)* have reported that significant metabolism occurs in the intestinal mucosa prior to passage into the portal circulation. However, saturation of intestinal absorption of the parent compound (to be discussed) is probably the major reason that maximal accumulation of 5-CH_3FH_4 is fourfold less after an oral dose of LV than after iv administration. As with the iv route, oral LV also gives rise to the more labile metabolites CH_2FH_4, FH_4, and 10-$CHOFH_4$. While there is less accumulation of these metabolites after oral vs iv administration, nevertheless, it is clear that significant amounts of all metabolites are present. 5-CH_3FH_4 exhibits peak accumulation at approx 3 h after oral administration of LV, whereas the more labile and transient pools achieve maximal elevation earlier.

The precise amount of LV needed for reversal of toxicity or 5FU modulation remains unclear. However, it can be seen in Fig. 4A that there is little saturation of maximal 5-CH_3FH_4 accumulation up to iv doses of LV as high as 500 mg/m^2. Likewise, there is little indication that the more transient CH_2FH_4 + FH_4 or 10-$CHOFH_4$ pools become saturated with regard to peak accumulation. Further, although not shown, total accumulation or AUC values for these metabolites were not saturable *(45)*. Hence, because there is little evidence of saturation after iv administration of LV, this route can be used to achieve very high plasma levels of all metabolites. On the other hand, in the case of oral administration, as doses of LV are increased there is clear saturation of 5-$CHOFH_4$ with regard to peak accumulation (Fig. 4B). Likewise, all metabolite pools also exhibit saturation. Again, AUC values were saturable in a manner similar to peak accumulation *(45)*. Hence, whereas iv doses as high as 500 mg/m^2 yield near proportional dose-dependent peak accumulation and AUC values for metabolites, when given orally, both plasma 5-$CHOFH_4$ itself and resultant metabolites increase little at doses of 250 mg/m^2 and beyond.

5.4. Tissue Disposition of Folates in Animals

Because it is difficult to obtain tissue samples from humans at sufficient frequency to determine kinetic profiles, animal models have been used as an alternative. Early models used both rats and mice but the exceptionally high supplementation of typical labo-

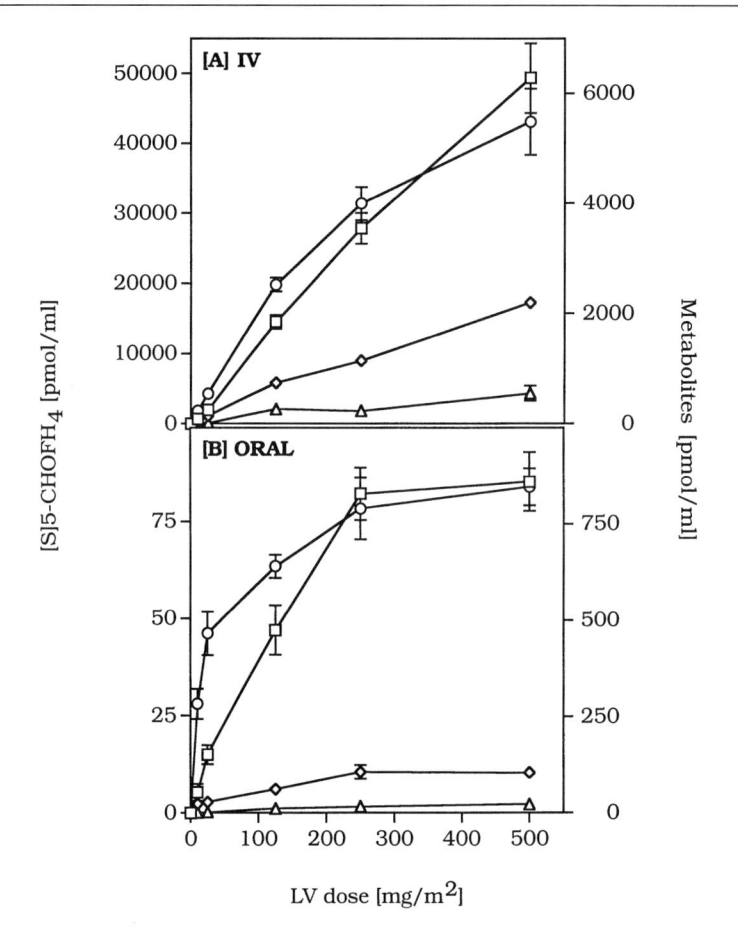

Fig. 4. Dose dependence of peak plasma accumulation of LV and metabolites thereof. Doses of 10, 25, 125, 250, and 500 mg/m² were administered iv (**A**) and 2 wk later orally (**B**) to healthy volunteers. The ternary complex assay was used to determine 5-CHOFH$_4$ (□), CH$_2$FH$_4$ + FH$_4$ (◇), 5-CH$_3$FH$_4$ (○), and 10-CHOFH$_4$ (△). Values are the mean ± SEM of duplicate analyses of samples from five volunteers.

ratory diets with FA (6 ppm) resulted in aberrantly high plasma and tissue folate levels compared to those in humans *(45,49,50)*. More recent models, using mice fed low FA laboratory chow, have yielded plasma folate levels 10-fold lower in these animals *(38,46,51,52)*. Additionally, these levels have been in the 10 n*M* range which is similar to those found in human plasma *(45)*.

A study of reduced folate accumulation in liver and sc implanted tumor tissue of mice fed a low FA diet was conducted after ip injection of LV (Figs. 5A, B) *(52)*. Plasma folate levels were also assayed and are included for comparison (Fig. 5C). Peak plasma elevation of all metabolites occurs more rapidly in mice than in humans. However, the same metabolites are present and they accumulate in nearly the same relative proportions as in humans. Interestingly, maximal accumulation of the presumed active metabolite,

Chapter 15 / Folates as Modulators

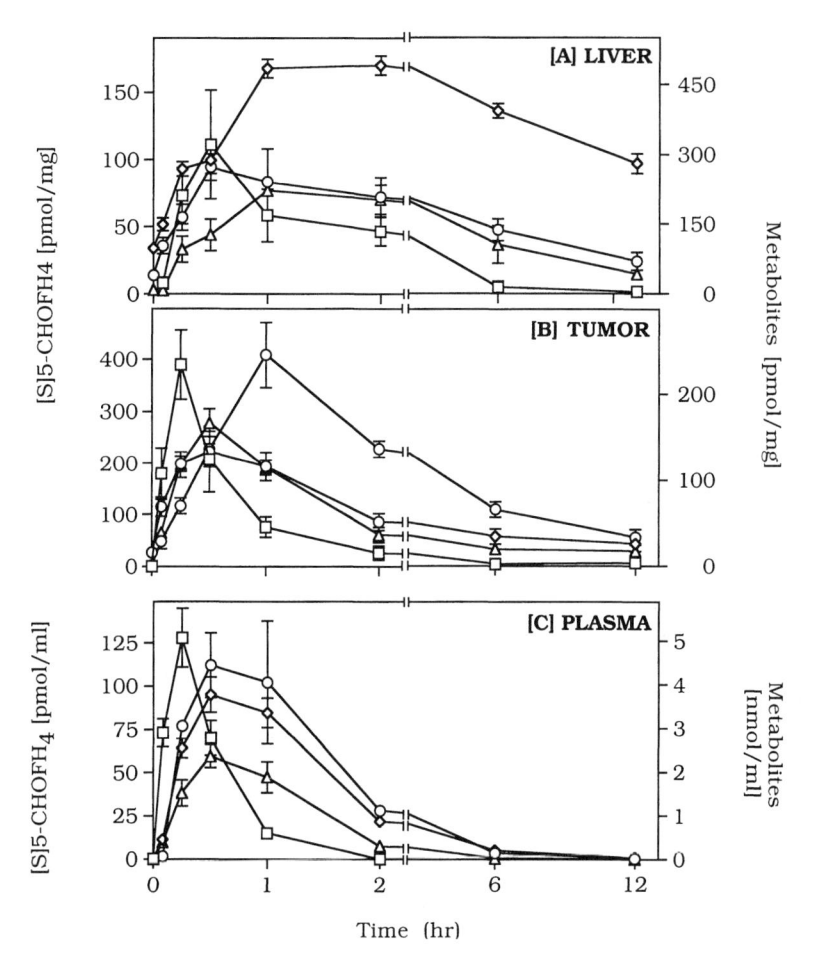

Fig. 5. Reduced folate metabolite accumulation in mice after LV administration. 5-CHOFH$_4$ (□), CH$_2$FH$_4$ + FH$_4$ (◇), 5-CH$_3$FH$_4$ (○), and 10-CHOFH$_4$ (△) were estimated by the ternary complex assay in liver (**A**), tumor (**B**), and plasma (**C**) of mice that had been maintained on a FA-deplete diet after ip injection of 90 mg/kg LV. Values are the mean ± SEM of duplicate analyses of samples from four mice.

CH$_2$FH$_4$, occurs in tumor and plasma at about the same time. This suggests plasma could be a major source of tumor CH$_2$FH$_4$ so that metabolism within the tumor itself may not be essential. Analysis of hepatic tissue shows higher metabolite accumulation compared to tumor. Likewise, lower levels of parent compound are present in liver. This indicates that liver more avidly metabolizes LV. Because peak accumulation of parent compound and essentially all metabolites occurs in tumor at essentially the same time as in plasma, estimation of folates in plasma could be useful as surrogate for accumulation of these folates in tumors. Once validated in other tumor systems and humans, this could provide the clinician with a valuable aid in determining the optimal interval between 5FU and LV administration.

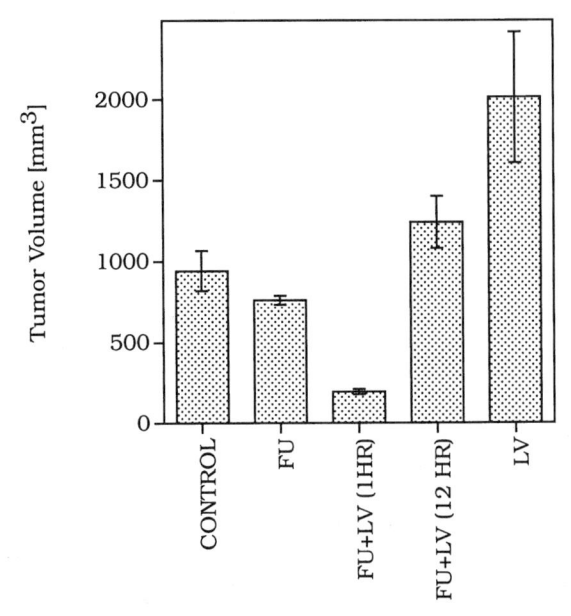

Fig. 6. Impact of time interval between LV and 5FU administration on tumor growth. Mice maintained on a FA-deplete diet for 2 wk were implanted subcutaneously with a mouse mammary tumor. One week later, 5FU and/or LV was administered ip daily for 9 d. On day 10, tumor volume was estimated and subtracted from estimates at the initiation of drug treatment. Values represent the mean ± SEM from five mice.

It has been presumed that the potentiation of 5FU antitumor activity requires elevation of LV metabolites in tumor tissue. To test this premise, 5FU was administered to FA-deficient mice 1 h after LV when metabolite levels were maximally elevated, and 12 h after LV when levels had returned to near baseline *(51)*. It can be seen in Fig. 6 that the 1-h interval resulted in tumor growth suppression to approx 80% compared with untreated controls. Alternatively, the 12-h interval not only did not result in inhibited growth, rather tumors grew 30% faster than in controls. This tumor growth enhancement effect was also seen when LV alone was administered to tumor-bearing animals. These results clearly demonstrate that 5FU potentiation can only be obtained when LV and/or its metabolites are elevated in the tumor. Possibly more important, failure to take into account the kinetic behavior of LV and its metabolites, could lead to deleterious tumor growth stimulation with this drug combination.

5.5. Comparison of Folic Acid Pharmacokinetics With Leucovorin

Folic acid has been considered as an alternative to LV for both antifolate toxicity reversal and as a potentiating agent for 5FU *(7,14,38,53)*. The primary impetus for use of LV rather than FA for modulation has been cell culture studies in which this fully reduced folate form does not have to undergo the relatively slow process of reduction via the enzyme DHFR that FA would require *(40,54)*. However, in animals and humans,

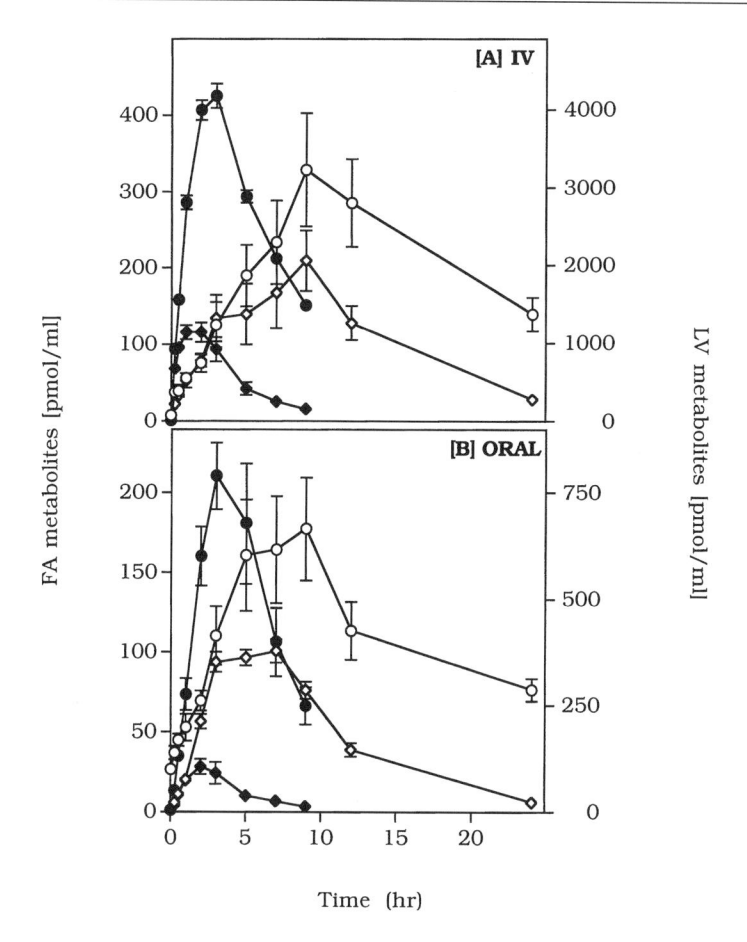

Fig. 7. Human plasma accumulation of metabolites after FA and LV administration. Folic acid (125 mg/m^2) and an equivalent dose of LV (250 mg/m^2 [R,S]LV) was administered iv **(A)** and 2 wk later orally **(B)** to healthy volunteers. Metabolite pools were estimated by the ternary complex assay. 5-CH$_3$FH$_4$ (○) and CH$_2$FH$_4$ + FH$_4$ (◇) resulting from FA are compared to 5-CH$_3$FH$_4$ (●) and CH$_2$FH$_4$ + FH$_4$ (◆) from LV. Values are the mean ± SEM of duplicate analyses of samples from five volunteers.

systemic metabolism can make reduced folate metabolites of FA available in plasma for uptake so that use of a fully reduced folate is not as necessary. Figure 7 shows a comparison of the pharmacokinetics of FA and LV administered to volunteers at equivalent doses *(55)*. It can be seen in Fig. 7A that iv administration of FA results in the same major as well as transient metabolite pools as LV. However, peak levels are somewhat lower. On the other hand, FA metabolites remain elevated much longer than LV metabolites. Oral administration of FA (Fig. 7B) also yields the same metabolites as oral LV, but in this case the difference in peak accumulation is not as great. This is probably because of the somewhat more avid uptake of FA into the circulatory system compared to LV. Again, metabolites remain elevated much longer after FA than after LV. Possible therapeutic advantages of the prolonged elevation of FA metabolites are a broader window for 5FU potentiation, and the ability to rescue patients with fewer doses of FA.

6. SUMMARY

Folates, particularly LV, have proven valuable as modulators of antitumor drugs from two perspectives. First, their ability to prevent or reverse excessive toxicities associated with antifolates has permitted higher doses to be achieved with concomitantly superior antitumor activity in many cases. Second, folates such as LV that can elevate tumor CH_2FH_4 are routinely used in combination with 5FU to stabilize the inhibitory ternary complex formed with this folate metabolite and the active metabolite of 5FU, resulting in diminished levels of the essential nucleotide, thymidylate.

Folates have been administered both orally and by iv injection. Following a bolus iv dose of LV the parent compound declines rapidly with the concomitant appearance of metabolites in plasma. Whereas $5\text{-}CH_3FH_4$ is the most abundant metabolite, CH_2FH_4, FH_4 and $10\text{-}CHOFH_4$ achieve significant levels but on a more transient basis. All metabolites achieve peak levels within the first 2 h and only marginal elevation remains several hours later. Peak levels and AUC values for each metabolite of LV are almost directly dependent on iv dose up to 500 mg/m^2. Oral administration of LV results in appearance of the same metabolites in generally the same proportions, but peak accumulation and AUC of metabolites is substantially less than after an iv dose. Unlike the iv route, oral administration shows saturation at doses of 250 mg/m^2 above. This is most likely caused by saturation of intestinal absorption because the parent compound LV also accumulates to only a limited extent in plasma. FA, administered orally or iv, remains in plasma for a much longer period than LV. Likewise, metabolites of FA, which are the same as after LV, remain elevated for a much longer period but do not achieve as high peak accumulation levels as metabolites of LV. Hence, although it is not clear that extremely high levels of parent compound or metabolites thereof are required for toxicity reversal or 5FU potentiation, high iv doses of LV can achieve more profound elevation than oral LV. On the other hand, FA given by either administration route results in more sustained elevation that could lead to superior results in some applications. Future studies need to address more precisely the dose and schedule requirements for toxicity reversal and 5FU potentiation for both LV and FA.

REFERENCES

1. Allegra CJ. Antifolates. In: (Chabner BA, Collins JM, eds) Cancer Chemotherapy: Principles and Practice. J.B. Lippincott, Philadelphia, 1990, pp. 110–153.
2. Rayl EA, Pizzorno G. Antifolates: current developments. *Cancer Treat Res* 1996; 87:197–223.
3. Priest DG, Bunni MA. Folates and folate antagonists in cancer chemotherapy. In: (Bailey LB, ed) Folate in Health and Disease. Marsel Dekker, New York, 1995, pp. 379–403.
4. Niemeyer CM, Hitchcock BS, Sallan SE. Comparative analysis of treatment programs for childhood acute lymphoblastic leukemia. *Semin Oncol* 1985; 12:122–130.
5. Schornagel JH, McVie JG. The clinical pharmacology of methotrexate. *Cancer Treat Rev* 1983; 10:53–75.

6. Jolivet J, Jansen G, Peters GH, Pinard MF, Schornagel JH. Leucovorin rescue of human cancer and bone marrow cells following edatrexate or methotrexate. *Biochem Pharmacol* 1994; 47:659–665.
7. Laohavinij S, Wedge SR, Lind MJ, Bailey N, Humphreys A, Proctor M, Chapman F, Simmons D, Oakley A, Robson L, Gumbrell L, Taylor GA, Thomas HD, Boddy AV, Newell DR, Calvert AH. A phase I clinical study of the antipurine antifolate lometrexol (DDATHF) given with oral folic acid. *Invest New Drugs* 1996; 14:325–335.
8. Gökbuget N, Hoelzer D. High-dose methotrexate in the treatment of adult acute lymphoblastic leukemia. *Ann Hematol* 1996; 72:194–201.
9. Pignon T, Lacarelle B, Duffaud F, Guillet P, Catalin J, Durand A, Monjanel S, Favre R. Pharmacokinetics of high-dose methotrexate in adult osteogenic sarcoma. *Cancer Chemother Pharmacol* 1994; 33:420–424.
10. Mini E, Trave R, Rustum YM, Bertino JR. Enhancement of the antitumor effects of 5-fluorouracil by folinic acid. *Pharmacol Ther* 1990; 47:1–9.
11. Sotos GA, Grogan L, Allegra CJ. Preclinical and clinical aspects of biomodulation of 5-fluorouracil. *Cancer Treat Rev* 1994; 20:11–49.
12. Jolivet J. Role of leucovorin dosing and administration schedule. *Eur J Cancer* 1995; 31:1311–1315.
13. Haas NB, Schilder RJ, Nash S, Weiner LM, Catalano RC, Ozols RF, O'Dwyer PJ. A phase II trial of weekly infusional 5-fluorouracil in combination with low-dose leucovorin in patients with advanced colorectal cancer. *Invest New Drugs* 1995; 13:229–233.
14. Smith GK, Amyx H, Boytos CM, Duch DS, Ferone R, Wilson HR. Enhanced antitumor activity for the thymidylate synthase inhibitor 1843U89 through decreased host toxicity with oral folic acid. *Cancer Res* 1995; 55:6117–6125.
15. Freisheim JH, Price EM, Ratnam M. Folate coenzyme and antifolate transport proteins in normal and neoplastic cells. *Adv Enz Reg* 1989; 29:13–36.
16. Shane B. Folypolyglutamate synthesis and its role in the regulation of one carbon metabolism. *Vitam Horm* 1989; 45:263–335.
17. McGuire JJ, Coward JK. Pteroypolyglutamate: biosynthesis, degradation, and function. In: (Blakely RL, Benkovic SJ, eds), Folates and Pterins. vol. 1, Wiley, New York, 1984, pp. 135–190.
18. Priest DG, Bunni MA, Romero-Fredes LR, Schmitz JC, Whiteley JM. A sensitive radioenzymatic assay for (S)-5-formyltetrahydrofolate. *Anal Biochem* 1991; 196:284–289.
19. Kisliuk RL. The biochemistry of folates. In: (Sirotnak FM, Burchall JJ, Enzminger WB, Montgomery JA, eds) Folate Antagonists as Therapeutic Agents. vol. 1, Academic, New York, 1984, pp. 2–68.
20. Bunni M, Doig MT, Donato H, Kesavan V, Priest DG. Role of methylenetetrahydrofolate depletion in methotrexate-mediated intracellular thymidylate synthesis inhibition in cultured L1210 cells. *Cancer Res* 1988; 48:3398–3404.
21. Baram J, Allegra CJ, Fine RL, Chabner BA. Effect of methotrexate on intracellular folate pools in purified myeloid precursor cells from normal human bone marrow. *J Clin Invest* 1987; 79:692–697.
22. Jackman AL, Calvert AH. Folate based TS inhibitors as anticancer drugs. *Ann Oncol* 1995; 6:871–881.
23. Clarke SJ, Jackman AL, Harrap KR. Antimetabolites in cancer chemotherapy. *Adv Exp Mol Biol* 1991; 309:7–13.
24. Rhee MS, Coward JK, Galivan J. Depletion of 5,10-methylenetetrahydrofolate and 10-formyltetrahydrofolate by methotrexate in cultured hepatoma cells. *Mol Pharmacol* 1992; 42:909–916.
25. Grant SC, Kris MG, Young CW, Sirotnak FM. Edatrexate, an antifolate with antitumor activity: a review. *Cancer Invest* 1993; 11:36–45.
26. Jackman AL, Farrugia DC, Gibson W, Kimbell R, Harrap KR, Stephens TC, Azab M, Boyle FT. ZD1694 (Tomudex): a new thymidylate synthase inhibitor with activity in colorectal cancer. *Eur J Cancer* 1995; 31:1277–1282.
27. Jackman AL, Kimbell R, Brown M, Brunton L, Harrap KR, Wardleworth JM, Boyle FT. The antitumor activity of ZD9331, a non-polyglutamatable quinazoline thymidylate synthase inhibitor. *Adv Exp Med Biol* 1994; 370:185–188.
28. Dash AK, Tyle P. Solid-state characterization of AG337 (Thymitaq), a novel antitumor drug. *J Pharm Sci* 1996; 85:1123–1127.
29. Shih C, Chen VJ, Gossett LS, Gates SB, Mackellar WC, Habeck LL, Shackelford KA, Mendelsohn LG, Soose DJ, Patel VF, Andis SL, Bewley JR, Rayl EA, Moroson BA, Beardsley GP, Kohler W, Ratnam

M, Schultz RM. LY231514, a pyrrolo[2,3-d]pyrimidine-based antifolate that inhibits multiple folate requiring enzymes. *Cancer Res* 1997; 57:1116–1123.
30. Matherly LH, Barlowe CK, Phillips VM, Goldman ID. The effects on 4-aminoantifolates on 5-formyltetrahydrofolate metabolism in L1210 cells. A biochemical basis of the selectivity of leucovorin rescue. *J Biol Chem* 1987; 262:710–717.
31. Galivan J, Nimec Z. Effects of folinic acid on hepatoma cells containing methotrexate polyglutamates. *Cancer Res* 1983; 43:551–555.
32. Goldman ID, Matherly LH. The cellular pharmacology of methotrexate. *Pharmacol Ther* 1985; 20:77–102.
33. Stromhaug A, Warren DJ, Slordal L. Effects of methotrexate on murine bone marrow cells *in vitro:* evidence of a reversible antiproliferative action. *Exp Hematol* 1995; 23:439–443.
34. Priest DG, Bunni M, Sirotnak FM. Relationship of reduced folate changes to inhibition of DNA synthesis induced by methotrexate in L1210 cells *in vivo. Cancer Res* 1989; 49:4204–4209.
35. Sirotnak FM, Donsbach RC, Moccio DM, Dorick DM. Biochemical and pharmacokinetic effect of leucovorin after high-dose methotrexate in a murine leukemia model. *Cancer Res* 1976; 36:4679–4686.
36. Balis FM, Holcenberg JS, Poplack DG. General principles of chemotherapy. In: (Pizzo PA, Poplack DG, eds) Principles and Practice of Pediatric Oncology. J.B. Lippincott, Philadelphia, 1989, pp. 165–205.
37. Lee JS, Murphy WK, Shirinian NH, Pang A, Hong WK. Alleviation by leucovorin of the dose-limiting toxicity of edatrexate: potential for improved therapeutic efficacy. *Cancer Chemother Pharmacol* 1991; 28:199–204.
38. Alati T, Worzalla JF, Shih C, Bewley JR, Lewis S, Moran RG, Grindey GB. Augmentation of the therapeutic activity of lometrexol [(6,R)5,10-dideazatetrahydrofolate] by oral folic acid. *Cancer Res* 1996; 56:2331–2335.
39. Danenberg PV, Danenberg KD. Effect of 5,10-methylenetetrahydrofolate on the dissociation of 5-fluoro-2'-deoxyuridylate from thymidylate synthetase: evidence for an ordered mechanism. *Biochemistry* 1978; 17:4018–4024.
40. Ullman B, Lee M, Martin DW, Santi DV. Cytotoxicity of 5-fluoro-2'-deoxyuridine: requirement for reduced folate cofactors and antagonism by methotrexate. *Proc Natl Acad Sci USA* 1978; 75:980–983.
41. Newman EM, Tsai JF. Microbiological analysis of 5-formyltetrahydrofolic acid and other folates using automatic 96-well plate reader. *Anal Biochem* 1986; 154:509–515.
42. Perry J, Chanarin I. Intestinal absorption of reduced folate compounds in man. *J Haematol* 1970; 18:329–339.
43. Wilson SD, Horne DW. High-performance liquid chromatographic determination of the distribution of naturally occurring folic acid derivatives in rat liver. *Anal Biochem* 1984; 142:529–535.
44. Duch DS, Bowers SW, Nichol CA. Analysis of folate cofactor levels in tissues using high-performance liquid chromatography. *Anal Biochem* 1983; 130:385–392.
45. Priest DG, Schmitz JC, Bunni MA, Stuart RK. Pharmacokinetics of leucovorin metabolites in human plasma as a function of dose administered orally and intravenously. *J Natl Cancer Inst* 1991; 83:1806–1812.
46. Schmitz JC, Grindey GB, Schultz RM, Priest DG. Impact of dietary folic acid on reduced folates in mouse plasma and tissues. Relationships to dideazatetrahydrofolate sensitivity. *Biochem Pharmacol* 1994; 48:319–325.
47. Trave R, Rustum YM, Petrelli NJ, Herrera L, Mittleman A, Frank C, Crease PJ. Plasma and tumor tissue pharmacology of intravenous leucovorin calcium in combination with fluorouracil in patients with advanced colorectal carcinoma. *J Clin Oncol* 1988; 6:1184–1191.
48. Whitehead VM, Pratt R, Viallet A, Cooper BA. Intestinal conversion of folinic acid to 5-methyltetrahydrofolate in man. *Br J Haematol* 1972; 22:63–67.
49. Martin DS, Stolfi RL, Colofiore JF. Failure of high-dose leucovorin to improve therapy with the maximally tolerated dose of 5-fluorouracil: a murine study with clinical relevance? *J Natl Cancer Inst* 1988; 80:496–501.
50. Carlsson G, Gustavsson B, Frosing R, Odin E, Hafstrom L, Spears CP, Larsson P. Antitumor effects of pure diastereoisomers of 5-formyltetrahydrofolate in hepatic transplants of a rodent colon carcinoma model. *Biochem Pharmacol* 1995; 50:1347–1351.

51. Raghunathan K, Schmitz JC, Priest DG. Impact of schedule on leucovorin potentiation of fluorouracil antitumor activity in dietary folic acid deplete mice. *Biochem Pharmacol* 1997; 53:1197–1202.
52. Raghunathan K, Schmitz JC, Priest DG. Disposition of leucovorin and its metabolites in dietary folic acid-deplete mice—comparison between tumor, liver and plasma. *Cancer Chemother Pharmacol* 1997; 40:126–130.
53. Asbury RF, Boros L, Brower M, Woll J, Chung A, Bennett J. 5-fluorouracil and high-dose folic acid treatment for metastic colon cancer. *Am J Clin Oncol* 1987; 10:47–49.
54. Evans RM, Laskin JD, Hakala MT. Effect of excess folates and deoxyinosine on the activity and site of action of 5-fluorouracil. *Cancer Res* 1981; 41:3288–3295.
55. Schmitz JC, Stuart RK, Priest DG. Disposition of folic acid and its metabolites: A comparison with leucovorin. *Clinical Pharmacol Therap* 1994; 55:501–508.

16 Antifolate Polyglutamylation in Preclinical and Clinical Antifolate Resistance

John J. McGuire

CONTENTS

INTRODUCTION
POLYGLUTAMYLATION AND PRECLINICAL RESISTANCE
POLYGLUTAMYLATION AND CLINICAL RESISTANCE
STRATEGIES FOR OVERCOMING RESISTANCE MEDIATED VIA
    DECREASED ACCUMULATION OF ANTIFOLATE POLYGLUTAMATES
ACKNOWLEDGMENT
REFERENCES

1. INTRODUCTION

1.1. Folylpoly(γ-Glutamate) Metabolites

1.1.1. Occurrence

The folates, a family of essential human vitamins, are cofactors in one-carbon transfer reactions, including those in the synthesis of serine, glycine, methionine, purines, and thymidylate. Across the phylogenetic spectrum, intracellular folates consist almost entirely of poly (γ-glutamyl) metabolites (Fig. 1; reviewed in refs. *1–3*). A distribution of lengths generally occurs that is cell type-specific; within a given source the distribution is generally the same for individual folate species containing different one-carbon units. In human cells, the usual range of lengths is 5–8 total glutamates with a total folate pool estimated to be 1–10 μM. Since polyglutamylation does not appear to be coupled directly to transport, monoglutamates (which are transport forms of the vitamin) must be present transiently, but intracellular levels are low or undetectable under physiological conditions. This suggests that transport, rather than the level of synthesis (below), is generally limiting to folylpolyglutamate synthesis.

From: *Anticancer Drug Development Guide: Antifolate Drugs in Cancer Therapy*
Edited by: A.L. Jackman © Humana Press Inc., Totowa, NJ

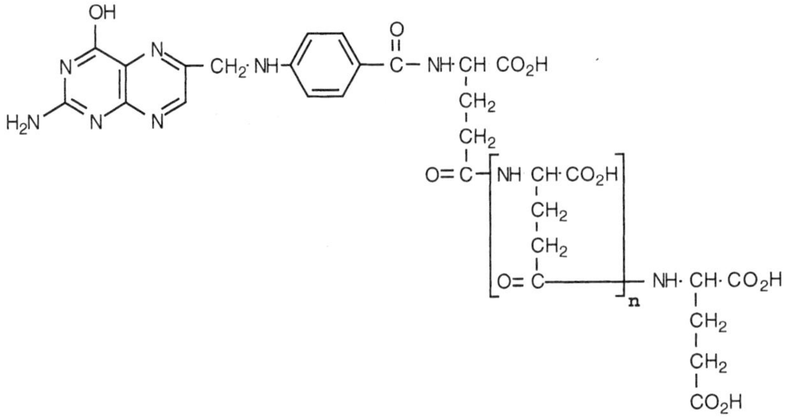

Fig. 1. General structure of folylpoly (γ-glutamates).

1.1.2. Functions

Folylpolyglutamates fulfill a number of functions in folate metabolism (reviewed in refs. *1–3*), but the main functions are: to retain folates at levels far in excess of the extracellular concentration (human plasma is approx 10 nM in folates [*4*]); and to serve as the kinetically preferred substrates for almost all folate-dependent reactions.

Two mechanisms contribute to polyglutamate retention. First, both systems known to transport folates (the reduced folate carrier [RFC] and the membrane-bound folate-binding protein [FBP]) transport monoglutamyl folates, but polyglutamyl folates are poorly transported (if at all), especially those containing more than two glutamates. Since folylpolyglutamates also cannot use these systems for efflux, and other known systems also do not efflux polyglutamates, facilitated efflux does not occur. Second, because of the high negative charge on folylpolyglutamates, they cannot passively diffuse through cell membranes.

Studies with isolated folate-dependent enzymes suggest that folylpolyglutamates are generally more catalytically efficient (up to 10^4-fold increased V_{max}/K_m) than monoglutamates. Often the K_m is substantially lower, but in some cases V_{max} is increased. Catalytic efficiency may also be enhanced by preferential channeling of polyglutamates in multifunctional folate-dependent enzymes. Although retention is essential at physiological extracellular folate concentrations, increased catalytic efficiency is apparently also essential since a cell line that transport folates normally, but cannot synthesize folylpolyglutamates, is unable to survive even in the presence of supraphysiological levels of reduced folates *(5)*. Thus at least one folate reaction cannot function well enough with a monoglutamate substrate to supply sufficient levels of a critical metabolite.

1.2. Antifolate Polyglutamate Metabolites

Poly(γ-glutamyl) metabolites of most glutamate-containing folate antagonists (antifolates) are important to their pharmacological actions. Generally, study of these metabolites utilizes radiolabeled drug and HPLC analytical methods. Cellular accumulation of antifolate polyglutamates and the lengths observed are a function of the drug used, the cell type studied, drug concentration, and drug exposure time. Drug exposures are generally $\leq$ 24 h because drug-induced cell lysis begins to occur unless protective metabolites are present. Polyglutamylation increases retention of all drugs that form at least triglutamates, but only increases target inhibitory potency of those drugs that are not intrinsically tight-binding as monoglutamates.

1.2.1. Occurrence/Function of Methotrexate Poly(γ-Glutamates) (MTXG$_n$)

Methotrexate (MTX) is the antifolate most extensively studied with regard to polyglutamyl metabolites (reviewed in refs. 6–8). Studies in human and murine cell lines and tissues show that MTXG$_n$ accumulate relatively slowly and that the distribution of lengths is often shorter than that of folylpolyglutamates in the same cell. For example, in human CCRF-CEM leukemia cells, the predominant lengths of folates are glu$_{6-8}$ (9), whereas MTXG$_{5-6}$ are the longest forms observed after a 24-h exposure to 10 μM MTX (10). These phenomena are related to the kinetics of the enzyme responsible for their synthesis (Subheading 1.3.).

MTX is itself a tight-binding yet reversible inhibitor of dihydrofolate reductase (DHFR). MTXG$_n$ are either equipotent or slightly more potent than MTX as DHFR inhibitors. Thus polyglutamate forms are not essential for obtaining maximum target inhibition with this drug. Since MTXG$_n$ are more potent inhibitors than MTX of other folate-dependent enzymes (e.g., thymidylate synthase [TMPS] and AICAR formyltransferase), it has been proposed that these enzymes act as alternate sites of MTX action. The primary intracellular target must be DHFR, however, since alteration of the level or MTX sensitivity of other enzymes occurs rarely if at all when selecting for resistance, whereas increased DHFR levels are common (11).

Although MTXG$_n$ are not required for potent DHFR inhibition, polyglutamylation is still required to retain intracellular drug at levels significantly above the extracellular concentration. This is especially true if extracellular MTX is removed after a short period of exposure ("pulse"), since MTX itself (if not bound to DHFR) rapidly effluxes from cells, whereas polyglutamates are retained. Retention is particularly high for MTXG$_{\geq 3}$. Numerous studies have shown that after pulse MTX exposure, MTXG$_n$ are critical to retaining an intracellular drug pool adequate to sustain the blockade of DHFR as required for prolonged DNA-synthesis inhibition and consequent cell death (8). Because of the tight-binding interaction of MTX with DHFR, however, MTXG$_n$ are not essential for cytotoxicity if extracellular drug is continuously present (12).

1.2.2. Occurrence/Function of Poly(γ-Glutamates) of Other Classical Antifolates

Other DHFR inhibitors have been characterized with respect to their metabolism to polyglutamates. These include aminopterin (AMT) (13), 10-ethyl-10-deazaAMT (10-EDAM) (13), and 8-deazaAMT and 8-deazaMTX (14). AMT and the 8-deaza analogs form shorter polyglutamates than MTX or 10-EDAM and this may effect the potency and/or selectivity observed between these two groups. Like MTXG$_n$, polyglutamates of these analogs are similar or identical in potency to their monoglutamates as tight-binding DHFR inhibitors. In each case examined, polyglutamates are more readily retained and the cytotoxic potency of these analogs in pulse exposure is related to their ability to accumulate longer (glu$_{\geq 3}$) forms.

Enzymes in the thymidylate and purine synthesis pathways are also targets for polyglutamylatable antifolates. Polyglutamylatable TMPS inhibitors have been of great interest recently (15). The first, the quinazoline CB3717 (5,8-dideaza-10-propargylpteroylglutamate), is a relatively poor substrate for polyglutamylation. CB3717 is a potent TMPS inhibitor as a monoglutamate, but polyglutamates are tight-binding and are well retained. Other quinazoline analogs are also accumulated as polyglutamates (e.g., ref. *16*). Structural modifications to increase solubility, transport efficiency, and ability to form polyglutamates subsequently led to two types of polyglutamylatable TMPS inhibitors *(15)*: One type requires polyglutamylation to potently inhibit TMPS (e.g., ZD1694) and one type is intrinsically tight-binding (e.g., BW1843U89). Both of these analogs are excellent substrates for polyglutamylation; ZD1694, however, can be readily converted to long ($glu_{\geq 3}$) metabolites, whereas BW1843U89 forms primarily (but not exclusively) glu_2. The purine biosynthesis inhibitor 5,10-dideazatetrahydrofolate (DDATHF) and related analogs are also extensively polyglutamylated *(17)* as is the multitargeted antifolate LY231514 *(18)*.

Polyglutamates of MTX and other antifolates are also accumulated in normal tissues (e.g., liver, bone marrow, intestine; ref. *6*). Their contribution to differential toxicity (selectivity) is beyond the scope of this review.

1.3. Synthesis and Degradation of Folate and Antifolate Poly(γ-Glutamates)

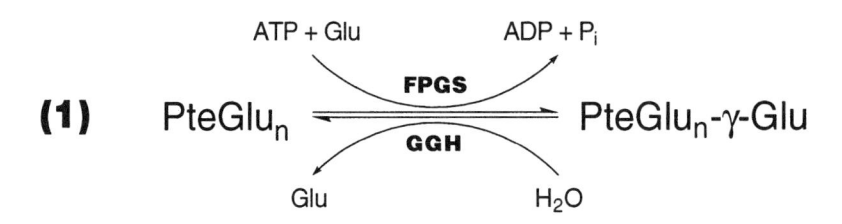

$$(1) \quad PteGlu_n \underset{GGH}{\overset{FPGS}{\rightleftharpoons}} PteGlu_n\text{-}\gamma\text{-}Glu$$

with ATP + Glu → ADP + P_i (forward, FPGS) and Glu + H_2O (reverse, GGH)

Steady-state levels of intracellular poly(γ-glutamates) of natural folates and antifolates are determined by their rate of synthesis, catalyzed by folylpolyglutamate synthetase (FPGS), and their rate of degradation, catalyzed by γ-glutamyl hydrolase (GGH; also called conjugase) (Reaction 1). Properties of these enzymes have been reviewed *(1,3,19)*. FPGS is found in the cytoplasm and mitochondria, and FPGS activity levels vary with cell type. Protein-bound (anti)folates are not FPGS substrates *(6)*. Two major forms of GGH have been described. One is on the small intestine brush border, has a neutral optimum, pH and hydrolyzes dietary folylpolyglutamates to absorbable monoglutamates; so far this GGH does not play a role in drug resistance. The activity of the second form varies with cell type, is a lysosomal glycoprotein, is also extensively secreted (although the significance of secretion is unclear at present), has an acidic optimum pH, and hydrolyzes intracellular polyglutamates by endo- and/or exopeptidase mechanisms depending on the source. Protein-bound (anti)folylpolyglutamates are not GGH substrates *(20)*. Recently, it was reported that prostate-specific membrane antigen has GGH activity *(21)*; the significance of this activity to the response of prostate tumors to antifolates remains to be elucidated.

1.4. Drug Resistance
1.4.1. Definitions of Intrinsic and Acquired Drug Resistance

Drug resistance is a relative term defined as a higher drug concentration (or dose) being required to achieve a biological effect in one system as compared to another. If one cell type never before exposed to drug requires a higher drug concentration than another cell type to achieve the same level of cytotoxicity, the first cell type displays natural (or intrinsic) resistance. Natural resistance is discussed further in Subheading 2.1.2. If cells are exposed to a cytotoxic drug level, a fraction of cells may survive and proliferate in that level of drug; such cells have acquired resistance. In vivo (either in preclinical models or the clinic) tumors are resistant when they do not respond at the maximum tolerated drug dose; in vivo resistance can either be natural or acquired. Biochemical and molecular mechanisms of natural and acquired resistance are probably the same.

1.4.2. Summary of Mechanisms of Antifolate Resistance

Based on the mechanisms of action of polyglutamylatable antifolates, many possible mechanisms of drug resistance exist *(8,22; see Chapter 3)*. These may occur either singly or as multiple mechanisms in the same cell. Many of these mechanisms have been identified preclinically and clinically. These mechanisms include:

1. Decreased access to the target of the antifolate, most often involving decreased activity of the active RFC or the FBP systems. Increased efflux is generally not observed.
2. Alterations of the target of the antifolate. Most commonly this involves increased expression of the target enzyme, often mediated by gene amplification. It less commonly involves a mutation decreasing the affinity of the target enzyme for drug.
3. Altered activity of secondary enzymes required for cytotoxicity. For example, TMPS activity in the absence of DHFR activity causes partial depletion of the reduced folate pool by conversion to dihydrofolates; this in turn inhibits both dTMP and purine synthesis. Low TMPS activity reduces the rate at which depletion occurs.
4. Increased folate pools *(17,23,24)* that can competitively reverse antifolate inhibition.
5. Decreased accumulation of polyglutamates of the drug. Decreased polyglutamate accumulation can lead to loss of retention and/or loss of potency against the target enzyme. This review will explore this resistance phenotype.

1.4.3. Decreased Antifolate Polyglutamate Accumulation as a Mechanism of Resistance

1.4.3.1. Secondary Effects Resulting in Decreased Antifolate Polyglutamate Accumulation.
Decreased antifolate polyglutamate accumulation may occur secondary to other resistance mechanisms. Decreased drug transport decreases the free intracellular drug concentration and hence decreases the substrate for polyglutamate accumulation. Thus, a breast-cancer cell line exhibiting a profound defect in MTX polyglutamylation *(25)* does so because of a profound decrease in net transport *(26)*. In whole cells known to have decreased transport, the difficulty of determining whether a primary polyglutamylation defect also occurs has been discussed *(27)*. Measurement of the metabolism or cytotoxic effect of a polyglutamylatable inhibitor that does not use the affected transporter has been suggested *(27,28)*. An alternative approach is to measure cell sensitivity in continuous exposure to a tight-binding monoglutamate inhibitor, such as MTX; cells with only a polyglutamylation defect will be sensitive. Another method *(29)* is to examine polyglutamylation at very high extracellular drug concentrations in which diffusion through the cell membrane overwhelms the transport defect and polyglutamylation can be directly compared to a sensitive counterpart. Since protein-bound antifolates are not FPGS substrates, an increase in target enzyme may also decrease polyglutamate accu-

mulation by decreasing the free drug level (e.g., ref. *27*). In whole cells known to have increased target levels, one approach to determining whether a primary polyglutamylation defect also occurs is to saturate the target with a lipophilic inhibitor prior to exposure of the cells to radiolabeled drug *(30)*. Decreased drug transport and/or increased target levels may be complicating factors in numerous examples in the literature in which decreased $MTXG_n$ accumulation was observed (e.g., refs. *30–34*). Although secondary decreases in antifolate polyglutamates may be important to the overall expression of resistance (since a decrease in polyglutamate accumulation will reinforce the primary mechanism), they will not be considered further here.

1.4.3.2. Primary Effects Resulting in Decreased Antifolate Polyglutamate Accumulation. Since steady-state polyglutamate levels are determined by the rates of synthesis and degradation (Subheading 1.3.), antifolate polyglutamate accumulation can be directly decreased by mutations or changes in regulation that decrease the activity of FPGS and/or increase GGH activity. Both mechanisms have been shown to occur.

Evidence to date indicates that decreased antifolate polyglutamate synthesis occurs through three mechanisms (which could also occur in combination): decreased expression of FPGS activity, arising either at the transcriptional or posttranscriptional level; mutation or polymorphisms in the FPGS coding sequence that decreases activity with the antifolate; and indirect factors decreasing FPGS activity with the antifolate, such as an increase in the folate pool that competes with the antifolate for polyglutamylation. Note that each mechanism must leave sufficient FPGS activity for the synthesis of the folylpolyglutamates that are essential for growth; however, since many natural folates are highly efficient FPGS substrates, only a portion of the constitutive FPGS level is actually required *(35,36)*. Decreased antifolate polyglutamate accumulation or decreased FPGS activity in extracts may be associated with either no change *(17,37–41)* or a decrease *(42–45)* in FPGS mRNA expression; no change in the DNA restriction fragment pattern or gene copy has been reported. Mutations or polymorphisms in the coding sequence that decrease FPGS activity have not been described to date, although kinetic differences in FPGS from resistant cell lines have been described that are consistent with their occurrence (e.g., refs. *35,46*). The effect of an increased folate pool on antifolate polyglutamate synthesis has been little studied, but in two cases of acquired antifolate resistance *(17,24)*, increased folylpolyglutamate pools were associated with decreased antifolate polyglutamylation. Since leukemic leukocytes have higher folate pools than normal leukocytes *(47)*, this mechanism could contribute to natural resistance.

Increased degradation of antifolate polyglutamates by increased GGH activity has been identified less often, but this may represent a bias in looking for this most recently discovered mechanism *(28)*. As noted *(19)*, increased GGH does not automatically mean decreased sensitivity to polyglutamylatable antifolates since the potential exists for hydrolysis of the folylpolyglutamate pool as well and this would tend to increase sensitivity. The situation is further complicated because the permease *(48)* that controls polyglutamate entry into lysosomes where GGH is located may be critical in establishing the effect that occurs. Molecular mechanisms behind increased GGH activity are not known, however, the recent cloning of rat and human GGH cDNAs by the Galivan and Ryan group *(49,50)* suggests that such data will soon be forthcoming.

1.4.3.3. Methods for Detecting Decreased Antifolate Polyglutamate Accumulation. Two indirect methods exist for detecting decreased polyglutamate accumulation in intact cells. One method measures inhibition in continuous and pulse exposure of *in situ* TMPS (*is*TMPS)-catalyzed metabolism of exogenously supplied [^{3}H]deoxyuridine by a panel of drugs that cover combinations of using (or not) the RFC and requiring (or not) polyglutamylation; the pattern of response compared to a known sensitive counterpart provides presumptive evidence for decreased polyglutamate accumulation *(51)*. This method has the advantage that it can be used on fresh tumor samples as well as cell lines. A second method uses a similar concept, but measures effects of an analogous panel of drugs on cell growth in continuous and pulse exposure *(27,52)*. Although both indirect methods also detect other mechanisms of antifolate resistance, at this point neither method differentiates between changes in FPGS or GGH as the source of decreased polyglutamate accumulation.

Direct biochemical measurements more precisely define the extent and mechanism of decreased polyglutamate accumulation. Quantitation of polyglutamate accumulation using radiolabeled drug can be performed, but is subject to possible complication if decreased transport or increased target levels are also present (Subheading 1.4.3.1.). Direct assay of FPGS *(35)* and GGH *(28)* activity in cell extracts can provide direct proof of the primary mechanism, but may not detect changes in regulation. Recent evidence suggests that measurement of both FPGS and GGH better predicts polyglutamate accumulation *(53)*. Since there is not a 1:1 relationship between FPGS or GGH activity and polyglutamate accumulation in whole cells, activity measurement of these enzymes in extracts dramatically underestimates the potential for decreased polyglutamate synthesis in most cases and also underestimates the level of resistance. Because of this, it is not yet clear whether enzyme activity measurements in extracts or polyglutamylation studies in whole cells will be most informative about antifolate sensitivity.

2. POLYGLUTAMYLATION AND PRECLINICAL RESISTANCE

2.1. Resistance in Vitro

2.1.1. Acquired Resistance in Vitro

2.1.1.1. MTX. Decreased MTXG$_n$ accumulation as a discrete resistance mechanism was not recognized until it was realized that a selection regimen must be used under which the retention function of MTXG$_n$ is paramount and only those cells that cannot synthesize them (and thus cannot retain drug) will survive (35,54). These conditions are met by using pulse drug exposures, generally ≤1 generation time, after which drug is removed. This exposure regimen also better mimics clinical MTX use in which it is given as a bolus or infusion (≤24 h). In addition, if high MTX concentrations are used in the selection, it will better mimic the high serum concentrations achieved in many clinical regimens. Pulse selection at low MTX concentrations may lead to other primary mechanisms of resistance (55). It is also now appreciated that pulse-exposure selection may be necessary for tight-binding monoglutamate enzyme inhibitors, but drugs that require polyglutamylation to be potent enzyme inhibitors may select for decreased polyglutamate accumulation even in continuous exposure.

The first well-characterized examples of acquired resistance as a result only of decreased MTXG$_n$ accumulation were the first selected by pulse exposure. Two populations of CCRF-CEM human leukemia cells were selected by 7 or 6 treatments for 24 h, respectively, with 3 μM (R3/7) or 30 μM (R30/6) MTX *(54)*. R3/7 and R30/6 are as sensitive as CCRF-CEM to continuous MTX exposure, but are highly resistant to exposures ≤24 h. The isTMPS inhibition assay (Subheading 1.4.3.3.) and biochemical assays indicate no alterations in transport or DHFR (levels or MTX sensitivity) in these sublines. The isTMPS inhibition assay and [^{3}H]MTX metabolism studies show that the sublines are defective in MTXG$_n$ accumulation. Extracts of each subline and R30dm (cloned from R30/6) show decreases in FPGS activity proportional to the deficiency of the cell line for MTXG$_n$ accumulation *(35)*. R30dm FPGS may also be kinetically altered relative to CCRF-CEM, but its low activity (≤10% of CCRF-CEM) precludes rigorous kinetic analysis *(35)*. Molecular analysis of these sublines shows no difference from parental CCRF-CEM in DNA restriction fragments or gene copy number and no difference in mRNA levels or size *(37)*. Recent data using a polyclonal antibody to FPGS in Western immunoblots shows that FPGS protein is expressed at levels proportional to reduced activity in each case *(56)*.

Acquired resistance as a result of decreased MTXG$_n$ accumulation was studied in a squamous-cell carcinoma of the head and neck cell line HNSCC-11B *(57)*, selected by either continuous (increasing stepwise from 10–400 nM) or pulse exposure (2 μM MTX for 24 h, 11 cycles). Continuous exposure selected for resistance primarily as a result of increased DHFR activity and decreased transport, but FPGS activity in extracts was decreased fourfold. This is an example of FPGS activity clearly decreased in a subline selected by continuous MTX exposure. The subline selected by pulse exposure had only a minor decrease in transport and was primarily resistant to pulse, but not continuous exposure, as a result of a sixfold decrease in FPGS activity. An additional variable in these studies was the use of parental cells grown in "physiological" folate concentrations (5 nM leucovorin and 5 nM folic acid), rather than 2.3 μM folic acid typical of cell-culture medium. The subline selected by pulse MTX exposure had qualitatively the same phenotype as other resistant lines (above) selected in folic acid-"rich" medium, suggesting that the medium folate concentration or type of folate may not be determinative for this mechanism of resistance.

MTX resistance was selected in the HCT-8 human ileocecal carcinoma *(58,59)* by pulse exposure with 100 μM MTX for 4 h (6 cycles) or continuous exposure to 0.1 μM MTX for 7 d (3 cycles). Pulse exposure selected for a subline with decreased transport; MTXG$_n$ accumulation is decreased, but this decrease could be secondary to decreased transport. Continuous exposure to low MTX selected for resistance as a result of decreased MTXG$_n$ accumulation; MTX transport and constitutive DHFR expression and DHFR sensitivity to MTX were unaltered. The resistance of this subline is puzzling since decreased synthesis and/or increased hydrolysis of MTXG$_n$ alone should not induce resistance to continuous MTX exposure.

2.1.1.2. Other Polyglutamylatable Antifolates. Decreased polyglutamate accumulation can contribute to acquired resistance to the polyglutamylatable TMPS inhibitor ZD1694, whether selected by continuous or pulse exposure. Continuous exposure selects for diverse phenotypes, including reduced transport, increased TMPS expression, and decreased polyglutamate accumulation. Thus far, which phenotype is selected seems to be stochastic and not related to cell type. In some cases, continuous exposure selected for other resistance phenotypes without affecting polyglutamylation *(27,39,60)*. Some resistant sublines appear to have decreased polyglutamate accumulation as their sole resistance mechanism. For example, following selection by continuous exposure to stepwise increasing ZD1694, the 1600-fold resistance of a MOLT-3 T-lymphoblastic leukemia subline results only from decreased polyglutamylation via decreased FPGS *(44)*. FPGS activity was not measured, but this subline expresses 60% of parental FPGS mRNA levels. A CCRF-CEM T-lymphoblastic leukemia subline selected similarly exhibited 11% of parental FPGS activity, but no change in FPGS mRNA levels *(40)*; decreased FPGS activity was the only defect noted and it led to >1000-fold ZD1694 resistance. In still other cases, continuous exposure selected for complex phenotypes that included decreased polyglutamylation, along with reduced uptake *(27,39)* and/or increased TS levels *(27,39)*. In a complex NCI H360 human colon tumor subline, FPGS activity was 2% of parental level, but FPGS mRNA level was unchanged *(39)*. Complex phenotypes are not necessarily seen at only very high levels of resistance *(27)*. Of note is that only small decreases in FPGS expression in cell lines exhibiting only that mechanism of resistance translate into decreased ZD1694 polyglutamate synthesis and very high levels of resistance. Interestingly, MTX-resistant sublines with similar decreases in FPGS activity show much lower levels of cross-resistance to ZD1694 *(9,44)*. There are other similar examples in the literature of apparently anomalous cross-resistance patterns. This effect is reminiscent of that seen in multidrug resistance where the selecting drug often gives the highest level of resistance, whereas other susceptible drugs exhibit lower levels of cross-resistance *(61)*. In polyglutamylation, this effect may represent selection of FPGS with specifically altered kinetics; DNA sequencing studies should be informative in this regard.

Selection for ZD1694 resistance by pulse exposure has been used less often. A 66-fold resistant HCT-8 subline, selected by 2-h pulse exposure to increasing (1–50 μM) ZD1694 concentrations, showed only 8% of the parental FPGS activity level and no change in FPGS mRNA level *(38)*; this subline does not have alterations in TMPS or transport. Intracellular pools of $H_4PteGlu_n$ and $5,10-CH_2-H_4PteGlu_n$ were measured in this subline; its pools were lower and the average chain length was shorter than in the parent. Changes in the folate pools consequent to decreased FPGS are also observed with other antifolates (e.g., DDATHF), but their significance in resistance is unclear. Treatment of MOLT-3 for 9 cycles at 1 μM ZD1694 for 24 h each cycle *(44)* yielded a 1300-fold resistant subline that, similar to the subline developed by the same lab by continuous exposure (above), showed only decreased polyglutamate accumulation and expressed only 40% of the FPGS mRNA level of the parent (activity was not measured).

Resistance to 5,10-dideazatetrahydrofolate (DDATHF), selected by continuous exposure, is associated with decreased polyglutamate accumulation in the cases examined thus far, although the phenotypes are all complex. In an 80-fold resistant H35 rat hepatoma subline, H35D, a sevenfold increase in GGH activity (with no change in FPGS activity) was correlated with decreased accumulation of antifolate polyglutamates and with resistance *(28)*; decreased uptake by the RFC also contributed to resistance, however. H35D represents the first example of acquired antifolate resistance as a result of increased GGH activity. The folate pool size and proportion of $H_4PteGlu_n$, $5,10-CH_2-H_4PteGlu_n$, and $10-HCO-H_4PteGlu_n$ are unchanged in H35D, but the average polyglutamate length was approx two residues shorter than in its parent *(62)*. Since shorter folylpolyglutamates may compete less effectively at target enzymes with antifolate polyglutamates, this shorter pool may undercut the degree of resistance resulting from decreased antifolylpolyglutamate synthesis. Three CCRF-CEM sublines were selected at increasing DDATHF concentrations *(17)*; the phenotype became more complex as the selecting concentration increased, but all showed decreased polyglutamylation with no evidence of decreased transport. The lowest level of resistance (24-fold) in subline R17 appeared to be related primarily to decreased FPGS activity (60% of parental); R17 FPGS had kinetic properties similar to parental FPGS. However, this subline had a twofold *increase* in total folates, almost all of which was 10-HCO-H$_4$PteGlu$_n$, but a decrease in the average length by about one residue. The contribution of these changes to resistance is unclear. At the highest level of resistance (5250-fold), multiple factors influenced resistance in subline R15, including decreased polyglutamate accumulation, which was a result of decreased FPGS (9% of parental) and increased GGH (200% of parental) activities. The total folate pool of R15 was decreased by twofold with most of the decrease coming from a 10-fold decrease in 10-HCO-H$_4$PteGlu$_n$, and a decrease in the average length by approx two residues; again the influence of the altered folate pool on resistance is unknown. There was no change in FPGS mRNA levels or size in any of the three sublines, consistent with change occurring posttranscriptionally.

Of note is the finding that FPGS activity and protein is overexpressed as a result of increased transcription with no change in gene copy number when resistance to the lipophilic, nonpolyglutamylatable antifolate metoprine is selected in low-folate medium *(43)*. Increased folate transport and enhanced polyglutamylation create an enlarged folate pool that reverses the effect of metoprine. The increase in transport and FPGS causes collaterally sensitive to MTX, as expected, although the magnitude of this effect is complicated by the enlarged folate pool, which should act to decrease MTX sensitivity. The FPGS in these lines had no change in its K_m value.

2.1.2. Natural Resistance In Vitro

A recurrent issue in natural resistance is establishing a standard against which resistance is defined and against which biochemical mechanisms may be causally related to that resistance. In one definition, tumor cells are naturally resistant when their EC$_{50}$ is >10% of the peak plasma concentration achieved in humans *(63)*. The number of tumors that fit this definition will depend on the exposure time chosen. Another definition involves use of the *is*TMPS inhibition assay (subheading 1.4.3.3.), which uses a set of exposure conditions to several drugs; the drugs, concentrations, and exposure times were defined so that a cell line representative of clinically sensitive disease tests as sensitive *(51)*. In many cases, practical definitions are used. One is a direct comparison of two or more cell lines; if one line is more resistant to a drug under any exposure condition, that line is considered naturally resistant. Finally, tumor-cell lines derived from tissues that are recognized as being clinically unresponsive to MTX are considered naturally resistant. The second problem is to relate a biochemical parameter, in this case polyglutamylation, to the observed natural resistance. The approach most often used is to correlate the sensitivity of the cell lines, as measured above, with their capacity for polyglutamylation of radiolabeled drug. However, this correlation is not trivial since multiple interrelated factors determine the level of polyglutamates of a drug that are required to inhibit a particular pathway, including the level of the target, the affinity of polyglutamates for the target, the competing folate pool, and the requirement for the end product of the pathway.

2.1.2.1. MTX. Natural resistance to MTX of AML compared to ALL has been studied in model systems. The AML cell line K562 synthesized fewer total MTXG$_n$ than did the ALL line CCRF-CEM; MTXG$_n$ in K562 were shorter as well *(46)*. These differences correlated with kinetic difference in the FPGS in these cell lines, which may represent a natural human polymorphism.

Diminished accumulation of MTXG$_n$ has also been studied in solid tumor models, including tumor types that are naturally sensitive and resistant to antifolates in the clinic. MTX sensitivity of three established HNSCC cell lines in continuous exposure was no different, but in pulse exposure (where polyglutamylation is expected to play a role) large differences were evident *(64)*. [^{3}H]MTX metabolism studies showed that lower MTXG$_n$ accumulation contributes to this natural resistance. The lower accumulation in the less-sensitive cell lines was not a result of decreased FPGS activity, as measured in crude extracts; GGH activity was not measured in this study. In another study of HNSCC *(65)*, seven established cell lines displayed similar sensitivity to continuous MTX exposure, but differences were again noted to sensitivity to pulse exposure. In the most resistant cell lines, FPGS activity in extracts was significantly lower *(65,66)*, but other determinants of response differed as well. Diminished MTXG$_n$ accumulation has been identified as the major mechanism of natural resistance in four recently established human soft tissue sarcoma cell lines *(67)*, but not in a methylcholanthrene-induced rat sarcoma *(68)*. Whether this represents a difference in subtype requires further exploration. The four resistant cell lines were derived from fresh patient tumors. The tumors from which two of these resistant cell lines were derived were tested when excised; one was resistant, but the other was sensitive, suggesting that in derivation a resistant subpopulation overgrew the initially sensitive population *(69)*. The FPGS level at saturating substrate in the four sarcoma lines was about the same as a sarcoma considered MTX sensitive, but in two of the lines the FPGS displayed a somewhat lower V_{max}/K_m, which may contribute to their lower polyglutamylation. In at least one of these sarcoma cell lines *(70)*, increased GGH activity, with no apparent change in FPGS activity, was identified as a mechanism of decreased accumulation of MTXG$_n$. Cervical squamous-cell carcinoma cell lines show resistance to 24-h exposures to MTX in outgrowth assays; the higher the level of the resistance in this group correlated with decreased accumulation of MTXG$_n$ (although an effect of transport could not be ruled out). Preliminary characterization of these cell lines *(42)* showed that reduced MTXG$_n$ accumulation correlated best with reduced FPGS activity consequent to decreased mRNA expression, but a role for observed GGH activity changes was not excluded.

2.2. Resistance In Vivo

In vivo resistance of L1210 leukemia to MTX was acquired much more rapidly than resistance to 10-EDAM *(71)*. Following MTX treatment, 20 distinct sublines exhibited changes in MTX transport or increased and/or altered DHFR; none showed a change in FPGS activity. Resistance to 10-EDAM in 20 sublines also appeared to be primarily a result of transport and/or DHFR alterations, but 7 sublines also exhibited low FPGS activity in extracts. When the 7 sublines were cloned and the FPGS studied in extracts, none displayed a change in K_m for AMT or 10-EDAM, but V_{max} was decreased by two- to 28-fold. All 7 clones showed decreased MTXG$_n$ accumulation when growing in mice.

The degree of decrease cannot be correlated with FPGS activity, however, since most clones had increased DHFR and/or decreased transport. However, one clone (in contradistinction to its parental subline) showed no change in transport, DHFR level or MTX/10-EDAM sensitivity of DHFR, but had only 4% of L1210 FPGS level; this clone synthesized <2% of the level of MTXG$_n$ compared to the parent in vivo. Thus, a direct correlation between the level of in vivo resistance, level of FPGS activity expressed, and decreased MTXG$_n$ accumulation in vivo was established. Further study *(41,72)* revealed that these 7 clones contained the same levels of 2.3-kb FPGS mRNA as the parent, but immunoblotting showed that they all expressed levels of FPGS (61 kDa) protein proportional to their reduced activity. There was no change in the half-life of FPGS (approx 4.3 h) in the resistant clones, as measured by FPGS activity. There was a substantial decrease in the ability of FPGS mRNA from the clones to support protein synthesis, suggesting a defect in translation was responsible for the low FPGS activity.

2.3. Clinical Relevance and Future Issues

Several features of decreased polyglutamate accumulation as a mechanism of drug resistance are of particular concern from a clinical viewpoint. First is the ease with which this resistance phenotype can be acquired. After as few as one pulse selection cycle, many resistant clones display the decreased polyglutamate accumulation phenotype, and some clones selected after only two cycles are as resistant as populations selected by six cycles *(37)*. Second, this phenotype is stable in vitro and in vivo once selected. A subline selected with pulse MTX exposure was stable for 68 wk in the absence of further MTX treatment *(35)*. Similar stability of this resistance phenotype has been observed in selection of other cell types and with other antifolates *(17,27,38,44)*. Third, relatively small decreases in FPGS activity may lead to high levels of resistance; this is seen especially with the newer non-DHFR targeted antifolates such as ZD1694 and DDATHF. It is also observed with MTX, however, since a subline selected with pulses of 30 µ*M* MTX, is resistant to pulse exposures as high as 300 µ*M* *(35)*. Thus exceptionally high levels of resistance by this mechanism may potentially be selected in the clinic.

Numerous issues remain to be addressed with respect to this phenotype, particularly in acquired resistance. These are probably best addressed at low levels of resistance, where possible, to avoid complications from other mechanisms and since low levels are more clinically relevant. Included among these issues are the following. How widespread is increased GGH as the biochemical mechanism for decreased polyglutamate accumulation? What effect does decreased FPGS and/or increased GGH activity have on folate pools and what is the effect of the folate pool on drug sensitivity? The data to date (above) do not present a unified picture, but the effect has not been fully evaluated. What factors influence the selection of this phenotype? This includes a wide array of interrelated topics. For example, the characteristics of the drug itself may have an effect based on numerous observations such as the finding that 10-EDAM selected for reduced polyglutamylation in vivo, whereas MTX did not *(71)*. Is this related to the lower K_m of 10-EDAM for FPGS relative to MTX or another characteristic? Is the frequency of this phenotype related to the constitutive level of FPGS? Is there an optimal pulse-exposure time or concentration that selects *against* this phenotype and is this optimum drug- and/or cell lineage-specific?

3. POLYGLUTAMYLATION AND CLINICAL RESISTANCE

3.1. Overview

Of the antifolates studied clinically, only MTX has been used widely enough to allow information about clinical resistance to be obtained. However, polyglutamylatable drugs that enter widespread clinical use in the future (e.g., ZD1694) may well encounter similar resistance mechanisms, even if the frequency of a particular mechanism is different. Each potential biochemical mechanism of MTX resistance discussed above (subheading 1.4.2.) may also occur clinically (reviewed in ref. *22,73*). Although natural and acquired clinical MTX resistance is widely recognized, the biochemical and molecular mechanisms involved are difficult to study experimentally. As noted by Bertino *(74)*, the relative ease of studying leukemias (compared to solid tumors) has led to the greatest knowledge in those diseases. Indeed, the inability to study resistance to any common chemotherapeutic agent readily in solid tumors is one of the barriers to increasing effective treatment in those diseases.

Study of clinical resistance presents some special issues in methodology. Since studies of patients are most often performed *ex vivo*, carefully standardized methods for cell isolation and biochemical testing must be employed *(75)*. When possible, repeated testing of the same patient should be done to provide data on experimental variation *(76)*. Although it is not done routinely, it would be good practice to include one "standard" cell line in each experiment to provide quality control. Since the number of patient cells is generally limiting, it would be useful to establish a common protocol for at least some tests so results from different labs could be compared. For example, *ex vivo* [^{3}H]MTXG$_n$ accumulation assays in patient samples routinely utilize a 24-h incubation period, but either 1 μM *(75)* or 10 μM *(69)* MTX concentrations have been used. Since MTXG$_n$ accumulation is concentration-dependent, these two schemes could lead to different conclusions. An argument could be made for the 10 μM level, since the higher level might at least partially overcome innate transport variations. If cell number is not limiting, it would also be useful to establish a standard efflux time in drug-free medium so that rapid turnover caused by elevated GGH could be detected. A number of other issues related to the conditions used in [^{3}H]MTXG$_n$ accumulation assays (e.g., peripheral blood lymphocytes vs marrow, incubation medium, presence of folic acid, serum type, and concentration) also need to be addressed.

Some general features have emerged from the studies to date. First, the levels of total drug and MTXG$_n$ in clinical samples are often only 10% that in established cell lines under similar exposure conditions (e.g., ref. *75*), however, this may not be as detrimental as it sounds, since DHFR levels are much lower in vivo than in cell-culture models *(77)*. A second and more important point is the extensive heterogeneity observed in any factor related to MTXG$_n$ accumulation. The heterogeneity occurs whether [^{3}H]MTXG$_n$ accumulation itself (e.g., refs. *75,78*), FPGS activity measurements (e.g., refs. *66,79*), or FPGS mRNA levels (by RT-PCR, refs. *80*) are measured. Although the median value of these parameters may vary between groups of patients with sensitive or resistant disease types (*see* Subheading 3.2.2.), heterogeneity in these values leads to significant overlap between the groups. In the worst case, this may indicate that these parameters will not be of use in prognosis or in making treatment decisions. However, if this heterogeneity simply parallels the heterogeneity of response seen even within sensitive disease types, and if higher values are associated with better response, this would indicate that we need to find ways to modulate the process to increase the number of patients obtaining higher values.

Only limited data is now available on acquired resistance and decreased polyglutamate accumulation (e.g., ref. 76). Most studies have focused on aspects of natural resistance.

3.2. Natural MTX Resistance

3.2.1. Recently Derived Cell Lines

A series of eight human small-cell lung carcinoma cell lines *(81)* isolated from untreated and MTX-treated patients showed a 100-fold variation in sensitivity to 24-h MTX exposure in vitro; the variation in sensitivity did not correlate with growth rate or previous chemotherapy. Although other resistance mechanisms were identified, the primary determinant leading to differential response in six of the eight was a lower level of polyglutamylation that did not allow retention of MTX above the level of DHFR once drug was removed at 24 h.

3.2.2. Fresh Patient Samples

3.2.2.1. Leukemias. The importance of MTXGn accumulation in the response of childhood ALL to standard regimens, which include MTX, has been addressed in a number of studies. Synthesis of MTXGn in samples from cancer patients was first described by Whitehead's group in bone marrow cells from pediatric ALL, AML, and non-Hodgkin's lymphoma patients (76,82,83); the levels of total drug and $MTXG_n$ accumulated were highly variable. In a larger prospective study (84) employing more sensitive methodology, a significant correlation emerged between 5-y event-free survival (EFS) in common (nonB-, nonT-cell) ALL and accumulation at diagnosis of >100 pmol $MTX/10^9$ blasts *and* >500 pmol $MTXG_n/10^9$ blasts after exposure *ex vivo* to 1 μM [^{3}H]MTX for 24 h. This correlation held only in patients with good risk factors (female or <7 yr old or $<20 \times/10^9$ blasts/L at presentation). Neither unmetabolized MTX levels nor $MTXG_n$ levels alone correlated significantly with EFS; paradoxically, the correlation between EFS and unmetabolized MTX levels (rather than $MTXG_n$ levels) was closest to significance, but this may have been a result of small sample size. Thus, even within a subtype of ALL considered chemosensitive, some patients may exhibit reduced $MTXG_n$ accumulation as a natural resistance mechanism which, rather than acquired resistance during treatment, may be responsible for treatment failure. Some poor risk patients who attained these levels of MTX and $MTXG_n$ did not achieve prolonged remission, suggesting that other factors are involved. A high degree of heterogeneity within groups was observed in this study.

The contribution of $MTXG_n$ accumulation to the clinical observation that childhood B-lineage. ALL responds better than T-lineage ALL has been studied. Early studies by Whitehead's group suggested that B-lineage cells accumulate higher levels of MTX and $MTXG_n$ and/or longer lengths *(84,85)*. Further studies by Göker et al. *(86)* and the St. Jude group *(78,87)* showed greater accumulation of $MTXG_n$ in B-lineage lymphoblasts than in those of T lineage. At low MTX dose, T-lineage blasts also tended to be slightly shorter in $MTXG_n$ length. Again there was considerable overlap in the ranges, indicating heterogeneity in the process. The study of Synold et al. *(78)* was of particular interest because of its unusual design. Patients were treated with high-dose (infusional) or low-dose (oral) MTX as a single agent immediately prior to standard induction therapy. The MTXG$_n$ pool synthesized in vivo were quantitated in bone marrow aspirates by an HPLC/enzyme inhibition assay 44 h after beginning treatment. Blasts were isolated at 4° in these studies to minimize efflux of MTX (and perhaps MTXG$_2$) as well as hydrolysis of MTXG$_n$ if GGH is present and active. In this type of study, it is not possible to control for bias introduced by loss of blasts following drug treatment *(87)*. B-lineage blasts accumulated higher levels of total MTXG$_n$ and MTXG$_{\geq 4}$ than did blasts of T-lineage ALL, regardless of MTX dose; the higher dose led to increased accumulation in both lineages. Of note, high-dose MTX treatment raised the level of MTXG$_n$ and MTXG$_{4-6}$ in T-lineage blasts to those achieved in B-lineage blasts at low-dose. The authors suggest that this provides a rationale for high-dose MTX treatment in ALL since T-lineage and those B-lineage subtypes that do not accumulate levels of MTXG$_n$>500 pmol/10^9 blasts (above) in standard therapy may do so during high-dose treatment. Furthermore, since there is considerable heterogeneity even within B-lineage blasts, high-dose MTX should ensure that a higher percentage of patients achieve cytotoxic intracellular pools. Further analysis of this study group showed that patients with the highest levels of MTXG$_n$, especially MTXG$_{3-6}$ achieved the greatest rate of blast reduction, the greatest total blast reduction in peripheral blood, and greatest inhibition of *de novo* purine synthesis in blasts following this single-agent therapy *(87)*. The mechanism for this differential MTXG$_n$ accumulation was studied *(79)*. There was no statistical difference in the constitutive expression of FPGS in T- and B-lineage ALL blasts because of extensive heterogeneity (20- to 50-fold range) in levels; however, the median activity of T-lineage ALL blasts was <33% that of B lineage. Furthermore, the authors noted a significant increase in FPGS activity in ALL blasts following MTX treatment and this increase was greater in B-lineage (188%) than T-lineage (37%) blasts; increased FPGS mRNA expression correlates with this increased activity in blasts *(88)*. Studies in two model cell lines indicate that a B-lineage line (NALM6) expresses higher constitutive FPGS activity than does a T-lineage line (diploid CCRF-CEM), the FPGS activity increases after MTX exposure and the increase is associated with an increase in FPGS mRNA greater in B-lineage than T-lineage cells *(88,89)*.

Other prognostic factors in ALL were also investigated in relation to MTXG$_n$ accumulation. In B-lineage ALL, hyperdiploidy (>50 chromosomes or DNA index >1.16) confers a more favorable prognosis. Whitehead et al. *(75)* showed that hyperdiploid B-lineage blasts accumulated significantly higher levels of MTXG$_n$ than do B-lineage blasts that are diploid or have other aneuploidy (45–47 chromosomes). Some hyperdiploid blasts accumulated exceptionally high levels of MTXG$_n$ (>2000 pmol/10^9 blasts). It is noteworthy that the distribution of lengths did not change appreciably, only the total levels. There was no correlation between MTXG$_n$ accumulation and other known prognostic factors, including S-phase cells (however, a later study did suggest a correlation of MTXG$_n$ with S-phase, ref. *(78)*. In these studies MTX itself was not analyzed because of methodological problems, however substantial heterogeneity in MTXG$_n$ accumulation was noted within each group that led to overlap between the groups. No biochemical or molecular studies of FPGS or GGH expression were undertaken in these cells. Other studies have confirmed that hyperdiploid B-lineage blasts accumulate higher levels of MTXG$_n$, especially of MTXG$_{\geq 3}$ *(78,86,87)*. Of interest is the finding that trisomy of chromosome 9, the location of human FPGS, was not observed *(75)* and no particular chromosomal duplication was correlated with higher MTXG$_n$ accumulation *(78)*. It would be of interest to reanalyze these data now that GGH has been assigned to chromosome 8, q12.23–13.1 *(90)*. ALL patients with translocations have unfavorable prognosis. Cells from five of five patients with a translocation, but normal ploidy, synthesized low (<500 pmol/10^9 blasts) levels of MTXG$_n$, whereas two of three with a translocation *and* hyperdiploidy (a favorable factor, above) accumulated high levels *(91)*. Response of individual patients was not documented in this preliminary publication. Of 52 nonhyperdiploid B-lineage ALL with karyotypic abnormalities, 13 exhibited a translocation involving 12p; blasts from these 13 patients accumulated low levels of MTXG$_n$ *ex vivo* compared to blasts with all other karyotypic abnormalities *(92)*. Interestingly, these patients were very responsive to therapy (which included MTX), suggesting that the 12p translocation may predispose to MTX sensitivity, so lower MTXG$_n$ pools are effective. Blasts from two adult B-lineage ALL patients with the t(4:11) translocation accumulated very low amounts of both total drug and MTXG$_n$ *(86)*; this subtype has a poor prognosis.

Göker et al. have proposed that the natural resistance of adult vs childhood ALL is related to lower accumulation of total drug and MTXG$_n$ in adult blasts of both T and B lineages *(86,93)*.

ALL is considered clinically sensitive to MTX-based therapy, whereas AML is not, despite *ex vivo* studies that often show similar MTX sensitivity in continuous exposure. The natural clinical resistance of AML has been postulated to be a result of less accumulation of MTXG$_n$, particularly MTXG$_{\geq 3}$, in AML cells *(74,94–97)*; this was a consistent finding, despite the use of different assay conditions in different studies. Although some early studies suggested that total drug accumulation was not different between ALL and AML (suggesting no difference in transport), more complete studies show that total drug is decreased in AML relative to ALL *(97)*, but at the long incubation times used this may reflect polyglutamylation and not transport differences. Significantly, the absolute levels of MTXG$_n$, particularly MTXG$_{3-6}$, are three- to fourfold higher in ALL than AML, although the percent of long MTXG$_{3-6}$ is only slightly higher *(97)*. Again there is great heterogeneity within both ALL and AML and wide overlap of the ranges between the two. The mechanism of this decrease has not been completely resolved, but several possibilities were explored. Whitehead et al. found that AML blasts have more rapid MTXG$_n$ turnover, presumably from increased GGH activity *(95)*. Lower constitutive expression of FPGS in AML relative to ALL may also play a role in this phenomenon *(79)*; this difference mirrors the difference observed in normal progenitors of these two lineages. In addition, as discussed above (subheading 2.1.2.1.), FPGS from AML blasts may have a lower V_{max}/K_m for MTX than does the FPGS of ALL blasts *(98)* suggesting that synthesis may also be less efficient in AML. Although AML as a group are considered naturally resistant to MTX, several recent studies from Bertino's group suggest that specific subclasses may in fact be sensitive because they are able to accumulate levels of MTXG$_n$ similar to ALL cells. These subclasses include acute monocytic leukemia (M5) *(97)* and acute megakaryocytic leukemia (M7) *(99)*. Similar to AML, CML has been briefly reported to synthesize low levels of MTXG$_n$ *(94)*, which may explain the insensitivity of this disease to MTX.

3.2.2.2. Solid Tumors. Cells isolated from soft-tissue sarcomas removed at surgery display a number of mechanisms of natural resistance to MTX, including decreased accumulation of $MTXG_n$ *(69)*. Direct biochemical studies verified decreased $MTXG_n$ synthesis in fresh specimens where it was indicated by the *is*TMPS inhibition assay (subheading 1.4.3.3.). This represents the first demonstration in fresh solid tumor samples that decreased $MTXG_n$ accumulation can be a mechanism of resistance. Cell lines were derived from some of these tumors; their characterization is described in subheading 2.1.2.1.

4. STRATEGIES FOR OVERCOMING RESISTANCE MEDIATED VIA DECREASED ACCUMULATION OF ANTIFOLATE POLYGLUTAMATES

Several strategies can be suggested for overcoming resistance mediated via decreased accumulation of antifolate polyglutamates. These strategies may be applicable to both natural and acquired resistance caused by this mechanism. At the present state of knowledge, it is not possible to empirically determine whether any strategy would selectively affect tumors and thus increase therapeutic selectivity. Fortunately, these strategies can be developed in in vitro (e.g., ref. 35) and in vivo *(71)* models to determine which have the greatest potential for benefit in the clinic.

4.1. Currently Feasible Strategies

4.1.1. Switch Drug Class

Polyglutamylation-deficient cell lines in vitro are not usually resistant to other commonly used agents such cisplatin *(9,100)*, carboplatin *(100)*, adriamycin, actinomycin D, etoposide, vincristine *(9)*. Some stochastic variations in sensitivity were noted to some agents under either continuous or pulse exposure *(9)*.

4.1.2. Alter Drug Dose or Scheduling

The data cited above (subheading 3.2.2.1.) with regard to leukemia, suggest that tumor cells that achieve higher levels of intracellular $MTXG_n$ may have a higher probability of being responsive to MTX. Since high-dose MTX increases the $MTXG_n$ pool in all leukemia cells, including those with naturally low $MTXG_n$ accumulation, high-dose MTX has been suggested as a general way of increasing $MTXG_n$ accumulation and response *(78)*. High-dose MTX may also overcome low transport, if it occurs. Sobrero et al. *(59)* have endorsed high-dose "up-front" to eliminate the maximum number of cells and thus lower the number of resistant cells remaining. It should be noted that the value of high-dose MTX has been questioned, citing evidence that higher doses may lead to both lower percent and lower absolute amounts of $MTXG_n$ accumulation in blasts *(101)*.

For MTX and other antifolates that are tight-binding inhibitors of their targets, extended infusions may be a second strategy. If the exposure time is long enough, even cells that do not accumulate $MTXG_n$ are as sensitive as cells that accumulate $MTXG_n$ well *(35)*, thus this resistance mechanism should be overcome by long infusions. In addition, since $MTXG_n$ accumulation is time-dependent, increased exposure time may allow a critical threshold to be passed in those that accumulate $MTXG_n$ less well. Increased tumor toxicity may be particularly hard to balance with host toxicity in this strategy, however.

4.1.3. Use an Alternate Polyglutamylatable Antifolate

Although many antifolates have similar determinants of action, including polyglutamylation, different tumor types may be clinically sensitive to treatment with different antifolates; in part this may be a result of enhanced polyglutamate accumulation. For example, MTX is ineffective against AML, but effective in ALL; this difference has been related to poorer accumulation in AML of total drug and of $MTXG_n$ (subheadings 2.1.2.1. and 3.2.2.1.). In contrast to MTX, AML cell lines accumulate more total ZD1694 more rapidly and convert it to longer polyglutamates than do ALL cell lines *(46,60)*. The greater accumulation of ZD1694 polyglutamates in AML models leads to sensitivity in pulse exposure similar to that of ALL models *(46)*. ZD1694 may thus be effective in overcoming the natural MTX resistance of AML. In addition, there is an intriguing observation *(60)* that no resistant cells could be selected from an AML cell line (K562) using pulse exposure, even at relatively low concentrations (50 n*M*), whereas they could be readily selected from a T-cell ALL cell line (MOLT-3). This may suggest that naturally MTX-resistant tumors may have a different resistance profile with different antifolates. Two naturally MTX-resistant soft tissue sarcoma lines displaying reduced $MTXG_n$ accumulation are more sensitive in terms of absolute concentration to pulse (24 h) ZD1694 or BW1843U89 (both of which are polyglutamylated to a greater extent than is MTX) than to MTX; in contrast, these lines are less sensitive to 24-h pulse DDATHF *(102)*. A series of HNSCC cell lines with varying natural sensitivity to pulse (24 h) MTX showed no or less difference to pulse exposures to 10-EDAM, ICI-198583 (a TMPS inhibitor related to ZD1694), or DDATHF, presumably because their more efficient transport and polyglutamylation allow cytotoxic levels of the drug to be synthesized during the drug exposure *(65)*.

Determination of which alternate antifolate is preferred or if the choice is case-specific or related to whether MTX resistance is natural or acquired will require careful evaluation since cross-resistance patterns are not consistent. For example, an HNSCC cell line with acquired MTX-resistance because of reduced FPGS expression retains full sensitivity to continuous or pulse DDATHF, but is cross-resistant to a polyglutamylatable TMPS inhibitor ICI-198583 *(57)*. However, a CCRF-CEM subline selected by pulse MTX exposure which has low FPGS activity is cross-resistant to DDATHF *(103)*.

4.1.4. Use a Nonpolyglutamylatable Antifolate

If polyglutamate accumulation is reduced, it may be efficacious to use an antifolate that does not require polyglutamylation for activity *(104)*. In this class would be lipophilic, nonclassical antifolates and "classical" antifolates that have been structurally modified to prevent polyglutamylation. The latter class consists primarily of analogs in which the glutamate appended to the heterocycle is replaced with an amino acid analog. Several of these replacements lead to loss of polyglutamylation, but do not alter other properties of the analog (e.g., refs. 12,15,105). One member of this class, ZD9331, is in an advanced state of testing *(15)*.

4.2. Future Prospects

4.2.1. FPGS Inhibitors

In cases in which acquired resistance (and perhaps natural resistance) is a result of decreased FPGS activity, the cells should be collaterally sensitive to FPGS inhibitors *(9)*.

It should be noted that cells apparently express at least 10-fold higher levels of FPGS than are required to maintain the folylpolyglutamate pools essential for normal growth *(35,36)*. This means that potent inhibitors will be required since FPGS activity will need to be fully suppressed. A second point is that FPGS inhibitors will require prolonged treatment to induce folate deficiency since the performed folate pool must be diluted out by cell division or by normal turnover (which is a slow process) *(106)*. The one class of specific, potent FPGS inhibitors reported to date are transported extremely poorly *(104)*; in this ornithine-containing class, potent FPGS inhibition and good transport may be mutually exclusive *(107)*. Studies on mechanism-based FPGS inhibitors offer a new approach to development of inhibitors of this enzyme *(115)*.

4.2.2. GGH Inhibitors

Specific inhibitors of GGH have the potential to increase polyglutamate accumulation by decreasing their degradation rate. Potential GGH inhibitors have been tested (early studies are reviewed in ref. *1*), including suramin (108), 2-mercaptomethylglutaric acid *(109)*, and diazo-oxo-norleucine(DON; ref. *110*), but as yet none appears to be specific or potent enough for use in other than preclinical models. Further studies in this area are clearly required.

4.3.3. Biochemical Modulation

Some biochemical means of effecting polyglutamate accumulation have been described, but none have been developed sufficiently for clinical use. For example, dipyridamole may enhance $MTXG_n$ synthesis *(111,112)*. Insulin treatment may promote greater $MTXG_n$ accumulation *(113)* as a result of decreased GGH activity *(114)*. As the regulation of FPGS and GGH activities are discovered, further opportunities for therapeutic intervention to alter their expression may be discovered.

ACKNOWLEDGMENT

Preparation of this review was supported by grants CA43500 and CA65755 to JJM and by Core Grant CA16056 to Roswell Park Cancer Institute.

REFERENCES

1. McGuire JJ, Coward JK. Pteroylpolyglutamates: biosynthesis, degradation, and function. In: (Blakley RL, Benkovic SJ, eds.) Folates and Pterins. Chemistry and Biochemistry of Folates. vol 1. Wiley, New York, 1984; pp. 135–190.
2. McGuire JJ, Bertino JR. Enzymatic synthesis and function of folylpolyglutamates. *Mol Cell Biochem* 1981; 38:19–48.
3. Shane B. Folylpolyglutamate synthesis and role in the regulation of one-carbon metabolism. *Vitam Horm* 1989; 45:263–335.
4. Cossins EA. Folates in biological materials. In: (Blakley RL, Benkovic SJ, eds.) Chemistry and Biochemistry of Folates. vol 1. Wiley, New York; 1984; pp 1–59.
5. McBurney MW, Whitmore GF. Isolation and biochemical characterization of folate deficient mutants of Chinese Hamster Cells. *Cell* 1974; 2:173–182.
6. Matherly LH, Seither RL, Goldman ID. Metabolism of the diamino-antifolates: biosynthesis and pharmacology of the 7-hydroxyl and polyglutamyl metabolites of methotrexate and related antifolates. *Pharmacol Ther* 1987; 35:27–56.
7. Chabner BA, Allegra CJ, Curt GA, Clendenin NJ, Baram J, Koizumi S, Drake JC, Jolivet J. Polyglutamation of methotrexate. Is methotrexate a prodrug? *J Clin Invest* 1985; 76:907–912.

8. Chu E, Allegra CJ. Antifolates. In: (Chabner BA, Longo DL, eds.) Cancer Chemotherapy and Biotherapy. 2nd ed. Lippincott-Raven, Philadelphia; 1996; pp. 109–148.
9. McGuire JJ, Heitzman KJ, Haile WH, Russell CA, McCloskey DE, Piper JR. Cross-resistance studies of folylpolyglutamate synthetase-deficient, methotrexate-resistant CCRF-CEM human leukemia sublines. *Leukemia* 1993; 7:1996–2003.
10. McGuire JJ, Mini E, Hsieh P, Bertino JR. Role of methotrexate polyglutamates in methotrexate- and sequential methotrexate-5-fluorouracil-mediated cell kill. *Cancer Res* 1985; 45:6395–6400.
11. Melera P. Acquired versus intrinsic resistance to methotrexate: diversity of the drug-resistant phenotype in mammalian cells. *Semin Cancer Biol* 1991; 2:245–255.
12. Galivan J, Inglese J, McGuire JJ, Nimec Z, Coward JK. γ-Fluoromethotrexate: synthesis and biological activity of a potent inhibitor of dihydrofolate reductase with greatly diminished ability to form poly-γ-glutamates. *Proc Natl Acad Sci USA* 1985; 82:2598–2602.
13. Samuels LL, Moccio DM, Sirotnak FM. Similar differential for total polyglutamylation and cytotoxicity among various folate analogues in human and murine tumor cells *in vitro*. *Cancer Res* 1985; 45:1488–1495.
14. Kuehl M, Brixner DI, Broom AD, Avery TL, Blakley RL. Cytotoxicity, uptake, polyglutamate formation, and antileukemic effects of 8-deaza analogues of methotrexate and aminopterin in mice. *Cancer Res* 1988; 48:1481–1488.
15. Jackman AL, Calvert AH. Folate-based thymidylate synthase inhibitors as anticancer drugs. *Ann Oncol* 1995; 6:871–881.
16. Sobrero AF, McGuire JJ, Bertino JR. Uptake and metabolism of 5,8-dideazaisofolic acid in human colon carcinoma cells. *Biochem Pharmacol* 1988; 37:997–1001.
17. Pizzorno G, Moroson BA, Cashmore AR, Russello O, Mayer JR, Galivan J, Bunni MA, Priest DG, Beardsley GP. Multifactorial resistance to 5,10-dideazatetrahydrofolic acid in cell lines derived from human lymphoblastic leukemia CCRF-CEM. *Cancer Res* 1995; 55:566–573.
18. Shih C, Chen VJ, Gossett LS, Gates SB, MacKellar WC, Habeck LL, Shackelford KA, Mendelsohn LG, Soose DJ, Patel VF, Andis SL, Bewley JR, Rayl EA, Moroson BA, Beardsley GP, Kohler W, Ratnam M, Schultz RM. LY231514, a pyrrolo[2,3-d]pyrimidine-based antifolate that inhibits multiple folate-requiring enzymes. *Cancer Res* 1997; 57:1116–1123.
19. Galivan J, Yao R, Rhee M, Schneider E, Ryan TJ. Glutamyl hydrolase. In: (Pfleiderer W, Rokos H, eds.) Proceedings of the 11th International Symposium on Folates Pterins. Blackwell, London; 1997; pp. 439–442.
20. Wang Y, Nimec Z, Ryan TJ, Dias JA, Galivan J. The properties of the secreted gamma-glutamyl hydrolases from H35 hepatoma cells. *Biochim Biophys Acta Protein Struct Mol Enzymol* 1993; 1164:227–235.
21. Pinto JT, Suffoletto BP, Berzin TM, Qiao CH, Lin S, Tong WP, May F, Mukherjee B, Heston WDW. Prostate-specific membrane antigen: a novel folate hydrolase in human prostate carcinoma cells. *Clin Cancer Res* 1996; 2:1445–1451.
22. Gorlick R, Goker E, Trippett T, Waltham M, Banerjee D, Bertino JR. Intrinsic and acquired resistance to methotrexate in acute leukemia. *N Engl J Med* 1996; 335:1041–1048.
23. Crosti P, Malerba M, Bianchetti R. A methotrexate-resistant line of Daucus carota with high levels of intracellular folates. *Plant Sci* 1993; 89:215–220.
24. Tse A, Moran RG. Control of the polyglutamation of 5,10-dideazatetrahydrofolate by intracellular folate pools: a novel mechanism of resistance to antifolates. *Proc Am Assoc Cancer Res* 1994; 35:304.
25. Cowan KH, Jolivet J. A methotrexate-resistant human breast cancer cell line with multiple defects, including diminished formation of methotrexate polyglutamates. *J Biol Chem* 1984; 259:10,793–10,800.
26. Pinard MF, Matherly LH, Jolivet J. Methotrexate resistance associated with a unique combination of influx and efflux defects. *Cell Pharmacol* 1993; 1:43–47.
27. Jackman AL, Kelland LR, Kimbell R, Brown M, Gibson W, Aherne GW, Hardcastle A, Boyle FT. Mechanisms of acquired resistance to the quinazoline thymidylate synthase inhibitor ZD1694 (Tomudex) in one mouse and three human cell lines. *Br J Cancer* 1995; 71:914–924.
28. Rhee MS, Wang Y, Nair MG, Galivan J. Acquisition of resistance to antifolates caused by enhanced gamma-glutamyl hydrolase activity. *Cancer Res* 1993; 53:2227–2230.

29. Galivan J, Balinska M. Control of methotrexate polyglutamate synthesis in cultured rat hepatoma cells. In: (Blair JA, ed.) Chemistry and Biology of Pteridines. Walter de Gruyter, Berlin, 1983; pp. 305–309.
30. Assaraf YG, Feder JN, Sharma RC, Wright JE, Rosowsky A, Shane B, Schimke RT. Characterization of the coexisting multiple mechanisms of methotrexate resistance in mouse 3T6 R50 fibroblasts. *J Biol Chem* 1992; 267:5776–5784.
31. Frei E, Rosowsky A, Wright JE, Cucchi CA, Lippke JA, Ervin TJ, Jolivet J, Haseltine WA. Development of methotrexate resistance in a human squamous cell carcinoma of the head and neck in culture. *Proc Natl Acad Sci USA* 1984; 81:2873–2877.
32. Curt GA, Jolivet J, Bailey BD, Carney DN, Chabner BA. Synthesis and retention of methotrexate polyglutamates by human small cell lung cancer. *Biochem Pharmacol* 1984; 33:1682–1685.
33. Koizumi S. Impairment of methotrexate (MTX)-polyglutamate formation of MTX-resistant K562 cell lines. *Jpn J Cancer Res. (Gann)* 1988; 79:1230–1237.
34. Koizumi S, Allegra CJ. Enzyme studies of methotrexate-resistant human leukemia (K562) subclones. *Leukemia Res* 1992; 16:565–569.
35. McCloskey DE, McGuire JJ, Russell CA, Rowan BG, Bertino JR, Pizzorno G, Mini E. Decreased folylpolyglutamate synthetase activity as a mechanism of methotrexate resistance in CCRF-CEM human leukemia sublines. *J Biol Chem* 1991; 266:6181–6187.
36. Shane B, Lowe K, Osborne C, Kim J, Lin B. Role of folylpolyglutamate synthetase in the regulation of folate and antifolate metabolism. In: (Curtius HC, Ghisla S, Blau N, eds.) Chemistry and Biology of Pteridines 1989. Walter de Gruyter, Berlin, 1989; pp. 891–895.
37. McGuire JJ, Haile WH, Russell CA, Galvin JM, Shane B. Evolution of resistance in the CCRF-CEM human leukemia cell line following intermittent exposure to methotrexate. *Oncol Res* 1995; 7:535–543.
38. Lu K, Yin MB, McGuire JJ, Bonmassar E, Rustum YM. Mechanisms of resistance to N-[5-[N-(3,4-dihydro-2-methyl-4-oxoquinazolin-6-ylmethyl)-N-methylamino]-2-thenoyl]-L-glutamic acid (ZD1694), a folate-based thymidylate synthase inhibitor, in the HCT-8 human ileocecal adenocarcinoma cell line. *Biochem Pharmacol* 1995; 50:391–398.
39. Drake JC, Allegra CJ, Moran RG, Johnston PG. Resistance to Tomudex (ZD1694): multifactorial in human breast and colon carcinoma cell lines. *Biochem Pharmacol* 1996; 51:1349–1355.
40. Barnes MJ, Estlin EJ, Taylor GA, Calvete JA, Newell DR, Lunec J, Hall AG, Pearson ADJ, Aherne W, Hardcastle A. The characterization of a Tomudex-resistant CCRF-CEM cell line. *Proc Amer Assoc Cancer Res* 1997; 38:99–99.
41. Roy K, Egan MG, Sirlin S, Sirotnak FM. Posttranscriptionally mediated decreases in folylpolyglutamate synthetase gene expression in some folate analogue-resistant variants of the L1210 cell—evidence for an altered cognate mRNA in the variants affecting the rate of de novo synthesis of the enzyme. *J Biol Chem* 1997; 272:6903–6908.
42. Barakat RR, Lovelace CIP, Li WW, Bertino JR. Decreased formation of methotrexate (MTX) polyglutamates in cervical carcinoma cell lines intrinsically resistant to MTX is associated with decreased expression of folylpolyglutamyl synthetase. *Proc Am Assoc Cancer Res* 1994; 35:305–305.
43. Roy K, Mitsugi K, Sirlin S, Shane B, Sirotnak FM. Different antifolate-resistant L1210 cell variants with either increased or decreased folylpolyglutamate synthetase gene expression at the level of mRNA transcription. *J Biol Chem* 1995; 270:26,918–26,922.
44. Takemura Y, Kobayashi H, Gibson W, Kimbell R, Miyachi H, Jackman AL. The influence of drug-exposure conditions on the development of resistance to methotrexate or ZD1694 in cultured human leukaemia cells. *Int J Cancer* 1996; 66:29–36.
45. Wang FS, Aschele C, Sobrero A, Chang YM, Bertino JR. Decreased folylpolyglutamate synthetase expression: a novel mechanism of fluorouracil resistance. *Cancer Res* 1993; 53:3677–3680.
46. Longo GSA, Gorlick R, Tong WP, Ercikan E, Bertino JR. Disparate affinities of antifolates for folylpolyglutamate synthetase from human leukemia cells. *Blood* 1997; 90:1241–1245.
47. Swendseid ME, Bethell FH, Bird OD. The concentration of folic acid in leucocytes. Observations on normal subjects and persons with leukemia. *Cancer Res* 1951; 11:864–867.
48. Barrueco JR, O'Leary DF, Sirotnak FM. Metabolic turnover of methotrexate polyglutamates in lysosomes derived from S180 cells. Definition of a two-step process limited by mediated lysosomal per-

meation of polyglutamates and activating reduced sulfhydryl compounds. *J Biol Chem* 1992; 267:15,356–15,361.
49. Yao R, Nimec Z, Ryan TJ, Galivan J. Identification, cloning, and sequencing of a cDNA coding for rat gamma-glutamyl hydrolase. *J Biol Chem* 1996; 271:8525–8528.
50. Yao R, Schneider E, Ryan TJ, Galivan J. Human gamma-glutamyl hydrolase: cloning and characterization of the enzyme expressed in vitro. *Proc Natl Acad Sci USA* 1996; 93:10,134–10,138.
51. Rodenhuis S, McGuire JJ, Narayanan R, Bertino JR. Development of an assay system for the detection and classification of methotrexate resistance in fresh human leukemic cells. *Cancer Res* 1986; 46:6513–6519.
52. Jackman AL, Kimbell R, Brown M, Brunton L, Boyle FT. Quinazoline thymidylate synthase inhibitors: methods for assessing the contribution of polyglutamation to their in vitro activity. *Anti-cancer Drug Design* 1995; 10:555–572.
53. Longo GSA, Gorlick R, Tong WP, Lin S, Steinherz P, Bertino JR. Gamma-glutamyl hydrolase and folylpolyglutamate synthetase activities predict polyglutamylation of MTX in acute leukemias. *Proc Am Assoc Cancer Res* 1997; 38:603–603.
54. Pizzorno G, Mini E, Caronnelo M, McGuire JJ, Moroson BA, Cashmore AR, Dreyer RN, Lin JT, Mazzei T, Periti P, and Bertino JR. Resistance to methotrexate in CCRF-CEM cells after short-term, high-dose treatment is associated with impaired polyglutamylation. *Cancer Res* 1988; 48:2149–2155.
55. Bernal SD, De Villa RS, Wong YC. Congruence of SQM1 protein expression with methotrexate sensitivity and transport. *Cancer Invest* 1995; 13:23–30.
56. McGuire JJ, Russell CA. Folylpolyglutamate synthetase (FPGS) expression in antifolate-sensitive and -resistant human leukemia cell lines. *Proc Am Assoc Cancer Res* 1997; 38:98.
57. van der Laan BFAM, Jansen G, Kathmann I, Schornagel JH, Hordijk GJ. Mechanisms of acquired resistance to methotrexate in a human squamous carcinoma cell line of the head and neck, exposed to different treatment schedules. *Eur J Cancer* 1991; 27:1274–1278.
58. Aschele C, Sobrero A, Faderan MA, Tong WP, Bertino JR. Mechanisms of resistance to different schedules of methotrexate in HCT-8 cells in vitro. *Proc Am Assoc Cancer Res* 1992; 33:410.
59. Sobrero AF, Aschele C, Rosso R, Nicolin A, Bertino JR. Rapid development of resistance to antifolates in vitro: possible clinical implication. *JNCI* 1991; 83:24–28.
60. Takemura Y, Gibson W, Kimbell R, Kobayashi H, Miyachi H, Jackman AL. Cellular pharmacokinetics of ZD1694 in cultured human leukemia cells sensitive, or made resistant, to this drug. *J Cancer Res Clin Oncol* 1996; 122:109–117.
61. Biedler JL. Drug resistance: genotype *versus* phenotype—thirty-second GHA Clowes Memorial Award Lecture. *Cancer Res* 1994; 54:666–678.
62. Yao R, Rhee MS, Galivan J. Effects of gamma-glutamyl hydrolase on folyl and antifolylpolyglutamates in cultured H35 hepatoma cells. *Mol Pharmacol* 1995; 48:505–511.
63. Li WW, Lin JT, Chang YM, Schweitzer B, Bertino B. Prediction of antifolate efficacy in a rat sarcoma model. *Int J Cancer* 1991; 49:234–238.
64. Pizzorno G, Chang YM, McGuire JJ, Bertino JR. Inherent resistance of human squamous cell lines to methotrexate as a result of decreased polyglutamylation of this drug. *Cancer Res* 1989; 49:5275–5280.
65. Van der Laan BFAM, Jansen G, Kathmann GAM, Westerhof GR, Schornagel JH, Hordijk GJ. *In vitro* activity of novel antifolates against human squamous carcinoma cell lines of the head and neck with inherent resistance to methotrexate. *Int J Cancer* 1992; 51:909–914.
66. Jansen G, Schornagel JH, Kathmann I, Westerhof GR, Hordijk GJ, van der Laan FAM. Measurement of folylpolyglutamate synthetase in head and neck squamous carcinoma cell lines and clinical samples using a new rapid separation procedure. *Oncol Res* 1992; 4:299–305.
67. Li WW, Lin JT, Schweitzer BI, Tong WP, Niedzwiecki D, Bertino JR. Intrinsic resistance to methotrexate in human soft tissue sarcoma cell lines. *Cancer Res* 1992; 52:3908–3913.
68. Li WW, Lin JT, Schweitzer BI, Bertino JR. Mechanisms of sensitivity and natural resistance to antifolates in a methylcholanthrene-induced rat sarcoma. *Mol Pharmacol* 1991; 40:854–858.
69. Li WW, Lin JT, Tong WP, Trippett TM, Brennan MF, Bertino JR. Mechanisms of natural resistance to antifolates in human soft tissue sarcoma. *Cancer Res* 1992; 52:1434–1438.
70. Li WW, Waltham M, Tong W, Schweitzer BI, Bertino JR. Increased activity of gamma-glutamyl hydrolase in human sarcoma cell lines: a novel mechanism of intrinsic resistance to methotrexate (MTX). *Adv Exp Med Biol* 1993; 338:635–638.

71. Rumberger BG, Schmid FA, Otter GM, Sirotnak FM. Preferential selection during therapy *in vivo* by edetrexate compared to methotrexate of resistant L1210 cell variants with decreased folylpolyglutamate synthetase activity. *Cancer Commun* 1990; 2:305–310.
72. Egan MG, Sirlin S, Rumberger BG, Shane B, Sirotnak FM. Molecular properties of edetrexate-resistant varaints of the L1210 cell with decreased folylpolyglutamate synthetase activity. *Proc Am Assoc Cancer Res* 1993; 34:275.
73. Sobrero AF, Bertino JR. Clinical aspects of drug resistance. *Cancer Surveys* 1986; 5:93–107.
74. Bertino JR, Lin JT, Pizzorno G, Li WW, Chang YM. The basis for intrinsic drug resistance or sensitivity to methotrexate. *Adv Enzyme Regul* 1989; 29:277–285.
75. Whitehead VM, Vuchich MJ, Lauer SJ, Mahoney D, Carroll AJ, Shuster JJ, Esseltine DW, Payment C, Look AT, Akabutu J, Bowen T, Taylor LD, Camitta B, Pullen DJ. Accumulation of high levels of methotrexate polyglutamates in lymphoblasts from children with hyperdiploid (>50 chromosomes) B-lineage acute lymphoblastic leukemia: a Pediatric Oncology Group Study. *Blood* 1992; 80:1316–1323.
76. Whitehead VM, Rosenblatt DS. Methotrexate metabolism by bone marrow cells from patients with leukemia. *Adv Exptl Med Biol* 1983; 163:287–303.
77. Kamen BA, Nylen PA, Whitehead VM, Abelson HT, Dolnick BJ, Peterson DW. Lack of dihydrofolate reductase in human tumor and leukemia cells in vivo. *Cancer Drug Delivery* 1985; 2:133–138.
78. Synold TW, Relling MV, Boyett JM, Rivera GK, Sandlund JT, Mahmoud H, Crist WM, Pui CH, Evans WE. Blast cell methotrexate-polyglutamate accumulation in vivo differs by lineage, ploidy, and methotrexate dose in acute lymphoblastic leukemia. *J Clin Invest* 1994; 94:1996–2001.
79. Barredo JC, Synold TW, Laver J, Relling MV, Pui CH, Priest DG, Evans WE. Differences in constitutive and post-methotrexate folylpolyglutamate synthetase activity in B-lineage and T-lineage leukemia. *Blood* 1994; 84:564–569.
80. Lenz HJ, Danenberg K, Schneiders B, Goeker E, Peters GJ, Garrow T, Shane B, Bertino JR, Danenberg PV. Quantitative analysis of folypolyglutamate synthetase gene expression in tumor tissues by the polymerase chain reaction: marked variation of expression among leukemia patients. *Oncology Res* 1994; 6:329–335.
81. Curt GA, Jolivet J, Carney DN, Bailey BD, Drake JC, Clendenin NJ, Chabner BA. Determinants of the sensitivity of human small-cell lung cancer lines to methotrexate. *J Clin Invest* 1985; 76:1323–1329.
82. Witte A, Whitehead VM, Rosenblatt DS, Vuchich M-J. Synthesis of methotrexate polyglutamates by bone marrow cells from patients with leukemia and lymphoma. *Dev Pharmacol Ther* 1980; 1:40–46.
83. Whitehead VM, Rosenblatt DS, Vuchich M-J, Beaulieu D. MTX polyglutamate synthesis in lymphoblasts from children with ALL. *Dev Chem Ther* 1987; 10:443–448.
84. Whitehead VM, Rosenblatt DS, Vuchich M-J, Shuster JJ, Beaulieu D. Accumulation of methotrexate and methotrexate polyglutamates in lymphoblasts at diagnosis of childhood acute lymphoblastic leukemia: a pilot prognostic factor analysis. *Blood* 1990; 76:44–49.
85. Whitehead VM, Vuchich MJ, Bernstein M, McClain K, Fort D, Shuster JJ, Lauer SJ, Akabutu J, Bowen T, Devine S, Payment C. Differences in chain-length of methotrexate polyglutamates in lymphoblasts from children with T- and B-lineage acute lumphoblastic leukemia. *Proc Am Assoc Cancer Res* 1992; 33:405–405.
86. Göker E, Lin JT, Trippett T, Ellisseyeff Y, Tong WP, Niedzwiecki D, Tan C, Steinherz P, Schweitzer BI, Bertino JR. Decreased polyglutamylation of methotrexate in acute lymphoblastic leukemia blasts in adults compared to children with this disease. *Leukemia* 1993; 7:1000–1004.
87. Masson E, Relling MV, Synold TW, Liu Q, Schuetz JD, Sandlund JT, Pui CH, Evans WE. Accumulation of methotrexate polyglutamates in lymphoblasts is a determinant of antileukemic effects in vivo—a rationale for high-dose methotrexate. *J Clin Invest* 1996; 97:73–80.
88. Galpin AJ, Schuetz JD, Masson E, Yanishevski Y, Synold TW, Barredo JC, Pui CH, Relling MV, Evans WE. Differences in folylpolyglutamate synthetase and dihydrofolate reductase expression in human B-lineage versus T-lineage leukemic lymphoblasts: Mechanisms for lineage differences in methotrexate polyglutamylation and cytotoxicity. *Mol Pharmacol* 1997; 52:155–163.
89. Synold TW, Willits EM, Barredo JC. Role of folylpolygutamate synthetase (FPGS) in antifolate chemotherapy; a biochemical and clinical update. *Leuk Lymphoma* 1996; 21:9–15.

90. Yao R. Studies of γ-glutamyl hydrolase: human tissue distribution and chromosome localization. In: (Pfleiderer W, Rokos H, eds.) Proceedings of the 11th International Symposium on Folates Pterins. Blackwell, London, 1997; pp. 475–478.
91. Whitehead VM, Vuchich MJ, Carroll AJ, Shuster JJ, Lauer SJ, Mahoney D, Akabutu J, Bowen T, Beardsley P, Leclerc J-M, Pullen DJ. Methotrexate metabolism in lymphoblasts with hyperdiploidy and/or translocations in children with acute lymphoblastic leukemia (ALL): a Pediatric Oncology Group Study. *Blood* 1990; 76(suppl. 1):335a.
92. Whitehead VM, Vuchich MJ, Cooley L, Lauer SJ, Mahoney D, Shuster JJ, Payment C, Bernstein M, Akabutu J, Bowen T, Kamen B, Ravindranath Y, Emami A, Beardsley P, Pullen J, Camitta B. Translocations involving chromosome 12p, methotrexate metabolism and outcome in childhood B-progenitor cell acute lymphoblastic leukemia (ALL): a Pediatric Oncology Group Pharmacology pilot study. *Proc Am Assoc Cancer Res* 1996; 37:381–381.
93. Gondo H, Harada M, Taniguchi S, Akashi K, Hayashi S, Teshima T, Takamatsu Y, Eto T, Nagafuji K, Yamasaki K, Shibuya T, Niho Y. Cyclosporine combined with methylprednisolone or methotrexate in prophylaxis of moderate to severe acute graft-versus-host disease. *Bone Marrow Transplant* 1993; 12:437–441.
94. Yamauchi H, Iwata N, Omine M, Maekawa T. In vitro methotrexate polyglutamate formation is elevated in acute lymphoid leukemia cells compared with acute myeloid leukemia and normal bone marrow cells. *Acta Haematol Japonica* 1988; 51:766–773.
95. Whitehead VM, Kalman TI, Rosenblatt DS, Vuchich M-J, Payment C. Regulation of methotrexate polyglutamate (MTXPG) formation in human leukemic cells. *Proc Am Assoc Cancer Res* 1988; 29:287–287.
96. Lin JT, Tong WP, Trippett T, Niedzwiecki D, Tao Y, Tan C, Steinherz P, Schweitzer BI, Bertino JR. Basis for the natural resistance to methotrexate in human acute non-lymphoblastic leukemia. *Leukemia Res* 1991; 15:1191–1196.
97. Göker E, Kheradpour A, Waltham M, Banerjee D, Tong WP, Elisseyeff Y, Bertino JR. Acute monocytic leukemia: A myeloid leukemia subset that may be sensitive to methotrexate. *Leukemia* 1995; 9:274–276.
98. Longo G, Gorlick R, Bertino JR. The thymidylate synthase inhibitors, tomudex and BW1843U89, are potent inhibitors of the growth of the myeloid leukemia cell line K562. *Proc Am Assoc Cancer Res* 1996; 37:384–384.
99. Argiris A, Longo GSA, Gorlick R, Tong W, Steinherz P, Bertino JR. Increased methotrexate polyglutamylation in acute megakaryocytic leukemia (M7) compared to other subtypes of acute myelocytic leukemia. *Leukemia* 1997; 11:886–889.
100. Kelland LR, Kimbell R, Hardcastle A, Aherne GW, Jackman AL. Relationships between resistance to cisplatin and antifolates in sensitive and resistant tumour cell lines. *Eur J Cancer* 1995; 31A:981–986.
101. Hum MC, Smith AK, Lark RH, Winick N, Kamen BA. If methotrexate polyglutamates are the answer, is high dose methotrexate the solution? *Proc Am Assoc Cancer Res* 1996; 37:370–370.
102. Li WW, Tong WP, Bertino JR. Antitumor activity of antifolate inhibitors of thymidylate and purine synthesis in human soft tissue sarcoma cell lines with intrinsic resistance to methotrexate. *Clin Cancer Res* 1995; 1:631–636.
103. Pizzorno G, Sokoloski JA, Cashmore AR, Moroson B, Cross AD, Beardsley GP. Intracellular metabolism of 5,10-dideazatetrahydrofolic acid in human leukemia cell lines. *Mol Pharmacol* 1991; 39:85–89.
104. McGuire JJ, Tsukamoto T, Hart BP, Coward JK, Kalman TI, Galivan J. Exploitation of folate and antifolate polyglutamylation to achieve selective anticancer chemotherapy. *Invest New Drugs* 1996; 14:317–323.
105. Rosowsky A, Bader H, Cucchi CA, Moran RG, Kohler W, Freisheim JH. Methotrexate analogues. 33. N^δ-Acyl-N^α-(4-amino-4-deoxypteroyl)-L-ornithine derivatives: synthesis and *in vitro* antitumor activity. *J Med Chem* 1988; 31:1332–1337.
106. McGuire JJ, Haile WH. Potent inhibition of human folylpolyglutamate synthetase by suramin. *Arch Biochem Biophys* 1996; 335:139–144.
107. Tsukamoto T, Haile WH, McGuire JJ, Coward JK. The synthesis and biological evaluation of N^α-(4-amino-4-deoxy-10-methylpteroyl)-DL-4,4-difluoroornithine. *J Med Chem* 1996; 39:2536–2540.
108. Rhee MS. Inhibition of γ-glutamyl hydrolase by levamisole and suramin. In: (Pfleiderer W, Rokos H,

eds.) Proceedings of the 11th International Symposium on Folates Pterins. Blackwell, London, 1997; pp. 467–470.
109. Whitehead VM, Kalman TI, Vuchich M-J. Inhibition of gamma-glutamyl hydrolases in human cells by 2-mercaptomethylglutaric acid. *Biochem Biophys Res Commun* 1987; 144:292–297.
110. Waltham MC, Li WW, Gritsman H, Tong WP, Bertino JR. γ-Glutamyl hydrolase from human sarcoma HT-1080 cells: characterization and inhibition by glutamine antagonists. *Mol Pharmacol* 1997; 51:825–832.
111. Kennedy DG, van den Berg HW, Clarke R, Murphy RF. Enhancement of methotrexate cytotoxicity towards the MDA.MB.436 human breast-cancer cell line by dipyridamole. The role of methotrexate polyglutamates. *Biochem Pharmacol* 1986; 35:3053–3056.
112. Chan CKC, Howell SB. Role of hypoxanthine and thymidine in determining methotrexate plus dipyridamole cytotoxicity. *Eur J Cancer* 1990; 26:907–911.
113. Kennedy DG, Clarke R, van den Berg HW, Murphy RF. The kinetics of methotrexate polyglutamate formation and efflux in a human breast cancer cell line (MDA.MB.436): the effect of insulin. *Biochem Pharmacol* 1983; 32:41–46.
114. Galivan J, Rhee MS. Insulin-dependent suppression in glutamyl hydrolase activity and elevated cellular methotrexate polyglutamates. *Biochem Pharmacol* 1995; 50:1659–1663.
115. Tsukamoto T, Haile WH, McGuire JJ, Coward JK. Mechanism-based inhibition of human folylpolyglutamate synthetase: design, synthesis, and biochemical characterization of a phosphapeptide mimic of the tetrahedral intermediate. *Arch Biochem Biophys* 1998; 355:109–119.

17 Antifolates in Combination Therapy

Stephen P. Ackland and Rosemary Kimbell

CONTENTS

INTRODUCTION
PRECLINICAL ANALYSIS OF COMBINED DRUG EFFECTS
DIHYDROFOLATE REDUCTASE INHIBITORS
THYMIDYLATE SYNTHASE INHIBITORS
CONCLUSIONS
REFERENCES

1. INTRODUCTION

In cancer chemotherapy, combinations of drugs are often necessary to achieve effective clinical response. Combinations were initially developed empirically in the late 1960s, in diseases such as leukemia and lymphoma. The basic principle in selection of these combinations was simple; drugs that were effective as single agents but had nonoverlapping normal tissue toxicity were chosen (e.g., vincristine and prednisone). If drugs had similar toxicities, specific schedules could be used so that toxicity was not compounded. If the drugs had different mechanisms of action, an additional bonus may occur because the tumor may be less able to develop resistance. This approach proved successful in acute leukemias, lymphoma, and testis cancer, where long-term survivors are few with single-agent therapy but commonplace after combination chemotherapy. In diseases such as breast cancer and small-cell lung cancer, combination chemotherapy increases responses from a paltry 15–30% for single agents to 40–70%.

In the quest for better combinations, and for effective combinations in the more common, less sensitive cancers (such as lung and colon cancer), scientists and clinicians have attempted to develop and apply logic and scientific principles to what was initially an empirical process. In vitro and in vivo preclinical studies have been undertaken, and the conclusions used to justify the clinical use of combinations. The identification of synergism (synergy) is the stated or implied aim in these explorations. Synergism or synergy is defined as the joint action of agents so that their combined effect is greater than the algebraic sum of their individual effects. Antagonism is the joint action of agents such that the combined effect is less than expected. Additivity is the boundary be-

From: *Anticancer Drug Development Guide: Antifolate Drugs in Cancer Therapy*
Edited by: A.L. Jackman © Humana Press Inc., Totowa, NJ

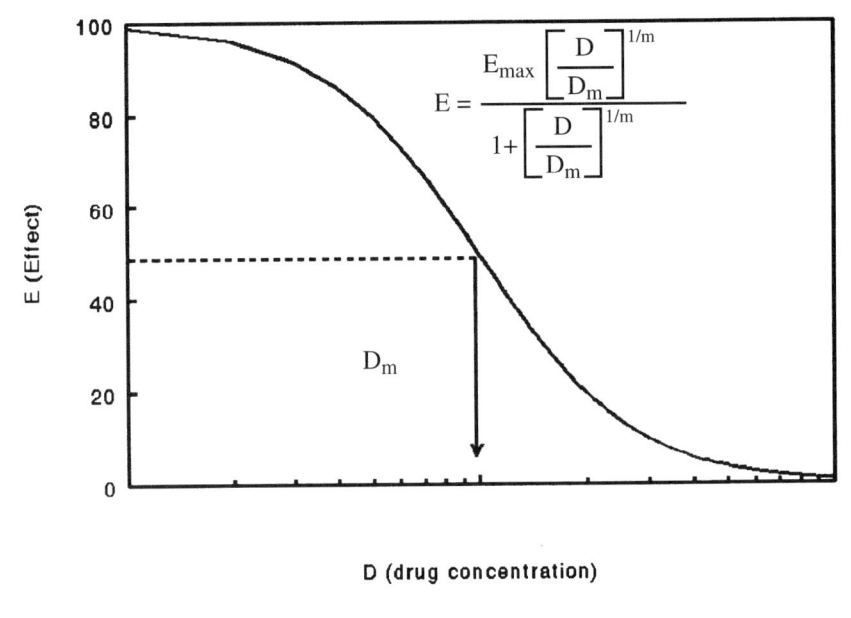

$$E = \frac{E_{max}\left[\dfrac{D}{D_m}\right]^{1/m}}{1+\left[\dfrac{D}{D_m}\right]^{1/m}}$$

Fig. 1

tween synergism and antagonism, where the agents concerned do not interact with each other, functioning independently to produce a result that is the sum of the individual effects of the drugs involved. These and other concepts have been imported from the fields of enzymology chemistry and basic pharmacology to develop models of drug behavior and interaction that have been applied to biological systems (especially in vitro cell cultures). This approach has resulted in a vast and sometimes confusing terminology, as well as a variety of simple and complex mathematical modeling techniques with which to analyze results.

This approach has been used extensively in the development of anticancer antimetabolites, where inhibition of pyrimidine or purine biosynthesis at multiple points in the pathways has the potential to result in synergistic cytotoxicity. This chapter will initially discuss the various methods available to analyze combined drug effects, indicating some of their pitfalls and limitations. Then we review preclinical data suggesting benefit from combinations of cytotoxic drugs including folate-based antimetabolites (but not including noncytotoxic modulators), and the clinical trials in which such combinations have been studied. The relevance of conclusions drawn from preclinical data to the treatment of human cancer is discussed.

2. PRECLINICAL ANALYSIS OF COMBINED DRUG EFFECTS

The design and analysis of preclinical studies to assess combined drug effects is exceedingly complex, and there is no consensus as to the best method. The primary reason for this complexity is because the relationship between concentration and effect (or dose and response) is not linear. Most drug concentration-effect relationships fit a sigmoidal curve, which is best modeled by the Hill model (Fig. 1) or the sigmoid E_{max} model (the same as the Hill model except that the maximum possible effect, E_{max}, is defined) *(1)*. As a consequence, two molecules of drug A do not have twice the effect of one molecule of drug A. Furthermore, the sigmoidal shape of the concentration-effect curve will vary from one drug to another; whereas the relative effects of two drugs can be normalized, the degree of sigmoidicity of the curve for each drug is unique. Also, and from a practical viewpoint, data from an experiment of a drug concentration-effect relationship may not fit a Hill model well, either because of variance in the experimental conditions or because that particular system is too complex for the model to apply. Other models that describe the relationship between dose and effect include exponential, exponential with shoulder, linear-quadratic, and log-log functions *(2)*. A complex system such as a cell or tumor, where there may be many physiological or biochemical steps between drug administration and action, and where the endpoint may be remote (e.g., percentage of control growth) may not fit a Hill model as easily as an isolated drug-target interaction.

As a consequence of this complexity, a vast number of mathematical modeling techniques have been designed to analyze the results of experiments examining combined drug effects (reviewed in ref. *3*). These models vary from simple to complex, and the vast number indicates a lack of consensus as to the best approach. Most models require specific experimental designs in order to analyze the data.

2.1. Isobolograms

This is an old established procedure that can be undertaken largely by hand and without the use of complex mathematics. Whereas the method is simple and flexible and generally accepted, it has several shortcomings so the biological interpretation and relevance of a result is uncertain. As a consequence, classical isobolograms have fallen from favor, but are still used by many investigators to consolidate conclusions drawn by using more complex methods.

2.2. Fractional Product Method of Webb

In this method *(4)* the measured effect of each drug alone is simply multiplied, and compared to the observed effect of the combination using the same doses of agents. This method assumes a linear dose-effect relationship for each drug and the combination, which is seldom the case.

2.3. Interaction Index of Berenbaum

This method *(5,6)* is the algebraic expression of the isobologram. If the interaction index, $I < 1$, synergism is concluded; if $I > 1$, antagonism is concluded. Whereas this is an adequate general method for many circumstances, its drawbacks are that the researcher must determine whether his data fit a dose-effect model adequately, and it is difficult to derive a good summary measure of the intensity of any interaction.

2.4. Method of Steele and Peckham

Steele and Peckham *(7)* proposed an envelope of additivity on an isobologram rather than a single additive line. Data points that fall between the two lines are considered to represent additivity. The mathematical methods for determining the two lines, and their significance, is controversial.

2.5. The Median-Effect Method of Chou and Talalay

This method *(8)* has a basic assumption that the dose-effect curves of each drug alone (drug 1, drug 2) as well as the combination of drug 1 and drug 2 fit the Hill model. A number of assumptions about the type of interaction of the two agents are made, and the analysis finally results in a single number called the combination index. A combination index, $CI < 1$ is said to represent synergism, and $CI > 1$ represents antagonism. The correctness of the assumptions and the mathematics that follow has been controversial *(2,3)*. However, in general, in studies of anticancer drug combinations this is the preferred model.

2.6. Response Surface Approach of Greco

This technique initially fits the data for both single agents to a concentration-effect model to gain initial parameter estimates *(3,9,10)*. The Hill model is generally applied, but other models may be used. Then a computer-modeling algorithm fits the data from an experiment to an equation, resulting in five estimated parameters (IC_{50}s for both drugs, dose-effect slopes for both drugs [assuming the Hill model] and the parameter, α). In addition the 95% confidence intervals for each parameter and the residuals can be estimated. This approach is mathematically complex, requiring computing power and statistical knowledge, and is difficult for most scientists to apply with confidence. As a consequence it has not found generalized application.

In summary, the analysis of combined drug effects in biological systems is complex and controversial. The various techniques developed each have shortcomings and pitfalls in their application. In cancer research, the median-effect method is used more frequently than any other method but its application to data and the interpretation of results need to be handled with caution.

3. DIHYDROFOLATE REDUCTASE INHIBITORS

DHFR is a pivotal enzyme involved in the maintenance of intracellular levels of reduced folates, which are essential for a number of biochemical reactions involving donation of one-carbon groups including production of dTMP from dUMP, and *de novo* synthesis of purine nucleotides. The consequence of these reactions is oxidation of tetrahydrofolates to dihydrofolate, which must then be converted back to tetrahydrofolates for participation in further one-carbon transfers (reviewed in ref. *11* and Chapters 2 and 3). Methotrexate is the most commonly used and best understood DHFR inhibitor in cancer management. Methotrexate is also a weak inhibitor of other folate-dependent enzymes, such as GARFT, AICAR, and TS. Accumulation of dihydrofolate polyglutamates as a consequence of DHFR inhibition can also directly inhibit folate-dependent enzymes *(12)*. Improved knowledge of the biochemistry and cellular pharmacology of methotrexate has led to the rational design of several new antifolate compounds with different pharmacological properties, including trimetrexate and edatrexate. In addition, modification of the primary structure of these antifolates has resulted in a number of GARFT inhibitors including lometrexol and AG2034 (*see* Chapter 13).

3.1. Methotrexate

The early discovery that leucovorin can be administered to leukemic cells in vitro several hours after treatment with methotrexate without preventing leukemic cell death represents one of the earliest discoveries that led to rational clinical use of combination therapy based on laboratory findings *(13)*. In clinical practice today, methotrexate with leucovorin rescue is seldom used, except when high doses of methotrexate are given, and even then the improvement in therapeutic index is questionable (reviewed in ref. *11*). Even so, the improved understanding of folate pharmacology, especially in relation to fluoropyrimidines, (*see* Chapter 3) has led to the development of a number of rationally designed, interesting, and clinically useful methotrexate combinations.

3.1.1. Methotrexate and 5FU

The combination of MTX and 5FU is predicated upon the observation that MTX-induced inhibition of *de novo* purine synthesis results in an increased concentration of phosphoribosyl pyrophosphate (PRPP). Enhanced anabolism of 5FU as a consequence of increased PRPP can result in increased incorporation of 5FU metabolites into RNA *(14,15)*. Sequential administration of MTX followed by 5FU is required, with a certain time lag to achieve significant accumulation of PRPP. The optimal time interval between drug treatment is 1–2 h in vitro, 4–12 h in mice, and theoretically approx 24 h in humans *(16,* reviewed in ref. *17)*. This time interval potentially allows rebound in tetrahydrofolate levels following recovery from DHFR inhibition, which may potentiate 5FU-induced TS inhibition. Clearly, simultaneous administration or otherwise inappropriate scheduling may be antagonistic.

In tumor-model systems the time interval between MTX and 5FU is critical for the best interaction of the two drugs *(16,18)*. In vitro studies with varying drug treatment intervals (3–22 h) and in various cell lines (leukemia, colon, and breast) have generally shown synergism or additivity, but in some studies antagonism has been demonstrated, particularly when prolonged 5FU exposure has been utilized (reviewed in ref. *19*). These studies of this combination have at best shown that appropriate scheduling gives greater cytotoxicity than either drug alone, but do not use any modeling to show synergism as defined above. Recent data by van der Wilt et al. in mice bearing colon cancers support the contention that the effectiveness of this combination is highly dependent on the time interval used *(20)*. A 17-h gap between MTX and 5FU gave a better therapeutic index than a 4-h gap. Moreover, LV did not enhance MTX/5FU and the addition of LV sometimes produced antagonism.

Phase II studies in colorectal cancer also suggest that the time interval in the sequence of MTX and 5FU is critical. Many early clinical trials of sequential MTX and 5FU used the wrong schedule and did not show greater benefit for the combination (reviewed in refs. *17,19,21*). Marsh et al. *(22)* compared a 1-h interval with a 24-h interval in this disease and showed a significantly better response rate (14 vs 29%) for the 24-h interval, with significantly better survival. Five randomized studies using a 12–24-h interval between MTX and 5FU in colorectal cancer have been performed (reviewed in refs. *19,21*). All involved small numbers of patients and three studies showed better response rate for MTX/5FU compared to 5FU alone or 5FU and leucovorin. Only one study comparing 5FU alone with MTX/5FU/LV demonstrated a survival benefit for the combination *(23)*. A meta-analysis of eight randomized trials comparing 5FU alone with MTX followed by 5FU (<4 to 24 h later) with or without leucovorin concluded that MTX/5FU was better than 5FU alone *(24)*.

Other studies have not generally supported the further exploration of this combination. A randomized study of sequential MTX and 5FU compared to simultaneous MTX-5FU in head and neck cancer showed greater toxicity but no difference in response between the two arms *(25)*. The time interval between MTX and 5FU in this study was 18 h, and leucovorin was given 24 h after MTX in each arm. In colorectal cancer, continuous infusion 5FU plus MTX was ineffective *(26)*, and sequential MTX and 5FU had marginal activity as second-line treatment *(27)*. The Nordic group compared MTX/5FU/LV with a 3 h and a 24 h interval to 5FU/LV and showed equivalence *(28)*.

In summary, although the sequential combination of MTX and 5FU has some pharmacological logic and is effective in vitro, its clinical application is not favored. Early studies used the wrong schedule and although more recent studies using the correct schedule have shown some benefit over single agent 5FU or 5FU plus leucovorin, there is a perception that 5FU modulation with LV has equivalent or better activity and greater convenience.

3.1.2. MTX plus Cisplatin

MTX and cisplatin are both highly active in a number of malignancies so their combination is empirically attractive. However, no plausible mechanism of interaction that may result in synergistic cytotoxicity is obvious. In vitro studies in the 1970s showed simple additive effects in a colon-cancer cell line *(29)*. An in vivo preclinical study suggested a better therapeutic index for this combination *(30)*. Whereas MTX plus cisplatin continues to be used in some malignancies (head and neck cancer and bladder cancer) a clear demonstration of improved efficacy has not been undertaken. Furthermore, since both drugs are potentially nephrotoxic and are excreted renally, there is concern about the toxicity of the combination.

3.2. Trimetrexate

Trimetrexate (TMQ), a quinazoline-based antifolate, is a more potent inhibitor of DHFR than MTX *(31)*. TMQ does not require active transport to enter cells and is not polyglutamated. As such, more prolonged exposures are required to produce antiproliferative activity *(32)*. Preclinical studies have shown broad activity against a variety of tumor cell lines, including those resistant to MTX on the basis of decreased active transport or decreased polyglutamation *(32,* reviewed in ref. *33)*. Clinical studies, mainly using iv bolus schedules, have demonstrated activity of TMQ in a variety of tumors, including head and neck, upper gastrointestinal, lung, and urothelial tumors.

Combinations of TMQ with other anticancer agents have been considered. In vitro studies of TMQ plus 5FU with LV using median effect analysis, have shown synergism of the two agents at one dose ratio, and have shown greater activity than MTX plus 5FU and LV *(34)*. The mechanism may be avoidance of competition between the reduced folate and its analog for cellular uptake. In a clinical study, a response rate of 20% in previously treated patients with GI cancer was achieved *(35)*. A more recent study of this combination, again with a 24-h interval between TMQ and 5FU showed a 50% response rate in advanced colorectal cancer but with considerable gastrointestinal toxicity *(36)*. A preliminary report of a similar study reported a 39% response rate *(37)*. These favorable results have led to two randomized trials comparing TMQ/5FU/LV to 5FU/LV alone, both of which are ongoing.

Other combinations with TMQ empirically tested in the clinic include cisplatin *(38,39)*, etoposide *(39)*, and cyclophosphamide *(40)*. It is not clear that these combinations are any improvement on the single agents involved.

3.3. Edatrexate (10-EDAM)

10-Ethyl-10-deaza-aminopterin (edatrexate, EDX, 10-EDAM) is structurally identical to MTX except for an ethylated C-10 instead of a methylated N-10 group. It is transported and polyglutamated more efficiently than MTX *(41)*, but appears to be more selectively accumulated in tumor cells than normal cells, which may account for its comparatively better therapeutic index in animal models (*see* Chapter 3). 10-EDAM polyglutamates are more potent DHFR inhibitors than MTX polyglutamates but have less activity against TS.

In in vitro studies combining 10-EDAM and cisplatin using median-effect analysis, synergism was observed at effect levels corresponding to greater than 60% inhibition of cell growth, but not at lower doses *(42)*. A similar study in A549 lung cancer cells using median-effect analysis suggested synergism only with the schedule of 10-EDAM followed by cisplatin *(43)*. Studies in murine mammary tumor model suggested greater therapeutic index using 10-EDAM with either cisplatin, cyclophosphamide melphalan, or 5FU than with any drug alone *(44)*. In this study a 7-h interval between 10-EDAM and 5FU was better than simultaneous treatment, similar to findings with MTX and TMQ. Similar results were seen in an intraperitoneal L1210 leukemia model, but not in an iv fibrosarcoma model. A later study of intraperitoneal 10-EDAM and cisplatin in a murine ovarian cancer showed a >160% increased life span compared to a 20% increased life span for cisplatin alone and 62% for 10-EDAM alone *(45)*. Early clinical studies of 10-EDAM with cisplatin or carboplatin are underway but as yet there is no evidence of clinical benefit.

Recent studies suggest possible benefit of combination of 10-EDAM with taxanes. In vitro studies in breast cancer cells using median-effect analysis show variable effects—synergism or antagonism *(46)*. Synergism was dependent on dose and schedule, occurring with 10-EDAM followed by taxane. This combination is currently the subject of clinical study.

Vinca alkaloids may possibly be effective in combination with 10-EDAM as suggested by a study in murine solid tumors, but clinical results are not yet available *(47)*.

4. THYMIDYLATE SYNTHASE INHIBITORS

Thymidylate synthase is a pivotal enzyme in DNA synthesis pathways, and converts dUMP by methylation to dTMP. This process is the only *de novo* source of dTMP, which is subsequently metabolized to dTTP, exclusively for incorporation into DNA during synthesis and repair. In general, tumor cells have a reduced ability to salvage pyrimidine nucleotides from extracellular fluid, so they are more sensitive than normal cells to the effects of TS inhibition. Therefore TS is an ideal target for anticancer therapy. The enzyme has two binding sites, for the substrate dUMP and for the methyl donor N^5,N^{10}-methylene tetrahydrofolate (CH_2-THF). These two binding sites are the targets for TS inhibition. Fluoropyrimidines (5-fluorouracil and 5'-deoxy-5-fluorouridine, FUdR) are the classical drugs that target the dUMP binding site. In the last decade, a number of groups have rationally developed several folate analog and other compounds that inhibit TS by binding to the folate pocket of the enzyme. The challenge for the future is to design effective combinations using these agents. With the expanding knowledge of their pharmacology and interactions, it should be possible to identify effective combinations in preclinical experiments.

4.1. Fluorouracil

5FU is the classical fluoropyrimidine which for decades has been the mainstay of the treatment of various types of cancer, including gastrointestinal, breast, and head and neck cancers. 5FU has remained pre-eminent despite its limited clinical activity as a single agent in most diseases (e.g., advanced colorectal cancer with objective response rates of <20%). Various modulators of 5FU cytotoxicity have been conceived and developed, which will retain the importance of this agent in cancer treatment.

One aim of modulating agents is to enhance inhibition of TS by the 5FU metabolite FdUMP. A variety of noncytotoxic agents have been developed which achieve this, including LV and α-interferon. In clinical studies the combination of 5FU with folate precursor LV has resulted in objective response rates of up to 40% *(48)*. The role of LV in conjunction with bolus 5FU treatment is now well established. Another approach to modulation of 5FU has been the development of specific inhibitors of DPD (dihydropyrimidine dehydrogenase), that are analogs of uracil including bromovinyldeoxyuridine (BVDU) *(49)*, 5-ethynyluracil (EU) *(50)*, and CDHP *(51)*. These agents are able to increase the bioavailability of 5FU (up to 100%) by inhibiting its catabolism resulting in a simulation of continuous infusion.

5FU is such an old drug that it has been empirically combined with many other cytotoxic agents over the years, with the understanding that anticancer activity may be additive but normal tissue toxicity is nonoverlapping. More recently, in vitro and in vivo preclinical studies have been undertaken in order to develop a rational basis for the clinical use of 5FU with various other cytotoxic drugs.

4.1.1. Cisplatin

Cisplatin and 5FU was an empirically developed clinical regimen which showed response rates far exceeding either single agent alone in metastatic head and neck cancers and in some other tumors *(52)*. Whether its clinical efficacy is a result of true synergism or just additivity is unclear, but subsequent preclinical studies have suggested a biochemical interaction may exist. Scanlon et al. showed increased TS expression in cisplatin-resistant cells, suggesting a link between TS and the action of cisplatin *(53)*. Johnston et al. *(54)* explored this combination in a human colon cancer cell line, and using median-effect analysis showed that a 24-h treatment with 5FU prior to cisplatin resulted in greater than additive cytotoxicity. Biochemical studies indicated a greater degree of DNA damage with the combination. Studies in mice have confirmed that the sequence of 5FU followed by cisplatin gives the best therapeutic index compared to simultaneous administration or the reverse sequence *(55,56)*. Another study by Shirasaka et al. *(57)* suggested that cisplatin inhibited intracellular L-methionine metabolism resulting in an increased pool of reduced folates in mammalian tumor models. Thus, the combination of 5FU and cisplatin is effective with a plausible metabolic basis. The sequence dependence seen in preclinical studies has not been obvious in the clinic; mostly cisplatin is given before 5FU for logistic reasons.

4.1.2. PALA (N-(phosphonacetyl)-L-aspartate)

PALA is an inhibitor of *de novo* pyrimidine synthesis which causes decreased intracellular pools of CTP, UTP, dCTP, and dTTP *(58)*. As a single agent PALA has no significant antitumor activity, probably because of the very high activity of the target enzyme (aspartate transcarbamylase) in tumor tissues compared to normal tissues. Preclinical studies indicate that PALA can modulate the cytotoxicity of 5FU, resulting in significantly increased anticancer response *(59)*. The potential mechanisms by which PALA may interact with 5FU are multiple, leading to a complicated interaction: PALA may cause depletion of orotic acid, an increase in PRPP, and depletion of uracil nucleotides (reviewed in ref. *58*). All of these mechanisms favor increased action of 5FU via either increased incorporation of FUTP into RNA or increased inhibition of TS. Such biochemical changes have been shown to occur in preclinical animal and human tumor model systems (reviewed in ref. *58*), supporting the clinical exploration of this combination. In mice bearing colon carcinoma 26B or leukemia L1210, van Laar et al. showed that pretreatment with PALA enhanced the antitumor activity of both 5FU and 5-fluoro-2'-deoxyuridine (FUdR) which was associated with reduced pools of CTP and UTP *(60)*.

Initial clinical phase II studies with the PALA/5FU combination demonstrated no significant benefit. These studies used high doses of PALA, often without a time interval before 5FU (reviewed in ref. *58*). However, subsequent studies based on the preclinical data of Martin et al. *(59)* have used low doses of PALA prior to an MTD dose of 5FU and shown high response rates. O'Dwyer et al. used 250 mg/m^2 PALA 24 h prior to a 24-h infusion of 5FU in patients with advanced colorectal cancer and produced a 43% response rate (95% CI 27–60%) in 37 patients *(61)*. Kemeny et al. gave PALA 250 mg/m^2 24 h before a bolus dose of 5FU to 42 patients with colorectal cancer, resulting in a 38% response rate (95% CI 23–53%) *(62)*. More recently, a report of the combination of PALA plus MTX 24 h before bolus 5FU in 26 patients with colorectal cancer gave a 23% response rate *(63)*. Whether or not these outcomes are significantly better than 5FU alone or 5FU/LV is unclear.

4.1.3. Taxanes

In view of their low toxicity, taxanes offer the promise of a greater therapeutic index when combined with many other agents including 5FU. Using isobologram analysis, Kano et al. showed schedule dependence of the interaction between paclitaxel and 5FU in four human carcinoma cell lines *(64)*. Simultaneous exposure showed subadditive effects in three of four cell lines. Sequential exposure to paclitaxel followed by 5FU was additive and the reverse sequence was antagonistic. In another study using median-effect analysis in breast-cancer cells, the sequence of paclitaxel followed by 5FU was confirmed as being optimal, but only proved more than additive when relatively high doses were used *(65)*. The basis for any interaction is not clear; in vitro neither drug appears to interfere with the cellular metabolic effects of the other *(65)*.

In phase II studies of paclitaxel, 5FU and LV in women with metastatic breast cancer the combination is active with overall response rates of 54–62% *(66,67)*. Whether this represents a real improvement over single agent therapy is not yet clear. Further clinical studies of this combination are awaited.

4.1.4. Other Agents

AZT (azidothymidine) is a thymidine analog that leads to incorporation of AZTTP into DNA blocking chain elongation during DNA synthesis. Incorporation can be increased when AZT is combined with TS inhibitors such as 5FU or MTX, resulting in increased DNA strand breaks and cytotoxicity *(68,69)*. Recently, in a panel of colon-carcinoma cell lines and using both the methods of Steele and Peckham and median-effect analysis, Andreuccetti and colleagues have shown strong evidence of synergism between these two agents when applied simultaneously for 72 h *(70)*. DNA damage was enhanced in the combination. Results of clinical studies are awaited.

Topoisomerase I inhibitors are a novel class of drugs with a unique mechanism of action, and are currently undergoing clinical evaluation in a variety of malignancies. Combinations are also being studied, mostly in an empirical fashion, without any hypotheses regarding biochemical interaction. In vitro studies in five different cell lines using various combinations of topotecan with other agents including 5FU and MTX, and using median-effect analysis, have shown mainly antagonism with antimetabolites, but the authors concluded that results can depend on the cell line examined *(71)*. Another study using an isobologram approach in two lung-cancer cell lines showed subadditive effects for the combination of SN38 and 5FU *(72)*. Others have shown sequence dependence *(73)* and lack of biochemical interaction *(74)* for the CPT-11/5FU combination, suggesting that if clinical development is to proceed there will not be a supporting biochemical rationale.

4.2. Tomudex

Tomudex is a folate-based TS inhibitor, which enters the cell via the reduced folate carrier, and can be converted to the pentaglutamate by folylpolyglutamate synthase, which is 100-fold stronger inhibitor of TS than the monoglutamate. Tomudex and its polyglutamates do not inhibit DHFR, GARFT, or AICARFT to any significant extent *(75)*. The effect of tomudex is therefore a pure and prolonged inhibition of TS allowing intermittent bolus treatment.

Tomudex has undergone phase II study in a number of malignancies including colon and breast cancer where it has modest activity (reviewed in ref. *21*). Phase III studies in colorectal cancer demonstrate activity similar to 5FU/LV *(76)*.

4.2.1. Cisplatin

Recently tomudex combinations have been studied in preclinical models by us and others. There are several potential points of interaction of cisplatin with folate-based TS inhibitors. Cisplatin has been shown to increase intracellular folates, possibly via reduced methionine *(53,57)*. Collateral sensitivity of cisplatin-resistant cell lines to fluoropyrimidines has been shown *(77,78)*. Cisplatin and fluoropyrimidines are synergistic in cell lines in vitro *(53)*, possibly as a consequence of increased DNA fragmentation *(54)*. Therefore we reasoned that tomudex and cisplatin might be synergistic. Kelland et al. *(79)* tested tomudex plus three platinum drugs in five pairs of cell lines, each consisting of a cisplatin-sensitive parent and a resistant subline. Median-effect analysis was used to assess cytotoxic interaction, and experiments were done multiple times so that a standard deviation could be given with the combination index at the IC_{50}. Additive effects were noted in all cell lines, with combination indices ranging from 1.35 ± 0.44 to 0.92 ± 0.13 in one pair of cell lines. Cross-resistance was not evident in these cells; nor did the cisplatin-resistant sublines have elevated TS activity. In our laboratory similar studies in ovarian cell lines using tomudex and cisplatin in a variety of schedules (simultaneous, tomudex before cisplatin, cisplatin before tomudex) have also shown additivity when assessed by median-effect analysis *(80)*. Examples are shown in Table 1 and

Table 1
Median-Effect Parameters for Four Experiments Combining Tomudex with Cisplatin

		Expt 1	Expt 2	Expt 3	Expt 4
Tomudex	Multiple r	0.94	0.97	0.99	0.99
	Intercept:	27.49	21.67	40.20	32.76
	Slope (m):	1.61	1.19	2.20	1.83
	Dm (μM):	0.038	0.013	0.012	0.017
	$n=$	8	7	5	6
Cisplatin	Multiple r	0.95	0.98	0.99	0.99
	Intercept:	19.14	22.45	18.08	16.59
	Slope (m):	1.42	1.51	1.23	1.13
	Dm (μM):	1.349	0.334	0.389	0.434
	$n=$	5	7	6	5
1:1 Combination	Multiple r	0.91	0.92	0.98	0.99
	Intercept:	17.98	24.73	34.88	37.91
	Slope (m):	1.07	1.42	1.95	2.19
	Dm (μM):	0.054	0.029	0.016	0.030
	$n=$	6	5	5	4

Method: A2780 human ovarian carcinoma cells were maintained in exponential growth as a monolayer in 25 cm^2 tissue-culture flasks in Dulbecco's minimal essential medium supplemented with 5% fetal calf serum, 1 mM L-glutamine in 5% CO_2 in air at 37°C. Cells were aliquotted into 96-well plates (3000 cells/well) and allowed to reach exponential phase growth (24–36 h) before drug addition. Tomudex, cisplatin or a 1:1 molar ratio were added to wells in triplicate in a non-random distribution across 96-well plates. For each experiment up to 8 dose-effect data points were used for each drug alone and the 1:1 combination. After 72-h incubation, wells were fixed and cell growth analyzed by the sulfrhodamine B assay. Surviving fraction (SF, or fraction unaffected) is calculated as the mean growth in drug treated wells ($n = 3$) compared to control wells. Median effect analysis is done on the raw data (SF vs dose) according to ref. 7.

Multiple r, correlation coefficient of log SF vs log dose; Dm, median or IC_{50} dose; n, number of experimental data points in linear regression analysis of log SF vs log dose.

Fig. 2, where the combination was applied in a 1:1 molar ratio simultaneously for 72 h to A2780 human ovarian carcinoma cells in vitro. Table 1 shows the median effect parameters estimated for each drug alone and the combination in each of four experiments. As can be seen in Fig. 2, the mean combination index for most fractions affected lies just

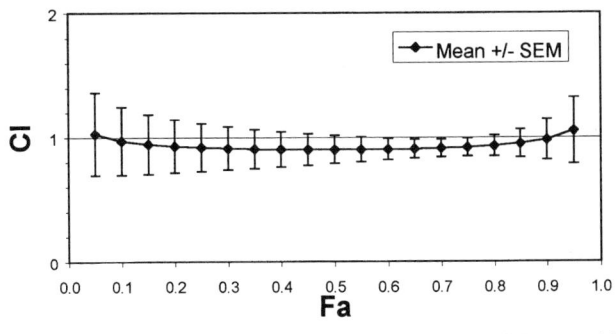

Fig. 2 Combination index v fraction affected plot showing mean $+/-$ SEM combination indices for a range of fractions affected in the four experiments of 1:1 ratio of tomudex and cisplatin.

below 1 (the line of additivity) and the standard error includes the line of additivity in each case. Thus this combination is clearly additive in its cytotoxic effects. Similar results were obtained in ADDP cells, a 40-fold cisplatin resistant subline of A2780, with one-seventh the TS activity of A2780. Furthermore, studies to elucidate any potential biochemical interaction have proved negative. Tomudex does not increase platination of DNA, DNA damage as assessed by a DNA unwinding assay is unaltered, and no effect of TS catalytic activity (A2780:ADDP = 12:1) was seen (data not published). We conclude that tomudex and cisplatin have additive effects.

No clinical studies of tomudex and cisplatin have yet been undertaken.

4.2.2. Fluorouracil

In a panel of six human colon-cancer cell lines, we studied the cytotoxic interaction of tomudex and 5FU using median-effect analysis *(81)*. In four cell lines the combination gave additive effects with continuous exposure to both drugs. Variable effects (antagonism or additivity, but not synergism) were seen with different sequences of the two drugs. These results suggest that this combination may have unpredictable effects in the clinic, and that a synergistic effect cannot be expected. Concomitant use of LV will tend to negate any cytotoxic effect of tomudex *(82)*.

A preliminary report of a phase I study of tomudex followed by 5FU suggests that the combination is tolerable, perhaps with less-than-additive toxicity *(83)*.

4.2.3. Topoisomerase I Inhibitors

We have studied the combination of tomudex with SN38, the active metabolite of CPT-11 (irinotecan) to ascertain the combined cytotoxic effects of these two agents *(84)*. These studies were undertaken in a panel of tumor cell lines with varying mechanisms of resistance to antifolates. Various durations and sequences of exposure to the two drugs were used and the results were analyzed using the median-effect method. Combinations of tomudex and SN38 at equitoxic doses (a fixed 1:1 ratio of their IC_{50}s under the relevant exposure conditions) showed antagonism, with combination indices of 1.2–1.5 at the IC_{50}, when exposure was concurrent for 5 d, and additivity when exposure was for 24 h. All other exposures at various relative doses and schedules proved either antagonistic or additive. However, synergistic effects were seen in all five colon cancer cell lines when 4 h exposure to SN38 was followed by 4 h exposure to tomudex (combination indices of 0.7–0.8 ± 0.1); the reverse sequence was antagonistic (combination indices of 1.0–1.3 ± 0.2). These findings were confirmed by isobologram analysis. Thus, the effects of tomudex plus SN38 are largely antagonistic, but variable and dependent on the cell line and schedule used. If these studies are applied in the clinic CPT-11 should be given before tomudex. Such a study in ongoing at the Royal Marsden Hospital.

Another study, reported in abstract form, used human HCT-8 colon cancer cells and the median-effect method *(85)*. The above findings were generally confirmed, although the rigour with which the median-effect method was applied is uncertain. In addition to schedule-dependence these investigators also suggested dose ratio dependence. Thus, this combination may be very tricky to use in the clinic.

4.2.4. Tomudex with Other Antifolates

Faessel et al. studied combinations of tomudex with TMQ, and AG2034 (a GARFT inhibitor) with TMQ in human HCT-8 cells *(86)*. They reasoned that super synergy may exist between nonpolyglutamatable DHFR inhibitors and polyglutamatable inhibitors of other folate-requiring enzymes. This concept of super synergy, wherein inhibition of more than one critical enzyme in a pathway may result in extraordinarily high degrees of synergism was first proposed by Gaumont et al. *(87)*. Using the response-surface approach *(3,9,10)* synergy was evident with both combinations and was enhanced by increasing the intracellular folate pools. Marked differences were observed between the FPGS-proficient parent and an FPGS-deficient subline, particularly in regard to the folic acid enhancement of synergy for the TMQ + tomudex combination. This study underscores the complex interactions in purine and pyrimidine synthetic pathways, and suggests that clinical application of multiple antifolates may be very unpredictable until further laboratory studies are undertaken.

4.2. Other Folate-Based TS Inhibitors

LY231514 is a multifunctional antifolate that inhibits mainly TS but also DHFR and GARFT (*see* Chapter 8). It has activity in a variety of tumor cell models (eg., lymphomas, lung, colon cancer) and is currently in the early phases of clinical development. Peters et al. studied gemcitabine and LY231514 combinations in lung-cancer cell lines using the median-effect method *(88)*. With a 4-h exposure marked synergism was seen. We have undertaken similar studies in ovarian cancer cell lines, using a 24-h simultaneous exposure and also shown marked synergism (Ackland et al., unpublished). A potential mechanism for synergistic interaction is bimodal TS inhibition, since one metabolite of gemcitabine is dFdUMP, which is an inhibitor of TS. Further studies are currently under way.

AG337 is a nonclassical TS inhibitor, which does not require carrier-mediated transport systems and is not polyglutamated (*see* Chapter 10). Raymond et al. studied the interaction of AG337 and cisplatin (simultaneous 48-h exposure and 1:1 molar concentration ratio) in HT29 human colon cancer cells and in 2008 ovarian cancer cells, and sublines made resistant to 5FU and cisplatin *(89)*. Using the median-effect method there was variable synergy, additivity, and antagonism according to the cell line and dose of drugs applied. However, at around the IC_{50} for the combination synergism was evident in three of the four cell lines. This combination warrants further exploration.

AG331 is similar to AG337. Pressacco et al. have added a "noncytotoxic" range of doses of AZT to a human bladder carcinoma cell line in conjunction with a fixed cytotoxic dose of AG331 *(90)*. The data clearly show an enhanced antitumor effect, but it is not possible to conclude from the data whether there is any interaction occurring between the two drugs; the data are consistent with either additive or synergistic effect. However, increased incorporation of AZTTP into DNA is shown, suggesting a mechanistic interaction. These findings are similar to those in a previous study by the same group using the combination of tomudex and AZT *(91)*.

5. CONCLUSIONS

There is now a wide range of new antifolate antimetabolites available for preclinical and clinical study. As a consequence there is a vast number of possible combinations of these agents with each other, with other antimetabolites, and with cytotoxic drugs with apparently unrelated mechanisms of action. Some of these combinations have been studied in vitro and/or in the clinic. In some cases a mechanistic hypothesis of interaction between the two or more agents has been developed, but in many cases the combination is empirical.

The correct method by which to study and analyze multiple drug effects in vitro is controversial; each method has its limitations and pitfalls. The median effect method is currently used most frequently in cancer research. Most in vitro studies of combined drug effects show variable interaction, which is cell-line dependent, schedule dependent, and often dependent on the relative concentrations of the agents employed and the dose. The most promising combinations for further study and clinical use are TMQ plus 5FU, SN38 plus tomudex, TMQ plus tomudex, and TMQ plus AG2034.

In spite of any optimism for a particular combination as a result of a preclinical study, it is difficult to extrapolate to the clinic. The human host with its cancer is a completely different environment to a tissue-culture dish containing monolayer cells in medium; the pharmacokinetics and distribution of the drugs need to be considered, as well as the heterogeneous biology of a solid tumour *in situ*. In addition the aim of combination therapy is to widen the therapeutic index between the tumor and normal tissues. Synergism in vitro is of no value if it occurs to an equal or greater extent in normal bone marrow or gut epithelial cells as in the tumor in the patient. In spite of their limitations, in vitro studies, including those discussed in this chapter do provide important insights to guide clinical application. Combinations that show antagonism in a range of tumor cell lines are unlikely to be effective. If synergism is dependent on the concentration ratio or exposure time, simulation of the laboratory situation in the patient may be possible to achieve. This latter situation is the case in MTX/5FU combinations, where the laboratory studies have shown that the time interval and duration of exposure is critical, and subsequent clinical studies taking these findings into account have proved beneficial. Laboratory studies of combinations also allow further unravelling of the complex interaction of the various components of the biosynthetic pathways involved in cell growth. Ultimately further scientific discoveries should point the way to optimal scheduling of a variety of antimetabolites with each other and with other DNA-interactive anticancer drugs to maximize tumor cell kill.

REFERENCES

1. Holford NHG, Scheiner LB. Understanding the dose-effect relationship: clinical applications of pharmacokinetic-pharmacodynamic models. *Clin Pharmacokinet* 1981; 6:429–453.
2. Berenbaum MC. What is synergy? *Pharmacol Rev* 1989; 41:93–141.
3. Greco WR, Bravo G, Parsons JC. The search for synergy: a critical review from a response surface perspective. *Pharmacol Rev* 1995; 47(2):331–385.
4. Webb JL. Effect of more than one inhibitor. In: Enzymes and Metabolic Inhibitors. Academic, New York, 1963, pp. 66–79, 486–512.
5. Berenbaum MC. Synergy, additivism and antagonism in immunosuppression. *Clin Exp Immunol* 1977; 28:1–18.
6. Berenbaum MC. Criteria for analyzing interactions between biologically active agents. *Adv Cancer Res* 1981; 35:269–335.
7. Steele GG, Peckham MJ. Exploitable mechanisms in combined radiotherapy-chemotherapy: the concept of additivity. *Int J Radiat Oncol Biol Phys* 1979; 5:85–91.
8. Chou TC, Talalay P. Quantitative analysis of dose-effect relationships: the combined effects of multiple drugs or enzyme inhibitors. *Adv Enzyme Reg* 1984; 22:27–55.
9. Greco WR, Park HS, Rustum YM. An application of a new approach for the quantitation of drug synergism to the combination of cis-diamminedichloroplatinum and 1-β-D-arabinafuranosylcytosine. *Cancer Res* 1990; 50:5318–5327.

10. Greco WR, Rustum YM. Reply to correspondence from Berenbaum MC, Suhnel J. re: Application of a new approach for the quantitation of drug synergism to the combination of *cis*-diamminedichloroplatinum and 1-β-arabinofuranosylcytosine. *Cancer Res* 1992; 52(August 15):4561–4565.
11. Ackland SP, Schilsky RL. High-dose methotrexate: a critical reappraisal. *J Clin Oncol* 1987; 5:2017–2031.
12. Allegra CJ, Fine RL, Drake JC, Chabner BA. The effect of methotrexate on intracellular folate pools in human MCF-7 breast cancer cells: evidence for direct inhibition of purine synthesis. *J Biol Chem* 1986; 261:6478–6485.
13. Goldin A, Venditti JM, Kline L, et al. Eradication of leukemic cells (L1210) by methotrexate and methotrexate plus citrovorum factor. *Nature* 1966; 212:1548–1550.
14. Pinedo HM, Peters GJ. 5-Fluorouracil: biochemistry and pharmacology. *J Clin Oncol* 1988; 6:1653–1664.
15. Cadman E, Heimer R, Benz C. The influence of methotrexate pretreatment on 5-fluorouracil metabolism on L1210 cells. *J Biol Chem* 1981; 256:1695–1704.
16. Bertino JR, Sawicki WL, Lindquist CA, et al. Schedule-dependent antitumor effects of methotrexate and 5-fluorouracil. *Cancer Res* 1977; 37:327–328.
17. Leyland-Jones B, O'Dwyer P. Biochemical modulation: application of laboratory models to the clinic. *Cancer Treat Rep* 1986; 70:219–229.
18. Benz C, Schoenberg M, Choti M, Cadman E. Schedule-dependent cytotoxicity of methotrexate and 5-fluorouracil in human colon and breast tumor cell lines. *J Clin Invest* 1980; 66:1162–1165.
19. Sobrero AF, Aschele C, Bertino JR. Fluorouracil in colorectal cancer—a tale of two drugs: implications for biochemical modulation. *J Clin Oncol* 1997; 15:368–381.
20. van der Wilt CL, Braakhuis BJM, Pinedo HM, et al. Addition of leucovorin in modulation of 5-fluorouracil with methotrexate: potentiating or reversing effect? *Int J Cancer* 1995; 61:672–678.
21. Kohne-Wompner C-H, Schmoll H-J, Harstrick A, Rustum YM. Chemotherapeutic strategies in metastatic colorectal cancer: an overview of current clinical trials. *Semin Oncol* 1992; 19(suppl 3):105–125.
22. Marsh JC, Bertino JR, Katz KH, Davis CA, Durivage HJ, Rome LS, et al. The influence of drug interval on the effect of methotrexate and fluorouracil in the treatment of advanced colorectal cancer. *J Clin Oncol* 1991; 9:371–380.
23. The Nordic Gastrointestinal Tumor Adjuvant Therapy Group. Superiority of sequential methotrexate, fluorouracil and leucovorin to fluorouracil alone in advanced symptomatic colorectal carcinoma: a randomized trial. *J Clin Oncol* 1989; 7:1437–1446.
24. The Advanced Colorectal Cancer Meta-Analysis Group. Meta-analysis of randomized trials testing biochemical modulation of fluorouracil by methotrexate in metastatic colorectal cancer. *J Clin Oncol* 1994; 12:960–969.
25. Browman GP, Levine MN, Goodyear MD, Russell R, Archibald SD, Jackson BS, et al. Methotrexate/fluorouracil scheduling influences normal tissue toxicity but not antitumor effects in patients with squamous cell head and neck cancer: results from a randomised trial. *J Clin Oncol* 1988; 6:963–968.
26. Lokich JJ, Phillips D, Green R, Paul S, Sonnerborn H, Zipoli TE, Curt G. 5-Fluorouracil and methotrexate administered simultaneously as a continuous infusion, a phase I study. *Cancer* 1985; 56:2395–2398.
27. Zaniboni A, LaBianca R, Martignoni G. Sequential methotrexate and 5-fluorouracil as second line chemotherapy for advanced colorectal cancer pretreated with 5-fluorouracil and leucovorin: a GISCAD study. *J Chemother* 1996; 8:82–85.
28. Grimelius B. Biochemical modulation of 5-fluorouracil: a randomized comparison of sequential methotrexate, 5-fluorouracil and leucovorin versus sequential 5-fluorouracil and leucovorin in patients with advanced symptomatic colorectal cancer. The Nordic Gastrointestinal Tumor Adjuvant Group. *Ann Oncol* 1993; 4:235–240.
29. Bergerat JP, Green C, Drewinko B. Combination chemotherapy in vitro IV. Response of human colon carcinoma cells to combinations using cis-diamminedichloroplatinum. *Cancer Biochem Biophys* 1979; 3(4):173–180.
30. Page RH, Talley RW, Buhagiar J. The enhanced antitumor activity of cis-diamminedichloroplatinum(II) against murine tumors when combined with other agents. *J Clin Hematol Oncol* 1977; 7:96.
31. Marshall JL, DeLap RJ. Clinical pharmacokinetics and pharmacology of trimetrexate. *Clin Pharm* 1994; 26:190–200.

32. Arkin H, Ohnuma T, Kamen BA, et al. Multidrug resistance in a human leukemic cell line selected for resistance to trimetrexate. *Cancer Res* 1989; 49:6556–6561.
33. Peters GJ, Ackland SP. New antimetabolites in preclinical and clinical development. *Exp Opin Invest Drugs* 1996; 5(6):637–679.
34. Romanini A, Li WW, Colofiore JR, et al. Leucovorin enhances cytotoxicity of trimetrexate/fluorouracil, but not methotrexate/fluorouracil in CCRF-CEM cells. *J Nat Cancer Inst* 1992; 84:1033–1038.
35. Conti JA, Kemeny N, Seiter K, et al. Trial of sequential trimetrexate, fluorouracil and high-dose leucovorin in previously treated patients with gastrointestinal carcinoma. *J Clin Oncol* 1994; 12:695–700.
36. Blanke CD, Kasimis B, Schein P, et al. Phase II study of trimetrexate, fluorouracil, and leucovorin for advanced colorectal cancer. *J Clin Oncol* 1997; 15:915–920.
37. Kreuser ED, Szelenyi H, Hohenberger P, et al. Trimetrexate, 5-fluorouracil, and folinic acid: an effective regimen in previously untreated patients with advanced colorectal carcinoma. *Proc Am Soc Clin Oncol* 1997; 16:294a.
38. Hudes GR, LaCreta F, Walczak J, et al. Pharmacokinetic study of trimetrexate in combination with cisplatin. *Cancer Res* 1991; 51:3080–3087.
39. Maroun JA, Natale RB, Robert F. Trimetrexate combined with cisplatin or etoposide in the treatment of non-small cell lung cancer: a pilot study. *Semin Oncol* 1988; 15:38–40.
40. Mattson K, Marsilta P, Tammilehto L, et al. Trimetrexate and cyclophosphamide for metastatic inoperable nonsmall cell lung cancer. *Semin Oncol* 1988; 15:32–37.
41. Westerhof GR, Schornagel JH, Kathmann I, Jackman AL, Rosowsky A, Hynes JB, Forsch RA, Peters GJ, Pinedo HM, Jansen G. Carrier- and receptor-mediated transport of folate antagonists targeting folate-dependent enzymes: correlates of molecular-structure and biological activity of inhibitors of dihydrofolate reductase, thymidylate synthase, glycinamide ribonucleotide transformylase and folylpolyglutamate synthetase. *Mol Pharmacol* 1995; 48:459–471.
42. Chou T-C, Tan Q-H, Sirotnak FM. Quantitation of the synergistic interaction of cisplatin and edatrexate in vitro. *Cancer Chemother Pharmacol* 1993; 31:259–264.
43. Perez EA, Hack FM, Webber LM, Chou C-T. Schedule-dependent synergism of edatrexate and cisplatin in combination in the A549 lung cancer cell line as assessed by median-effect analysis. *Cancer Chemother Pharmacol* 1993; 33:245–250.
44. Schmid FA, Sirotnak FM, Otter GM, DeGraw JI. Combination chemotherapy with a new folate analog: activity of 10-ethyl-10-deaza-aminopterin compared to methotrexate with 5fluorouracil and alkylating agents against advanced metastatic disease in murine tumor models. *Cancer Treat Rep* 1987; 71:727–7323.
45. Sirotnak FM, Schmid FA, DeGraw JI. Intracavitary therapy of murine ovarian cancer with cis-diamminedichloroplatinum(II) and 10-ethyl-10-deaza-aminopterin incorporating systemic leucovorin protection. *Cancer Res* 1989; 49:2890–2893.
46. Chou T-C, Otter GM, Sirotnak FM. Schedule-dependent synergism of taxol or taxotere with edatrexate against human breast cancer cells in vitro. *Cancer Chemother Pharmacol* 1996; 37:222–228.
47. Otter GM, Sirotnak FM. Effective combination therapy of metastatic murine solid tumors with edatrexate and the vinca alkaloids, vinblastine, navelbine and vindesine. *Cancer Chemother Pharmacol* 1994; 33:286–290.
48. Peters GJ, Van Groeningen CJ. Clinical relevance of biochemical modulation of 5-fluorouracil. *Ann Oncology* 1991; 2:469–480.
49. De Clerq E. Antiviral agents: characteristic activity spectrum depending on the molecular target with which they interact. *Adv Virus Res* 1993; 43:1–55.
50. Spector T, Porter DJT, Nelson DJ, et al. 5-Ethynyluracil (776C85), a modulator of the therapeutic activity of 5-fluorouracil. *Drugs Future* 1994; 19:565–571.
51. Shirasaka T, Fukushima M, Shimamoto Y, Kimura K. Preclinical studies on S-1, a new oral tegafur plus modulators: optimal molar ratio and antitumor activity. *Recent Adv Chemother* 1993; (Proc 18th Int Congr Chemotherapy):927.
52. Rooney M, Kish J, Jacobs J, et al. Improved complete response rate and survival on advanced head and neck cancer after three-course induction therapy with 120-hour 5-FU infusion and cisplatin. *Cancer* 1985; 55:1123.
53. Scanlon KJ, Newman EM, Lu Y, Priest DG. Biochemical basis for cisplatin and fluorouracil synergism in human ovarian carcinoma cells. *Proc Natl Acad Sci USA* 1986; 83:8923–8925.

54. Johnston PG, Geoffrey F, Drake J, Voeller D, Grem JL, Allegra CJ. The cellular interaction of 5-fluorouracil and cisplatin in a human colon carcinoma cell line. *Eur J Cancer* 1996; 32A(12):2148–2154.
55. Kuroki M, Nakano S, Mitsugi K, et al. In vivo comparative therapeutic study of optimal administration of 5-fluorouracil and cisplatin using a newly established HST-1 human squamous-carcinoma cell line. *Cancer Chemother Pharmacol* 1993; 29:273–276.
56. Pratesi G, Gianni L, Manzotti C, Zunino F. Sequence dependence of the antitumor and toxic effects of 5-fluorouracil and cis-diamminedichloroplatinum combination on primary colon tumors in mice. *Cancer Chemother Pharmacol* 1988; 21:237–240.
57. Shirasaka T, Shimamoto Y, Ohshimo H, et al. Metabolic basis of the synergistic antitumor activities of 5-fluorouracil and cisplatin in rodent tumor models in vivo. *Cancer Chemother Pharmacol* 1993; 32:167–172.
58. Grem JL, King SA, O'Dwyer PJ, Leyland-Jones B. Biochemistry and clinical activity of N-(phosphonacetyl)-L-aspartate: a review. *Cancer Res* 1988; 48:4441–4454.
59. Martin DS, Stolfi RL, Sawyer RC, et al. Therapeutic utility of utilizing low doses of N-(phosphonacetyl)-L-aspartate in combination with 5-fluorouracil: a murine study of clinical relevance. *Cancer Res* 1983; 43:2317–2321.
60. van Laar JAM, Durrani FA, Rustum YM. Antitumor activity of the weekly intravenous push schedule of 5-flouro-2'-deoxyuridine ± N-(phosphonacetyl)-L-aspartate in mice bearing advanced colon carcinoma 26. *Cancer Res* 1993; 53:1560–1564.
61. O'Dwyer PJ, Paul AR, Walczak J, et al. Phase II study of biochemical modulation of fluorouracil by low dose PALA in patients with colorectal cancer. *J Clin Oncol* 1990; 8:1497–1503.
62. Kemeny N, Conti JA, Seiter K, et al. Biochemical modulation of bolus fluorouracil by PALA in patients with advanced colorectal cancer. *J Clin Oncol* 1992; 10:747–752.
63. Kohne C-H, Harstrick A, Hiddemann W, et al. Modulation of 5-fluorouracil with methotrexate and low-dose N-(phosphonacetyl)-L-aspartate in patients with advanced colorectal cancer. Results of a phase II study. *Eur J Cancer* 1997; 33:1896–1899.
64. Kano Y, Akutsu M, Tsunoda S, et al. Schedule-dependent interaction between paclitaxel and 5-fluorouracil in human carcinoma cell lines in vitro. *Br J Cancer* 1996; 74:704–710.
65. Geoffroy F, Patel M, Ren Q-F, Grem J. Interaction of fluorouracil and paclitaxel in MCF-7 human breast carcinoma. *Proc Am Assoc Cancer Res* 1994; 35:330.
66. Johnson DH, Paul D, Hande KR. Paclitaxel, 5-fluorouracil and folinic acid in metastatic breast cancer: BRE-26, a phase II trial. *Semin Oncol* 1997; 24(suppl 3):22–25.
67. Klaassen U, Harstrick A, Wilke H, Seeber S. Paclitaxel combined with weekly high dose 5-fluorouracil/folinic acid and cisplatin in the treatment of metastatic breast cancer. *Semin Oncol* 1996; 23(suppl 11):32–37.
68. Tosi P, Calabresi P, Goulette FA, et al. Azidothymidine-induced cytotoxicity and incorporation into DNA in the human colon tumor cell line HCT-8 is enhanced by methotrexate in vitro and in vivo. *Cancer Res* 1992; 52:1797–1805.
69. Brunetti I, Falcone A, Calabresi P, et al. 5-Fluorouracil enhances azidothymidine cytotoxicity: in vitro, in vivo and biochemical studies. *Cancer Res* 1990; 50:4026–4031.
70. Andreuccetti M, Allegrini G, Antonuzzo A, et al. Azidothymidine in combination with 5-fluorouracil in human colorectal cell lines; in vitro synergistic cytotoxicity and DNA-induced strand-breaks. *Eur J Cancer* 1996; 32A:1219–1226.
71. Kaufmann SH, Peereboom D, Buckwalter CA, et al. Cytotoxic effects of topotecan combined with various anticancer agents in human cancer cell lines. *J Nat Cancer Inst* 1996; 88:734–741.
72. Pei XH, Nakanishi Y, Takayama K, et al. Effect of CPT-11 in combination with other anticancer agents in lung cancer cells. *Anti-Cancer Drugs* 1997; 8:231–237.
73. Grivicich I, Mans DRA, da Rocha AB, et al. The cytotoxicity of the irinotecan (CPT-11)-5-fluorouracil (5-FU) combination in human colon carcinoma cell lines is related to the sequence dependent introduction of DNA lesions. *Proc Am Assoc Cancer Res* 1997; 38:318.
74. Harstrick A, Vanhoefer U, Muller C, et al. Combination of CPT-11 and 5-FU in colorectal cancer: preclinical rationale and initial phase I results. *Proc Am Assoc Cancer Res* 1997; 38:318.
75. Jackman AL, Taylor GA, Gibson W, et al. ICI D1694, a quinazoline antifolate thymidylate synthase inhibitor that is a potent inhibitor of L1210 tumor cell growth *in vitro* and *in vivo*: a new agent for clinical study. *Cancer Res* 1991; 51:5579–5581.

76. Cunningham D, Zalcberg JR, Rath U, et al. Tomudex (ZD1694): results of a randomised trial in advanced colorectal cancer demonstrate efficacy and reduced mucositis and leucopoenia. *Eur J Cancer* 1995; 31A:1945–1954.
77. Ohe Y, Sugimoto Y, Saijo N. Collateral sensitivity of cisplatin-resistant human lung cancer cell lines to thymidylate synthase inhibitors. *Cancer J* 1990; 3:332–336.
78. Fram RJ, Woda BA, Wilson JM, Robichaud N. Characterization of acquired resistance to cis-di-amminedichloro platinum(II) in BE human colon carcinoma cells. *Cancer Res* 1990; 50:72–77.
79. Kelland LR, Kimbell R, Hardcastle A, et al. Relationships between resistance to cisplatin and antifolates in sensitive and resistant tumour cell lines. *Eur J Cancer* 1995; 31A:981–986.
80. Ackland SP, Kuiper CM, Garg M, et al. Variable effects of the combination of tomudex (ZD1694) and cisplatin in ovarian cancer cell lines. *Ann Oncol* 1996; 7(suppl 1):87.
81. Kimbell R, Brunton L, Jackman AL. Combination studies with tomudex and 5-fluorouracil in human colon tumour cell lines. *Br J Cancer* 1996; 73(suppl XXVI):29.
82. Rees C, Kimbell R, Valenti M, et al. Effects of leucovorin (LV) and folic acid (FA) on the cytotoxicity of the thymidylate synthase (TS) inhibitors, tomudex (ZD1694) and ZD9331. *Proc Am Assoc Cancer Res* 1997; 38:3184.
83. Schwartz GK, Kemeny N, Saltz L, et al. Phase I trial of sequential Tomudex® (TOM) and 5-fluorouracil (5-FU) in patients with advanced colorectal carcinoma. *Proc Am Soc Clin Oncol* 1997; 16:208a.
84. Kimbell R, Jackman AL. In vitro studies with ZD1694 (Tomudex) and SN38 in human colon tumour cell lines. In: (Pfleiderer and H Rokos, eds.) Proceedings of International Symposium on the Chemistry and Biology of Pteridines and Folates Blackwell Wissenschafts-Verlag, Berlin, 1997.
85. Aschele C, Baldo C, Guglielmi A, et al. Sequence dependent synergism between Tomudex and irinotecan in human colon cancer cells in vitro. *Ann Oncol* 1996; 7(suppl 1):88.
86. Faessel H, Lu K, Slocum HK, et al. Comparisons of the synergistic growth inhibition by trimetrexate (TMQ) + AG2034 and TMQ + tomudex (ZD1694) of human ileocecal HCT-8 cells and DW2, a subline deficient in folylpolyglutamate synthetase (FPGS). *Proc Am Assoc Cancer Res* 1997; 38:98.
87. Gaumont Y, Kisliuk RL, Parsons JC, Greco WR. Quantitation of folic acid enhancement of antifolate synergism. *Cancer Res* 1992; 52:2228–2235.
88. Peters GJ, Van Moorsel CJA, Veerman G, et al. Synergism of gemcitabine (GEM) with etoposide (VP), mitomycin C (MMC) and LY231514 (LY). *Proc Am Assoc Cancer Res* 1997; 38:319.
89. Raymond E, Djelloul S, Buquet-Fagot C, et al. Synergy between the non-classical thymidylate synthase inhibitor AG337 (Thymitaq) and cisplatin in human colon and ovarian cancer cells. *Anti-Cancer Drugs* 1996; 7:752–757.
90. Pressacco J, Mitrovski B, Ehrlichman C. Cytotoxic and biochemical consequences of combining AZT and AG331. *Cancer Chemother Pharmacol* 1995; 35:387–390.
91. Pressacco J, Ehrlichman C. Combination studies with 3'-azido-3'-deoxythymidine (AZT) plus ICI D1694: cytotoxic and biochemical effects. *Biochem Pharmacol* 1993; 46:1989.

18 Pharmacodynamic Measurements and Predictors of Response to Thymidylate Synthase Inhibitors

David Farrugia and Patrick G. Johnston

CONTENTS

    INTRODUCTION
    IMPORTANCE OF TS INHIBITION
    DETERMINANTS OF RESISTANCE TO TS INHIBITORS
    QUANTITATION OF TS IN HUMAN TUMORS
    CLINICAL RELEVANCE OF THYMIDYLATE SYNTHASE (TS) EXPRESSION
    TS INHIBITORS AND OTHER TARGETS: DIHYDROPYRIMIDINE DEHYDROGENASE
    PLASMA DEOXYURIDINE AS A PHARMACODYNAMIC MARKER OF TS INHIBITION
    FUTURE DIRECTIONS
    REFERENCES

1. INTRODUCTION

The use of chemotherapy in patients with advanced metastatic cancer has been suboptimal and despite several decades of active investigation 5-fluorouracil remains one of the most active agents in the treatment of diseases such as colorectal, breast, and head and neck cancer. Attempts to biomodulate the activity of 5-fluorouracil have focused primarily on enhancing its ability to inhibit the target enzyme thymidylate synthase which is essential for the *de novo* synthesis of pyrimidine nucleotides. Recent clinical trials have focused on the development of other novel inhibitors of thymidylate synthase in an attempt to improve therapeutic strategies aimed at inhibiting this important enzyme. In this chapter we will explore the importance of thymidylate synthase and its clinical relevance in the development of novel therapeutic strategies.

From: *Anticancer Drug Development Guide: Antifolate Drugs in Cancer Therapy*
Edited by: A.L. Jackman © Humana Press Inc., Totowa, NJ

2. IMPORTANCE OF TS INHIBITION

Thymidylate synthase (TS) is a folate-dependent enzyme that catalyzes the methylation of 2′ deoxyuridine 5′ monophosphate (dUMP) using 5,10-methylene tetrahydrofolate which serves as a one-carbon donor for the reductive methylation to deoxythymidine monophosphate (dTMP), which is required for *de novo* pyrimidine nucleotide synthesis, DNA replication, and repair *(1)*. TS is also a critical target for the fluoropyrimidine drugs which are widely used in the treatment of breast, gastrointestinal, and head and neck cancers *(2,3)*. 5-Fluorouracil (5FU) is converted intracellularly to fluorodeoxyuridine monophosphate (FdUMP) and in the presence of 5,10-methylene tetrahydrofolate forms a stable covalent TS ternary complex (TS-FdUMP-5,10 methylene tetrahydrofolate) resulting in TS inhibition *(4,5)*. In addition to 5FU, recent work has focused on the development of other inhibitors of TS with a structure that is similar to that of 5,10-methylene tetrahydrofolate. Several novel antifolate inhibitors of thymidylate synthase have been synthesized and found to have potent antitumor activity in vitro and in vivo. Initial compounds such as CB3717 (N10-propargyl-5, 8 dideazafolate) were tested clinically and found to be associated with unpredictable and severe nephrotoxicity *(6)*. The life-threatening nephrotoxicity was presumed to be caused by precipitation of the relatively insoluble parent compound in the urine. This ultimately resulted in the decision to discontinue its further development. A newer generation 2-desamino-2-methyl-N10-substituted-5-8 dideazafolate ZD1694 (raltitrexed) was a more water-soluble analog of CB3717 designed to circumvent unpredictable nephrotoxicity *(7)*. Jackman and coworkers carefully characterized a series of 2-desamino-2-methyl-N10-substituted-5-8 dideazafolates *(7)*. From this group of 15 compounds ZD1694 (raltitrexed) was found to be the most potent. Raltitrexed structurally resembles the physiological folates and hence requires active transmembrane transport to gain intracellular access. It also undergoes metabolism to the polyglutamated forms that are approx 100-fold more potent as inhibitors of TS when compared with the unmetabolized monoglutamate form. Raltitrexed has demonstrated activity in a variety of preclinical models and has been administered safely to patients in a series of clinical trials. Several international Phase I–III clinical studies have now been completed in a variety of malignancies. These studies would suggest that raltitrexed (Tomudex) is an active drug in several solid tumors including colorectal, breast, ovarian, and non-small cell lung cancer *(8–10)*. Two other compounds AG331 and AG337 were synthesized to bind specifically to the 5,10-methylene tetrahydrofolate binding site of TS by using X-ray crystallography and computer modeling of this site. They do not depend on a folate carrier for influx like ZD1694 and its analog and are not polyglutamated intracellularly *(11)*. Thus the central role of TS in the *de novo* synthesis of dTMP and DNA synthesis has made it a major target for antitumour drug development.

3. DETERMINANTS OF RESISTANCE TO TS INHIBITORS

The major limitations to the use of these TS-directed chemotherapeutic agents has been the development of clinical resistance. The ability of the 5FU active metabolite fluorodeoxyuridine monophosphate (FdUMP) to inhibit TS is influenced by several factors including the concentration of TS enzymes, the amount of FdUMP formed and its rate of breakdown, the amount of competing normal substrate dUMP, the level of 5-10-

methylene tetrahydrofolate and the extent of its polyglutamation. In tumor-bearing mice receiving 5FU, Myers et al. showed that expansion of the intracellular dUMP pools could compete with FdUMP for newly synthesized TS which lead to the reduction of the cytotoxic effect of 5FU by reducing FdUMP inhibition of dTMP synthesis *(12)*. In separate studies Klubes and colleagues also noted that the persistence of FdUMP in rodent tumors correlated best with sensitivity to 5FU although the indigenous dUMP pools were greater and expanded somewhat more rapidly in nonresponsive solid rat Walker 256 carcinomas in which DNA synthesis correlated with a more rapid decrease in the intracellular FdUMP concentration *(13)*. Other studies have confirmed that the more rapid decline in FdUMP concentration may be a more important determinant of 5FU-resistant neoplasms *(14)*. Thus the basis for resistance in some cells may be explained by the rate of nucleotide inactivation.

Over the last decade, evidence has accumulated suggesting that insufficient inhibition of TS may be a major resistance mechanism to 5FU as well as the newer folate TS inhibitors both in preclinical models and in patients. Using TS biochemical assays Swain and colleagues measured TS enzyme levels prior to and 24 h following 5FU therapy in tumors from patients with advanced breast cancer with cutaneous metastatic deposits *(15)*. In this study they observed that TS levels were increased approx threefold in tumor biopsies specimens taken 24 h following 5FU. Since the level of TS appeared to be an important determinant of sensitivity to 5FU, these investigators felt that this induction may serve as an efficient mechanism by which malignant cells develop acute resistance to fluoropyrimidines. Further studies by Chu and colleagues demonstrated a 2.8-fold increase in TS enzyme activity in vitro after 24 h of exposure to 5FU in H630 colon carcinoma cells *(16)*. Moreover, they also noted that simultaneous exposure to nongrowth-inhibitory concentrations of gamma interferon completely abrogated 5FU-mediated induction of TS *(17)*. Similar observations were also made by Spears et al. when they measured the degree of TS inhibition in solid tumor and normal liver biopsies obtained 20–240 min following administration of 5FU. TS inhibition was maximal after 90 min, with 70–80% inhibition in tumor tissues compared to 50% inhibition in histologically normal tissue. Patients whose tumors were responsive to 5FU had greater inhibition of TS, moreover, TS inhibition was greater when the tumor concentration of FdUMP was 75 pmol/gm or more, and the FdUMP/dUMP ratio was greater than 10 *(18)*. Amplification of the TS gene with increased TS mRNA expression and Ts enzyme content has been found in cell lines resistant to 5FU or fluorodeoxyuridine (FdUrd) *(19,20)*. Moreover, alterations in TS have also been noted in cell lines resistant to fluoropyrimidines. Berger and colleagues have reported a colon-cancer cell line with intrinsic resistance to FdUrd which contains an altered structural form of TS with decreased affinity for both FdUMP and 5,10-methylene tetrahydrofolate *(21)*. These investigators isolated and sequenced a DNA clone specific for the altered TS and identified two point mutations, one of them in the 3' untranslated region and the second a substitution of histidine for tyrosine in codon 33 of the protein-coding region. Although the function of the tyrosine remains uncertain, it is one of the five residues that are invariant among eight species in which TS has been examined.

Increased TS expression would also appear to play a significant role in the development of resistance to the folate-based TS inhibitors. Resistance to folate TS inhibitors such as CB3717 had earlier been described in mouse L1210 leukemia cells and human lymphoblastoid cells and appeared to be caused by increased TS expression *(22)*. In addition to increased TS expression, more recent studies would suggest that decreased folylpolyglutamate synthase (FPGS) activity may also be a determinant of response. Jackman and colleagues have studied the mechanisms of resistance to Tomudex in four cell lines, the mouse L1210 leukemia line, the human W1L2 lymphoblastoid line, and two human ovarian lines CH1 and 41M *(23)*. In the W1L2 lymphoblastoid line and the CH1 ovarian line, the primary mechanism of resistance was increased TS expression. In contrast, the 41M ovarian cells did not accumulate ZD1694 because of a defective transport through the reduced folate carrier, whereas the L1210 leukemia cell line did not accumulate the polyglutamated species of ZD1694 and had a 13% reduction in FPGS activity. In ZD1694-resistant MCF-7 breast cell lines Drake and colleagues found that TS levels were increased 52-fold, whereas, in ZD1694-resistant NCI H630 colon cells FPGS activity was decreased by 48-fold *(24)*. Thus in the newer generation of folate-based TS inhibitors both FPGS and TS expression levels would appear to be important determinants of activity given that the inability to form polyglutamated antifolates may result in decreased TS inhibition.

Taken together these observations support the critical role of TS in defining the activity of fluoropyrimidines and folate-based TS inhibitors and suggest that the determination of TS levels in tumor tissues may also help clarify the relationship between pretreatment TS levels, prognosis, and/or response to TS-directed therapies.

4. QUANTITATION OF TS IN HUMAN TUMORS

The quantitation and detection of TS in human tissues has traditionally been performed by enzymatic biochemical assays that either measure catalytic activity or the amount of radiolabeled FdUMP binding to TS following extraction of the enzymes from cells and tissues *(25,26)*. These assays have several limitations when applied to the measurement of TS activity in human tissue samples. Whereas these assays have the required sensitivity for quantitating enzymes in pure populations of rapidly dividing malignant cells in vitro, they lack adequate sensitivity to measure the lower levels of enzyme activity in human tumors. Previous investigations measuring TS levels in breast tumor biopsy specimens have revealed that large quantities of tumour (>50 mg) are required to carry out these studies *(15)*. Both the catalytic and FdUMP binding assays require that the enzyme is active, therefore only fresh frozen tissues can be assayed, thus limiting these assays to prospective studies with the caveat that no proteolytic enzyme degradation has occurred during the preparation of the samples. In addition, the biochemical assays do not discriminate between areas of the tumor with differing morphologies and cannot measure TS on a cell-by-cell basis. Since tissues and cell preparations are a composite of a heterogeneous population, any measurement of TS enzymes using biochemical techniques is confounded by the degree of contamination by cells other than those of interest. Whereas these assays are extremely useful for preclinical studies, their application to clinical tumor samples has been limited and their methodology cannot be applied to archival material such as paraffin-embedded tissues. Recently several new assays have been developed for the quantitation of TS protein and TS gene expression that appear to be highly sensitive. Horikoshi et al. developed a polymerase chain reaction (PCR)-based method to quantitate the expression of TS in clinical tumor samples

(27). Because of its exquisite sensitivity this PCR technique provided the means for detecting and quantitating TS in small tumor biopsy samples. In addition, a panel of human monoclonal antibodies capable of detecting human TS using immunological assays such as ELISA, Western immunoblotting, and flow cytometric analysis have recently been developed *(28)*. These antibodies are highly specific and have been demonstrated to be highly sensitive and accurately quantitative using these immunological techniques *(29)*. Moreover, two of these antibodies are capable of detecting TS by immunohistochemical staining in human colon cancer cell lines and tissues *(28)*. Immunological quantitation of TS in 5FU-sensitive and resistant tumor cell lines has shown an excellent correlation with biochemical assays with a lower limit of sensitivity of 0.3 fmol TS protein. Moreover, these studies have demonstrated a direct correlation between the level of TS protein expression and 5FU sensitivity *(29)*. These immunological and RT-PCR techniques have been independently applied to the quantitation of TS gene and TS protein expression in human colon and gastric tumours and found to correlate closely *(30)*. Thus both assay systems have the ability to quantitate TS levels in patient tumor samples pre-and postchemotherapy and have now laid the basis for studies examining the clinical role of TS in the development of new therapeutic strategies focused on the inhibition of this critical enzyme.

5. CLINICAL RELEVANCE OF THYMIDYLATE SYNTHASE (TS) EXPRESSION

Considerable variation in TS expression has been reported among clinical tumor specimens from both primary tumors *(30–32)* and metastatic disease *(33–35)* in the same way that differences have been demonstrated between sensitive and resistant tumor cell lines in vitro *(29)*. TS would appear to be highly expressed in tumor tissues compared to the normal tissues from which they have arisen. In colorectal cancer, tumor-to-normal gastrointestinal mucosal ratios have ranged from 2 to 10 *(32,36–38)*. Recent studies examining the level of TS expression in clinical tumor samples suggest that TS expression predicts for overall clinical outcome and response to cytotoxic therapy. Using the TS 106 antibody immunohistochemical technique on paraffin-embedded sections, Johnston et al. have shown that TS protein expression, predicts for disease-free and overall survival in patients with rectal cancer independent of Dukes stage *(30)*. Disease-free and overall survival was significantly better in patients whose tumors stained less intensely for TS. Similarly Pestalozzi et al. have found that lower TS protein expression in patients with node-positive primary breast cancer correlates with improved disease-free and overall survival independent of other established prognostic factors in this disease *(39)*. In both of these studies, adjuvant chemotherapy had the greatest impact on survival in tumors expressing higher TS levels.

Several other studies have suggested that the level of TS staining in primary tumor sections may not necessarily correlate with chemosensitivity of subsequent metastases, suggesting that changes in TS expression may occur with tumor evolution. In a study of colorectal tumors, TS staining in sections of primary tumor failed to predict for response of subsequent advanced disease to palliative chemotherapy *(32)*. TS expression may also vary depending on the site of metastatic disease, and this may be one explanation for the differential response to TS inhibitor therapy sometimes encountered between different disease sites in the same patient. Evidence to support this has recently come from Gorlick and colleagues *(40)* who have shown that lung metastases have a higher mean TS mRNA expression compared to hepatic metastasis. In this study, the lung and liver biopsies were not paired samples from the same patients but obtained from separate patients. The predictive value of TS overexpression may be further enhanced if combined with other molecular characteristics. Lenz et al. reported that increased pretreatment TS expression together with expression of mutant p53 identified a subgroup of primary stage II colon cancer with a poorer prognosis *(41)*. In addition to the association with fluoropyrimidine resistance, Kitchens et al. found higher TS expression, in colon cancer cell lines which also expressed a mismatch repair deficient (RER+) phenotype *(42)*.

In the setting of advanced metastatic disease, both high TS mRNA, quantified by RT-PCR, and high TS protein expression, have been shown to predict for a poor response to fluoropyrimidine-based therapy in colorectal *(33–36)*, gastric *(31,43)*, and head and neck cancer *(44)*. Considerable overlap between responders and nonresponders was often present in the low TS category, but patients with TS levels above the median tended not to respond. In the metastatic disease setting the presence of mutant p53 has also been associated with higher TS expression and also predicts for failure of therapy *(45)*.

In the adjuvant and advanced disease studies, TS predicted outcome of therapy not only for TS inhibitors such as 5FU but also when other agents were used that are cytotoxic through other mechanisms. That such a correlation should emerge is interesting, and suggests that TS may be a marker of overall tumor sensitivity to a number of therapeutic approaches. Although TS expression does not directly correlate with other markers of tumor proliferation such as expression of Ki-67 antigen *(39)*, it does correlate with tumor stage *(30)*, RER+ status *(42)*, as well as p53 status *(41)* with higher TS expression being reported with later tumor stage and mutant p53 status. This suggests that changes in TS expression may accompany the increasing genetic instability in more advanced tumors, which in turn may not only be associated with resistance to TS-directed therapy but also to other chemotherapeutic approaches.

The advent of new folate-based specific TS inhibitors such as ZD1694 has stimulated interest in the role of TS not only as a marker of tumor behavior and prognosis, but also as a predictor of treatment toxicity in normal tissues. The influence of TS expression on response to therapy can now be studied in the context of treatment with agents which are pure inhibitors of TS. This eliminates an important and potentially confounding property of 5FU, that of its schedule-dependent effects upon RNA and DNA *(46)*. Because novel folate-based TS inhibitors such as ZD1694 are also substrates for folate-uptake mechanisms and polyglutamation, the expression of the corresponding membrane carriers and polyglutamating enzymes may also influence treatment outcome. Preliminary data from a ongoing study of ZD1694 in advanced colorectal cancer *(34)*, has suggested that tumors with higher expression of the polyglutamating enzyme FPGS have higher ZD1694 levels. Correlation of these parameters with tumor response to folate-based TS inhibitors is awaited.

This study has also evaluated the expression of TS and other markers of ZD1694 metabolism in normal bowel tissue and their relation to toxicity. In eight patients in whom pretreatment TS mRNA was quantified from rectal biopsies, higher TS expression was associated with more severe bowel toxicity. Rectal biopsies were repeated 5 after the first dose of ZD1694 and those patients experiencing more severe bowel toxicity had a twofold higher median tomudex levels ($n = 10$) in the rectal mucosa. Thus TS levels may prove useful as a determinant of risk of toxicity in patients treated with these cytotoxic agents.

These studies evaluating the expression of TS in human tumors would suggest that the ability to predict response and outcome based upon TS expression in human tumors may provide the opportunity in the future to select patients most likely to benefit from TS-directed therapy.

6. TS INHIBITORS AND OTHER TARGETS: DIHYDROPYRIMIDINE DEHYDROGENASE

5FU has poor oral bioavailability and is rapidly cleared from plasma ($t_{1/2} = 10$–20 min). Both of these properties result from the rapid degradation of 5FU to fluoro-β-alanine, the rate-limiting enzyme in this catabolic pathway, being dihydropyrimidine dehydrogenase (DPD,EC1.5.1.3) *(47)*. This catabolic pathway accounts for elimination of at least 80% of an administered dose of 5FU, and has received considerable attention as a potential target for pharmacological manipulation *(48)*. DPD is primarily found in the liver, but is also present in bowel, pancreas, lung, kidney, lymphocytes, and other tissues as well as a broad spectrum of tumor types. DPD activity in tumors has been shown to be higher than that of the corresponding normal tissues from which the tumor has arisen *(49)*. DPD activity in peripheral blood mononuclear cells has been found to correlate with that found in a normal functioning liver, so that peripheral-blood mononuclear DPD activity measurements have been applied to population studies *(50)*. Such studies have shown that levels of this enzyme vary among individuals, and between sexes. Etienne et al. *(51)* in a study of 185 consecutive cancer patients reported an eightfold difference in enzyme activity in this population, and a 15% lower mean level of enzyme activity in females, but no variation with age. However, peripheral-blood mononuclear DPD activity correlated poorly with 5FU clearance and the incidence of toxicity in this group and consequently could not be used for 5FU dose adaptation.

An uncommon severe genetic deficiency of DPD, thought to follow an autosomal-recessive inheritance pattern, has been identified and is characterized by severe 5FU toxicity *(52)*. Confirmation of suspected deficiency by means of peripheral blood mononuclear DPD measurements (activity < 0.1 nmol/min/mg protein) would require marked reductions in 5FU dose or even alternative chemotherapy regimens. More recently with the advent of potent inhibitors of the enzyme, peripheral-blood mononuclear DPD activity have been used to monitor the biochemical efficacy of these agents *(53)*. Studies on biopsy material from head and neck cancer showed that patients with lower tumor-to-normal-tissue DPD ratios were more likely to respond to 5FU-based regimens *(54)*, raising the possibility that selective inhibition of tumoral DPD may make tumor cells more susceptible to 5FU.

DPD activity in normal tissues exhibits diurnal variation with an inverse relationship with plasma 5FU, the latter varying up to fivefold over 24 h during-continuous infusion *(48,55)*. Thus DPD activity in normal tissues is increased at night with peak activity at approx 1:00 A.M.. Cell division in normal proliferating tissues also exhibits cyclical variations in activity with peak activity during day time *(56)*. Similar studies in tumor cells harvested from patients have shown that tumors also possess circadian fluctuations in proliferative activity, but tumor cycles are out of phase with those of normal tissues *(56)*. These observations have given rise to the concept that a cycle-specific drug metabolized by DPD, such as 5FU, would affect normal tissues less if given at night when DNA synthesis and cell proliferation are lower, and the catabolic pathway for the drug is more active. Conversely, tumor cells would be more susceptible if exposure coincided with periods of increased cell division. Hence the net result of infusing 5FU at night might be to reduce dose-limiting toxicity in normal tissues, allowing dose escalation, and hopefully greater tumor-cell kill.

Two relatively novel approaches in the development of 5FU therapy are under evaluation. The first involves attempts to increase 5FU oral bioavailability either by synthesizing DPD-resistant prodrugs, or the design of DPD inhibitors that can be coadministered with oral 5FU. The second approach has been the use of chronomodulated infusions of 5FU in order to take advantage of diurnal variations in enzyme activity. A number of orally stable 5FU prodrugs such as tegafur are in various stages of clinical evaluation *(57,58)*. These have also been combined with uracil in molar ratios of 1:4 which result in saturation of DPD, and a greatly enhanced oral bioavailability. These agents have made oral 5FU dosing an attractive alternative for the future and trials are under way comparing established regimens of iv infusional 5FU with oral formulations. Combinations of 5FU and inhibitors of DPD such as ethinyluracil *(53)* have also greatly enhanced the oral bioavailability of the former. The use of protracted infusion schedules of 5FU through indwelling central venous catheters has produced response rates superior to those of bolus 5FU alone *(59)*, and equivalent to those of leucovorin-modulated bolus 5FU *(60)*. Chronomodulation of infusional 5FU was designed to compliment the diurnal fluctuations in 5FU catabolism described above. This involves the administration of 5FU at a variable rate following a sinusoidal pattern through a programmable portable infusion pump, so that infusion rate is maximal at night, and is followed by a drug-free period during day time. Results from randomized clinical studies have supported this rationale with less toxicity and higher response rates reported for chronomodulated therapy compared to a constant-rate infusion *(61)*. In these studies, 5FU was combined with the platinum analog oxaliplatin, which was also chronomodulated but with a peak infusion time at 4:00 P.M. Greater neurotoxicity from oxaliplatin in the chronomodulated arm was attributed to a drug interaction reducing the efficacy of this drug in the constant-rate infusion arm and therefore subsequent studies incorporated the use of a pump with separate infusion ports for each drug. Response rates were impressive with 53% responding to chronomodulated treatment compared to 32% to constant-rate infusions *(62)*. The main limitation of this approach is the dependence on specialized pumps and indwelling central lines.

7. PLASMA DEOXYURIDINE AS A PHARMACODYNAMIC MARKER OF TS INHIBITION

Deoxyuridine (dUrd) is a byproduct of the intracellular accumulation of dUMP following TS inhibition. Accumulation of dUMP occurs both as a direct consequence of TS inhibition, and also as a result of increased activity of other enzymes including ribonucleotide reductase which converts UDP to dUDP, and deoxycytidylate deaminase which converts dCMP to dUMP *(63)*. These enzymes may be suppressed by negative feedback from the cellular levels of TTP, and are therefore activated when TTP levels fall during TS inhibition *(64)*. dUMP is catabolized intracellularly to dUrd which effluxes from cells and can be measured in plasma. Preclinical studies in mice, using HPLC *(65)*, have demonstrated rises in plasma dUrd during a course of five daily boluses of the specific TS inhibitor CB717, followed by rapid normalization after termination of exposure *(66)*. Transient changes were also observed in patients undergoing treatment in the phase I study of CB3717 *(66)*. These studies suggested a potential role for this metabolite as a pharmacodynamic indicator of TS inhibition in normal tissues.

Earlier estimates of human plasma dUrd reported values of 600 ± 300 nM using RIA *(67)*, but these high values may have reflected lack of specificity of the antibodies used. Taylor et al. *(66)* reported pretreatment plasma dUrd concentrations of approx 100 nM using HPLC in a small group of cancer patients. Clinical measurements of plasma dUrd were made in a phase I study of the nonclassical antifolate AG337 *(68)*. Pretreatment dUrd levels were of the order of 100 nM and consistent two to threefold were observed at the end of a 24-h infusion of AG337, above a "threshold dose." Within 24 h of cessation of the infusion, plasma dUrd levels returned to baseline. Further dose escalations above the threshold dose at which dUrd elevations occurred, were not accompanied by a greater magnitude of dUrd elevation.

Farrugia et al. *(34)* studied changes in plasma dUrd following administration of ZD1694 in patients with advanced colorectal cancer. A novel HPLC method was used that incorporated fluorimetric detection of dUrd derivatized with a fluorescent agent 4-bromomethyl-6,7-dimethoxycoumarin (BrMdmc) *(69)*. BrMdmc was specific in its binding to nucleosides, fatty acids, and carboxylic acids and therefore reduced the number of interfering peaks so that only a single HPLC step was required. The plasma dUrd in healthy volunteers was approx 60 nM, whereas the mean pretreatment level in 11 patients with advanced colorectal cancer was 50 nM (range 19–82 nM).

The profile of plasma dUrd was measured in the same patients on days 1, 5, and 14 following a first dose of ZD1694 (day 0). Results are shown in Fig. 1. In all patients, a rise in dUrd was seen on day 1 (24 h posttreatment) which ranged from 1.5-to 5.8-fold over the pretreatment level, and which returned to baseline by day 5 in all but one patient. Intermediate time points between days 1 and 5 are currently under study to determine more accurately the rapidity of normalization of plasma dUrd following ZD1694.

The observed rise in dUrd in these clinical studies is evidence of TS inhibition in normal tissues. The correlation of TS inhibition with normal tissue toxicity is currently under evaluation.

Current studies are addressing whether plasma dUrd measurements may help to optimize the scheduling of treatment with TS inhibitors. An ongoing phase I study of the novel quinazoline nonpolyglutamable TS inhibitor ZD9331 *(70)* is evaluating the role of plasma dUrd as a pharmacodynamic guide to dose escalation.

8. FUTURE DIRECTIONS

Future Directions has been a major focus for the development of novel therapeutic strategies. The biomodulation of 5FU by leucovorin, the inhibition of 5FU degradation by DPD inhibitors, and the clinical introduction of rationally designed TS inhibitors have begun to show great clinical promise. More recently the introduction of quantita-

Profiles in 10 patients

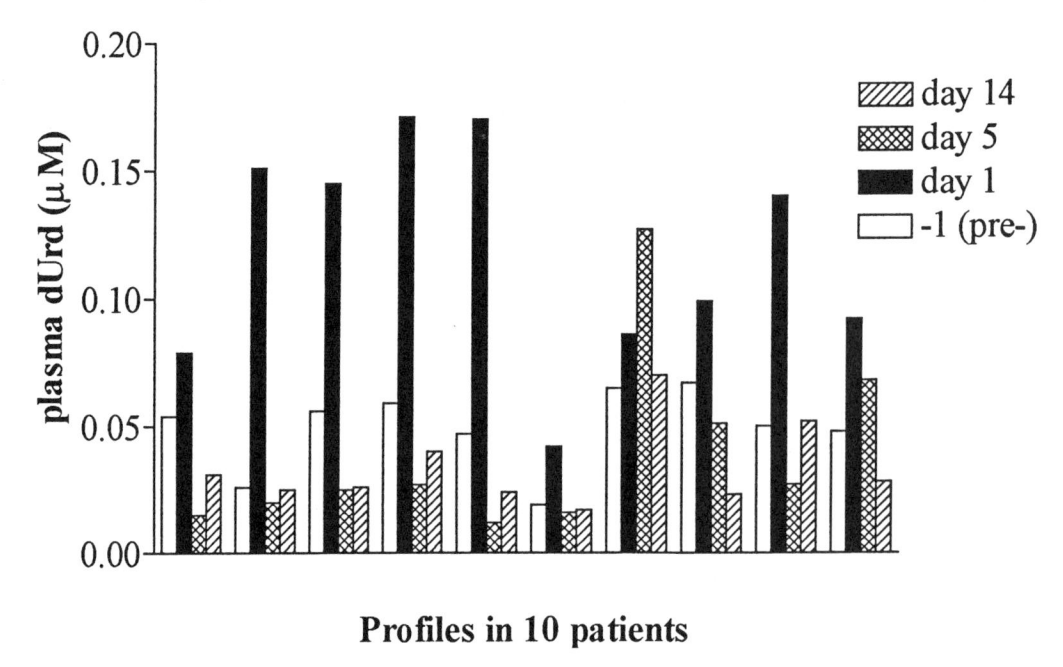

Fig. 1. Changes in plasma dUrd with time in cycle 1 after ZD1694 3.0 mg/m^2.

tive TS assays that facilitate measurement of TS expression in clinical tumor. The ability to determine the effects of TS-directed therapies on TS expression in patient tumor samples will aid in the determination of the importance of TS in clinical drug resistance and will ultimately lead to improved therapeutic strategies aimed at inhibiting this critical enzyme. The relationship between TS expression in normal tissues and toxicity of TS inhibitors, as well as the significance of changes in plasma dUrd may also shed more light on the effect of these agents on normal proliferating tissues.

REFERENCES

1. Grem JL. Fluorinated pyrimidines. In: (Chabner BA, Collins JM, eds.) Cancer Chemotherapy, Principles and Practice. Philadelphia, Lippincott, 1990; pp. 180–224.
2. Danenberg PV. Thymidylate synthase—a target enzyme in cancer chemotherapy. *Biochem Biophys Acta* 1977; 473:73–92.
3. Moertel CC. Chemotherapy for colorectal cancer. *N Engl J Med* 1994; 330:1136–1143.
4. Santi DV, McHenry CS, Sommer M. Mechanisms of interaction of thymidylate synthase with 5-fluorodeoxyuridylate. *Biochemistry* 1974; 13:471–480.
5. Lockshin A, Danenberg PV. Biochemical factors affecting the tightness of 5-fluorodeoxyuridylate binding to human thymidylate synthase. *Biochem Pharmacol* 1981; 30:247–257.
6. Cantwell BMJ, Macauley V, Harris AL, Kaye SB, Smith IE, Milsted RAV, Calvert AH. Phase II study of the antifolate N10-propargyl-5.8-dideazafolic acid (CB3713) in advanced breast cancer. *Eur J Clin Oncol* 1988; 24:733–736.
7. Jackman AL, Taylor GA, Gibson W, Kimbell R, Brown M, Calvert AH, Judson IR, Hughes LR. ICI D1694, a quinazoline antifolate thymidylate synthase inhibitor that is a potent inhibitor of L1210 tumour growth in vitro and in vivo. A new agent for clinical study. *Cancer Res* 1991; 51:5579–5586.
8. Jodrell DI, Newell DR, Calvert JA, Stephens TC, Calvert AH. Pharmacokinetics and toxicity studies with the novel quinazoline thymidylate synthase inhibitor D1694. *Proc Am Assoc Cancer Res* 1990; 31:31–34.

9. Sorenson JM, Jordan E, Grem JL, Hamilton JM, Arbuck SG, Johnston P, Allegra CJ. Phase I trial of D1694. A pure thymidylate synthase inhibitor. *Proc Am Soc Clin Oncol* 1993; 12:158 (abstract).
10. Zalcberg JR, Cunningham D, Van Cutsem E, Francois E, Schornagel J, Adenis A, Green M, Iveson A, Azab M, Seymour I. ZD 1694: a novel thymidylate synthase inhibition with substantial activity in the treatment of patients with advanced colorectal cancer. *J Clin Oncol* 1996; 14:716–721.
11. Jackson RC, Johnston AL, Shetty BV, Varney MD, Webber S, Webber SE. Molecular design of thymidylate synthase inhibitors. *Proc Am Assoc Cancer Res* 1993; 34:566–567.
12. Myers CE, Young RC, Chabner BA. Biochemical determinants of 5-fluorouracil response in vivo: the role of deoxyuridylate pool expansion. *J Clin Invest* 1975; 56:1231–1238.
13. Klubes P, Connelly K, Cerna I, Mandel HG. Effects of 5-fluorouracil on 5-Fluorodeoxyuridine 5-monophosphate and 2-deoxyuridine 5-monophosphate pools and DNA synthesis in solid mouse L1210 and rat Walker 256 tumours. *Cancer Res* 1978; 38:2325–2330.
14. Aschele C, Sobrero A, Faderan MA, Bertino JR. Novel mechanisms of resistance to 5-Fluorouracil in human colon cancer (HCT-8) sublines following exposure to two different clinically relevant schedules. *Cancer Res* 1992; 52:1855–1862.
15. Swain SM, Lippman ME, Egan EF, Drake JC, Steinberg SM, Allegra CJ. 5-Fluorouracil and high-dose leucovorin in previously treated patients with metastatic breast cancer. *J Clin Oncol* 1989; 7:890–899.
16. Chu E, Zinn S, Boarman D, Allegra CJ. The interaction of g interferon and 5-fluorouracil in the H630 human colon carcinoma cell line. *Cancer Res* 1990; 50:5834–5840.
17. Chu E, Koeller D, Johnston PG, Zinn S, Allegra CJ. The regulation of thymidylate synthase in human colon cancer cells treated with f-fluorouracil and interfeton gamma. *Mol Pharmacol* 1993; 43:527–533.
18. Spears CP, Gustavsson BG, Mitchel MS. Thymidylate synthetase inhibition in malignant tumours and normal liver of patients given intravenous 5-fluorouracil. *Cancer Res* 1984; 44:4144–4150.
19. Clark JL, Berger SL, Mittelmann A, Berger FG. Thymidylate synthase gene amplification in a colon tumor resistant to fluoropyrimidine chemotherapy. *Cancer Treat Rep* 71:261–265.
20. Washtein WL. Increased levels of thymidylate synthase in cells exposed to 5-fluotouracil. *Mol Pharmacol* 1984; 25:171–177.
21. Berger SH, Barbour KW, Berger FG. A naturally occurring variation in thymidylate synthase structure is associated with a reduced response to 5 "fluoro-2" deoxyuridine in a human tumor cell line. *Mol Pharmacol* 1988; 34:480–488.
22. Jackman AL, Alison DL, Calvert AH, Harrap KR. Increased thymidylate synthase in L1210 cells possessing acquired resistance to N^{10} propargyl-58-dideaza folic acid (CB3717). Development, characterization and cross resistance studies. *Cancer Res* 1986; 46:2810–2815.
23. Jackman AL, Kelland LR, Kimbell R, Brown M, Gibson W, Aherne GW, Hardcastle A, Boyle FT. Mechanisms of acquired resistance to the quinazoline thymidylate synthase inhibitor 2D1694 (Tomudex) in one mouse and three human cell lines. *B J Cancer* 1995; 71:914–924.
24. Drake JC, Allegra CJ, Moran RG, Johnston PG. Resistance to tomudex (ZD1694). Multifactorial in human breast and colon carcinoma cell lines. *Biochem Pharmacol* 1996; 51:10,1349–1355.
25. Roberts D. An isotopic assay for thymidylate synthetase. *Biochemistry* 1966; 5:3546–3548.
26. Moran RG, Spears CP, Heidelberger C. Biochemical determinants of tumor sensitivity to 5-fluorouracil; ultrasensitive methods for the determination of 5-fluoro-2-deoxyuridylate and thymidylate synthase *Proc Natl Acad Sci* 1979; 76:3,1456–1460.
27. Horikoshi T, Danenberg KD, Stadlbauer THW, Volkenandt M, Shea LCC, Aigner K, Gustavsson B, Leichman L, Frosing R, Ray M, Gibson NW, Spears CP, Danenberg PV. Quantitation of thymidylate synthase. Dihydrofolate reductase and DT-diaphorase gene expression human tumours using the polymerase chain reaction. *Cancer Res* 1992; 52(1):108–116.
28. Johnston PG, Liang CM, Henry S, Chabner BA, Allegra CJ. The production and characterization of monoclonal antibodies that localize human thymidylate synthase in the cytoplasm of human cells and tissues. *Cancer Res* 1991; 51:6668–6676.
29. Johnston PG, Drake JC, Trepel J, Allegra CJ. Immunological quantitation of thymidylate synthase using the monoclonal antibody TS 106 in 5-fluorouracil-sensitive and resistant human cancer cell lines. *Cancer Res* 1992; 52:4306–4312.
30. Johnston PG, Fisher ER, Rockett HE, Fisher B, Wolmark N, Drake JC, Chabner BA, Allegra CJ. The role of thymidylate synthase expression prognosis and outcome of adjuvant chemotherapy in patients with rectal cancer. *J Clin Oncol* 1994; 12:2640–2647.

31. Lenz HJ, Leichman CJ, Danenberg KD, Danenberg PV, Groshen S, Cohen L, Laine L. Crookes P. Silberman H, Baranda J, Garcia Y, Li J, Leichman L. Thymidylate synthase mRNA level in adenocarcinoma of the stomach: a predictor for primary tumour response and overall survival. *J Clin Oncol* 1995; 14(1):176–182.
32. Findlay MPN, Cunningham D, Morgan G, Clinton S, Hardcastle A, Aherne GW. Lack of correlation between thymidylate synthase levels in primary colorectal tumours and subsequent response to chemotherapy. *Br J Cancer* 1997; 75(6):903–909.
33. Johnston PG, Lenz HJ, Leichman CG, Danenberg KD, Allegra CJ, Danenberg PV, Leichman L. Thymidylate synthase gene and protein expression correlate and are associated with response to 5-fluorouracil in human colorectal and gastric tumors. *Cancer Res* 1995; 55:1407–1412.
34. Farrugia DC, Cunningham D, Mitchell F, et al. A pharmacodynamic study of the antifolate thymidylate synthase inhibitor tomudex™ in advanced colorectal cancer. In: (Pfeiderer W, Rokos H, eds.) Chemistry and Biology of Pteridines and Folates 1997. Blackwell Science, Berlin; 1997, pp. 241–244.
35. Leichman CG, Lenz H, Leichman L, Danenberg KD, Baranda J, Groshen S, Boswell W, Mitzger R, Tan M, Danenberg PV. Quantitation of Intratumoral thymidylate synthase expression predicts for disseminated colorectal cancer response and resistance to protracted-infusion fluorouracil and weekly leucovorin. *J Clin Oncol* 1997; 15:3223–3229.
36. Parise Jr O, Janot F, Luboinski B, Massaad L, Albin N, Toussaint C, Verjus MA, Bonnay M, Gouyette A, Chabot GG. Thymidylate synthase activity, folates, and glutathione system in head and neck carcinoma and adjacent tissues. *Head & Neck* 1994; 16:158–164.
37. Ardalan B, Dang Z. Thymidylate synthase gene expression in normal and malignant colorectal tissues: relation to in vivo response and survival. *Proc Amer Assoc Cancer Res* 1996; 37:201.
38. Davis RA, Sticca RP, Dunlap RB, Berger FG, Berger SH. Thymidylate synthase variation in human colonic tissues. *Proc Amer Assoc Cancer Res* 1996; 37:175.
39. Pestalozzi BC, Peterson HF, Gelber RD, Goldhirsch A, Fusterson BA, Trihia H, Lindtner J, Cortes-Funes H, Simmoncini E, Hyrne MJ, Golouh R, Rudenstam CM, Castiglione-Gertsch M, Allegra CJ, Johnston PG. Prognostic importance of thymidylate synthase expression in early breast cancer. *J Clin Oncol* 1997; 15(5):1923–1931.
40. Gorlick R, Banerjee D, Miles JS, Mezger R, Salonga D, Danenberg K, Danenberg P, Kemeny N, Bertino JR. Higher levels of thymidylate synthase gene expression are observed in pulmonary as compared to hepatic metastases of colorectal adenocarcinoma. *Proc Amer Assoc Cancer Res* 1997; 38:615.
41. Lenz H, Danenberg KD, Leichman CG, Florentine B, Johnston PG, Groshen S, Danenberg PV, Leichman LP. p53 and thymidylate synthase (TS) expression in untreated stage II colon cancer: association with recurrence, survival and tumour site. *Proc Amer Assoc Cancer Res* 1997; 38:614.
42. Kitchens ME, Berger FG. The relationships between mismatch repair defects and expression of thymidylate synthase in fluoropyrimidine-sensitive and -resistant colon tumour cell lines. *Proc Amer Assoc Cancer Res* 1997; 38:614.
43. Alexander HR, Grem JL, Hamilton JM, Pass HI, Hong M, McAtee N, et al. Thymidylate synthase protein expression is associated with response following neoadjuvant chemotherapy and resection for locally advanced gastric cancer. *Cancer J* 1995; 1:49–54.
44. Johnston PG, Mick R, Recant W, Behan KA, Dolan E, Ratain M, Beckmann E, Weichselbaum RR, Allegra CJ, Vokes EE. Thymidylate synthase expression predicts for response to neoadjuvant induction chemotherapy in advanced head and neck cancers. *J Natl Cancer Inst* 1997; 89:308–313.
45. Lenz H, Danenberg KD, Leichman CG, Hayashi K, Metzger R, Salonga D, Kortes V, Banerjee D, Bertino JR, Groshen S, Leichman L, Danenberg PV. p53 status and thymidylate synthase levels are predictors of chemotherapy efficacy in patients with advanced colorectal cancer. *Proc Am Soc Clin Oncol* 1996; 15:216.
46. Sobrero AF, Aschele C, Bertino JR. Fluorouracil in colorectal cancer—a tale of two drugs: implications for biochemical modulation. *J Clin Oncol* 1997; 15(1):368–381.
47. Pinedo HM, Peters GJ. Fluorouracil: biochemistry and pharmacology. *J Clin Oncol* 1988; 6(10):1653–1664.
48. Harris BE, Song R, Soong S, Diasio RB. Relationship between dihydropyrimidine dehydrogenase activity and plasma 5-fluorouracil levels with evidence for circadian variation of enzyme activity and plasma drug levels in cancer patients receiving 5-fluorouracil by protracted continuous infusion. *Cancer Res* 1990; 50:197–201.

49. Daher G, Harris BE, Diasio RB, Powis G, eds. Anticancer Drugs: Antimetabolite Metabolism and Natural Anticancer Agents. 2, Metabolism of Pyrimidine Analogues and Their Nucleosides. Pergamon Cambridge, 1994; pp. 55–94.
50. Chazal M, Etienne MC, Renee N, Bourgeon A, Richelme H, Milano G. Link between dihydropyrimidine dehydrogenase activity and peripheral blood mononuclear cells and liver. *Clin Cancer Res* 1996; 2:507–510.
51. Etienne MC, Lagrange JL, Dassonville O, Fleming R, Thyss A, Renee N, Schneider M, Demard M, Milano G. Population study of dihydropyrimidine dehydrogenase in cancer patients. *J Clin Oncol* 1994; 12(11):2248–2253.
52. Takimoto CH, Lu Z, Zhang R, Liang MD, Larson LV, Cantilena Jr RL, Grem JL, Allegra CJ, Diasio RB, Chu E. Severe neurotoxicity following 5-fluorouracil-based chemotherapy in a patient with dihydropyrimidine dehydrogenase deficiency. *Clin Cancer Res* 1996; 2:477–481.
53. Baker SD, Khor SP, Adjei AA, Doucette M, Spector T, Donehower RC, Grochow LB, Sartorius SE, Noe DA, Hohneker JA, Rowinsky EK. Pharmacokinetic, oral bioavailability, and safety study of fluorouracil in patients treated with 776C85, an inactivator of dihydropyrimidine dehydrogenase. *J Clin Oncol* 1996; 14(12):3085–3096.
54. Etienne MC, Cheradame S, Fischel JL, Formento P, Dassonville O, Renee N, Schneider M, Thyss A, Demard F, Milano G. Response to fluorouracil therapy in cancer patients: the role of tumoral dihydropyrimidine dehydrogenase activity. *J Clin Oncol* 1995; 13(7):1663–1670.
55. Etienne MC, Milano G, Lagrange JL, Bajard F, Francois E, Thyss A, Schneider M, Renee N, Fety R. Marked fluctuations in drug plasma concentrations caused by use of portable pumps for fluorouracil continuous infusion. *J Natl Cancer Inst* 1993; 85(12):1005–1007.
56. Hrushesky WJM, Bjarnason GA. Circadian cancer therapy. *J Clin Oncol* 1993; 11(7):1403–1417.
57. Pazdur R, Lassere Y, Rhodes V, Ajani JA, Sugarman SM, Patt YZ, Jones DV, Markowitz AB, Abbruzzese JL, Bready B, Levin B. Phase II trial of uracil and tegafur plus oral leucovorin: an effective oral regimen in the treatment of metastatic colorectal carcinoma. *J Clin Oncol* 1994; 12(11):2296–2300.
58. Saltz LB, Leichman CG, Young CW, Muggia FM, Conti JA, Spiess T, Jeffers S, Leichman LP. A fixed-ratio combination of uracil and ftorafur (UFT) with low dose leucovorin. An active oral regimen for advanced colorectal cancer. *Cancer* 1995; 75(3):782–785.
59. Lokich JL, Ahlgren JD, Gullo JL, Philips JA, Fryer JG. A prospective randomized comparison of continuous infusion fluorouracil with a conventional bolus schedule in metastatic colorectal carcinoma: A mid-atlantic oncology program study. *J Clin Oncol* 1989; 7(4):425–432.
60. Advanced colorectal cancer metanalysis project. Modulation of fluorouracil by leucovorin in patients with advanced colorectal cancer: evidence in terms of response rate. *J Clin Oncol* 1992; 10(6):896–903.
61. Levi F, Giacchetti S, Adam R, Zidani R, Metzger G, Misset JL. Chronomodulation of chemotherapy against metastatic colorectal cancer. *Eur J Cancer* 1995; 31A(7/8):1264–1270.
62. Bertheault-Cvitkovic F, Jami A, Ithzaki M, Brummer PD, Brienza S, Adam R, Kunstlinger F, Bismuth H, Misset JL, Levi F. Biweekly intensified ambulatory chronomodulated chemotherapy with oxaliplatin, fluorouracil, and leucovorin in patients with metastatic colorectal cancer. *J Clin Oncol* 1996; 14(11):2950–2958.
63. Maybaum J, Cohen MB, Sadee W. In vivo rates of pyrimidine nucleotide metabolism in intact mouse T-lymphoma (S-49) cells treated with 5-fluorouracil. *J Biol Chem* 1981; 256(5):2126–2130.
64. Jackson RC, Jackman AL, Calvert AH. Biochemical effects of a quinazoline inhibitor of thymidylate synthetase, *N*-(4-(*N*-((2-amino-4-hydroxy-6-quinazolinyl)methyl)prop- 2-ynylamino)benzoyl)-L-glutamic acid (CB3717), on human lymphoblastoid cells. *Biochem Pharmacol* 1983; 32(24):3783–3790.
65. Taylor GA, Dady PJ, Harrap KR. Quantitative high performance liquid chromatography of nucleosides and bases in human plasma. *J Chromat* 1980; 183(4):421–431.
66. Taylor GA, Jackman AL, Calvert AH, et al. Plasma nucleoside and base levels following treatment with the new thymidylate synthase inhibitor CB3717. In: (De Bruyn CHMM, Simmonds HA, Muller MM, eds.) Purine Metabolism in Man *IV*, Part B: Biochemical, Immunological and Cancer Research. Plenum, New York; 1984, pp. 379–82.
67. Traut TW. Physiological concentrations of purines and pyrimidines. *Mol Cell Biochem* 1994; 140:1–22.
68. Rafi I, Taylor GA, Calvete JA, Boddy AV, Balmanno K, Bailey N, et al. Clinical pharmacokinetic and pharmacodynamic studies with the nonclassical antifolate thymidylate synthase inhibitor 3,4-dihydro-

2-amino-6-methyl-4-oxo-5-(4-pyridylthio)-quinazolone dihydrochloride (AG337) given by 24-hour continuous intravenous infusion. *Clin Cancer Res* 1995; 1:1275–1284.
69. Mitchell F, Farrugia D, Rees C, Cunningham D, Judson I, Jackman AL. Estimation of 2'-deoxyuridine (dUrd) in human plasma by HPLC with fluorimetric detection; a pharmacodynamic marker for thymidylate synthase (TS) inhibition. *Br J Cancer* 1997; 75(suppl. 1):25.
70. Rees C, Judson I, Beale P, Mitchell F, Smith R, Mayne K, Averbuch S, Jackman A. Phase I trial of ZD9331, a non-polyglutamatable thymidylate synthase (TS) inhibitor given as a five-day continuous infusion. *Proc Am Soc Clin Oncol* 1997; 16:208a.

19 Molecular Regulation of Expression of Thymidylate Synthase

Edward Chu, Jingfang Ju, and John C. Schmitz

CONTENTS

INTRODUCTION
GENE AMPLIFICATION OF THYMIDYLATE SYNTHASE
TRANSCRIPTIONAL REGULATION OF THYMIDYLATE SYNTHASE
TRANSLATIONAL REGULATION OF TS
INTERACTION OF TS WITH CELLULAR RNAS
CONCLUSIONS
ACKNOWLEDGMENTS
REFERENCES

INTRODUCTION

Thymidylate synthase (TS) is a folate-dependent enzyme that catalyzes the reductive methylation of 2′-deoxyuridine-5′-monophosphate (dUMP) by the reduced folate 5, 10-methylenetetrahydrofolate (CH_2-THF) to 2′-deoxythymidine-5′-monophosphate (dTMP, thymidylate) and dihydrofolate *(1,2)*. Once synthesized, dTMP is then metabolized intracellularly to the dTTP triphosphate form, an essential precursor for DNA biosynthesis (*see* Fig. 1). Whereas dTMP can also be formed through the salvage pathway via phosphorylation of thymidine by thymidine kinase, the TS-catalyzed reaction provides the sole intracellular *de novo* source of dTMP. Given its central role in dTMP and DNA biosynthesis and given the observation that inhibition of this reaction results in cessation of cellular proliferation and growth, TS represents an important target for cancer chemotherapy *(2–4)*.

There are several lines of evidence that offer further support to the concept that TS is an important chemotherapeutic target. First, various in vitro studies have demonstrated a strong association between the level of intracellular expression of TS enzyme activity and fluoropyrimidine sensitivity *(5–8)*. Thus, neoplastic cell lines and tumors with in-

From: *Anticancer Drug Development Guide: Antifolate Drugs in Cancer Therapy*
Edited by: A.L. Jackman © Humana Press Inc., Totowa, NJ

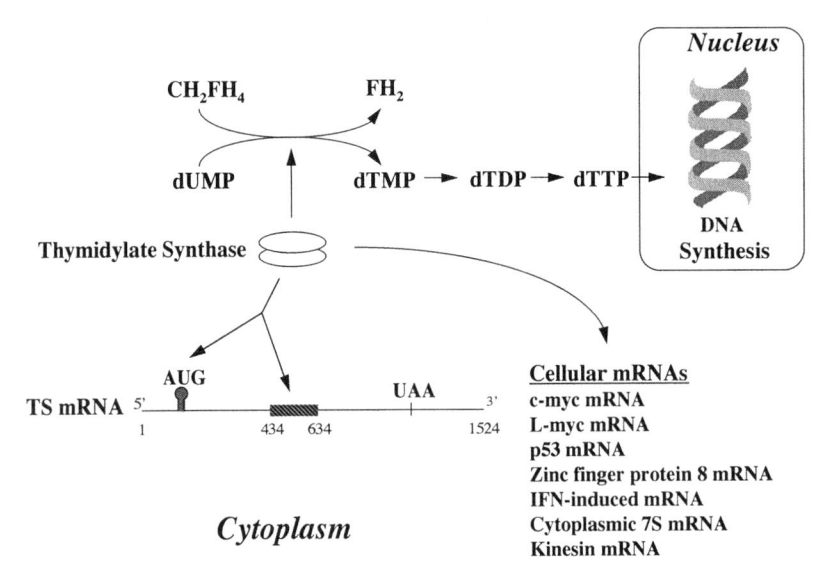

Fig. 1. Cellular functions of thymidylate synthase—the role of TS in *de novo* synthesis of thymidylate and in regulating the expression of cellular mRNAs as an RNA binding protein.

creased TS enzyme activity have been shown to be relatively more resistant to the cytotoxic effects of the fluoropyrimidines. Second, clinical studies have shown a strong correlation between the level of TS enzyme inhibition within patient tumor samples after 5-fluorouracil (5FU) treatment and eventual clinical response to 5FU-based chemotherapy *(9,10)*. Third, using cell-free systems, it was shown that the TS enzyme ternary complex with 5-fluoro-2'-deoxyuridine-5'-monophosphate (FdUMP) and CH$_2$-THF was significantly more stable in the presence of increasing concentrations of the reduced folate CH$_2$-THF. These cell-free studies were then extended to the in vitro setting where it was shown that 5FU cytotoxicity was enhanced upon addition of leucovorin (LCV) in various human malignant cell lines *(11–17)*. Based on these preclinical investigations, the concept of enhancement of 5FU cytotoxicity by LCV was directly applied into the clinical setting where it has been used in the treatment of various human malignancies including advanced colorectal, breast, and head and neck cancer. In several randomized trials, the overall response rate to 5FU/LCV combination therapy was superior (30–35%) to treatment with 5FU alone (10–15%) in the treatment of advanced colorectal cancer *(18–22)*. Finally, recent clinical studies conducted in Europe and in North America have shown that the antifolate analog ZD1694, a specific inhibitor of TS, has relatively good activity against advanced colorectal cancer with an overall response rate of 25–30% *(23–25)*. In at least one randomized study performed under the auspices of the EORTC, this compound was associated with improved overall response rates when compared to the 5FU/LCV combination as well as with a decreased incidence of host toxic events *(23)*.

GENE AMPLIFICATION OF THYMIDYLATE SYNTHASE

Gene amplification is a well-characterized mechanism for increased gene expression, and its role in mediating drug resistance has been particularly well-established. Schimke et al. *(26)* were the first to identify amplification of the dihydrofolate reductase (DHFR) gene in Chinese hamster ovary cells made resistant to the antifolate analog methotrexate (MTX). There is now evidence that the process of DHFR gene amplification with resultant overexpression of the DHFR protein may have clinical relevance. With regard to TS, amplification of the TS gene has been observed in cultured malignant cells treated with the fluoropyrimidines 5FU and FdUrd *(5,27)* or with the TS inhibitor antifolate compounds such as CB3717 *(28,29)* and D1694 *(30)*. In each of these studies, a strong association between the level of TS expression and relative fluoropyrimidine and/or antifolate sensitivity was observed. Thus, malignant cell lines and tumors with higher levels of TS protein are more resistant to the cytotoxic effects of these agents. TS gene amplification has now been well-documented in various in vitro systems. However, there remains little evidence to directly link this process as a relevant mechanism for the development of clinical drug resistance. Whereas Clark et al. *(31)* reported a four to six-fold increased level in the TS gene copy number in a tumor sample obtained from a patient with progressive colon cancer relative to other tumor specimens following treatment with 5FU and leucovorin chemotherapy, a pretreatment biopsy sample was not obtained to determine the baseline tumor TS gene copy number. Thus, this clinical study provides only suggestive evidence that the process of TS gene amplification may play a clinically important role in the acquisition of resistance following fluoropyrimidine therapy.

TRANSCRIPTIONAL REGULATION OF THYMIDYLATE SYNTHASE

The majority of the initial studies on the regulation of expression of TS focused on cell-cycle-directed events. As has been well-described, TS enzyme activity increases dramatically and appears to be maximal at the G1/S-phase boundary of the cell cycle in eukaryotic cells *(32)*. Whereas the expression of TS, as it relates to the yeast system, is controlled primarily by transcriptional events *(33)*, regulation of mouse and human TS appears to be significantly more complicated. In quiescent cells, the levels of TS mRNA and TS protein are present at relatively low levels. However, when resting cells are stimulated to proliferate upon addition of serum, both TS mRNA and TS protein levels increase by more than 10- to 20-fold as cells progress from the G1- to S-phase *(34,35)*. These initial findings suggested that the expression of TS as it relates to growth stimulation and the cell cycle may be regulated at the transcriptional level.

Several *cis*-acting regulatory elements have been identified in both the murine and human TS gene as controlling TS expression at the transcriptional level. With regards to the mouse TS gene, sequences in the 5′-flanking region as well as in various intronic sequences have been identified as essential regulatory elements. In the 5′ flanking region, sequences between -119 and -75 relative to the AUG codon of the mouse TS gene are critical for TS expression *(36)*. Careful analysis revealed that this region contains an Sp1 binding site, two GGAAG motifs (potential binding sites for members of the Ets family of transcription factors), and an E2F binding site *(36,37)*. A similar analysis of the human TS 5′ flanking sequence was recently performed showing that an Sp1 consensus sequence is also present in the promoter region of the human TS gene. Subsequent mutational and deletional analysis has shown that this binding motif is, in fact, critical for the promoter activity of the human TS gene *(38)*. Comparison of the Sp1-binding motif (GAGGCGGA) in the promoter region of human and mouse TS revealed an extremely high degree of homology (90%). Taken together, these findings suggest the importance of the Sp1 motif in maintaining the promoter activity of the TS gene.

Another important regulatory element is the CACCC motif (CCACACCC) located at nucleotide positions -228 to -221 in the 5′ flanking region of the human TS gene *(35)*. By itself, the CACCC box does not seem to be a promoter element. However, it appears to play an important role in optimizing the TS promoter activity. Whereas a CACCC consensus sequence is present in the 5′ flanking regions of both the mouse and rat TS gene, its location is further upstream of the Sp1 binding motif. At the present time, the precise role for the CACCC motif in the regulated expression of either the mouse and/or rat TS remains to be characterized.

For the expression of several essential S-phase-specific genes including dihydrofolate reductase, thymidine kinase, ribonucleotide reductase, and DNA polymerase α, the E2F consensus sequence has been implicated as playing an essential regulatory role *(39)*. In the mouse TS gene, a putative E2F binding element is present in the TS 5′ flanking region. However, deletion of this E2F element did not alter TS promoter activity nor did it abolish growth-regulated expression of the TS gene *(40)*. These findings suggest that the E2F binding site may not play a role in the regulation of mouse TS expression. As for the human TS gene, the role of E2F in determining the expression of TS at the transcriptional level remains to be defined.

Recent studies have suggested that intronic sequences may play an important role in controlling the expression of TS, primarily at the posttranscriptional level. Johnson and colleagues have shown that the regulation of the mouse TS minigene, devoid of any intronic sequences, was completely abolished in mouse ST6 cells *(41)*. Unfortunately, it remains unclear as to which specific intron or which sequence element within a given intron is necessary for regulation. However, these initial results suggest that the presence of an efficiently spliced intron is required for optimal expression of TS. With regard to the human TS gene, the presence of the first intron has been shown to be important for controlling its expression *(42)*. However, the potential role of other introns in determining the expression of human TS remains to be characterized. Clearly, further studies must be performed to investigate the potential role of other introns and to identify the specific sequences within these introns that control TS expression.

As has been described above, transcriptional and posttranscriptional events play a critical role in the expression of TS during the cell cycle. In addition to cell-cycle-related events, chronic exposure of malignant cells to various anticancer agents can lead to increased expression of TS that is controlled at the transcriptional level. Work by Scanlon et al. *(6)* demonstrated that selection of human ovarian cancer cells in cisplatin led to the development of cross-resistance to 5FU. They found that cisplatin-resistant cells expressed three- to four-fold higher levels of TS when compared to wild-type parental cells. Moreover, the increased level of expression of TS was not associated with TS gene amplification but rather was the direct result of an increased transcriptional rate. A series of adriamycin-resistant human breast cancer MCF-7 and human colon cancer DLD-1 cells were established, and characterization of these cell lines revealed that they were cross-resistant to the fluoropyrimidines 5FU and FdUrd *(7)*. Of note, these resistant cell lines had not previously been exposed to either of these fluoropyrimidine compounds. Further evaluation revealed that the development of fluoropyrimidine resistance was associated with an increased expression of TS protein. The increased expression of TS was not the result of gene amplification but was caused by enhanced transcription of the TS gene. Whereas the precise molecular mechanism(s) by which this process occurs remains to be characterized, these two studies *(6,7)* suggest that the ability to increase the expression of TS in response to chronic exposure to cytotoxic agents other than fluoropyrimidines may serve as an important adaptive response mechanism for malignant cells to circumvent the effects of various cytotoxic stress and thereby maintain cellular synthetic function.

TRANSLATIONAL REGULATION OF TS

Several investigators have described acute elevations of TS enzyme activity in both in vitro and in vivo systems after short-term administration of TS inhibitor compounds such as MTX and 5FU. The initial observation of TS enzyme induction was made by Labow and coworkers *(43)* who measured a 10-fold increase in TS enzyme activity following partial hepatectomy of rats with an additional 10- to 15-fold increase in response to MTX treatment. Subsequent to that observation, various groups using a host of in vitro and in vivo animal model systems observed a similar induction of TS enzyme activity following exposure to the fluoropyrimidines 5FU and/or FUdR *(9,10,44,45)*. Although the mechanism(s) by which the induced expression of TS in response to exposure to these antimetabolites had not been characterized at that time, several possibilities were proposed including enhanced TS transcription, enhanced stability of TS mRNA, enhanced translation of TS mRNA, and enhanced stability of TS protein.

In each of these earlier studies, it had been suggested that the enhanced expression of TS in response to TS inhibitor compounds might, in some manner, be important in the development of cellular drug resistance. Given this theoretic possibility, significant research efforts were placed on characterizing the biochemical and molecular mechanisms involved in mediating this acute response to drug treatment. Using normal mammary epithelial 70N and human breast cancer MCF-7 cells, Keyomarsi and Pardee *(46)* showed that TS enzyme activity increased by more than 40-fold in response to treatment with the folate-based TS inhibitor, Tomudex, whereas TS mRNA levels remained constant. Addition of cycloheximide, an inhibitor of protein synthesis, prevented the drug-induced increase in TS enzyme activity whereas 5, 6-dichlorobenzimidazole, a well-characterized inhibitor of transcription, had absolutely no effect on Tomudex-induced TS elevation. These findings implicated the role of a posttranscriptional regulatory event in mediating the increased expression of TS. However, it remained unclear as to whether the induction of TS enzyme activity was mediated by a translational or posttranslational process. Studies from our own laboratory using a human colon cancer H630 cell line showed that the levels of both TS protein and TS enzymatic activity increased in response to 5FU exposure while the levels of TS mRNA remained unchanged *(47)*. Furthermore, pulse-chase labeling and immunoprecipitation studies revealed that the increased expression of TS resulted from new protein synthesis and not from enhanced stability of the TS protein. It is noteworthy that this 5FU-mediated induction of TS was effectively repressed in the presence of the cytokine gamma-interferon (IFN), at concentrations that were nongrowth inhibitory. This effect of IFN on downregulating the expression of TS appeared to be biologically relevant as it resulted in a nearly 20-fold increase in the cytotoxic effects of 5FU in the H630 cell line *(47)*. Thus, this study provided the first direct evidence for the role of translational regulation in controlling TS expression in an intact biological system and supported the biological relevance of this regulatory process. These findings suggested that the ability to regulate the expression of TS at the translational level represents an important mechanism by which normal cellular synthetic function can be tightly controlled during various phases of the cell cycle. Moreover, this autoregulatory process may provide an efficient defense mechanism for the development of cellular drug resistance in response to anticancer drugs targeted against TS so that cellular synthetic function can be properly maintained.

The potential for translational control of TS was initially postulated by Belfort et al. *(48)* after identification and analysis of the sequence and structural features of the *E. coli thyA* gene. Subsequently, Kisliuk and coworkers *(49)* made the interesting observation that TS isolated from an MTX-resistant *Streptococcus faecium* species was bound to a poly-G tetraribonucleotide sequence. Whereas the precise nature of this RNA–protein interaction was not further characterized, it was suggested that this short RNA sequence might, in some manner, be part of a longer RNA sequence with a potential regulatory function. Upon cloning and sequencing of the human TS cDNA, Takeishi et al. *(50)* suggested the potential for translational control given the presence of three tandem repeats in the 5′-untranslated region (UTR) of the human TS cDNA. Their initial secondary structure analysis suggested that these 28–34 nt repeat sequences might be able to base pair and form stable stem-loop structures. Additional experiments revealed that deletion of all three tandem repeats significantly increased translational efficiency of TS by two- to three-fold *(51)*. Thus, this study was the first to demonstrate the in vivo biological relevance of translational regulation of TS mRNA. Whereas the precise mechanism(s) by which TS mRNA translation was directly controlled remained to be defined, these initial studies suggested the possibility of a *trans*-acting protein and/or other cellular factor interacting with the TS mRNA to repress translation.

Since the expression of TS appeared to be controlled by a translational regulatory process during the cell cycle as well as in response to cytotoxic agents, an extensive series of experiments were undertaken to more precisely characterize the regulation of TS mRNA translation. Using a rabbit reticulocyte lysate in vitro translation system, it was shown that translation of human TS mRNA was repressed in the presence of human recombinant TS protein *(52)*. This interaction was specific in that this same human recombinant TS protein was unable to repress the translation of several, unrelated mRNAs including human chromogranin A, human folate receptor, human preplacental lactogen, yeast, and brome mosaic virus. Further, the native state of the protein appeared to be essential for the inhibitory effect as TS protein that had been enzymatically cleaved with proteinase K or heat-denatured was ineffective at repressing TS mRNA translation. This initial set of experiments suggested the possibility of a direct interaction between TS protein and its own mRNA. RNA gel mobility-shift assays confirmed that human recombinant TS protein did indeed form a ribonucleoprotein (RNP) complex with its own human TS mRNA. This interaction was shown to be specific and one of high affinity with binding affinities in the range of 1 to 3 nM. Moreover, no other cellular cofactor or protein appeared to be required for binding of TS protein to its cognate TS mRNA as RNA binding activity was preserved when different preparations of human recombinant TS, ranging in purity from partially pure to homogeneously pure were employed. Despite these initial in vitro findings, it remains to be determined whether other cellular cofactors or proteins may be required in the in vivo setting for maximal effect.

Two different regions on TS mRNA were identified that interact with high affinity to TS protein *(53)* (*see* Fig. 1). The first site is contained within the first 188 nucleotides of the TS mRNA and can be narrowed down to a core 30-nt sequence that includes the AUG translational start site. The second site is located within the protein-coding region and corresponds to 434 to 634. Since previous investigations had identified sequences in the 5'-UTR as playing a critical role in regulating the translation of several other mRNAs *(54,55)*, much of the initial research efforts focused on the 5' upstream binding site. Using an Zuker RNA-fold secondary structure algorithm, analysis of the first site predicted a stable stem-loop structure with the loop domain being composed of the sequence GCCAUG. Further mutational analysis revealed that this sequence was essential as a recognition element for TS protein binding.

With regards to the RNA binding activity of the TS protein, RNA gel-shift experiments have shown that the redox state of the protein is an important determinant factor *(56)*. In the presence of reducing agents such as 2-mercaptoethanol and/or dithiothreitol, the RNA binding activity of TS is significantly enhanced. In contrast, the presence of an oxidizing agent such as diamide or N-ethylmaleimide significantly inhibits RNA binding in a dose-dependent manner. In addition to the redox state, it is clear that the protein must be ligand-free for optimal RNA binding activity. When TS is bound by either of its physiologic substrates dUMP and/or CH_2-THF or bound by the 5FU metabolite FdUMP, TS is unable to interact with its own mRNA. The end-result of this disruption in RNA binding is relief of translational repression with resultant new synthesis of TS protein. The inability of substrate-bound TS protein to bind mRNA is most likely caused by a conformational change in TS protein after substrate binding, making the true RNA binding domain no longer accessible. An alternative possibility that has yet to be ruled out is that the substrate and RNA binding domains of the protein may overlap one another.

Recently, efforts have focused on identifying the specific domain(s) on the TS protein that is essential for RNA binding. For these initial studies, various mutant *E. coli* TS proteins were analyzed for their ability to interact with TS mRNA *(57)*. Proteins with point mutations in the nucleotide-binding region with the exception of the highly conserved cysteine (C146S) maintained their ability to bind RNA. In contrast, proteins with point mutations in the folate-binding region completely lost their RNA-binding activity suggesting that this region may represent an important domain for RNA binding. Since the nucleotide- and folate-binding region mutant proteins were both catalytically inactive, these findings also indicate that the functions of RNA binding and enzyme catalysis are not mediated by a common domain on the TS protein.

As a first step towards more precisely defining the region(s) on TS responsible for RNA binding, intact native TS was digested with cyanogen bromide to generate six peptide fragments *(58)*. RNA gel-shift experiments were subsequently performed to identify TS proteolytic fragments that retained RNA-specific binding activity. One such 12,000-kDa fragment was isolated. Peptide sequencing revealed that this fragment corresponded to amino acids 35–140 of the folate-binding domain. Various peptides within this region were chemically synthesized and analyzed for their RNA binding activity. A short 29-amino acid fragment corresponding to amino acids 35–63 was identified that binds TS mRNA with relatively high affinity, albeit 10-fold lower than either *E. coli* or human recombinant TS. Additional studies will be necessary to identify the specific amino acid contact points that directly interact with the TS mRNA.

INTERACTION OF TS WITH CELLULAR RNAs

There is growing evidence in the literature demonstrating that a given RNA-binding protein has the potential to specifically interact with more than one cellular mRNA species. One of the best examples is the iron-responsive factor that binds to at least three different mRNAs, ferritin, transferrin receptor, and erythroid aminolevulinate synthase, and is involved in the coordinate regulation of these genes *(59,60)*. In order to determine whether TS, in its capacity as an RNA-binding protein, could interact with other cellular mRNAs, an immunoprecipitation:RNA-random PCR (rPCR) was developed in our laboratory *(61)*. Using this approach, nine different cellular RNAs were shown to form a ribonucleoprotein (RNP) complex with TS in intact human colon cancer H630 cells *(61)*. Several of these isolated RNA sequences display a high degree of homology to those encoding the human p53 tumor suppressor protein, the c- and L-*myc* family of transcription factors, and the human zinc finger 8 transcription factor, all of which have been felt to play a role in cell growth and metabolism (*see* Fig. 1). Both p53 and c-*myc* encode nuclear phosphoproteins that play essential roles in the regulation of cell cycle progression, DNA synthesis, and apoptosis. Previous studies from this lab showed that TS specifically interacts with the C-terminal coding region of c-*myc* mRNA resulting in its translational repression *(62)*. More recently, we have confirmed the interaction between TS and a 489-nt sequence in the protein-coding region of the human p53 mRNA *(63)*. Whereas the biological significance of this RNA–protein interaction remains to be characterized, preliminary results suggest that p53 mRNA translation is repressed upon binding of TS. These studies suggest that TS may be involved in the coordinate regulation of expression and/or function of genes in addition to its own. This may be especially relevant given the central role of TS in providing the requisite nucleotide substrate for DNA biosynthesis and given that TS, p53, and c-*myc* are critically involved in the regulation of cellular growth and proliferation. Taken together, a model is now beginning to emerge whereby TS appears to serve as an important regulator of certain key aspects of cellular metabolism.

CONCLUSIONS

Thymidylate synthase plays a central role in the biosynthesis of thymidylate, an essential precursor for DNA biosynthesis. It is well-established that transcriptional, posttranscriptional, and translational events are all involved in regulating TS expression as it relates to cell-cycle-associated events and growth proliferation. With regard to the mechanisms underlying the expression of TS in response to chronic drug exposure, gene amplification and enhanced transcription have been shown to play major roles. Translational regulation appears to be the principle mechanism underlying the acute expression of TS in response to treatment with various TS inhibitor compounds. The ability to increase the expression of TS in response to growth stimuli and/or to exposure to cytotoxic agents either on an acute or chronic basis serves as an important adaptive response mechanism that allows for normal cellular synthetic function to be maintained. Recent investigations have shown that in addition to its well-established role in enzyme catalysis, TS can also function as an RNA-binding protein. In this capacity, TS can regulate its own synthesis and that of other critical cellular genes at the translational level (*see* Fig. 1). Clearly, an enhanced understanding of each of these basic regulatory events should provide new insights as to how the expression of TS is controlled. Moreover, these molecular-based investigations may provide important leads for the rational design and development of novel therapeutic approaches that aim to inhibit TS expression.

ACKNOWLEDGMENTS

The authors wish to thank Bruce Chabner, Carmen Allegra, and Frank and Gladys Maley for their valued collaborations, insightful discussions, encouragement, and support throughout this work. We also wish to thank members of our laboratory, both past and present, for their dedicated research efforts and contributions to this work.

REFERENCES

1. Friedkin M, Kornberg A. The enzymatic conversion of deoxyuridylic acid to thymidylic acid and the participation of tetrahydrofolic acid. In: *Chemical Basis of Heredity* (McElroy WO, Glass B, eds.). John Hopkins Press, Maryland, 1957, pp. 609–614.
2. Santi DV, Danenberg PV. Folates in pyrimidine nucleotide biosynthesis. In: *Folates and Pteridines* Vol. 1 (Blakely RL, Benkovic SJ, eds.) Wiley, New York, 1984, pp. 345–398.
3. Danenberg PV. Thymidylate synthase: a target enzyme in cancer chemotherapy. *Biochem Biophys Acta* 1977; 473:73–79.
4. Hardy LW, Finer-Moore JS, Montfort WR, Jones MO, Santi DV, Stroud RM. Atomic structure of thymidylate synthase: target for rational drug design. *Science* 1987; 235:448–455.
5. Berger SH, Jenh CH, Johnson LF, Berger F. Thymidylate synthase overproduction and gene amplification in fluorodeoxyuridine-resistant human cells. *Mol Pharmacol* 1985; 28:461–467.
6. Scanlon KJ, Kashani-Saabet M. Elevated expression of thymidylate synthase cycle genes in cisplatin-resistant human ovarian carcinoma A2780 cells. *Proc Natl Acad Sci USA* 1988; 85:650–653.
7. Chu E, Drake JC, Koeller DM, Zinn S, Jamis-Dow CA, Yeh GC, Allegra CJ. Induction of thymidylate synthase associated with multidrug resistant in human breast and colon cancer cell lines. *Mol Pharmacol* 1991; 39:136–143.
8. Johnston PG, Drake JC, Steinberg SM, Allegra CJ. Quantitation of thymidylate synthase in human tumors using an ultrasensitive enzyme-linked immunoassay. *Biochem Pharm* 1993; 45:2483–2486.
9. Swain SM, Lippman MC, Egan EF, Drake JC, Steinberg SM, Allegra CJ. 5-Fluorouracil and high-dose leucovorin in previously treated patients with metastatic breast cancer. *J Clin Oncol* 1989; 7:890–899.
10. Van der Wilt CL, Pinedo HM, Smit K, Peters GJ. Elevation of thymidylate synthase following 5-fluorouracil treatment is prevented by the addition of leucovorin in murine colon tumors. *J Clin Oncol* 1994; 12:2035–2042.
11. Langebach RJ, Danenberg PV, Heidelberger C. Thymidylate synthetase: mechanism of inhibition by 5-fluoro-2'-deoxyuridylate. *Biochem Biophys Res Commun* 1972; 48:1565–1571.
12. Santi DV, McHenry CS, Sommer H. Mechanism of interaction of thymidylate synthetase with 5-fluorodeoxyuridylate. *Biochemistry* 1974; 13:471–480.
13. Evans RM, Laskin JD, Hakala MT. Effect of excess folates and deoxyinosine on the activity and the site of action of fluorouracil. *Cancer Res* 1981; 41:3288–3295.
14. Houghton JA, Schmidt C, Houghton PJ. The effect of derivatives of folic acid on the fluorodeoxyuridine-thymidylate synthetase covalent complex in human colon xenografts. *Eur J Cancer Clin Oncol* 1982; 18:347–354.

15. Radparvar S, Houghton PJ, Houghton JA. Effect of polyglutamation of 5,10-methylenetetrahydrofolate on the binding of 5-fluoro-2'-deoxyuridylate to thymidylate synthase purified from a human colon adenocarcinoma xenograft. *Biochem Pharmacol* 1989; 38:335–342.
16. Keyomarsi K, Moran RG. Folinic acid augmentation of the effects of fluoropyrimidines on murine and human leukemic cells. *Cancer Res* 1988; 46:5229–5235.
17. Mini E, Mazzei T, Coronnello M. Effects of 5-methyltetrahydrofolate on the activity of fluoropyrimidines against human leukemia (CCRF-CEM) cells. *Biochem Pharmacol* 1987; 36:2905–2911.
18. Petrelli N, Douglas HO Jr, Herrera L, Rusell D, Stablein DM, Bruckner HW, Schinella R, Green MD, Muggia RM, Megibow A, Greenwald ES, Levin B, Gaynor E, Loutfi A, Kalser MH, Barkin JS, Benedatta P, Woolley PV, Nauta R, Weaver DW, Leichman LP. The modulation of fluorouracil with leucovorin in metastatic colorectal carcinoma: a prospective randomized phase III trial. *J Clin Oncol* 1989; 7:1419–1426.
19. Erlichman C, Fine S, Wong A, Elhakim T. A randomized trial of fluorouracil and folinic acid in patients with metastatic colorectal carcinoma. *J Clin Oncol* 1988; 6:469–475.
20. Doroshow JH, Multhauf P, Leong L, Margolin K, Litchfield T, Akman S, Carr B, Bertrand M, Goldberg D, Blayney D. Prospective randomized comparison of fluorouracil versus fluorouracil and high-dose continuous infusion leucovorin calcium for the treatment of advanced colorectal cancer in patients previously unexposed to chemotherapy. *J Clin Oncol* 1990; 8:491–501.
21. Poon MA, O'Connell MJ, Moertel CG, Wieand HS, Cullinan SA, Everson LK, et al. Biochemical modulation of fluorouracil: evidence of significant improvement of survival and quality of life in patients with advanced colorectal carcinoma. *J Clin Oncol* 1989; 7:1407–1418.
22. Advanced colorectal cancer meta-analysis project. Modulation of fluorouracil by leucovorin in patients with advanced colorectal cancer: evidence in terms of response rate. *J Clin Oncol* 1992; 10:896–903.
23. Cunningham D, Zalcberg JR, Rath U, Olver I, Van Cutsem E, Svensson C, et al. 'Tomudex' Colorectal Cancer Study Group. 'Tomudex' (ZD1694): results of a randomized trial in advanced colorectal cancer demonstrate efficacy and reduced mucositis and leucopenia. *Eur J Cancer* 1995; 12:1945–1954.
24. Zalcberg JR, Cunningham D, Van Cutsem E, Francois E, Schornagel J, Adenis A, Green M, Iveson A, Azab M, Seymour I. ZD1694: a novel thymidylate synthase inhibitor with substantial activity in the treatment of patients with advanced colorectal cancer. *J Clin Oncol* 1996; 14:716–721.
25. Pazdur R, Vincent M. Raltrixed (Tomudex) versus 5-fluorouracil and leucovorin (5-FU + LV) in patients with advanced colorectal cancer (ACC): results of a randomized multicenter, North American trial. *Proc Am Soc Clin Oncol* 1997; 22:228a.
26. Schimke RT. Gene amplification in cultured animal cells. *Cell* 1984; 37:705–513.
27. Copur S, Aiba K, Drake JC, Allegra CJ, Chu E. Thymidylate synthase gene amplification in human colon cancer cell lines resistance to 5-fluorouracil. *Biochem Pharmacol* 1995; 49:1419–1426.
28. Danenberg KD, Danenberg PV. Activity of thymidylate synthetase and its inhibition by 5-fluorouracil in 10-propargyl-5,8-dideazafolate. *Mol Pharmacol* 1989; 36:219–223.
29. Imam A, Crossley PH, Jackman AL, Little P. Analysis of thymidylate synthase gene amplification and of mRNA levels in the cell cycle. *J Biol Chem* 1989; 36:219–223.
30. Drake JC, Allegra CJ, Moran RG, Johnston PG. Resistance to Tomudex (ZD1694) is multifactorial in human breast and colon carcinoma cell lines. *Biochem Pharm* 1996; 51:1349–1355.
31. Clark JL, Berger SH, Mittleman A, Berger F. Thymidylate synthase gene amplification in a colon tumor resistant to fluoropyrimidine chemotherapy. *Cancer Treat Rep* 1987; 71:261–265.
32. Conrad AH. TS activity in cultured mammalian cells. *J Biol Chem* 1971; 246:1318–1323.
33. McIntosh EM, Ord RW, Storms RK. Cell cycle-dependent expression of thymidylate synthase in Saccharomyces cerevisiae. *Mol Cell Biol* 1988; 8:4616–4624.
34. Navalgund LG, Rossana C, Muench AL, Johnson JL. Cell cycle regulation of thymidylate synthetase gene expression in cultured mouse fibroblasts. *J Biol Chem* 1980; 255:7386–7390.
35. Ayusawa D, Shimizu K, Koyama H, Kaneda S, Takeishi K, Seno T. Cell cycle-directed regulation of thymidylate synthase messenger RNA in human diploid fibroblasts stimulated to proliferate. *J Mol Biol* 1986; 190:559–567.
36. Li D, Osborn K, Johnson LF. The 5'-flanking region of the mouse TS gene is necessary but not sufficient for normal regulation in growth stimulated cells. *Mol Cell Biol* 1991; 11:1023–1029.
37. Horie N, Takeishi K. Identification of functional elements in the promoter region of the human gene for thymidylate synthase and nuclear factors that regulate the expression of the gene. *J Biol Chem* 1997; 272:18,375–18,381.

38. Joliff K, Li Y, Johnson LF. Multiple protein-DNA interaction in the TATAA-less mouse thymidylate synthase promoter. *Nucleic Acids Res* 1991; 19:2267–2274.
39. Farnham PJ, Slansky JE, Kollmar R. The role of E2F in the mammalian cell cycle. *Biochem Biophys Acta Rev Cancer* 1993; 1155:125–131.
40. Ash J, Liao W, Ke Y, Johnson LF. Regulation of mouse thymidylate synthase gene expression in growth-stimulated cells: upstream S phase control elements are indistinguishable from the essential promoter elements. *Nucleic Acid Res* 1995; 23:4649–4656.
41. Ash J, Ke Y, Korb M, Johnson LF. Introns are essential for growth-regulated expression of the mouse thymidylate synthase gene. *Mol Cell Biol* 1993; 13:1565–1571.
42. Takayanagi A, Kaneda S, Ayusawa D, Seno T. Intron 1 and the 5'-flanking region of the human thymidylate synthase genes as a regulatory determinant of growth-dependent expression. *Nucleic Acids Res* 1992; 20:4021–4025.
43. Labow R, Maley GF, Maley F. The effect of methotrexate on enzymes induced following partial hepatectomy. *Cancer Res* 1969; 29:366–372.
44. Washtein WL. Increased levels of thymidylate synthetase in cells exposed to 5-fluorouracil. *Mol Pharmacol* 1984; 25:171–177.
45. Keyomarsi K, Moran RG. Mechanism of the cytotoxic synergism of fluoropyrimidines and folinic acid in mouse leukemic cells. *J Biol Chem* 1998; 263:14,402–14,409.
46. Keyomarsi K, Samet J, Molnar G, Pardee AB. The thymidylate synthase inhibitor, ICI D1694, overcomes translational detainment of the enzyme. *J Biol Chem* 1993; 268:15,142–15,149.
47. Chu E, Koeller DM, Johnston PG, Zinn S, Allegra CJ. Regulation of thymidylate synthase in human colon cancer cells treated with 5-fluorouracil and interferon-gamma. *Mol Pharmacol* 1993; 43:527–533.
48. Belfort M, Maley G, Pedersen-Lane J, Maley F. Primary structure of the *Escherichia coli thyA* gene and its thymidylate synthase product. *Proc Natl Acad Sci USA* 1983; 80:4914–4918.
49. Thorndike J, Kisliuk RL. Identification of poly G bound to thymidylate synthase. *Biochem Biophys Res Commun* 1986; 139:461–465.
50. Takeishi K, Kaneda S, Ayusawa D, Shimizu K, Gotoh O, Seno T. Nucleotide sequence of a functional cDNA for human thymidylate synthase. *Nucleic Acids Res* 1985; 13:2035–2043.
51. Kaneda S, Takeishi K, Ayusawa D, Shimizu K, Seno T, Altman S. Role in translation of a triple tandemly repeated sequence in the 5'-untranslated region of human thymidylate synthase mRNA. *Nucleic Acids Res* 1987; 15:1259–1270.
52. Chu E, Koeller DM, Casey JL, Drake JC, Chabner BA, Elwood PC, Zinn S, Allegra CJ. Autoregulation of human thymidylate synthase messenger RNA translation by thymidylate synthase. *Proc Natl Acad Sci USA* 1991; 88:8977–8981.
53. Chu E, Voeller D, Koeller DM, Drake JC, Takimoto CH, Maley GF, Maley F, Allegra CJ. Identification of an RNA binding site for human thymidylate synthase. *Proc Natl Acad Sci USA* 1993; 90:517–521.
54. Kozak M. Structural features in eukaryotic mRNAs that modulate the initiation of translation. *J Biol Chem* 1991; 266:19,867–19,870.
55. McCarthy JEG, Kolimus H. Cytoplasmic mRNA-protein interactions in eukaryotic gene expression. *Trends Biochem Sci* 1995; 20:191–197.
56. Chu E, Voeller DM, Morrison PF, Jones KL, Takechi T, Maley GF, Maley F, Allegra CJ. The effect of reducing reagents on binding of thymidylate synthase protein to thymidylate synthase messenger RNA. *J Biol Chem* 1994; 269:20,289–20,293.
57. Voeller DM, Changchien L, Maley GF, Maley F, Takechi T, Turner RE, Montfort WR, Allegra CJ, Chu E. Characterization of a specific interaction between *Escherichia coli* thymidylate synthase and *Escherichia coli* thymidylate synthase mRNA. *Nucleic Acids Res* 1995; 23:869–875.
58. Voeller DM, Maley GF, Maley F, Changchien L, Allegra CJ, Chu E. Identification of an RNA-binding domain of *E. coli* thymidylate synthase (TS). *Proc Am Assoc Cancer Res* 1996; 37:406.
59. Klausner RD, Rouault TA, Harford JB. Regulating the fate of mRNA: the control of cellular iron metabolism. *Cell* 1993; 72:19–28.
60. Melefors O, Hentze MW. Translational regulation by mRNA/protein interactions in eukaryotic cells: ferritin and beyond. *BioEssays* 1993; 15:85–90.
61. Chu E, Cogliati T, Copur, SM, Borre A, Voeller DM, Allegra CJ, Segal S. Identification of *in vivo* target RNA sequences bound by thymidylate synthase. *Nucleic Acids Res* 1996; 24:3222–3228.

62. Chu E, Takechi T, Jones KL, Voeller DM, Copur SM, Maley GF, Maley F, Segal S, Allegra CJ. Thymidylate synthase binds to *c-myc* RNA in human colon cancer cells and *in vitro*. *Mol Cell Biol* 1995; 15:179–185.
63. Chu E, Copur S, Jones KL, Khleif S, Voeller D, Maley GF, Maley F, Allegra CJ. Thymidylate synthase binds to p53 RNA. *Proc Am Assoc Cancer Res* 1995; 36:563.

20 The Role of Uracil Misincorporation in Thymineless Death

G. Wynne Aherne and Sherael Brown

CONTENTS
INTRODUCTION
EVIDENCE FOR URACIL MISINCORPORATION
CONCLUSIONS
REFERENCES

1. INTRODUCTION

The biochemical consequences of thymidylate synthase (TS) inhibition are well known and shown diagramatically in Fig. 1. TS catalyzes the reductive methylation of dUMP to form thymidylate (dTMP), which is a rate-limiting step for the *de novo* synthesis of dTTP the only deoxynucleotide required exclusively for DNA synthesis. The methyl group involved in the reaction is donated by 5,10-methylene tetrahydrofolic acid. When the enzyme is inhibited dTMP pools (and subsequently dTTP pools) are depleted and dUMP accumulates behind the enzyme block because of loss of feedback inhibition by dTTP on three enzymes, ribonucleotide reductase, deoxycytidylate deaminase, and thymidine kinase *(1)*.

The term "thymineless death" was first coined in 1954 and used to describe the biochemical status of an *Escherichia coli* thymine-requiring mutant that lost viability within one generation when placed in medium lacking thymine *(2)*. Later studies showed that the bacteriostatic effects of sulfanilamide were caused by an induced thymineless and purineless state. However if a source of purines was provided the drug was bactericidal and a state of "unbalanced growth" occurred in which there was continued synthesis of protein and RNA even though DNA synthesis was inhibited and cells had arrested in S-phase *(3)*. The characteristics of thymineless death have since been reviewed *(4,5)*. It is widely accepted that unbalanced growth is a feature of cells treated with antifolates and other compounds that inhibit TS, causing depletion of intracellular dTTP pools. Unbalanced growth needs to persist for some time (approx one generation time) before cells are committed to loss of viability *(6–8)*, but precise molecular mechanisms and events

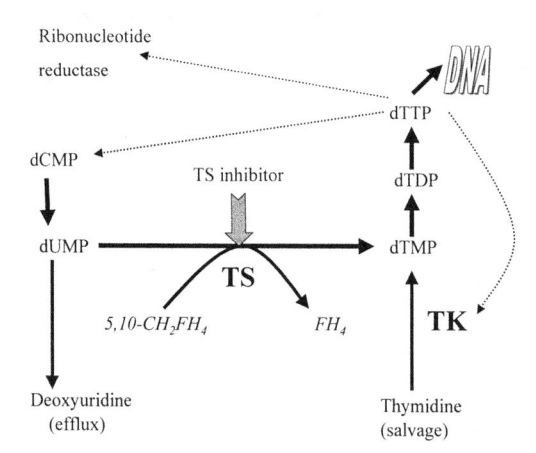

Fig. 1. The reaction catalyzed by thymidylate synthase. Dotted lines show negative feedback effects of dTTP pools. Inhibition of the enzyme causes depletion of dTTP pools and elevation of dUMP pools.

downstream of TS inhibition that explain cell death are still unclear (9–12 and Chapter 21 this volume).

Inhibition of TS results in a series of complex biochemical events. Through various feedback and regulatory mechanisms, dTTP depletion causes marked perturbations in other intracellular deoxynucleotide (dCTP, dGTP, and dATP) pools (13). The profound effects of imbalances in DNA precursor pools on genetic stability and cytotoxicity have recently been reviewed (14). Inhibition of TS by fluorodeoxyuridine (FUdR), for example, in mouse FM3a cells (15) caused depletion of intracellular dTTP pools with subsequent inhibition of DNA synthesis. An imbalance of dNTP pools (elevation of dATP and depletion of dTTP and dGTP) was also observed leading to DNA damage. It was concluded that this dNTP pool imbalance was the event that triggered cell death by the induction of endonuclease activity (16). Later work also showed that treatment of L1210 cells with methotrexate (MTX) (17) and CB3717 (18) resulted in a marked perturbation of the dTTP/dATP ratio leading to cytotoxicity. Similar observations were made in human colon-carcinoma cell lines (GC3/cl and a clonally derived TS$^-$ mutant) treated with 5-fluorouracil and leucovorin (19). It was concluded that elevated dATP pools maintained during TTP depletion were essential for cells to commit to thymineless death. dUTP was not detected in these drug-treated cells.

Another mechanism of cell death in TS inhibited cells that is now widely accepted is that of uracil misincorporation. Although DNA polymerases (20) can utilize dTTP and dUTP with equal efficacy, uracil is not normally found in DNA. This is primarily because of the activity of two enzymes: the pyrophosphatase dUTPase (21) (EC 3.6.1.23) limits the amounts of dUTP found intracellularly and uracil-DNA glycosylase (UDG)(22) (EC 3.2.2.3) rapidly excises any uracil that is found in DNA. However, TS inhibition can lead to the formation of significantly increased quantities of dUMP (23–25). If not effluxed from the cell as deoxyuridine, dUMP is converted to dUTP, which if present in sufficient quantity can overwhelm dUTPase, resulting in misincorporation of uracil into DNA. The fraudulent base is rapidly removed from DNA by UDG but in the presence of a greatly increased dUTP/dTTP ratio the apyrimidinic site is likely

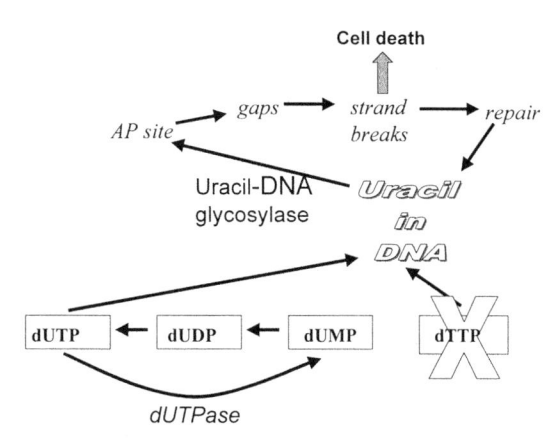

Fig. 2. The uracil misincorporation pathway.

to be refilled by uracil. This leads to a futile cycle of misincorporation, excision, repair, and further misincorporation resulting in DNA strand breaks and eventually cell death (Fig. 2). This process has been used to explain DNA damage and mutagenic events that occur during nutritional folate deficiency *(26,27)* and following spontaneous deamination of cytosine residues in DNA *(28,29)*.

In this chapter the evidence for uracil misincorporation as a mechanism of cell death in TS inhibited cells will be reviewed and the role of cellular expression of dUTPase examined.

2. EVIDENCE FOR URACIL MISINCORPORATION

2.1. Studies on Prokaryotypic Systems

The hypothesis that uracil misincorporation could lead to cell death in TS-inhibited cells was originally based on the study of bacterial mutants. An apparent increase in short, Okazaki DNA fragments was detected in dUTPase deficient mutants of *E. coli* *(30)* compared with revertants that had regained dUTPase activity. Subsequent studies using various bacterial dUTPase or UDG mutants showed that the increase in short DNA fragments was related to increasing levels of dUTP and subsequent excision repair *(31–33)*. These studies also suggested that the presence of some of the small Okazaki-sized DNA precursors in normal (wild-type) cells were caused by this repair mechanism *(30)*. Also it was shown that DNA with as much as 30% replacement of thymine by uracil was transcriptionally functional provided the DNA is not repaired by UDG *(34)*.

The isolation of UDG from human cells *(35)*, implied that DNA damage in mammalian cells could be caused by uracil misincorporation. Even very small amounts of dUTP (2.5%) in the presence of dTTP in an in vitro system that synthesised polyoma DNA in isolated cell nuclei, caused a transient accumulation of Okazaki fragments *(36)*. Uracil misincorporation into DNA was determined by including radioactive deoxyuridine into the cell system. Radiolabeled dNTP was almost completely recovered from the DNA fragments and addition of uracil (an inhibitor of UDG) increased total synthesis of DNA and produced longer strands of daughter DNA. The interpretation of these results was that an excision-repair mechanism for removing uracil from DNA existed in mammalian cells and that the process caused damage to DNA resulting in increased formation of small (4s) fragments of DNA. Similar conclusions were drawn from results obtained using lysates of human cultured lymphocytes *(37)*, i.e., high levels of dUTP relative to dTTP could interfere with the synthesis of DNA. Such observations led the way to studies in mammalian tumor cells exposed to compounds that resulted in thymineless death.

2.2. Early Studies in Mammalian Cells

Because of the wide interest in and clinical use of TS inhibitors for the treatment of malignancy it became increasingly important to elucidate the biochemical mechanisms underlying their cytotoxicity. The development of specific TS inhibitors *(38)* later allowed the cytotoxic effects of reduced dTTP pools to be investigated without the complications in interpretation that the use of compounds with more than one locus of action, such as MTX and fluorouracil, presented.

In the early 1980s there were a number of publications that examined the role of uracil misincorporation in cells treated with compounds known to deplete dTTP pools. Thus treatment of cells with MTX (in the presence of radioactive deoxyuridine) was shown to result in the measurement of radioactivity in DNA whereas none could be measured in untreated cells *(39)*. Again the addition of uracil increased the amount of radioactivity present in DNA, allowing the conclusion that one of the mechanisms of excluding dUTP from DNA was being inhibited by addition of the nucleoside. The same authors *(40)* also showed that in cultured human lymphoblasts treated with MTX, TTP pools were substantially depleted, dUMP pools increased 1000-fold, and that dUTP was measured in treated but not untreated cells resulting in markedly increased dUTP/dTTP ratios. Further evidence in support of uracil misincorporation following treatment of human lymphoblastic and leukemic cell lines with antifolates was also reported, for example with metoprim *(41)*, FUdR *(42)*, and piritrexim *(43)*. Indirect evidence that uracil misincorporation has a role to play in the damaging effects of antifolates was also presented in this latter paper. Drug resistance was established in cells (MOLT-4) treated with the piritrexim alone although it was not possible to establish resistance when cells were coexposed to the antifolate and deoxyuridine (10 μM).

In 1986 Fraser and Pearson expressed a note of caution despite the increasing evidence that uracil misincorporation was a mechanism of cell death *(44)*. They could not detect any uracil in DNA in either HeLa or CCRF-HSB2 human lymphoblastoid cells treated with MTX in either the presence or absence of 10 mM uracil. In another study, L1210 cells treated for 16 h at growth-inhibitory concentrations with the specific TS inhibitor CB3717, accumulated only traces of dUTP (1–2 pmol/10^6; undetected in untreated cells) even though dTTP was depleted and dUMP elevated 23-fold compared to control cells. In addition, cytotoxicity was not potentiated as would be expected in the presence of exogenous deoxyuridine or reduced by blocking the accumulation of deoxyuridylate with either PALA or pyrazofurin *(23)*. In a later study using the same cell line and the specific TS inhibitor ZD1694, a similar amount of dUTP was formed in spite of substantially reduced dTTP and elevated pools of dUMP *(25)* even though the cells were treated with doses equivalent to 50–100X IC$_{50}$. In general, cell lines of hemapoetic origin appear to accumulate very little or no dUTP (and express high levels of dUTPase). This may represent a mechanism for protecting the stem cells during hematopoesis.

"Why do antifolate-treated cells die?" This question was addressed in 1987 *(45)*. In the author's opinion, DNA lesions caused by the uracil misincorporation excision/repair process presented a plausible explanation for cell death in antifolate-treated cells, but two pieces of evidence were missing. It was vitally important to show that DNA damage and cytotoxicity was related to the accumulation of dUTP. Also the relationship between variations in dUTPase and UDG activity or expression and cytotoxicity had not been addressed. As most of the work at this time had been carried out using human cells of hemopoetic origin, cells from a variety of other tissues needed to be studied to obtain a wider perspective on the importance of uracil misincorporation.

2.3. dUTP Accumulation and dUTPase Expression

The importance of salvage mechanisms to the growth inhibitory and cytotoxic effects of antimetabolites is well known *(46)*. Of relevance to the present discussion, exogenous thymidine was shown to provide protection from the antitumor properties of the specific TS inhibitor CB3717 and prevent its growth inhibitory effects *(47,48)*. In tissue culture, nontoxic doses of dipyridamole (a nucleoside transport inhibitor) could reverse this protection *(48)*. As the effect was greater than could be achieved by limiting thymidine in the medium it was thought that dipyridamole also prevented efflux of deoxyuridine, thereby helping to maintain deoxyuridine nucleotide pools. Essentially the same conclusion was reached when increased dUMP pools were observed following treatment of cells with fluorouracil and dipyridamole *(49)*.

It could be predicted from these observations that in the presence of dipyridamole intracellular pools of dUTP following TS inhibition would be further enhanced over those formed in the absence of dipyridamole thus potentiating cytotoxicity. This study showed that dUTP accumulation, measured by specific radioimmunoassay *(50)*, was dose- and time-related and dipyridamole enhanced dUTP formation in A549 human lung carcinoma cells treated with CB3717 (1X and 10X IC_{50}) *(51)*. dUTP accumulation was an early event. By 4 h, dUTP pools in cells treated at the IC_{50} were approx 3 times higher than untreated controls and dipyridamole (10 μM) potentiated these 10-fold. These increased dUTP pools correlated not only with growth-inhibitory effects but also with DNA damage measured by alkaline elution. An increase in damage in nascent DNA was detectable following a 4 h exposure to CB3717, showing that DNA damage was also an early event. When all results of CB3717 alone and CB3717 with dipyridamole were combined, there was a significant correlation between dUTP pools and DNA strand breaks. Newly synthesized DNA was more sensitive to the effects of CB3717 than mature DNA, an observation that may have been expected from previous observations on the effect of increased dUTP/dTTP ratios on Okazaki fragment formation. The damaging effects of CB3717 on mature DNA would result from the inability to repair apyrimidimic sites when the cell is deplete in dTTP but fortified with dUTP.

Compelling evidence for the importance of the uracil misincorporation pathway in TS-inhibitor-mediated cell death has been presented more recently in three key papers. Firstly, DNA damage patterns in three human colorectal-tumor cell lines treated with FUdR or CB3717 exhibited marked variation *(52)*. Similarly sized DNA fragments were obtained in HT29 and SW620 cells although the latter line was less sensitive to the drugs. Either longer exposure times or increased drug concentrations were required to obtain the same degree of DNA damage as occurred in HT29 cells. As TS was equally inhibited in both cell lines, it was proposed that some event following enzyme inhibition, e.g., in the uracil misincorporation pathway was responsible for conferring this resistance.

A subsequent study *(53)* compared in detail the effects of TS inhibition by FUdR in these two human colorectal-tumor cell lines by measurement of dUTPase activity, dUTP accumulation, DNA damage, and loss of colony formation. It was concluded that the resistance of SW620 cells, as measured by clonogenic assay and DNA damage, was caused by a 4.4-fold higher dUTPase activity than in HT29 cells. This resulted in a 45-fold lower accumulation of dUTP (2.0 ± 0.7 pmol/10^6 cells) compared with HT29 cells (90.4 ± 27.3 pmol/10^6 cells). This not unexpected finding highlighted the importance of biochemical events downstream of TS inhibition and the role of dUTPase in determining cytotoxicity in cells in which TS is effectively inhibited, i.e., in the thymineless state.

Thirdly, the most convincing evidence that dUTPase is critically involved in mediating a cytotoxic event in TS-inhibited cells has come from studies using cells transfected with the enzyme *(54)*. The HT29 human colorectal-tumor cell line transfected with *E. coli* dUTPase was protected from FUdR-induced DNA damage and cytotoxicity. Compared to the neotransfected control cells this protection was afforded by a four- to five-fold higher enzyme activity. These results are similar to our own obtained with ZD9331, a nonpolyglutamatable specific TS inhibitor *(55)*. The neotransfected cells lost the ability to form colonies 4–24 h following drug exposure (1 μM ZD9331). This compares to the dUTPase transfected cells in which a cytotoxic effect was not observed until 24–48 h *(56)*. We also showed that the accumulation of dUTP was significantly attenuated in the dUTPase-transfected cells (27.8 ± 8.4 vs 41.7 ± 2.6 pmol/10^6 cells).

The recent use of cells transfected with antisense dUTPase cDNA represents an elegant approach to exemplifying the importance of dUTPase activity *(57)*. HT29 cells were transfected with either sense or antisense expressing constructs of human nuclear dUTPase. Transfected cells that underexpress dUTPase (antisense) were more sensitive to FUdR than overexpressing cells (sense). This evidence of sensitisation to the effects of TS inhibition is a convincing demonstration of the role of dUTPase in promoting resistance to TS inhibitors.

However, evidence in support of mechanisms of cell death other than that of uracil misincorporation continues to be presented. Thymineless death has been compared in HCT-8 human colorectal cells and MOLT4 leukemic cells. Although both cell lines die in an apoptotic process following treatment with the specific antifolate TS inhibitor 1843U89, DNA fragmentation patterns were different *(58)*. It was shown that only HCT-8 cells accumulated dUTP and incorporated uracil in DNA in a dose-dependent way. It was concluded that uracil misincorporation was not a factor in cell death and that apoptosis was initiated by increased dATP pools in the dTTP depleted state (*see* Chapter 21).

Following from earlier results *(54)*, dUTPase transfected cells and neotransfected control cells were exposed to MTX and CB3717 for 24 h *(59)*. Significant resistance to DNA damage and cytotoxicity in the transfected cell line was demonstrated over 24 h. However after longer exposure times, there was no difference in survival even though DNA damage was greater in the neotransfected controls. It was suggested that DNA damage caused by uracil misincorporation is time-dependent and that longer exposure periods result in cytotoxic events caused by alternative mechanisms (presumably those initiated by dTTP depletion).

Our own work using several human tumor cell lines, has shown that the amount of dUTP accumulated over 24 h following exposure to ZD9331 was inversely related to dUTPase expression *(60)* or activity *(61)*. But dUTP accumulation did not correlate with growth inhibition determined using the 5-d MTT assay. ZD9331 (1 μM) was more cytotoxic to A549 human lung carcinoma cells over 24 h (approx 8% survival) compared with MOR lung carcinoma cell lines (approx 60% survival). A549 cells accumulate significant pools of dUTP (66 ± pmol/10^6 cells) but no dUTP was formed in the MOR cells in this period. However the A549 cell line (IC_{50} 70nM) was less sensitive to ZD9331 than the MOR cells (IC_{50} 7.3 nM) as determined by MTT assay. These results imply that DNA damage because of uracil misincorporation in those cells that can accumulate dUTP is an early event and that other events as a consequence of pool perturbations secondary to dTTP depletion may initiate later cell death mechanisms.

2.4. dUTPase Characterisation and Expression

dUTPase is a ubiquitous enzyme, largely conserved throughout evolution, whose main function is to maintain low intracellular levels of dUTP. It is a pyrophosphatase, converting dUTP to dUMP and pyrophosphate. Earliest studies on dUTPase were carried out in bacterial systems and it has since been determined that it is an essential enzyme in *E. coli* and *S. cerevisiae (62,63)*. The effects of functional mutations in *E. coli* dUTPase have already been described. The human enzyme from several cell types has been purified and characterized *(64–66)*. The latter report showed that the enzyme has a molecular size of 45,000 daltons and consists of two identical monomers that associate in the presence of divalent cations such as Mg^{2+}. The enzyme (K_m 2.5 μM) is specific for dUTP although FdUTP is also converted to the monophosphate form by this enzyme *(67)*. Further characterization has been achieved using cDNA probes *(68,69)* and by resolution of the crystal structure of the enzyme complexed to deoxyuridine nucleotides *(70,71)*. The latter studies showed that the enzyme was a homotrimer with three active sites. The discrepancy between the reported dimeric and trimeric structures of dUTPase has not been explained. The amino acid sequences for dUTPase from several species including viral sequences have been compared *(72)*. Two distinct forms of dUTPase have been identified in human cells *(69,73)*: A more abundant but smaller enzyme that is localized in the nucleus and a mitochondrial form with slightly higher mass. These isoforms have the same K_m for dUTP, and are encoded by the same gene. The sequence of the cDNAs is identical except for slight differences in the amino terminus.

Evidence has accumulated to show that dUTPase activity is cell-cycle dependent *(74–76)*. Stimulation of peripheral blood lymphocytes results in phosphorylation of dUTPase at the onset of DNA synthesis *(77)* and recent evidence has shown that phosphorylation occurs on a single serine residue on the nuclear form of dUTPase. The phosphorylation site corresponded to the target sequence for cyclin-dependent phosphorylation by p34^{cdc2} *(78)*. At the onset of DNA synthesis, the nuclear form of the enzyme is induced but expression of the mitochondrial form is not effected by cell cycle changes *(79)*.

Immunological studies have shown that dUTPase is widely distributed in the tissues *(79,80)* with higher levels of expression in more rapidly dividing tissues. There was strong association between the extent of dUTPase nuclear staining and the staining obtained for the proliferation marker *Ki* 67. This was also true when a variety of neoplastic tissues were studied.

There is now strong evidence that the cellular expression of dUTPase can vary dramatically. We have shown considerable variation in dUTPase expression across human ovarian, colorectal, and lung tumor cell line panels using immunoblotting (unpublished results). This is in accord with previous results obtained on 46 cell lines in which dUTPase activity was shown to vary 70-fold. Parenthetically there was a similarly wide range in UDG activity *(81)*. Preliminary studies in our laboratory have indicated that dUTPase may be under selective pressure in TS inhibited cells. In two W1L2 human lymphoblastoid cell lines with acquired resistance to either ZD9331 (unpublished results) or ZM24914 *(82)* there was 40- and 20-fold increased TS activity compared to the parent cell line. However both resistant lines also showed increased expression (and activity) of dUTPase by immunoblotting (two- to threefold) compared to the parent cell line. Whether increased dUTPase expression following exposure to TS inhibitors occurs clinically remains to be determined.

Because of the protective effect high dUTPase expression may have on the clinical response to TS inhibitors and its cell-cycle-regulated activity, the enzyme has often been proposed as a target for the development of chemotherapeutic agents *(72)*. However very few inhibitors have been described. Six uracil analogs inhibited the enzyme in either intact cells or crude cell extracts and increased the DNA-damaging effects of MTX when used at a concentration of 0.1 m*M (81)*. Several mercury (II) compounds were found to inhibit dUTPase, but potency against the human enzyme was low *(83)*. A series of substrate analog inhibitors of dUTPase showed a time- and dose-dependent growth inhibition of human tumor cell lines that was selective compared with a nontransformed fibroblast control *(84)*. The future availability of potent selective inhibitors of dUTPase may provide the tools to further investigate the importance of dUTPase although their use as therapeutic agents or modulators of TS inhibitors remains to be determined.

3. CONCLUSIONS

Undoubtedly there is now a large body of evidence that in principle supports uracil misincorporation as a mechanism of promoting DNA damage and cell death in TS-inhibited cells. This evidence includes the dose- and time-related accumulation of dUTP and the correlation of intracellular dUTP pools with both DNA damage and loss of clonogenicity. The ability to accumulate dUTP during inhibition of TS is largely determined by the activity of dUTPase. But this pathway is not the only mechanism by which cells die following exposure to TS inhibitors.

The evidence suggests that another pathway plays a major role in the cytotoxic effects of TS inhibitors. Inhibition of TS *per se* resulting in TTP depletion and subsequent cellular perturbations in deoxynucleotide ratios is a lethal event. The cells will be arrested at the G1/S border by checkpoint controls within a period of time that may approximate to a generation (cell-cycle) time. Subsequent perturbations in dNTP pools (e.g., dATP/dTTP ratio) and cessation of DNA synthesis will initiate downstream events leading to cell death. As long as TS can be inhibited in the cells for this critical time, the consequence will be cell death. Thus is DNA damage caused by dUTP accumulation important? Several studies have shown that DNA damage because of uracil misincorporation occurs during the first 24 h of drug exposure when (with cells in culture) a substantial proportion will be actively replicating DNA. But it has also been shown that the differential effect of uracil misincorporation on cell death (as measured clonogenically) is short-lived. When cells that accumulate dUTP and those that do not are compared over longer exposure periods, differences in survival are not evident. In the clinical situation in which the duration of TS inhibition is not as easy to control as in cell culture, this early damage to the viability of the cell may become an important event. It is likely that cells die by a combination of the effects of dTTP depletion and uracil misincorporation. In addition the complexities of the many downstream events controlling apoptosis and cell-cycle arrest that are frequently disrupted in malignant cells will also be of enormous importance.

Thus almost half a century after antifolates were introduced into the clinic, precise mechanisms of cell death in thymineless cells have not been defined. Further studies using genetically characterized cell lines may facilitate our understanding of these processes and those of other downstream events. In spite of compelling evidence in favor of uracil misincorporation, it should not be assumed that this is the mechanism by which TS-inhibited cells die. Rather it is likely that cells die because of the combined effect of dTTP depletion and uracil misincorporation and the importance of the latter will depend on the specific expression of the major enzymes (dUTPase and UDG) involved in the process.

4. REFERENCES

1. Jackson RC. The regulation of thymidylate biosynthesis in Novikoff hepatoma cells and the effects of amethopterin, 5-fluorodeoxyuridine and 3-deazauridine. *J Biol Chem* 1978; 253:7440–7446.
2. Cohen SS, Barner HD. Studies on unbalanced growth in *Escherichia coli. Proc Natl Acad Sci USA* 1954; 40:885–893.
3. Cohen SS, Barner HD. Studies on the induction of thymine deficiency and on the effects of thymidine and thymidine analogues in *Escherichia coli. J Bacteriol* 1956; 71:588–596.
4. Cohen SS. On the nature of thymineless death. *Ann NY Acad Sci* 1971; 186:292–301.
5. Barclay BJ, Kunz BA, Little JG, Haynes RH. Genetic and biochemical consequences of thymidylate stress. *Can J Biochem* 1982; 60:172–193.
6. Rueckert RR, Mueller GC. Studies on unbalanced growth in tissue culture: induction and consequences of thymidine deficiency. *Cancer Res* 1960; 20:1584–1591.
7. Yin M-B, Guimaraes MA, Zhang Z-G, Arrendondo MA, Rustum YM. Time dependence of DNA lesions and growth inhibition by ICI D1694, a new quinazoline antifolate thymidylate synthase inhibitor. *Cancer Res* 1992; 52:5900–5905.
8. Smith SG, Lehman NL, Moran RG. Cytotoxicity of antifolate inhibitors of thymidylate and purine synthesis to WiDr colonic carcinoma cells. *Cancer Res* 1993; 53:5697–5706.
9. Houghton JA, Harwood FG, Houghton PJ. Cell cycle processes determine cytostasis or cytotoxicity in thymineless death of colon cancer cells. *Cancer Res* 1994; 54:4967–4973.
10. Harwood, FG, Frazier MW, Krajewski S, Reed, JC, Houghton JA. Acute and delayed apoptosis induced by thymidine deprivation correlates with expression of p53 and p53-regulated genes in colon carcinoma cells. *Oncogene* 1996; 12:2057–2067.
11. Matsui S-I, Arredondo, MA, Wrzosek C, Rustum YM. DNA damage and p53 induction do not cause ZD1694-induced cell cycle arrest in human colon carcinoma cells. *Cancer Res* 1996; 56:4715–4723.
12. Houghton JA, Harwood FG, Tillman DM. Thymineless death in colon carcinoma cells is mediated via Fas signalling. *Proc Natl Acad Sci USA* 1997; 94:8144–8149.

13. Jackson RC, Grindey GB. The biochemical basis for methotrexate cytotoxicity. In: (Sirotnak FM, Burchall JJ, Ensminger WD, Montgomery JA, eds.) Folate Antagonists as Therapeutic Agents. 1, Biochemistry, Molecular Actions, and Synthetic Design. Academic, New York, 1984; pp. 289–315.
14. Kunz BA, Kohalmi SE, Kunkel TA, Mathews CK, McIntish EM Reidy JA. Deoxyribonucleoside triphosphate levels: a critical factor in the maintenance of genetic stability. *Mutation Res* 1994; 318:1–64.
15. Yoshioka A, Tanaka S, Hiraoka O, Koyama Y, Hirota Y, Ayusawa D, Seno T, Garrett C, Wataya Y. Deoxyribonucleoside triphosphate imbalance. 5-fluorodeoxyuridine-induced DNA double strand breaks in mouse FM3A cells and the mechanism of cell death. *J Biol Chem* 1987; 262:8235–8241.
16. Wataya Y, Hwang H-S, Nakazawa T, Takahashi K, Otani M, Igawi T. Molecular mechanism of cell death induced dNTP pool imbalance. *Nucleic Acids Symposium Series* 1993; 29:109–110.
17. Kwok JB, Tattersall MNH. DNA fragmentation, dATP pool elevation and potentiation of antifolate cytotoxicity in L1210 cells by hypoxanthine. *Br J Can* 1992; 65:503–508.
18. Chong L, Tattersall MHN. 5,10-dideazatetrahydrofolic acid reduces toxicity and deoxyadenosine triphosphate pool expansion in cultured L1210 cells treated with inhibitors of thymidylate synthase. *Biochem Pharmacol* 1995; 49:819–827.
19. Houghton JA, Tillman DM. Harwood FG, Ratio of 2′-deoxyadenosine-5′-triphosphate/thymidine-5′-triphosphate influences the commitment of human colon carcinoma cells to thymineless death. *Clin Cancer Res* 1995; 1:723–730.
20. Richardson CC, Schildkraut CL, Kornberg A. Studies on the replication of DNA by DNA polymerases. *Cold Spring Harbor Symp Quant Biol* 1963; 28:9–19.
21. Bertani E, Häggmark A, Reichard P. Enzymatic synthesis of deoxyribonucleotides: II Formation and interconversion of deoxyuridine phosphates. *J Biol Chem* 1963; 238:3407–3413.
22. Lindahl T. An N-glycosidase from Escherichia coli that releases free uracil from DNA containing deaminated cytosine residues. *Proc Natl Acad Sci USA* 1974; 71:3449–3653.
23. Jackson RC, Jackman AL, Calvert AH. Biochemical effects of a quinazoline inhibitor of thymidylate synthetase, *N*-(4-(*N*-((2-amino-4-hydroxy-6-quinazolinyl)methyl)prop- 2ynyl amino)benzoyl)-L-glutamic acid (CB3717), on human lymphoblastoid cells. *Biochem Pharmacol* 1983; 32:3783–3790.
24. Mitrovski B, Pressacco J, Mandelbaum S, Erlichman C. Biochemical effects of folate-based inhibitors of thymidylate synthase in MGU-U1 cells. *Cancer Chemother Pharmacol* 1994; 35:109–113.
25. Aherne GW, Hardcastle A, Raynaud, F, Jackman AL. Immunoreactive dUMP and TTP pools as an index of thymidylate synthase inhibition; effect of Tomudex (ZD1694) and a nonpolyglutamated quinazoline antifolate (CB30900) in L1210 mouse leukaemia cells. *Biochem Pharmacol* 1996; 51:1293–1301.
26. Wickramasinghe SN, Fida S. Misincorporation of uracil into cells into the DNA of folate- and B_{12}-deficient HL60 cells. *Eur J Haematol* 1993; 50:127–132.
27. Blount BC, Mack MM, Wehr CM, MacGregor JT, Hiatt RA, Wang G, Wickramasinghe SN, Everson RB, Ames BN. Folate deficiency causes uracil misincorporation into DNA and chromosome breakage: Implications for cancer and neuronal damage. *Proc Natl Acad Sci USA* 1997; 94:3290–3295.
28. Lindahl T. DNA glycosylases, endonucleases for apurinic/apyrimidinic sites, and base excision-repair. *Prog Nucleic Acid Res Mol Biol* 1979; 22:135–192.
29. James SJ, Miller BJ, Basnakian AG, Pogribny IP, Pogribna M, Muskhelishvili L. Apoptosis and proliferation under conditions of deoxynucleotide pool imbalance in liver of folate/methyl deficient rats. *Carcinogenesis* 1997; 18:287–293.
30. Tye B-K, Nyman P-O, Lehman, IR, Hochhauser S, Weiss B. Transient accumulation of Okazaki fragments as a result of uracil incorporation into nascent DNA. *Proc Nat Acad Sci USA* 1977; 74:154–157.
31. Tye B-K, Lehman IR. Excision repair of uracil incorporated in DNA as a result of a defect in dUTPase. *J Mol Biol* 1977; 117:293–306.
32. Tamanoi F, Okazaki T. Uracil incorporation into nascent DNA of thymine-requiring mutant of *Bacillus subtlilis* 168. *Proc Natl Acad Sci USA* 1978; 75:2195–2199.
33. Olivero BM. DNA intermediates at the *Escherichia coli* replication fork: effect of dUTP, *Proc Natl Acad Sci USA* 1978; 75:238–242.
34. Warner HR, Duncan BK. *In vivo* synthesis and properties of uracil-containing DNA, *Nature* 1978; 272:32–34.
35. Sekiguchi M, Hayakawa H, Makino F, Tanaka K, Okada Y. A human enzyme that liberates uracil from DNA. *Biochem Biophys Res Commun* 1976; 73:293–299.

36. Brynolf K, Eliasson R, Reichard P. Formation of Okazaki fragments in polyoma DNA synthesis caused by misincorporation of uracil. *Cell* 1978; 13:573–580.
37. Grafstrom R, Tseng B, Goulian M. The incorporation of uracil into animal cell DNA in vitro. *Cell* 1978; 15:131–140.
38. Jackman AL, Calvert AH. Folate-based thymidylate synthase inhibitors as anticancer drugs. *Ann Oncol* 1995; 6:871–881.
39. Goulian M, Bleile B, Tseng BY. Methotrexate-induced misincorporation of uracil into DNA. *Proc Natl Acad Sci USA* 1980; 77:1956–1960.
40. Goulian M, Bleile B, Tseng BY. The effect of methotrexate on levels of dUTP in animal cells. *J Biol Chem* 1980; 255:10,630–10,637.
41. Sedwick, WD, Kutler M, Brown OE. Anti-folate-induced misincorporation of deoxyuridine monophosphate into DNA: inhibition of high molecular weight DNA synthesis in human lymphoblastoid cells. *Proc Natl Acad Sci* 1981; 78:917–921.
42. Ingraham HA, Tseng BY, Goulian M. Nucleotide levels and incorporation of 5-fluorouracil and uracil into DNA of cells treated with 5-fluorodeoxyuridine. *Mol Pharmacol* 1982; 21:211–216.
43. Richards RG, Brown OE, Gillison ML, Sedwick WD. Drug concentration-dependent DNA lesions are induced by the lipid-soluble antifolate, Piritrexim (BW301U). *Mol Pharmacol* 1986; 30:651–658.
44. Fraser DC, Pearson CK. Is uracil misincorporation into DNA of mammalian cells a consequence of methotrexate treatment? *Biochem Biophys Res Commun* 1986; 135:886–893.
45. Jackson RC. Unresolved issues in the biochemical pharmacology of antifolates, *NCI Monographs* 1987; 5:9–15.
46. Fox M, Boyle JM, Kinsella AR. Nucleoside salvage and resistance to antimetabolite anticancer agents. *Br J Cancer* 1991; 64:428–436.
47. Jackman AL, Taylor GA, Calvert AH, Harrap KR. Modulation of anti-metabolite effects: effects of thymidine on the efficacy of the quinazoline-based thymidylate synthetase inhibitor, CB3717. *Biochem Pharmacol* 1984; 33:3269–3275.
48. Curtin NJ, Harris AL. Potentiation of quinazoline antifolate (CB3717) toxicity by dipyridamole in human lung carcinoma, A549, cells. *Biochem Pharmacol* 1988; 37:2113–2120.
49. Grem JL, Mulcahy RT, Miller EM, Allegra CJ, Fischer PH. Interaction of deoxyuridine with fluorouracil and dipyridamole in a human colon cancer cell line. *Biochem Pharmacol* 1989; 38:51–59.
50. Piall EM, Curtin NJ, Aherne GW, Harris AL, Marks V. The quantitation by radioimmunoassay of 2'-deoxyuridine-5'-triphosphate in extracts of thymidylate synthase inhibited cells. *Anal Biochem* 1989; 177:347–352.
51. Curtin NJ, Harris AL, Aherne GW. Mechanism of cell death following thymidylate synthase inhibition: 2'-deoxyuridine-5'-triphosphate accumulation, DNA damage and growth inhibition following exposure to CB3717 and dipyrdamole. *Cancer Res* 1991; 51:2346–2352.
52. Canman CE, Tang H-Y, Normolla DP, Lawrence TS, Maybaum J. Variations in patterns of DNA damage induced in human colorectal tumour cells by 5-fluorodeoxyuridine: implications for mechanisms of resistance and cytotoxicity. *Proc Natl Acad Sci USA* 1992; 89:10,474–10,478.
53. Canman CE, Lawrence TS, Shewach DS, Tang H-Y, Maybaum J. Resistance to 5-fluorodeoxyuridine-induced DNA damage and cytotoxicity correlates with an elevation of deoxyuridine triphosphatase activity and failure to accumulate deoxyuridine triphosphate. *Cancer Res* 1993; 53:5219–5224.
54. Canman CE, Radany EH, Parsels LA, Davis MA, Lawrence TS, Maybaum J. Induction of resistance to 5-fluorodeoxyuridine cytotoxicity and DNA damage in human tumor cells by expression of *Escherichia coli* deoxyuridine triphosphatase. *Cancer Res* 1994; 54:2296–2298.
55. Jackman AL, Kimbell R, Aherne GW, Brunton L, Jansen G, Stephens TC, Smith MN, Wardleworth JM, Boyle FT. Cellular pharmacology and in vivo activity of a new anticancer agent, ZD9331: a water soluble, nonpolyglutamatable, quinazoline-based inhibitor of thymidylate synthase. *Clin Cancer Res* 1997; 3:911–921.
56. Brown SD, Hardcastle A, Aherne GW. Deoxyuridine triphosphatase (dUTPase) expression and cellular response to thymidylate synthase (TS) inhibitors. In: (Pfleiderer W, Rokos H, eds) Chemistry and Biology of Pteridines and Folates 1997. Blackwell Science, Berlin, 1997, pp. 271–274.
57. Ladner R, Caradonna S. Lowering dUTPase levels through antisense induces sensitivity to 5-fluorodeoxyuridine in HT29 cells. *Proc Am Assoc Cancer Res* 1997; 38:614.
58. Sundseth R, Singer S, Yates B, Smith G, Ferone R, Dev I. Thymineless apoptotic death induced by 1843U89 in human tumour cell lines is independent of dUTP accumulation and misincorporation of dUMP into DNA. *Proc Am Assoc Cancer Res* 1997; 38:476.

59. Parsels LA, Loney TL, Maybaum J. Expression of *E. coli* dUTPase partially protects HT29 cells from DNA fragmentation and cytotoxicity induced by CB3717 or MTX. *Proc Am Assoc Cancer Res* 1995; 36:406.
60. Brown S, Hardcastle A, Kelland L, Jackman A, Ladner RD, Aherne W. Deoxyuridine triphosphate (dUTPase): its relevance in cell sensitivity to thymidylate synthase (TS) inhibitors. *Br J Cancer* 1996; 73(suppl. XXVI):13.
61. Brown SD, Hardcastle A, Ladner RD, Aherne GW. Components of the uracil misincorporation pathway: their influence on cellular response to thymidylate synthase (TS) inhibitors. *Br J Cancer* 1997; 75(suppl. 1):25.
62. El-Hajj HH, Zhang H, Weiss B. Lethality of a *dut* (deoxyuridine triphosphatase mutation in *Escherichia coli. J Bacteriol* 1988; 170:1069–1075.
63. Gadsden MH, McIntosh EM, Game JC, Wilson EM, Haynes RH. dUTP pyrophosphatase is an essential enzyme in *Saccharomuces cerevisiae. EMBO J* 1993; 12:4425–4431.
64. Williams MV, Cheng Y-C. Human deoxyuridine triphosphate nucleotidohydrolase: purification and characterization of the deoxyuridine triphosphate nucleotidohydrolase from acute lymphocytic leukaemia. *J Biol Chem* 1979; 254:2897–2901.
65. Ingraham HA, Goulian M. Deoxyuridine triphosphatase: a potential site of interaction with pyrimidine nucleotide analogues. *Biochem Biophys Res Commun* 1982; 109:746–752.
66. Caradonna SJ, Adamkiewicz DM. Purification and properties of the deoxyuridine triphosphate nucleotidohydrolase enzyme derived from HeLa S3 cells. *J Biol Chem* 1984; 259:5459–5464.
67. Caradonna SJ, Cheng Y-C. The role of deoxyuridine triphosphate nucleotidohydrolase, uracil DNA glycosylase and DNA polymerase α in the metabolism of 5-fluorodeoxyuridine in human tumor cells. *Mol Pharmacol* 1980; 18:513–520.
68. McIntosh EM, Ager DD, Gadsden MH, Haynes RH. Human dUTPpyrophosphatase: cDNA sequence and potential biological importance of the enzyme. *Proc Natl Acad Sci USA* 1992; 89:8020–8024.
69. Ladner RD, McNulty DE, Carr SA, Roberts GD, Caradonna SJ. Characterization of distinct nuclear and mitochondrial forms of human deoxyuridine triphosphate nucleotidohydrolase. *J Biol Chem* 1996; 271:7745–7751.
70. Larsson G, Svensson LA, Nyman PO. Crystal structure of the *Escherichia coli* dUTPase in complex with a substrate analogue (dUDP). *Nature Struct Biol* 1996; 3:532–538.
71. Mol CD, Harris JM, McIntosh EM, Tainer JA. Human dUTP pyrophosphatase, uracil recognition by a β hairpin and active sites formed by 3 separate subunits. *Structure* 1996; 4:1077–1092.
72. McIntosh EM Haynes RH. dUTP pyrophosphatase as a potential target for chemotherapeutic drug development. *Acta Biochimica Polonica* 1997; 44:159–172.
73. Ladner RD, Caradonna SJ. The human dUTPase gene encodes both nuclear and mitochondrial isoforms. *J Biol Chem* 1997; 272:19,072–19,080.
74. Vilpo JA, Autio-Harmainen H. Uracil-DNA glycosylase and deoxyuridine triphosphatase: studies of activity and subcellular location in human normal and malignant lymphocytes, *Scand J Clin Lab Invest* 1983; 43:583–590.
75. Duker NJ, Grant CL. Alterations in the levels of deoxyuridine triphosphatase, uracil-DNA glycosylase and AP endonuclease during the cell cycle. *Exp Cell Res* 1980; 125:493–497.
76. Hokari S, Hasegawa M, Tanaka M, Sakagishi Y, Kikuchi G. Deoxyuridine triphosphate nucleotidohydrolase: Distribution of the enzyme in various rat tissues. *J Biochem* 1988; 104:211–214.
77. Strahler JR, Zhu X-X, Hora N, Wang YK, Andrews PC, Roseman NA, Neel JV, Turka L, Hanash SM. Maturation stage and proliferation-dependent expression of dUTPase in human cells. *Proc Natl Acad Sci USA* 1993; 90:4991–4995.
78. Ladner RD, Carr SA, Huddleston MJ, McNulty DE, Caradonna SJ. Identification of a consensus cyclin-dependent kinase phosphorylation site unique to the nuclear form of human deoxyuridine triphosphate nucleotidohydrolase. *J Biol Chem* 1996; 271:7752–7757.
79. Ladner R, Lynch F, Caradonna S. Differential expression and immunohistochemical localization of human dUTPase isoforms. *Proc Am Assoc Cancer Res* 1997; 38:156.
80. Hokari S, Horikawa S, Tsukada K, Sakagishi Y. Expression of deoxyuridine triphosphatase during liver regeneration in rat. *Biochem Mol Biol Intl* 1995; 37:583–590.
81. Beck WR, Wright GE, Nusbaum NJ, Chang JD, Isselbacher EM. Enhancement of methotrexate cytotoxicity by uracil analogues that inhibit deoxyuridine triphosphate nucleotidohydrolase (dUTPase) activity. *Adv Exp Med Biol* 1986; 195B:97–104.

82. Kobayashi H, Takemura Y, Miyachi H, Skelton L, Jackman AL. Effect of hammerhead ribozyme against human thymidylate synthase on the cytotoxicity of thymidylate synthase inhibitors. *Jpn J Cancer Res* 1995; 86:1014–1018.
83. Williams MV. Effects of mercury (II) compounds on the activity of dUTPases from various sources. *Mol Pharmacol* 1986; 29:288–292.
84. Zalud P, Wachs WO, Nyman PO, Zeppezauer MM. Inhibition of the proliferation of human cancer cells in vitro by substrate-analogous inhibitors of dUTPase. *Adv Exp Med Biol* 1995; 370:135–138.

21 Thymineless Death

Peter J. Houghton

CONTENTS

INTRODUCTION
THYMINELESS STRESS
MOLECULAR REGULATION OF THYMINELESS DEATH
TRANSLATION OF DNA DAMAGE CAUSED BY THYMINELESS STRESS
  TO THYMINELESS DEATH
FUTURE PROSPECTS
REFERENCES

1. INTRODUCTION

Conceptually, certain classes of anticancer agents that inhibit DNA replication would be anticipated to cause cytostasis rather than cytotoxicity. These include antimetabolite drugs that either directly or indirectly inhibit formation of essential deoxynucleotides for DNA replication and repair. Within this class are 5-fluoropyrimidines, antifolates, and inhibitors of pyrimidine biosynthesis such as PALA, each of which restricts synthesis of dTMP *de novo*. Of importance is that agents that induce "thymineless death," through restriction of dTMP represent major chemotherapeutic classes used for palliative treatment of carcinomas of colon, breast, head and neck, and certain lung tumors, as well as certain hematopoietic malignancies. However, molecular events controlling the cell cycle that influence or control the commitment process in thymineless death are poorly understood.

Over the past several years a new concept of how drugs exert cytotoxicity, and some of the molecular events controlling this, have been elucidated. One current model suggests that damage to DNA induced by genotoxic agents is recognized by protein complexes, in which the tumor suppressor, p53, is though to be part. Damage signaled through p53 results in arrest of cells in G1 or G2-phase of the cell cycle. If damage is below some critical threshold, cells will re-enter the cell cycle after repair, or if that threshold is exceeded, cells will initiate apoptosis. Although undoubtedly an oversimplification, the model allows a conceptually different view of how anticancer drugs kill cells, and indeed how these agents may be somewhat tumor selective in their

From: *Anticancer Drug Development Guide: Antifolate Drugs in Cancer Therapy*
Edited by: A.L. Jackman © Humana Press Inc., Totowa, NJ

action. Thus, cell death is not the result of damage *per se,* but how the cell processes the damage. If this is correct, then understanding the molecular framework that links specific forms of DNA damage to initiation of cellular programs that initiate apoptosis becomes critical in understanding how drugs really work. Clearly, it has been established that defects in signaling downstream of the DNA lesion prevent apoptosis. Consequently, one can now understand why measurements of drug uptake, activation, levels of target enzymes, DNA breaks, and so on frequently fail to predict sensitivity of cells to antimetabolite drugs. The application of such assays to predict clinical responses of tumors would seem even more futile without adequate characterization of molecular events that link specific types of DNA damage to the apoptotic cascade. In this article we review some of the information that links thymineless death through dTTP restriction to cellular machinery that initiates cell death through the process of apoptosis.

2. THYMINELESS STRESS

2.1. Use of Mutant Cells Deficient in Thymidylate Synthase

One disadvantage of using drugs to inhibit thymidylate synthase, is that there are invariably secondary targets that may complicate interpretation of the results. Thus, it is well established that 5-fluorinated pyrimidines may exert cytotoxicity through inhibition of thymidylate synthase, incorporation of fraudulent nucleotide into RNA, with effects on processing of transcripts, or direct incorporation into DNA. Almost certainly secondary sites of action of all of the other thymidylate synthase inhibitors will be identified at some point in time. The response to agents that deplete cellular pools of dTTP can be specifically studied in cells deficient in thymidylate synthase *(1–3).* Such cells require exogenous nucleoside to maintain DNA synthesis. Consequently, withdrawal of dThd recapitulates the effect of pharmacologic inhibition of thymidylate synthase without potential confounding effects such as incorporation of fraudulent nucleotides into nucleic acids, or effects in the purine biosynthetic pathway. The system has advantage, also, in that by readdition of dThd irreversible commitment to reproductive cell death may be determined by an inability to rescue cells.

2.2. Perturbation of Deoxyribonucleoside Triphosphate Pools During Thymineless Death

Thymidylate-synthase-deficient mammalian cells have been used to understand alterations in deoxyribonucleoside triphosphate pools (dNTP) and their biological significance following dThd withdrawal. In thymidylate-synthase-negative (TS$^-$) murine FM3A cells, withdrawal of dThd was associated with rapid loss of clonogenic potential and DNA fragmentation ($t_{1/2}$ approx 6 h), associated with a rapid loss of dTTP, dGTP, and a modest elevation of dATP. In these cells it was concluded that the imbalance between dGTP and dATP may be the signal for cell death *(4).* However, the kinetics for cell death appear to be cell-line specific, and may be controlled, to some extent, by conditions of cell growth (i.e., suspension or adherent monolayer culture). For example, human colon-adenocarcinoma cells (GC$_3$/TS$^-$) lacking thymidylate synthase lost colony formation relatively slowly after dThd withdrawal *(5).* In asynchronous populations of cells 50% could not be rescued (i.e., had lost clonogenic potential) when dThd was added after 65 h of dThd starvation. Measurement of dNTP pools demonstrated charac-

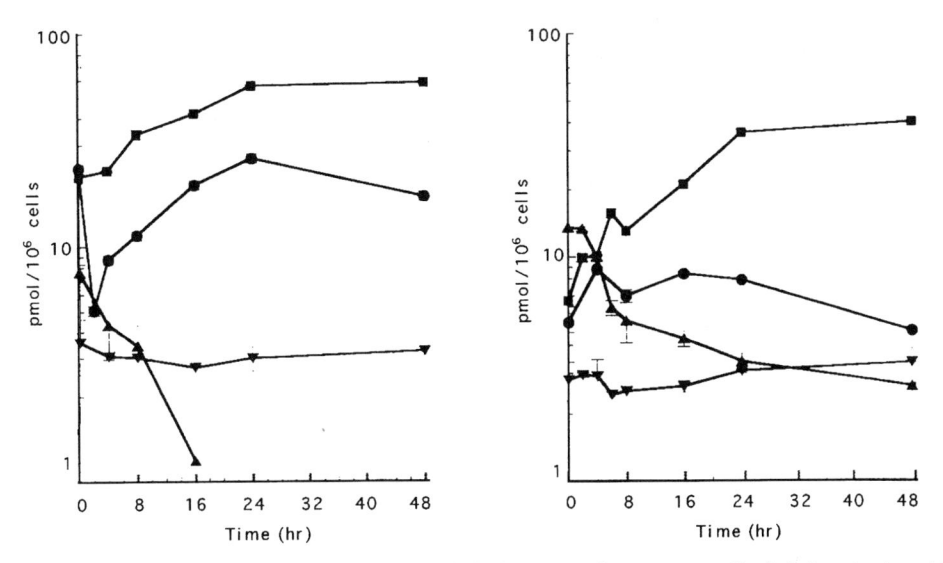

Fig. 1. Effect of dThd withdrawal on dNTP pools in human colon cancer cells deficient in thymidylate synthase. Following dThd deprivation, changes in dNTP pools were determined in asynchronously growing TS⁻ cells for periods up to 48 h. Data represent mean ± SD of two to four determinations per point (■) dATP; (▲) dTTP; (●) dCTP; (▼) dGTP. Basal levels of dNTP pools were 21 ± 0.7, 22 ± 0.2, and 3 ± 1 pmol/10⁶ cells, respectively. (From ref. 5, with permission).

teristics different from those in murine models following induction of the thymineless state. In the human model, dGTP pools were not depleted, and after a brief decline, dCTP pools recovered to control levels within 24 h, Fig. 1. Thymineless death, as determined by internucleosomal DNA fragmentation and loss in clonogenic survival, correlated with a temporally associated decrease in dTTP and elevation in the dATP pool. Where dUTP (or FdUTP following treatment with FUra or FdUrd) has been considered to play an important role in the mechanism of induction of thymineless death, dUTP has been detected at relatively high levels within cells (90–338 pmol/10⁶ cells). However, in GC$_3$/TS⁻ cells dUTP was not detectable following dThd withdrawal *(5)*.

3. MOLECULAR REGULATION OF THYMINELESS DEATH

3.1. The Role of the Tumor Suppressor Gene p53 in Anticancer Drug Response

There is considerable evidence that the p53 tumor suppressor gene is involved in the control of cell growth, being involved in both G1, G2, and possibly mitotic checkpoint function. Several studies have shown that overexpression of functional p53 may sensitize cells to certain classes of cytotoxic drugs *(6–8)*. The most extensively studied function of p53 is as a G1 cell-cycle checkpoint, where the protein becomes elevated in response to DNA-damaging agents *(9,10)*. Inactivation of p53 by mutation or deletion results in genomic instability *(11,12)*. In part, this may be a consequence of mutants of p53 being unable to increase expression of the cyclin-dependent kinase inhibitor, p21^{cip1}. Loss of p21^{cip1} expression is associated with G2 arrest after DNA damage (gamma radiation), and rereplication of DNA without cytokinesis *(13)*. Of interest is that p53-deficient mice have normal fetal development, but these animals are predisposed to the development of several different types of neoplasm *(14,15)*. The loss of G1-checkpoint control in movement of cells from G1 to S-phase has also reduced cellular sensitivity to cytotoxic agents *(6)* and ionizing radiation *(16–18)*.

The functional activity of wild-type p53 (wtp53), which is frequently lost following mutation, is mediated via transcriptional activation or downregulated expression of genes involved in growth arrest, survival, or cell death responses, through sequence-specific interactions with DNA *(19–21)*. These genes include a 21-kDa protein ($p21^{Waf1/Cip1}$) that binds to and inhibits G1 cyclin-dependent kinases, thereby preventing entry of cells from G1 to S-phase *(22)*; the Bax gene, which is also directly transcriptionally activated by wtp53 *(23)*, and is a proapoptotic protein in response to toxic stress *(24–29)*; and the homologous protein, Bcl-2, which opposes the function of Bax, and can prolong cell survival *(24,30)*. Expression of the Bcl-2 gene, which contains a p53-dependent negative response element *(21)*, may be downregulated by wtp53, and the coordinate regulation of Bax and Bcl-2 can occur simultaneously *(26)*. Both Bax and Bcl-2 are expressed in the normal colon. Bax is expressed at higher levels in the epithelial cells of the upper portions of the crypts *(31)*, and Bcl-2, in the lower crypt cells *(32,33)*. During neoplastic progression, deregulated expression of Bcl-2 has been reported *(33)*. Constitutive expression of Bcl-2 may result in protection from p53-induced apoptosis *(34,35)*, and the cytotoxicity of some anticancer agents *(36–39)*. These include drugs that inhibit thymidylate synthase *(40,41)*.

3.2. p53 and the Cellular Response to Antimetabolite Agents

The initial work by Lowe et al. *(6)* demonstrated p53-dependent cytotoxicity for several anticancer agents in murine-embryo fibroblasts (MEFs) that expressed the E1A or were transformed with E1A plus T24-*ras* oncogenes. MEFs derived from $p53^{+/+}$, $p53^{+/-}$, or $p53^{-/-}$ animals were quite resistant to ionizing radiation, FUra, and topoisomerase II poisons. However, when cells were transfected with the viral E1A oncogene cells from $p53^{+/+}$ or $p53^{+/-}$ embryos became sensitive to these agents, whereas MEFs from $p53^{-/-}$ embryos were resistant. In cells expressing E1A and E1B genes, the latter of which counteracts wtp53 *(42)*, $p53^{+/+}$ cells were also resistant. Further, studies where MEFs were transformed with E1A and T24-*ras* also demonstrated p53-dependent sensitivity to radiation, FUra, and topoisomerase II inhibitors. In contrast, cell killing by sodium azide, a respiratory poison that uncouples mitochondrial oxidative phosphorylation and depletes ATP, was p53-dependent. Whereas these studies are seminal in defining p53-dependent sensitivity to various cytotoxic agents, including the antimetabolite FUra, the role of p53 is complicated by an enhanced rate of spontaneous apoptosis in E1A-expressing $p53^{+/+}$ cells. Further, the biochemical lesion responsible for initiating apoptosis (incorporation into RNA, DNA, or thymineless death) is unclear from this study, as the ability of dThd to protect cells was not examined. Thus, the induction of apoptosis observed could have been a consequence of any of several mechanisms of action discussed previously. However, that p53 may be implicated in determining the cytotoxic response to antimetabolites is now established. Using an inhibitor of carbamoylphosphate synthetase (PALA), it was found that Li-Fraumeni fibroblasts ($p53^{+/-}$), and murine fibroblasts that expressed mutant alleles, but transfected with a wtp53 allele, growth arrested in presence of drug. In contrast, cells lacking wtp53 proceeded from G1 to S-phase, resulting in amplification of the CAD gene (encoding the trifunctional enzyme carbamoyl-phosphate synthetase, aspartate transcarbamylase, dihydroorotase) and drug resistance *(11)*. Similar results were reported by Yin et al. *(12)*, in which arrest of cell-cycle progression in the presence of PALA occurred only in cells expressing a wtp53 allele. These data indicate that wtp53 was involved in establishing a G1 checkpoint that arrests cells in response to PALA treatment. Results obtained in clones expressing mutant and wtp53 alleles where entry into S-phase was partially inhibited, suggests that the ratio of mutant to wt protein, rather than the absolute level of wtp53, is the critical determinant of PALA-induced G1 arrest *(12)*. The antimetabolite PALA depletes both pyrimidines and purines, including UTP, CTP, dCTP, dGTP, and dTTP *(43)*, it is not possible to attribute the cytostatic effect to depletion of any particular nucleotide pool, or to extrapolate to the actions of thymidylate synthase inhibitors, or antifols. For example, growth arrest in cells exposed to the dihydrofolate reductase inhibitor methotrexate is less clear, as cells with either wild-type *(11,44)* or mutant *(12)* p53 alleles arrested in G1.

3.3. p53 and the Cellular Response to Thymidylate Synthase Inhibitors

Preliminary clinical studies have implicated p53 in influencing the responses of patients with advanced colon cancer to treatment with FUra administered with leucovorin *(45)*. Since the p53 gene is mutated in high frequency (>75%) in colon carcinomas, occurring during progression from adenoma to carcinoma *(46)*, this observation is of considerable importance. The basis for modulation of FUra with a reduced folate is to increase the level of thymidylate synthase inhibition by promoting efficient and tight binding of the proximal metabolite FdUMP to the enzyme. This is achieved by increasing the concentration of higher polyglutamate forms of CH_2-H_4PteGlu (reviewed in ref. *47*). In the clinical study reported, 43% (6 of 14) of patients had mutated p53 alleles, and of these 4 of 5 did not respond to treatment. In contrast, of 9 patients with tumors that expressed wtp53, 7 demonstrated response to therapy. Although used less frequently in patients, FdUrd is converted to FdUMP by thymidine kinase, and is a potent inhibitor of thymidylate synthase (reviewed in refs. *48,49*). Transfection of wtp53 into HL60 leukemic cells that lack p53 expression was found to sensitize cells approx 10-fold to FdUrd. Additional studies, in which cells were synchronized in G1 showed a further 10-fold sensitization, as cells appeared to remain blocked in G1, whereas $p53^{-/-}$ cells proceeded into S-phase *(50)*. It remains unclear whether such arrested cells maintain proliferative potential, or whether they are reproductively dead. In the model proposed by Lane *(51)*, the p53 tumor-suppressor gene is not required during a normal cell cycle; this is supported by the relative lack of a phenotype in knockout mice in which p53 has been disrupted *(52)*. The suppressor p53 is considered to cause G1 arrest, only after the cell has been stressed by exposure to radiation or other genotoxic agents. Arrest may be followed by repair, or apoptosis. According to this model, cells lacking p53 would not arrest in G1, but would progress through DNA synthesis which would lead to additional mutations, and death.

3.4. p53 and Cellular Response to dTTP Depletion

Whereas the biological significance of G1 arrest of irradiated cells has not been established as a mechanism to promote survival of cells that have reproductive capacity, there is accumulating evidence that p53 may determine the fate of cells exposed to antimetabolites that target thymidylate synthase *(45,50)*. However, in the clinical studies reported it is assumed that responses to the combination of FUra and leucovorin is mediated by inhibition of thymidylate synthase, and although probable, is not possible to confirm. On the other hand, laboratory studies impose artificial conditions, for example, where either wt or dominant-negative p53 alleles are overexpressed in cells. This presents concern, as the transgene is not under control of the endogenous promoter, hence regulation may not recapitulate the endogenous gene. Consequently, it can only be assumed that the gene product acts in a physiologic manner. In most studies, exogenous genes are expressed from viral promoters, which results in very high levels of expression that potentially may lead to observations that have limited utility when applied to clinical cancer.

3.5. Regulation of p53 in Commitment

Despite the concerns raised, more direct evidence suggests that thymineless death, the end-product involved in targeting thymidylate synthase with inhibitors, is a p53-dependent process *(53)*. As discussed above, cells deficient in thymidylate synthase (TS$^-$) commit to reproductive death upon withdrawal of exogenous dThd. The human colon-cancer cell line GC$_3$/TS$^-$ variant loses the ability to be rescued by dThd with a t$_{1/2}$ approx 65 h. We subsequently selected a TS$^-$ variant (designated Thy4) that was resistant to thymineless death, anticipating that comparison between this variant and the TS$^-$ cells would be valuable in defining important regulatory steps in thymineless death *(54)*.

As shown in Fig. 2, the loss of clonogenic potential was similar in TS$^-$ and Thy4 populations when dThd was withdrawn from asynchronous populations of cells. This suggested that Thy4 cells were not resistant to the induction of apoptosis when deprived of dTTP during DNA replication. However, when cells were first synchronized in G1-phase by leucine block, then released in the absence of exogenous dThd, Thy4 cells maintained clonogenic potential for up to 5 d in the absence of dThd. In contrast, there was >90% loss of clonogenic potential in TS$^-$ cells, Fig. 2. Loss of clonogenicity in both TS$^-$ and Thy4 cells was associated with internucleosomal cleavage of DNA, characteristic of apoptosis, and uptake of the vital dye trypan blue. These data suggest that Thy4 cells are able to arrest in G1-phase (or possibly very early S-phase), and maintain viability for at least 5 d, after which time there is a precipitous loss of viability, indicating delayed apoptosis. Further studies with these cells indicated that acute and delayed apoptosis induced by dThd deprivation correlated with expression of p53 and p53-regulated genes *(53)*. Both TS$^-$ and Thy4 are derived from GC$_3$/c1 colon carcinoma cells, and each is heterozygous for p53, expressing both mutant (240 Ser to Arg) and wt alleles. Examination of p53 proteins in TS$^-$ and Thy4 cells released from G1 block in the absence of dThd showed that in TS$^-$ cells, which commit to acute apoptosis, wtp53 predominated. In Thy4, which commits to apoptosis much later, levels of mutant protein exceeded those of wt for up to 5 d (Fig. 3). Functional activity of p53 only in TS$^-$ cells was supported by the ability of wild-type p53 to activate a p53 reporter plasmid. Consistent with these data, levels of MDM2 expression increased in TS$^-$ cells within 24 h, and con-

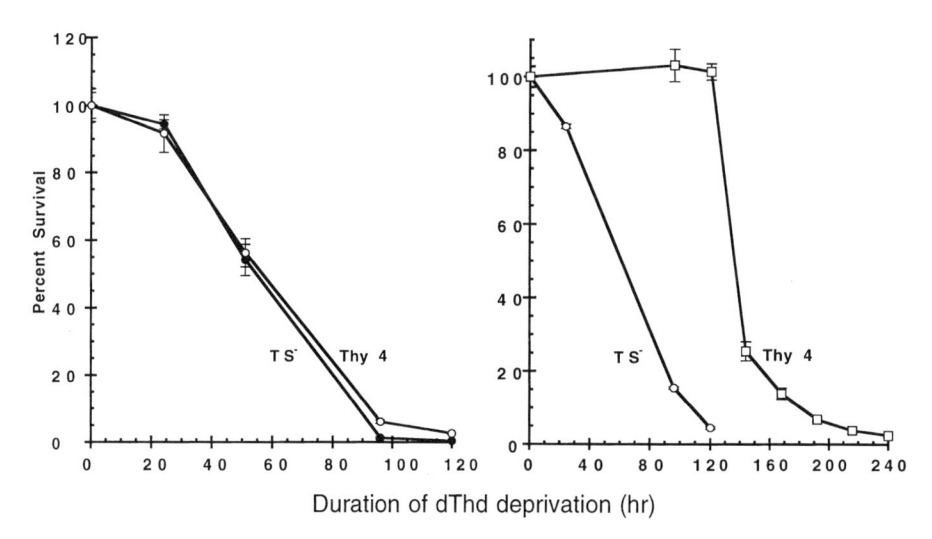

Fig. 2. Left panel: Clonogenic survival of asynchronous populations of TS⁻ (●) and Thy4 (○) cells following dThd withdrawal. Right panel: Clonogenic survival of G0 synchronized TS⁻ (○) and Thy4 (□) cells following leucine restoration and dThd withdrawal. Cells were rescued with dThd (20 μM) for intervals up to 10 d, and clonogenic survival was determined 11 d after rescue (from ref. *54* with permission).

tinued to increase over the time course of the experiment in cells released from G1 block in the presence or absence of dThd. Of note was the change in the ratio of wt to mutant p53 protein in Thy4 cells as they committed to delayed apoptosis. In these cells, the level of mutant protein decreased, whereas the level of wt protein demonstrated a lesser fall resulting in wild-type:mutant ratio >1 just prior to loss of clonogenic potential. Upon onset of delayed apoptosis, levels of MDM2 increased approx fourfold, consistent with functional p53. These results support the contention that the effect of p53 on cellular response may be defined by the ratio of wt to mutant protein, as proposed by Yin et al. *(12)*.

4. TRANSLATION OF DNA DAMAGE CAUSED BY THYMINELESS STRESS TO THYMINELESS DEATH

4.1. The Link Between DNA Damage and Apoptosis

As discussed above, it is now considered that cytotoxic agents cause cellular damage, and that such damage initiates programmed cell death (apoptosis). The molecular characterization of elements that link these processes are as yet poorly defined. Because expression of p53 increases the sensitivity of cells to undergo apoptosis in response to cytotoxic agents, it has been postulated as an intermediary in linking DNA damage to the apoptotic machinery. Apoptosis may be initiated through activation of autocrine death-loops. Four cell-surface death receptors have been identified (Fas, Wsl/DR-3, DR-4, and TNFR-1). Of these the best characterized involves binding of Fas ligand (FasL)

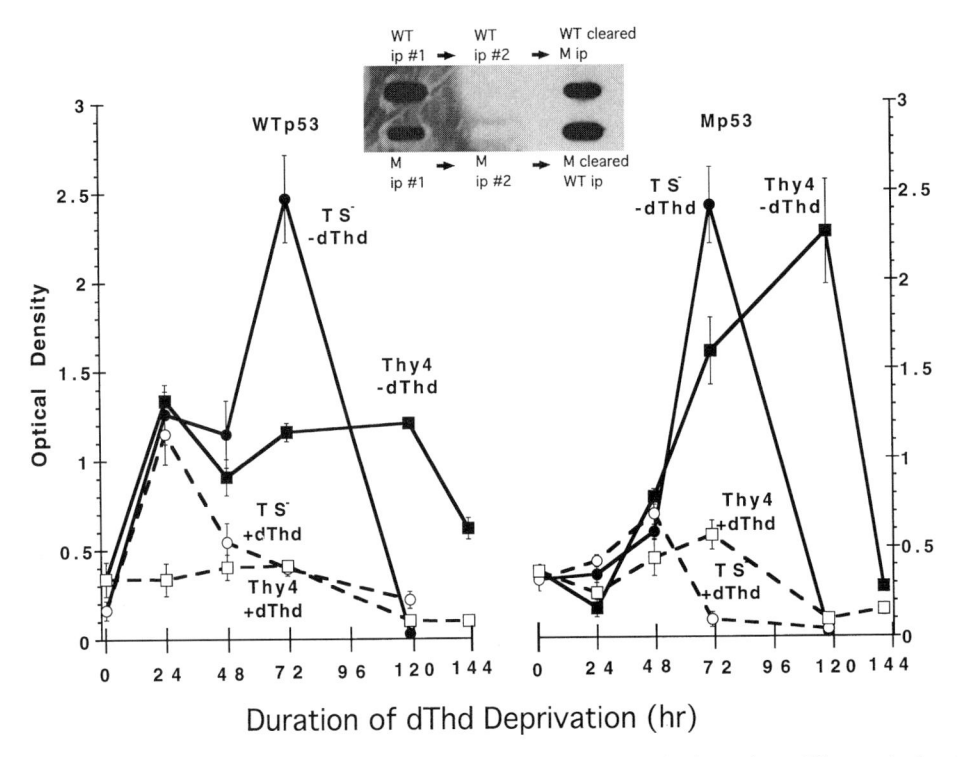

Fig. 3. (A) Slot-blot analysis showing quantitative immunoprecipitation of wtp53 protein by the PAb1620 antibody, and of mutant p53 (mp53) protein by the PAb240 antibody in extracts derived from TS⁻ cells. Lysates were immunoprecipitated twice using PAb1620 then further immunoprecipitated with PAb240 (upper panel), or alternatively, precipitated twice to remove mutant p53 (PAb240) and then with PAb1620 specific for wtp53 (lower panel). Immunoprecipitated proteins were detected following slot-blot analysis on nitrocellulose membranes, using the pan p53 antibody DO-I (which recognizes both wtp53 and mutant p53) conjugated to horseradish peroxidase, and ECL reagents. No cross reactivity between antibodies and proteins was evident. (B) Quantitative immunoprecipitation of wtp53 and mutant p53 proteins from TS⁻ and Thy4 cells following release from G0 synchrony in the absence or presence of dThd. After immunoprecipitation, proteins were quantitated following slot-blot analysis. Data represent the mean ± SD of 2–4 determinations from two independently derived sets of samples for each of the p53 proteins. Extracts derived from equivalent cell numbers were analyzed (from ref. 53 with permission).

to a cell-surface receptor, Fas (55–57). Fas is a type I integral membrane protein characterized by cysteine-rich residues. It belongs to the tumor-necrosis-factor receptor superfamily, and it contains an intracellular domain required for downstream signaling. FasL is a type II transmembrane protein homologous to tumor necrosis factor and related cytokines (58). This initiates a complex involving protein–protein interactions mediated through so-called death-domains. Thus, Fas interacts with FADD, and the death-effector domain of FADD interacts with a similar domain of proteases (FLICE, FLICE-2). These proteases exist in cells as zymogens and are rapidly cleaved to form activated proteases. These caspases then degrade both structural and other proteins (e.g., poly-ADP ribose polymerase) within the nucleus, as well as activate endonucleases. Fas is consti-

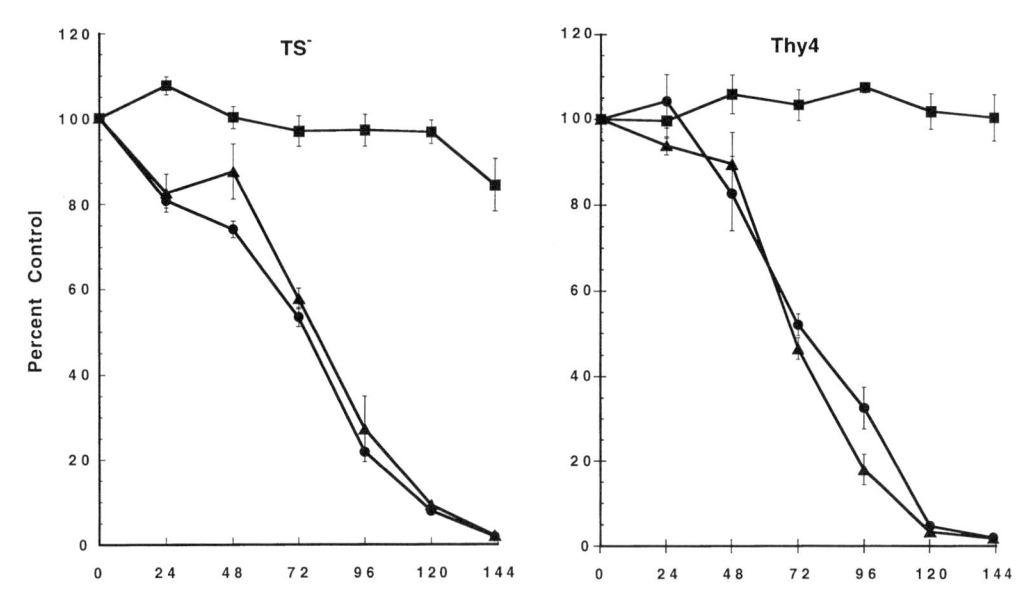

Fig. 4. Protection from apoptosis induced by dThd deprivation in asynchronously growing cultures of TS⁻ and Thy4 by a Fas-inhibiting antibody that binds to FasL. Cells were plated and treated with NOK-1 monoclonal antibody (100 ng/mL; ■), a mouse IgG1 isotype-matched control antibody (100 ng/mL; ▲), or no antibody (●) at the time of plating. Following afternight attachment, cells were washed, and deprived of dThd by refeeding with dThd-free medium containing the respective antibodies. At various times for up to 6 d, cells were rescued with dThd (20 μM), and colony formation was determined after a further 11 d. Data represent the mean ± SD of triplicate determinations (from ref. 60 with permission).

tutively expressed in human colonic epithelium, both in cytoplasm and on the basolateral membrane (59), suggesting that it may play a role in normal tissue homeostasis. Expression was found to be reduced in colon adenocarcinoma, and variable levels have been reported in cell lines established in vitro from colon tumors (59). Thus, one possible conduit for translating DNA damage induced by thymineless stress to apoptosis could be activation of the Fasl-Fas apoptotic pathway through a p53-dependent pathway.

4.2. Activation Fas-Mediated Apoptosis by Thymineless Stress

One approach to determining whether dThd withdrawal activates the Fas autocrine loop is to block the Fas receptor using the monoclonal antibody NOK-1 (60). As discussed above, when dThd is withdrawn from asynchronous cultures of TS⁻ or Thy4 cells, there is a similar rapid rate of commitment to apoptosis. However, withdrawal of dThd in the presence of NOK-1 almost completely protected cells from loss of clonogenic potential, Fig. 4. Blocking the Fas receptor also protected cells when released from G1/G0 synchrony. Further studies showed that onset of commitment to apoptosis (i.e., the point at which cells could not be rescued by dThd), was associated with expression of FasL. This occurred more rapidly in TS⁻ cells than in Thy4 cells, and thus correlated with acute or delayed apoptosis. These results clearly implicate initiation of an autocrine death loop in the process of thymineless death, and may have important implication in treatment of colon adenocarcinoma. These studies demonstrate that DNA damage caused by drugs that restrict dTTP is a proximal event, and that deficiencies in downstream signaling pathways that link DNA damage to initiating apoptotic cascades may result in drug resistance. Such downstream events may limit the predictive value of biochemical measurements of drug action such as the level of thymidylate synthase inhibition, or incorporation of fraudulent nucleotides into DNA, or DNA strand breaks.

5. FUTURE PROSPECTS

The finding that thymineless stress activates the FasL-Fas death pathway reinforces the notion that drug-induced DNA damage is a proximal event that initiates a process in which the cell commits suicide. Increasing information suggests that cellular resistance to drugs may occur through defects in this signaling system, in which the cell cannot complete the process. It would be anticipated, therefore, that cells unable to undergo apoptosis subsequent to attempting replication under thymineless conditions, would accumulate mutations at a high frequency, possibly accelerating the process of tumor progression. One potential concern would be that such a predisposition (i.e., failure to execute the death program) within a normal cell, during some phase of differentiation, could result in transformation.

We can now divide resistance to agents targeted at thymidylate synthase into at least two components: events proximal to DNA damage, and events distal to damage. In the former group drug transport, metabolism, sequestration, and levels of target enzyme may be included. These have been the major focus for pharmacologic studies, and have served as a basis for designing modulation regimens. For example, the combination of FUra and reduced folates, or combination with inhibitors of dihydropyrimidine dehydrogenase. Clearly, for inhibitors of thymidylate synthase to exert cytotoxicity, enzyme inhibition must lead to dTTP depletion, thus modulation to increase this effect is important. However, once that is accomplished the resistance mechanisms distal to damage may determine cellular response. It will now be of importance to determine the frequency with which the FasL-Fas pathway is activated by thymineless stress in different tumor types. However, the Fas loop may be one of several known pathways, and potentially unknown pathways, to be involved in translation of thymineless-DNA damage to apoptosis. Potentially Fas and other pathways may be the targets for modulation strategies that enhance translation of thymineless stress into thymineless death.

REFERENCES

1. Li IC, Chu EHY. Mutants of chinese hamster cells deficient in thymidylate synthetase. *J Cell Physiol* 1984; 120:109–116.
2. Ayusawa D, Shimizu K, Koyama H, Takeishi K, Seno T. Accumulation of DNA strand breaks during thymineless death in thymidylate synthase-negative mutants of mouse FM3A cells. *J Biol Chem* 1983; 258:12,448–12,454.
3. Houghton PJ, Germain GS, Hazelton BJ, Pennington JW, Houghton JA. Mutants of human colon adenocarcinoma selected for thymidylate synthase deficiency. *Proc Natl Acad Sci USA* 1989; 86:1377–1381.
4. Yoshioka A, Tanaka S, Hiraoka O, Koyama Y, Hirota Y, Ayusawa D, Seno T, Garrett C, Wataya Y. Deoxyribonucleoside triphosphate imbalance: 5-fluorourdeoxyuridine-induced DNA double-strand breaks in mouse FM3A cells and the mechanism of cell death. *J Biol Chem* 1987; 282:8235–8241.

5. Houghton JA, Tillman DM, Harwood FG. Ratio of 2'-deoxyadenosine-5'-triphosphate/thymidine-5'-triphosphate influences commitment of human colon carcinoma cells to thymineless death. *Clin Cancer Res* 1995; 1:723–730.
6. Lowe SW, Ruley HE, Jacks T, Housman DE. p53-dependent apoptosis modulates the cytotoxicity of anticancer agents. *Cell* 1993; 74:957–967.
7. Fan S, El-Deiry WS, Bae I, Freeman J, Jondle D, Bhatia K, Fornace AJ, Magrath I, Kohn KW, O'Connor PM. p53 gene mutations are associated with decreased sensitivity of human lymphoma cells to DNA damaging agents. *Cancer Res* 1994; 54:5824–5830.
8. Lowe SW, Bodis B, McCarthy A, Remington LH, Ruley HE, Fisher D, Housman DE, Jacks T. p53 status and the efficacy of cancer therapy in vivo. *Science* 1994; 266:807–810.
9. Kastan MB, Onyekwere O, Sidransky D, Vogelstein B, Craig RW. Participation of p53 protein in the cellular response to DNA damage. *Cancer Res* 1991; 51:6304–6311.
10. Kuerbitz SJ, Plunkett BS, Walsh WV, Kastan MB. Wild-type p53 is a cell cycle checkpoint determinant following irradiation. *Proc Natl Acad Sci USA* 1992; 89:7491–7495.
11. Livingstone LR, White A, Spouse J, Livanos E, Jacks T, Tlsty TD. Altered cell cycle arrest and gene amplification potential accompany loss of wild-type p53. *Cell* 1992; 70:923–935.
12. Yin Y, Tainsky MA, Bischoff FZ, Strong LC, Wahl GM. Wild-type p53 restores cell cycle-control and inhibits gene amplification in cells with mutant p53 alleles. *Cell* 1992; 70:937–948.
13. Waldman T, Lengauer C, Kinzler KW, Vogelstein B. Uncoupling of S phase and mitosis induced by anticancer agents in cells lacking p21. *Nature* 1996; 381:713–716.
14. Donehower LA, Harvey M, Slagle BL, McArthur MJ, Montgomery CA, Butel JS, Bradley A. Mice deficient for p53 are developmentally normal but susceptible to spontaneous tumours. *Nature* 1992; 356:215–221.
15. Jacks T, Remington L, Williams BO, Schmitt EM, Halachmi S, Bronson RT, Weinberg RA. Tumor spectrumanalysis in p53-mutant mice. *Curr Biol* 1994; 4:1–7.
16. Lee JL, Bernstein A. p53 mutations increase resistance to ionizing radiation. *Proc Natl Acad Sci USA* 1993; 90:5742–5746.
17. McIlwrath AJ, Vasey PA, Ross GM, Brown R. Cell cycle arrests and radiosensitivity of human tumor cell lines: dependence on wild-type p53 for radiosensitivity. *Cancer Res* 1994; 54:3718–3722.
18. Yount GL, Haas-Kogan DA, Vidair CA, Haas M, Dewey WC, Israel MA. Cell cycle synchrony unmasks the influence of p53 function on radiosensitivity of human glioblastoma cells. *Cancer Res* 1996; 56:500–506.
19. El-Deiry WS, Kern SE, Pietenpol JA, Kinzler KW, Vogelstein B. Definition of a consensus binding site for p53. *Nature Genet* 1992; 1:45–49.
20. Pietenpol JA, Papadopoulos N, Markowitz S, Willson JKV, Kinzler, KW. Vogelstein B. Paradoxical inhibition of solid tumor cell growth by bcl2. *Cancer Res* 1994; 54:3714–3717.
21. Miyashita T, Harigai M, Hanada M, Reed JC. Identification of a p53-dependent negative response element in the bcl-2 gene. *Cancer Res* 1994; 54:3131–3135.
22. El-Deiry WS, Tokino T, Velculescu VE, Levy DB, Parsons R, Trent JM, Lin D, Mercer WE, Kinzler KW, Vogelstein B. WAF1, a potential mediator of p53 tumor suppression. *Cell* 1993; 75:817–825.
23. Miyashita T, Reed JC. Tumor suppressor p53 is a direct transcriptional activator of the human bax gene. *Cell* 1995; 80:293–299.
24. Oliver FJ, Marvel J, Collins MKL, Lopez-Rivas A. Bcl-2 oncogene protects a bone marrow-derived pre-B-cell line from 5'-flour,2'-deoxyuridine-induced apoptosis. *Biochem Biophys Res Commun* 1993; 194:126–132.
25. Oltvai ZN, Milliman CL, Korsmeyer SJ. Bcl-2 heterodimerizes in vivo with a conserved homolog, Bax, that accelerates programmed cell death. *Cell* 1993; 74:609–619.
26. Miyashita T, Krajewski S, Krajewska M, Wang HG, Lin HK, Liebermann DA, Hoffman P, Reed JC. Tumor suppressor p53 is a regulator of bcl-2 and bax gene expression in vitro and in vivo. *Oncogene* 1994; 9:1799–1805.
27. Oltvai ZN, Korsmeyer SJ. Checkpoints of dueling dimers foil death wishes. *Cell* 1994; 79:189–192.
28. Selvakumaran M, Lin H-K, Miyashita T, Wang HG, Krajewski S, Reed C, Hoffman B, Liebermann D. Immediate early up-regulation of bax expression by p53 but not TGF beta 1: a paradigm for distinct apoptotic pathways. *Oncogene* 1994; 9:1791–1798.

29. Zhan Q, Fan S, Bae I, Guillouf C, Liebermann DA, O'Connor PM, Fornace AJ. Induction of bax by genotoxic stress in human cells correlates with normal p53 status and apoptosis. *Oncogene* 1994; 9:3743–3751.
30. Reed JC. Bcl-2 and the regulation of programmed cell death. *J Cell Biol* 1994; 124:1–6.
31. Krajewski S, Krajewski M, Shabaik A, Wang H-G, Irie S, Fong L, Reed JC. Immunohistochemical analysis of in vivo patterns of Bcl-X expression. *Cancer Res* 1994; 54:5501–5507.
32. Lu Q-L, Poulsom R, Wong L, Hanby AM. Bcl-2 expression in adult and embryonic non-haematopoietic tissues. *J Pathol* 1993; 169:431–437.
33. Bronner MP, Culin C, Reed JC, Furth EE. The bcl-2 proto-oncogene and the gastrointestinal epithelial tumor progression model. *Am J Pathol* 1995; 146:20–26.
34. Chiou S-K, Rao L, White E. Bcl-2 blocks p53-dependent apoptosis. *Mol Cell Biol* 1994; 14:2556–2563.
35. Wang Y, Szekely L, Okan I, Klein G, Wiman KG. Wild-type p53-triggered apoptosis is inhibited by bcl-2 in a v-myc-induced T-cell lymphoma line. *Oncogene* 1993; 8:3427–3431.
36. Dole M, Nunez G, Merchant AK, Maybaum J, Rode CK, Bloch CA, Castle VP. Bcl-2 inhibits chemotherapy-induced apoptosis in neuroblastoma. *Cancer Res* 1994; 54:3253–3259.
37. Miyashita T, Reed JC. bcl-2 gene transfer increases relative resistance of S49.1 and WEHI7.2 lymphoid cells to cell death and DNA fragmentation induced by glucocorticoids and multiple chemotherapeutic drugs. *Cancer Res* 1992; 52:5407–5411.
38. Walton MI, Whysong D, O'Connor PM, Hockenberry D, Korsmeyer SJ, Kohn KW. Constitutive expression of human Bcl-2 modulates nitrogen mustard and camptothecin induced apoptosis. *Cancer Res* 1993; 53:1853–1861.
39. Kamesaki S, Kamesaki H, Jorgensen TJ, Tanizawa A, Pommier Y, Cossman J. bcl-2 protein inhibits etoposide-induced apoptosis through its effects on events subsequent to topoisomerase II-induced DNA strand breaks and their repair. *Cancer Res* 1993; 53:4251–4256.
40. Fisher TC, Milner AE, Gregory CD, Jackman AL, Aherne GW, Hartley JA, Dive C, Hickman JA. bcl-2 modulation of apoptosis induced by anticancer drugs: resistance to thymidylate stress is independent of classical resistance pathways. *Cancer Res* 1993; 53:3321–3326.
41. Oliver FJ, Marvel J, Collins MKL, Lopez-Rivas A. Bcl-2 oncogene protects a bone marrow-derived pre-B-cell line from 5'-fluor,2'-deoxyuridine-induced apoptosis. *Biochem Biophys Res Commun* 1993; 194:126–132.
42. Debbas M, White E. Wild-type p53 mediates apoptosis by E1A, which is inhibited by E1B. *Genes Dev* 1993; 7:546–554.
43. Moyer JD, Smith PA, Levy EJ, Handschumacher RE. Kinetics of N-(phosphonacetyl)-L-aspartate and pyrazofurindepletion of pyrimidine ribonucleotide and deoxyribonucleotide pools and their relationship to nucleic acid synthesis in intact and permeabilized cells. *Cancer Res* 1992; 42:4525–4531.
44. Tltsy T. Replication of the dihydrofolate reductase genes on double minute chromosomes in a murine cellline. *Proc Natl Acad Sci USA* 1992; 87:3132–3136.
45. Lenz H-J, Danenberg KD, Leichman L, Leichman C, Danenberg PV. *Proc Am Assoc Cancer Res* 1995; 36:3332A.
46. Fearon ER, Vogelstein B. A genetic model for colorectal tumorigenesis. *Cell* 1990; 61:759–767.
47. Tew KD, Houghton PJ, Houghton JA. Modulation of 5-fluorouracil. In: Preclinical and Clinical Modulation of Anticancer Drugs. CRC Press, Boca Raton, 1993, pp. 197–321.
48. Danenberg PV. Thymidylate synthetase—a target enzyme in cancer chemotherapy. *Biochim Biophys Acta* 1977; 473:73–92.
49. Houghton JA, Houghton PJ. 5-Halogenated pyrimidines and their nucleosides. In: (Fox B, Fox M, eds.) Antitumor Drug Resistance—Handbook of Experimental Pharmacology. Springer-Verlag, Berlin. 1984, pp. 515–549.
50. Lenz H-J, Ju J-F, Danenberg KD, Banergee D, Bertino JR, Danenberg PV. Effect of p53 activity on the cytotoxicity of 5-fluoro-2'-deoxyuridine and its inhibition of thymidylate synthase. *Proc Am Assoc Cancer Res* 1995; 36:121A.
51. Lane DP. Cancer. p53, guardian of the genome. *Nature* (London) 1992; 358:15–16.
52. Jacks T, Remington L, Williams B, Scmitt E, Halachmi S, Bronson R, Weinberg R. Tumor spectrum analysis in p53-mutant mice. *Curr Biol* 1994; 4:1–7.
53. Harwood FG, Frazier MW, Krajewski S, Reed JC, Houghton J. Acute and delayed apoptosis induced by thymidine deprivation correlates with expression of p53 and p53-regulated genes in colon carcinoma cells. *Oncogene* 1996; 12:2057–2067.

54. Houghton JA, Harwood FG, Houghton PJ. Cell cycle control processes determine cytostasis or cytotoxicity in thymineless death of colon cancer cells. *Cancer Res* 1994; 54:4967–4973.
55. Debatin KM, Suss D, Krammer PH. Differential expression of APO-1 on human thymocytes: implications for negative selection? *Eur J Immunol* 1994; 24:753–758.
56. Watanabe-Fukanaga R, Brannan CI, Copeland NG, Jenkins NA, Nagata S. Lymphoproliferation disorder in mice explained by defects in Fas antigen that mediates apoptosis. *Nature* (London) 1992; 356:314–317.
57. Rozzo SJ, Eisenberg RA, Cohen PL, Kotzin BL. Development of the T cell receptor repertoire in lpr mice. *Semin Immunol* 1994; 6:19–26.
58. Smith CA, Farrah T, Goodwin RG. The TNF receptor superfamily of cellular and viral proteins: activation, costimulation, and death. *Cell* 1994; 76:959–962.
59. Moller P, Koretz K, Leithauser F, Bruderlein S, Henne C, Quentmeier A, Krammer PH. Expression of APO-1(CD95), a member of the NGF/TNF receptor superfamily, in normal and neoplastic colon epithelium. *Int J Cancer* 1994; 57:371–377.
60. Houghton JA, Harwood FG, Tilman DM. Thymineless death in colon carcinoma cells is mediated via Fas signaling. *Proc Natl Acad Sci USA* 1997; 94:8144–8149.

22   Genetic Determinants of Cell Death and Toxicity

D. Mark Pritchard and John A. Hickman

CONTENTS
- INTRODUCTION
- APOPTOSIS AND ITS GENETIC REGULATION
- THE RELATIONSHIP BETWEEN DRUG-INDUCED APOPTOSIS AND THERAPEUTIC RESPONSE
- SPECIFIC EXAMPLE—THE GASTROINTESTINAL TRACT
- CONCLUSIONS
- REFERENCES

1. INTRODUCTION

Current chemotherapeutic drugs used for the treatment of disseminated cancer impose cytotoxicity to tumor cells but also to normal tissues, toxicities that are often dose limiting. All of the antitumor drugs, regardless of their modes of action, induce apoptosis or programmed cell death, a process which is under genetic control (reviewed in ref. *1*). This suggests that the cytotoxicity of these agents is an active cellular response to perturbation rather than a direct consequence of a particular type of perturbation or damage (a fall in nucleotide pools or DNA strand breaks, for example). The particular menu of gene expression controlling programmed cell death, of genes which can either promote or suppress deletion of "damaged" cells, is different in different cell types. This determines the "threshold" at which perturbation to the cell may engage cell death. Put simply, some cells will die more readily than others with the same load of damage. It is therefore reasonable to hypothesize that the expression patterns of genes that alter the threshold of cells to undergo apoptosis will contribute not only to the efficacy of chemotherapy in terms of tumor response *(2,3)*, but also to determining host toxicity. Is this hypothesis proven?

The precise relationship between observations of the acute induction of apoptosis by anticancer drugs and the long-term therapeutic or toxic outcome is not entirely clear. There is conflicting data, particularly from some in vitro experiments, concerning the relationship between apoptotic cell death and clonogenic survival, a valuable measure of the long-term capability of cells to survive and proliferate. In this chapter, we will give an overview of apoptosis and its genetic control. We will discuss the controversies that currently exist concerning the relationship between apoptosis and therapeutic response. This will be illustrated by describing one model system in detail, the apoptosis and toxicity induced by 5-fluorouracil (5FU) and Tomudex (ZD1694) in the intestinal epithelium of various transgenic mice. Surprisingly, the mechanisms of action of these two drugs appear to be very different in these normal epithelial cells.

The epithelia of the gut are not only particularly sensitive to the perturbations induced by this class of antimetabolite drug, causing dose-limiting toxicity at this site, but these epithelia also give rise to tumors to which the drugs 5-fluorouracil and Tomudex (ZD1694) are targeted. We suggest that understanding the controls and determinants of survival and death in these normal epithelia may aid understanding of the same events in tumors of the colon and rectum. By using mice in which a particular gene has been removed (knockouts) the influence of the gene product on the induction of acute apoptosis and long-term outcome (histopathology) can be monitored. Our results illustrate that the relationship between drug-induced damage, the induction of apoptosis, and long-term fate of a tissue is complex. This reflects the complexity of function of some of these gene products and demonstrates that apoptosis is only one factor determining overall drug response. Most importantly however, our data show that in vivo, expression of a gene that controls what are commonly termed "downstream" events, is an absolute determinant of 5-fluorouracil-induced gastrointestinal toxicity. Downstream events are those that are beyond the biochemical perturbation or damage itself, such as damage "sensing" and signaling, prior to a commitment to die.

2. APOPTOSIS AND ITS GENETIC REGULATION

Apoptosis is a regulated process for the removal of unnecessary, aged, or damaged cells and is thus crucial to many events during the development and homeostasis of multicellular organisms. Defects in apoptosis can lead to disease, including cancer (in which DNA-damaged cells are not deleted), autoimmune disease, and degenerative disorders.

Apoptosis was originally described on the basis of distinctive cell morphology *(4,5)*. The cytoplasm shrinks and the cell becomes detached from its neighbors; chromatin becomes condensed at the nuclear membrane; the cell membrane takes on a 'blebbed' appearance, and the cell fragments. The resulting 'apoptotic bodies' are then phagocytosed. In contrast to necrosis, in which membrane integrity is not maintained, apoptosis usually occurs asynchronously in single cells and does not cause an inflammatory response or result in tissue destruction.

The process of apoptosis can be subdivided into three different phases: initiation, in which damage signals are integrated; an effector stage in which the cell becomes irreversibly committed to apoptosis; and execution, in which proteins and DNA are cleaved (*see* Fig. 1). Initiation can be triggered by a range of disparate stimuli either physiological (such as binding of glucocorticoids or Fas ligand to their receptors) or pharmacological (by for example radiation, anticancer drugs, or noxious stimuli). The effector stage is complex. In the case of apoptosis initiated by the death-inducing Fas receptor there appears to be direct activation of components of a protease (caspase) cascade involved in the execution phase. This occurs via the proteolytic FLICE component of the

Chapter 22 / Genetic Determinants

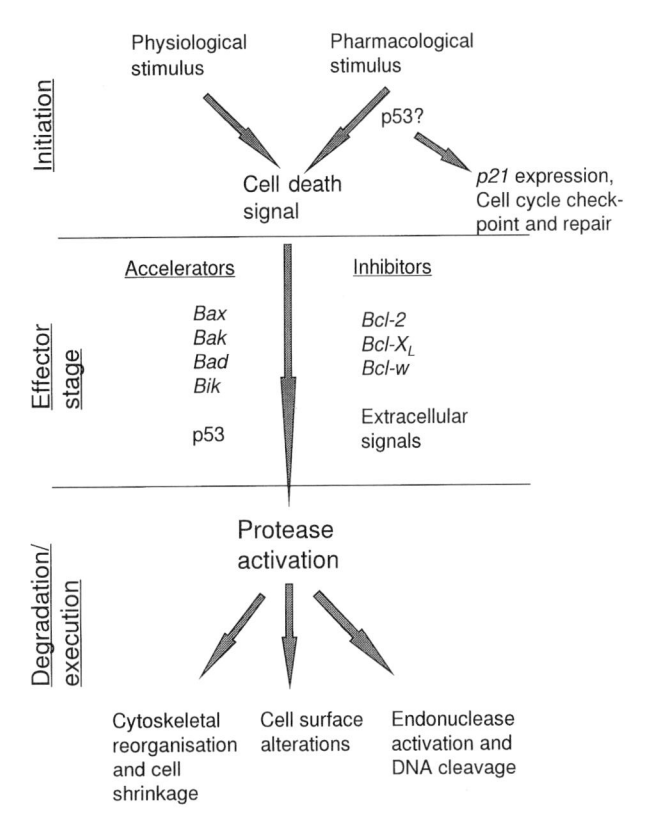

Fig. 1. Schematic representation of the general pathway of apoptosis. Details of the pathway vary according to cell phenotype and context.

Fas receptor (reviewed in ref. 6). Death induced by other stimuli, which does not involve proximal activation of the caspase-mediated proteolytic cascade, is suppressed by the expression of bcl-2, bcl-w, and bcl-X_L and accelerated by the homologous proteins bax, bak, and bik (reviewed in ref. 7). In the case of genomic damage, the tumor supressor p53 may, according to cellular background, become activated as a promoter of apoptosis. The nature of the signals, for example arising from DNA damage, which activate members of the bcl-2 family of proteins is unknown as is the nature of the biochemical event that irreversibly commits the cell to die. Recent evidence suggests that "commitment to die" occurs prior to caspase activation and is distinct from the degradative events that characterize execution (8).

The execution phase exhibits common features regardless of the initiating stimulus. Whereas the effector stage is still subject to (genetic) regulation and manipulation, execution/degradation is not regulatable. Degradative events include the proteolysis of key cellular proteins including nuclear lamins, elements of the cytoskeleton, polyADPribose polymerase (*see* ref. 9 for recent review), and the cleavage of DNA, first into 50-kb fragments then commonly to internucleosomal fragments (multiples of 200 bp; the DNA ladder). Apoptosis, as distinct from commitment to death appears to be integrated and/or initiated by events in mitochondria, including a change in membrane potential, the release of cytochrome c, and the activation of caspases via the activation of an adapter protein apaf-1, which uses cytochrome c to activate caspase-3 *(10)*.

As mentioned above, the effector stage is regulated by the products of a number of genes, most notably by p53 and members of the bcl-2 family. A full discussion of these gene products is beyond the scope of this chapter (for recent reviews *see* refs *7,10–12*) but a few remarks are pertinent for the discussion which follows: p53 can both promote apoptosis and/or cause cell-cycle arrest (a cell-cycle checkpoint) via expression of the cyclin dependent-kinase inhibitor *p21$^{WAF1/CIP1}$*. This critical "choice" of apoptosis vs survival at a cell-cycle checkpoint depends on the stimulus and upon cellular context (Fig. 1). These contextual elements are complex: signals from survival factors, the stoichiometry of the members of the bcl-2 family, the expression and status of other proteins controlling the progression through the cell cycle (for example the retinoblastoma protein) all impact upon what may be viewed as an iterative assessment of the integrity of the cell and its ultimate response to damage. Knockout transgenic mouse models of many of the cell-death regulating genes now exist to allow study of their in vivo function (e.g., *p53 [13]*; *p21$^{WAF1/CIP1}$ [14]*; *bcl-2 [15,16]*; *bax [17]*, and *bcl-x [18*, although in this last case it proved to be embryonic lethal]). These studies in vivo have the advantage of allowing an analysis of the contribution of a particular gene in a cell within its proper context.

The morphology of apoptosis in vivo can be assessed by light and electron microscopy and by biochemical techniques that detect cleaved DNA *(19)*. These are events at or beyond the degradation stage. Discrepancy is sometimes seen between the results of different methods (e.g., between light microscopy and TUNEL labeling of DNA cleavage in the intestine *[20]*), hence careful analysis of the published data is essential. A number of other considerations are also important for obtaining accurate and meaningful quantitative estimates of apoptotic events, as the rate of degradation and extent of fragmentation into apoptotic bodies may be tissue dependent. Very often the evidence for apoptosis comes from the detection of apoptotic bodies or fragments rather than whole apoptotic cells. The question arises as to whether these represent a single apoptotic cell or have arisen from several. The problem of being unable to accurately estimate the quantity of apoptosis and to integrate it with time is very considerable. Lack of attention to such details is likely to give misleading data when investigators attempt to define an apoptotic index analogous to a mitotic index (reviewed in ref. *21*).

3. THE RELATIONSHIP BETWEEN DRUG-INDUCED APOPTOSIS AND THERAPEUTIC RESPONSE

As stated above, all chemotherapeutic agents induce apoptosis and there are many in vitro and in vivo examples showing that this acute apoptosis (an apoptotic morphology within 36 h) is genetically regulated. However, the relationship between this acute apoptosis and the therapeutic effects of a drug as demonstrated by clonogenic assays in vitro and by the efficacy of tumor therapy in human patients remains to be clarified. Early studies showed the p53 dependence of radiation and cytotoxic drug-induced acute apoptosis in thymocytes and fibroblasts in vitro *(22–24)* and radiation-induced intestinal apoptosis in vivo (*see* Subheading 4.1.) *(25,26)*. However, analysis of long-term survival by clonogenic assays in vitro has been controversial. For example, Slichenmeyer *(27)* showed no increase in survival of embryonic fibroblasts from *p53*-null mice, compared to their *p53* wild-type counterparts, following radiation or camptothecin treatment. A number of studies have shown resistance, no change or drug sensitization using clonogenic assays of cancer cells in which the half life of the p53 protein has been reduced by transfection with human papilloma virus E6. The different results depended on the cellular background and the particular drug *(27–30)*. Similarly, in vivo, whereas p53 activation following radiation is important for apoptosis in certain tissues such as the thymus and intestine, it seems to have little importance in others such as liver, skeletal muscle, and brain *(31)*. Even in those tissues in which there is almost complete dependence on p53 for acute radiation-induced apoptosis, such as the small intestine, no clonogenic crypt survival has been demonstrated in $p53^{-/-}$ (knockout) animals after radiation, although the doses used were high (10 Gy) *(32)*. In the clinical setting, with particular reference to colorectal cancer, p53 expression has been shown to affect the apoptotic index in a small series of colorectal cancers given preoperative radiotherapy *(33)*. The response rates but not survival patterns of patients with colonic cancers treated with modulated 5-fluorouracil chemotherapy were also changed according to p53 status *(34)*. Clearly there are p53-independent mechanisms of cell death and paradoxically, as noted above, the checkpoint function of p53 may promote a cessation of the cell cycle and subsequent survival, according to cellular background (Fig. 1).

Bcl-2 expression has also been shown to affect acute apoptosis in vitro; for example fluorodeoxyuridine treatment of a B-cell lymphoma cell line transfected with *bcl-2* showed significant survival of DNA-damaged cells in comparison to cells transfected with vector alone *(35)*. However, the study by Yin and Schimke *(36)* showed no difference in clonogenic survival of *bcl-2*-transfected HeLa cells treated with aphidocolin, yet there was a significant difference in the kinetics of the onset of apoptosis. Such differences may reflect the different cellular contexts. For example, lack of extracellular signals (modulating cellular background) may influence bcl-2 function. Walker et al. *(37)* have shown that *bcl-2* transfection delayed apoptosis but had no effect on clonogenicity of Burkitt's lymphoma cells grown under conventional culture conditions, yet when the milieu of the germinal center was provided by ligation of CD40 and stromal signals, a significant clonogenic survival was observed. *Bcl-2* expression has also been shown to affect acute radiation-induced apoptosis in the colon in vivo as discussed in Subheading 4.1., but to date no attempts have been made to see whether such apoptosis translates into a clonogenic type difference in crypt survival *(20)*. In the clinical setting *bcl-2* expression in colorectal cancers is associated with improved patient survival even within a particular Duke's stage *(38,39)*. In contrast, *bcl-2* expression has often been associated with a poorer prognosis in lymphoma and a range of other tumors *(40)*.

There are a number of potential explanations for some of the discrepancies described above. As discussed, in vitro clonogenic experiments, although important, do reflect a grossly artificial situation, and the presence of other survival signals might alter results considerably.

The question remains as to whether altering the expression of those genes that are known to be important in controlling the process of apoptosis will allow the development of more effective treatment regimes for patients. We will discuss this below in detail with particular reference to one system—the effects of antimetabolites in the mouse intestinal tract. Here, normal cells are in their normal extracellular and contextual envi-

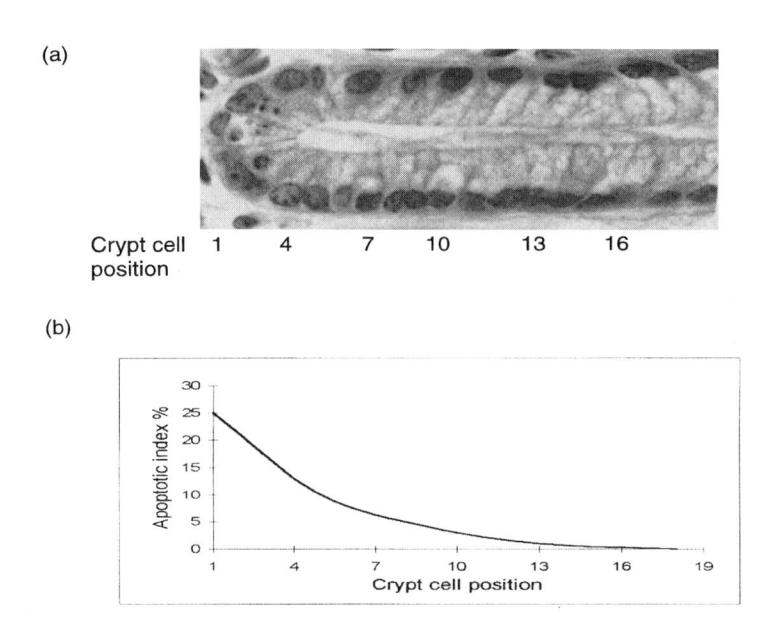

Fig. 2. (A) Photomicrograph of a murine colonic crypt with apoptotic bodies at cell positions 1 and 2. The cell positions are numbered. (B) Analysis of 200–300 half crypts from 4–6 mice can give plots of cell positional apoptotic index percentage. The plot shown is a hypothetical distribution for a population in which the crypt shown in the photomicrograph would represent a typical example.

ronment; transgenic models potentially allow the investigation of the effects of single genes; apoptosis can be easily and accurately scored and histological changes can be readily seen as the tissue is rapidly renewing and the consequences of drug toxicity (i.e., diarrhea) can be measured and are clinically important. We will show that expression of the *p53* gene in this setting is a crucial determinant of both apoptosis and cumulative drug response. The data also demonstrate the complex relationship between apoptosis and therapeutic response and provide insights that might explain some of the conflicting data described above.

4. SPECIFIC EXAMPLE—THE GASTROINTESTINAL TRACT
4.1. Cell Death in the Intestine

The intestinal epithelium is constantly renewing itself—cells originate from a small number of stem cells located near the base of the crypts of Lieberkühn; these cells proliferate rapidly within the crypt compartment and differentiate as they migrate upwards. In the small intestine, cells pass onto the villus and are eventually shed from the villus tip; the colon does not have villi and cells are shed from the colonic table region. This tissue architecture allows for the precise analysis of spontaneous and induced apoptosis that can be related to other cellular parameters such as mitosis, proliferation, or differentiated phenotype and also the position of the cell along the crypt-villus axis. Morphologically apoptotic cells can be readily detected in the crypt compartment of intestinal epithelium by light microscopy of hematoxylin and eosin-stained cross sections and statistically valid results can be obtained from counting 200–300 well-oriented half crypts from groups of 4–6 mice *(20,41)* (Fig. 2). An alternative method for quantifying apoptosis is the *in situ* TdT-mediated dUTP-biotin nick end-labeling technique (TUNEL) *(42)*. However, this method shows staining at the villus tip and colonic table regions, where morphologically apoptotic cells are very rarely seen. In the intestinal tract therefore this technique is generally considered to be less useful than conventional morphological criteria, as a result of the false-negative and false-positive results obtained *(20,41,43)*.

Morphological evidence of spontaneous apoptosis can be observed in the intestinal crypts of healthy mice at a frequency of one cell in every fifth longitudinal small intestinal crypt section. This apoptosis occurs predominantly at the presumed stem-cell zone (cell positions 4–6) in the murine small intestine, but at cell positions above the presumed stem-cell zone in the murine colon. *p53*-null mice *(13)* show similar levels of spontaneous apoptosis to their wild-type counterparts *(25,26)*, whereas *bcl-2*-null mice *(15)* show similar levels of spontaneous apoptosis to their wild-type counterparts in the small intestine, but elevated levels specifically at the presumed stem-cell positions (cell positions 1–2) at the colonic crypt base where immunohistochemical bcl-2 expression has also been detected *(20)*. As already mentioned, very few morphologically apoptotic cells are observed by electron microscopy at the villus tips, where effete cells are known to be shed *(44)*. However, recent evidence *(45–47)* has suggested that a specialized form of apoptosis does occur at this site.

The use of γ-radiation to induce apoptosis in the intestine has been widely studied *(48,49)*. Apoptosis is induced readily, rapidly (peak incidence at 4–6 h) and predominantly at the stem-cell zone of mouse small intestine by γ-radiation. The dose threshold for apoptosis induction is greater in the colon and this response is not concentrated in the stem cell zone. Radiation-induced apoptosis is strongly affected by the expression of *p53* and *bcl-2* genes. *p53*-null mice show greatly suppressed levels of cell death at all times following 1 Gy. A late wave of apoptosis is observed at 24 h following the administration of 8 Gy, these late p53-independent deaths appearing to occur at G2/M phase *(25,26,32,50)*. *Bcl-2*-null mice show elevated levels of apoptosis following γ-radiation but, as with spontaneous apoptosis in these animals, this response is specifically concentrated at the stem-cell zone at the base of colonic crypts *(20)*. These differences between murine small and large intestine are summarized in Table 1.

4.2. 5-Fluorouracil-Induced Acute Apoptosis in the Mouse Intestine

A number of chemotherapeutic drugs have been shown to induce apoptosis in the normal murine small intestinal epithelium within 12 h of bolus intraperitoneal administration. Different agents target different cell positions within the crypt hierarchy. The significance of this finding remains unclear *(51,52)*. It is possible that it reflects either the selective imposition of damage in cells at these different positions, differences in repair capacity and/or differences in the qualitative response for the engagement of apoptosis according to the nature of the damage/perturbation. Apoptotic bodies have also been shown in colonic biopsy specimens of patients suffering from 5-fluorouracil (5FU)-induced colitis *(53,54)*.

The regulation of the acute apoptosis induced by 5FU in mouse intestinal epithelium has been studied by us in considerable detail *(55)*. The administration of 40 mg/kg 5FU by bolus intraperitoneal injection to wild-type mice induces apoptosis as early as 4.5 h and with a peak at 24 h in both the small intestinal and colonic crypts. It targets the early

Table 1
Differences in Genetic Control of Spontaneous and γ-Radiation Induced Apoptosis in Murine Small and Large Intestine

Parameter	Small intestine	Colon
Human tumor incidence	Low	High
Proposed stem-cell positions	Cell positions 4–6	Cell positions 1–2
Cell position of spontaneous apoptosis	At stem-cell zone	At cell positions above stem-cell zone
Threshold of radiation-induced apoptosis	Low	High
Cell position of radiation-induced apoptosis	At stem-cell zone	At cell positions above stem-cell zone
p53-null mice	Suppressed radiation-induced apoptosis	Suppressed radiation-induced apoptosis
bcl-2-null mice	Minor effects on apoptosis only	Increased spontaneous and radiation-induced apoptosis at stem-cell zone

transit cells (maximum at cell positions 6–8) in the small intestine, and cells in the putative stem-cell zone (cell positions 1–2) in the colon (Fig. 3). We have shown that this response is p53-dependent both by immunohistochemistry and by showing a suppressed response in *p53*-null mice (Fig. 3A,B).

Bcl-2 null animals showed a wave of apoptosis restricted to the stem-cell zone at the base of colonic crypts 4.5 h following 40 mg/kg 5FU. This was not seen in wild-type animals (Fig. 3C). However, by 24 h no differences were observed between wild-type and null mice (Fig. 3D), suggesting either that *bcl-2* is acting to delay rather than prevent apoptosis completely or that apoptosis at this time is *bcl-2* independent (Pritchard et al., submitted). These findings suggest that 5FU induces its cellular damage soon after administration (4.5 h), but that the apoptotic response is normally suppressed in the colonic stem cell zone by *bcl-2* expression.

The mechanism of action of 5FU in this in vivo setting can also be studied by administering modulators of drug action along with the drug. We have shown that the apoptotic response to 40 mg/kg 5FU in the intestine was not altered by administration of thymidine. Thymidine given in the same schedule could suppress the thymidylate synthase inhibitor Tomudex induced apoptosis as discussed in Subheading 4.4. However, apoptosis was significantly reduced by administration of 3500 mg/kg uridine 2 h following 5FU *(55)*. This uridine-dosing schedule has previously been shown to rescue 5FU-induced intestinal toxicity in mice and rats *(56–58)*. Provocatively, this suggests that 5FU is acting predominantly via an RNA damaging mechanism of action to activate p53 rather than as a thymidylate synthase inhibitor. Whereas this agrees with previously published data *(59)*, it raises important questions about what damage is being sensed by p53 if RNA metabolism is perturbed. It is possible that secondary changes in DNA integrity, which are subsequent to alterations in RNA metabolism are sensed by p53. Experiments in a 5-fluorouracil-treated colon-carcinoma cell line have shown DNA to be intact at the time of the appearance of p53 protein (DMP, unpublished data).

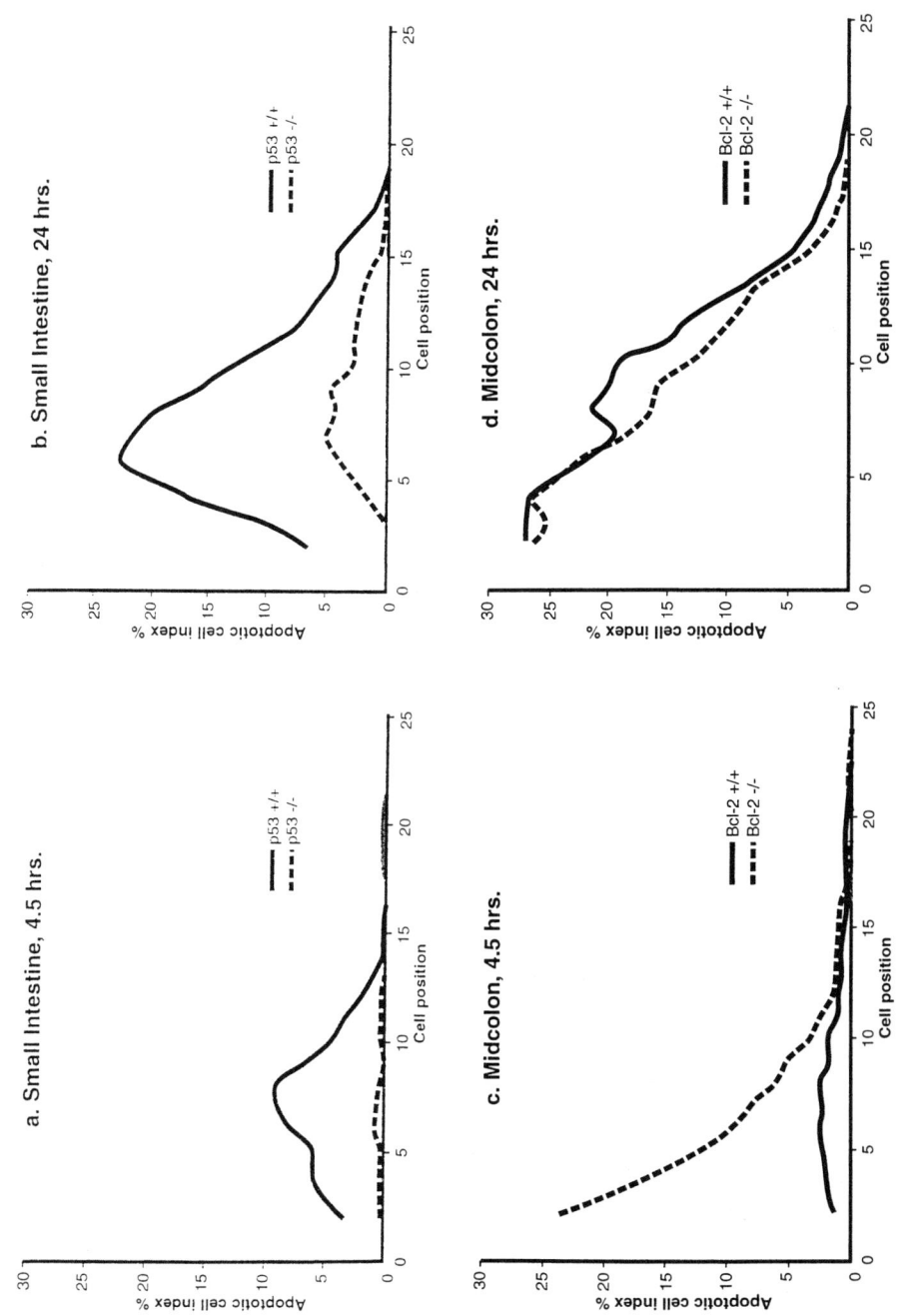

Fig. 3. Cell-positional distribution of apoptosis following ip administration of 40 mg/kg 5FU (four mice in each experimental group): **(A)** Small intestine after 4.5 h of *p53* wild-type and homozygously null mice, **(B)** small intestine after 24 h of *p53* wild-type and homozygously null mice, **(C)** midcolon after 4.5 h of *bcl-2* wild-type and homozygously null mice, **(D)** midcolon after 24 h of *bcl-2* wild-type and homozygously null mice. **A** and **B** from ref. 55, **C** and **D** from Pritchard et al., submitted.

4.3. Relationship Between Acute 5-Fluorouracil-Induced Apoptosis and Gastrointestinal Toxicity

As discussed above, 5FU-induced acute apoptosis in the gastrointestinal epithelium is strongly influenced by the expression of p53. Since 5FU also causes toxicity to the gastrointestinal epithelium when given in high or multiple doses, this system provides a useful in vivo model to test the correlation between p53 expression, acute apoptosis, and subsequent histopathology indicative of toxicity. We have compared 5FU-induced changes in gut morphology and function in *p53* wild-type and *p53*-null mice in which patterns of acute apoptosis were significantly different according to genotype (Pritchard et al., submitted).

5FU was first administered to groups of BDF1 wild-type mice as a single dose or two doses given 6 h apart either of 40 or 400 mg/kg. Mouse weights and survival were monitored and groups of four mice were sacrificed at times ranging from 4.5 h to 14 d after drug administration. Hematoxylin and eosin stained sections of intestines were examined on a cell positional basis by light microscopy for apoptosis, mitosis, and tritiated thymidine labeling (as a proliferation marker) as outlined in Fig. 2. Cell counts and area measurements provided data on crypt and villus integrity and histopathology. The 400 mg/kg doses were toxic, inducing weight loss and death with changes in gut histology (crypt destruction and villus shortening) maximum at 96 h. The 40 mg/kg doses, by contrast, were well tolerated and caused none of the above changes. Surprisingly, the peak apoptotic index percentage, in which we scored accumulating apoptotic events (NB *not* only single apoptotic cells but also apoptotic fragments), measured after 24 h was only marginally higher at 400 compared to 40 mg/kg *(55)*. This suggests that events in addition to apoptosis are required for toxicity. Toxicity was described by changes in cellularity of the crypt (numbers of cells per crypt length) and by gross losses of morphological integrity. What are these other events, in addition to apoptosis, that give rise to subsequent toxicity?

There was a more profound suppression of proliferation and mitosis observed at the higher (400 mg/kg) drug doses. As noted above (*see* Fig. 1) one of the functions of p53 is cell cycle checkpoint control, via $p21^{WAF1/CIP1}$ expression. The suppression of progression through the cell cycle and the subsequent loss of mitotic cells as a consequence of this may be short or long term: In mesenchymal-cells the expression of $p21^{WAF1/CIP1}$ was associated with senescence *(60)*. We are currently investigating the fates of the cells that have escaped apoptosis and instead of undergoing a transient checkpoint, may go into a long-term arrest that is sufficient to prevent maintenance of tissue architecture.

When the toxic 400 mg/kg ×2 dose was administered to *p53*-null animals, suppression of apoptosis at timepoints up to 24 h was found as noted previously *(55)*, although some late p53-independent apoptosis was observed at 54 h. Crucially, these animals showed significant preservation of intestinal histology at times (78 and 102 h) when their wild-type counterparts showed maximum gut toxicity based on histological measurements (Pritchard et al., submitted). Thus, loss of p53 function in vivo effectively abrogated the toxicity of 5FU to otherwise normal cells in their normal cellular environment. The data illustrates that the regulation of 5FU-induced apoptosis and toxicity in the otherwise normal cells of the mouse intestine by p53 is complex and suggests that the measurement of an apoptotic index alone is not a helpful predictor of subsequent toxicity. This may partially explain why data relating the expression of a single gene product (with multiple functions) to the outcome of human cancers that have a heterogeneous array of other mutations is likely to be ambiguous. However, the important observation is that, despite the complexities of mechanism (apoptosis/checkpoint/ long-term cell-cycle arrest) contributing to toxicity, it is determined by downstream events modulated by a gene product, in this case p53.

4.4. Tomudex Induces Apoptosis in the Mouse Intestine with a Pattern Different From 5FU

The new antifolate thymidylate synthase inhibitors such as Tomudex (ZD1694) (for review, *see* ref. *61*) are proving to be as efficacious as folinic acid-modulated 5FU in the treatment of advanced colorectal cancer, but with a generally more favorable toxicity profile *(62)*. However, Tomudex can cause severe and unpredictable gastrointestinal toxicity in humans. A model of this has been developed by us using two mouse strains that have greatly differing susceptibilities to intestinal toxicity following Tomudex administration: DBA/2 mice are relatively resistant, whereas Balb/c mice are relatively sensitive (Jackman, unpublished data). We have investigated whether there are any important differences between 5FU- and Tomudex-induced apoptosis in the murine intestine.

Following bolus administration, Tomudex induces apoptosis predominantly in the small intestine of wild-type BDF1 mice with few effects in the colon. This is different from 5FU (*see* Subheading 4.2). Furthermore, differentiated cells, higher up the small intestinal crypt, (maximum at cell positions 10–14) are targeted by Tomudex in comparison to 5FU which caused cell death maximally at cell positions 6–8. Apoptosis is not induced as early by Tomudex as following administration of 5FU, but the peak incidence of apoptosis for both drugs is at 24 h. As with 5FU, there is a plateau in response to drug doses above a particular dose level, in the case of Tomudex 10 mg/kg (DMP, unpublished observations). Whereas 5FU causes cell death in the intestine predominantly by its RNA-damaging mechanism of action as discussed in Subheading 4.2., Tomudex-induced apoptosis could be abrogated by coadministration of 500 mg/kg thymidine, strongly suggesting that it resulted from thymidylate synthase inhibition *(55)*.

We have observed statistically significant differences in the apoptotic yield in the small intestine of DBA/2 mice compared to Balb/c mice following Tomudex. This is a pattern congruent with the amount of toxicity caused by this agent in these two different strains (Fig. 4). The relationship between Tomudex-induced apoptosis and toxicity in the intestine is currently under active investigation using the model system devised for 5FU described in Subheading 4.3. Intriguingly, we have also demonstrated that Tomudex-induced apoptosis in the murine intestinal epithelium is p53-independent, again unlike 5FU, since no differences were observed in apoptotic yield between *p53* wild-type and null mice (DMP, unpublished observation). This observation is surprising considering the drug's proposed mechanism of action, which is to induce damage to nascent strands of DNA as a result of thymidylate synthase inhibition *(55)*. However, a Tomudex-induced p53-independent cell death is not without precedent: Although Tomudex has been shown to induce p53 and WAF1 expression in HCT-8 colon carcinoma cells *(63)*, the cell-cycle arrest caused by this agent seems to occur via an alternative pathway to DNA damage and p53 induction *(64)* and the expression of p53 in these cells appears to be coincidental rather than contributing to death.

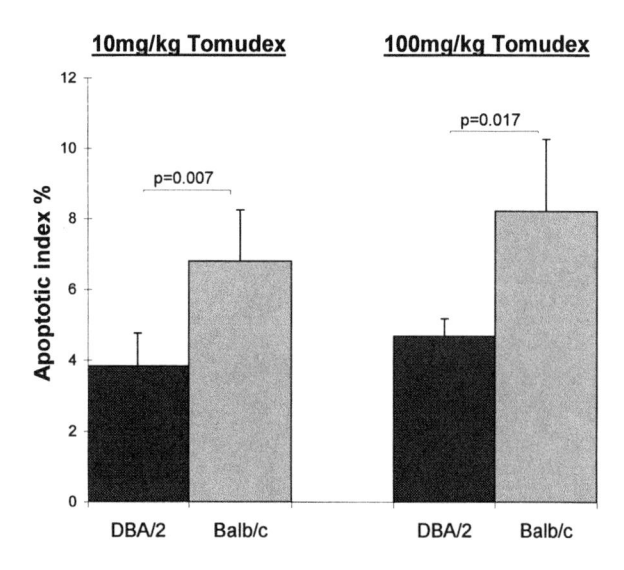

Fig. 4. Apoptotic indices in DBA/2 and Balb/c mice 24 h after ip administration of 10 and 100 mg/kg Tomudex (five animals in each experimental group). Statistical analysis by two tailed Student's *t*-test assuming unequal variance of the groups being compared.

These are important differences in the cell positional details, mechanisms, and genetic regulation of Tomudex-and 5FU-induced intestinal apoptosis in the epithelia of the murine gastrointestinal tract. This was surprising to us. It suggests that mechanistically, these two agents are quite different. After 5FU, an RNA-driven p53-dependent perturbation induces cell death and inhibition of proliferation. After Tomudex, an undefined thymidylate synthase-driven event initiates apoptosis in a p53-independent manner, suggesting that DNA damage is *not* the event responsible for death. Further investigation may help to elucidate the relevance of these findings to the gastrointestinal toxicity induced by these drugs and their efficacy against tumors.

5. CONCLUSIONS

We have demonstrated in the murine intestine in vivo that p53 expression can affect the response of the epithelium to 5FU. The expression of apoptosis-modulating genes has the *potential* to affect the outcome of therapy although we point out that p53 also has downstream effects on cell proliferation because of its cell-cycle checkpoint role. These results to our knowledge, arise from the first comprehensive in vivo experiments to study acute changes in apoptosis and subsequent histopathological changes, including changes in proliferation and mitosis. Whether they can be generalized remains to be determined. This is a particularly pertinent question with respect to cells with a transformed phenotype. Our studies also caution against the use of static measurements of apoptotic index as predictors of response, since the process of apoptosis is exquisitely dynamic and because such data does not take account of other vital parameters such as the capacities of a tissue to repair and regenerate.

REFERENCES

1. Thompson CB. Apoptosis in the pathogenesis and treatment of disease. *Science* 1995; 267:1456–1462.
2. Dive C, Hickman JA. Drug target interactions: only the first step in the commitment to a programmed cell death. *Br J Cancer* 1991; 64:192–196.
3. Fisher DE. Apoptosis in cancer therapy: crossing the threshold. *Cell* 1994; 78:539–542.
4. Kerr JFR, Wyllie AH, Currie AR. Apoptosis: a basic biological phenomenon with wide ranging implications in tissue kinetics. *Br J Cancer* 1972; 26:239–257.
5. Arends MJ, Wyllie AH. Apoptosis: mechanisms and roles in pathology. *Int Rev Expt Pathol* 1991; 32:223–254.
6. Mariani SM, Matiba B, Krammer PH. CD95 (APO-1/Fas) and its ligand in the mouse immune system. *Behring Inst Mitt* 1996; 97:12–23.
7. Reed JC. Double identity for proteins of the bcl-2 family. *Nature* 1997; 387:773–776.
8. McCarthy NJ, Whyte MKB, Gilbert CS, Evan GI. Inhibition of Ced-3/ICE-related proteases does not prevent cell death induced by oncogenes, DNA damage, or the Bcl-2 homologue Bak. *J Cell Biol* 1997; 136:215–227.
9. Takahashi A, Earnshaw WC. ICE-related proteases in apoptosis. *Curr Opinion Genetics Devel* 1996; 6:50–55.
10. Vaux DL. CED-4—the third horseman of apoptosis. *Cell* 1997; 90:389–390.
11. Harris CC. Structure and function of the p53 tumor suppressor gene: clues for rational cancer therapeutic strategies. *J Natl Cancer Inst* 1996; 88:1442–1455.
12. Kroemer G. The proto-oncogene bcl-2 and its role in regulating apoptosis. *Nature Medicine* 1997; 3:614–620.
13. Donehower LA, Harvey M, Slagle BL, McArthur MJ, Montgomery Jr, CA, Butel JS, Bradley A. Mice deficient for p53 are developmentally normal but susceptible to spontaneous tumours. *Nature* 1992; 356:215–221.
14. Deng C, Zhang P, Harper JW, Elledge SJ, Leder P. Mice lacking p21$^{CIP1/WAF1}$ undergo normal development, but are defective in G1 checkpoint control. *Cell* 1995; 82:675–684.
15. Nakayama K, Nakayama K, Negishi I, Kuida K, Shinkai Y, Louie MC, Fields LE, Lucas PJ, Stewart V, Alt FW, Loh DY. Disappearance of the lymphoid system in Bcl-2 homozygous mutant chimeric mice. *Science* 1993; 261:1584–1588.
16. Veis DI, Sorenson CM, Dhutter JR, Korsmeyer SJ. Bcl-2 deficient mice demonstrate fulminant lymphoid apoptosis, polycystic kidneys and hypopigmented hair. *Cell* 1993; 75:229–240.
17. Knudson CM, Tung KSK, Tourtellotte WG, Brown GAJ, Korsmeyer SJ. Bax-deficient mice with lymphoid hyperplasia and male germ cell death. *Science* 1995; 270:96–99.
18. Motoyama N, Wang F, Roth KA, Sawa H, Nakayama K, Nakayama K, Negioshi I, Senju S, Zhang Q, Fujii S, Loh DY. Massive cell death of immature haematopoietic cells and neurons in Bcl-x-deficient mice. *Science* 1995; 267:1506–1510.
19. Cotter TG, Martin SJ. Techniques in Apoptosis. Portland Press, London.
20. Merritt AJ, Potten CS, Watson AJM, Loh DY, Nakayama K, Nakayama K, Hickman JA. Differential expression of bcl-2 in intestinal epithelia-correlation with attenuation of apoptosis in colonic crypts and the incidence of colonic neoplasia. *J Cell Science* 1995; 108:2261–2271.
21. Potten CS. What is an apoptotic index measuring? A commentary. *Br J Cancer* 1996; 74:1743–1748.
22. Clarke AR, Purdie CA, Harrison DJ, Morris RG, Bird CC, Hooper ML, Wyllie AH. Thymocyte apoptosis induced by p53-dependent and independent pathways. *Nature* 1993; 362:849–852.
23. Lowe SW, Ruley HE, Jacks T, Housman DE. p53-dependent apoptosis modulates the cytotoxicity of anticancer agents. *Cell* 1993; 74:957–967.
24. Lowe SW, Schmitt EM, Smith SW, Osborne BA, Jacks T. p53 is required for radiation-induced apoptosis in mouse thymocytes. *Nature* 1993; 362:847–849.
25. Merritt AJ, Potten CS, Kemp CJ, Hickman JA, Ballmain A, Lane DP, Hall PA. The role of p53 in spontaneous and radiation-induced apoptosis in the gastrointestinal tract of normal and p53-deficient mice. *Cancer Res* 1994; 54:614–617.
26. Clarke AR, Gledhill S, Hooper ML, Bird CC, Wyllie AH. p53 dependence of early apoptotic and proliferative responses within the mouse intestinal epithelium following γ-irradiation. *Oncogene* 1994; 9:1767–1773.
27. Slichenmeyer WJ, Nelson WG, Slebos RJ, Kastan MB. Loss of p53-associated G1 checkpoint does not decrease cell survival following DNA damage. *Cancer Res* 1993; 53:4164–4168.

28. Hawkins DS, Demers GW, Galloway DA. Inactivation of p53 enhances sensitivity to multiple chemotherapeutic agents. *Cancer Res* 1993; 56:892–898.
29. Fan S, Smith ML, Rivet DJ, Duba D, Zhan Q, Kohn KW, Fornace Jr, AJ, O'Connor PM. Disruption of p53 function sensitizes breast cancer MCF-7 cells to cisplatin and pentoxifylline. *Cancer Res* 1995; 55:1649–1654.
30. Fan S, Chang JK, Smith ML, Duba D, Fornace Jr, AJ, O'Connor PM. Cells lacking CIP1/WAF1 genes exhibit preferential sensitivity to cisplatin and nitrogen mustard. *Oncogene* 1997; 14:2127–2136.
31. MacCallum DE, Hupp TR, Midgley CA, Stuart D, Campbell SJ, Harper A, Walsh FS, Wright EG, Balmain A, Lane DP, Hall PA. The p53 response to ionising radiation in adult and developing murine tissues. *Oncogene* 1996; 13:2575–2587.
32. Merritt AJ, Allen T, Potten CS, Hickman JA. Apoptosis in small intestinal epithelia from p53-null mice: evidence for a delayed, p53-independent G2/M-associated cell death after γ-irradiation. *Oncogene* 1997; 14:2759–2766.
33. Hamada M, Fujiwara T, Hizuta A, Gochi A, Naomoto Y, Takakura N, Takahashi K, Roth JA, Tanaka N, Orita K. The p53 gene is a potent determinant of chemosensitivity and radiosensitivity in gastric and colorectal cancers. *J Cancer Res Clin Oncol* 1996; 122:360–365.
34. Brett MC, Pickard M, Green B, Howel-Evans A, Smith D, Kinsella A, Poston G. p53 protein overexpression and response to biomodulated 5-fluorouracil chemotherapy in patients with advanced colorectal cancer. *Eur J Surg Oncol* 1996; 22:182–185.
35. Fisher TC, Milner AE, Gregory CD, Jackman AL, Aherne GW, Hartley JA, Dive C, Hickman JA. bcl-2 modulation of apoptosis induced by anticancer drugs: resistance to thymidylate stress is independent of classical resistance pathways. *Cancer Res* 1993; 53:3321–3326.
36. Yin DX, Schimke RT. Bcl-2 expression delays drug-induced apoptosis but does not increase clonogenic survival after drug treatment in HeLa cells. *Cancer Res* 1995; 55:4922–4928.
37. Walker A, Taylor ST, Hickman JA, Dive C. Germinal center-derived signals act with bcl-2 to decrease apoptosis and increase clonogenicity of drug-treated human B lymphoma cells. *Cancer Res* 1997; 57:1939–1945.
38. Ofner D, Riehemann K, Maier H, Riedmann B, Nehoda H, Totsch M, Bocker W, Jasani B, Schmid KW. Immunohistochemically detectable bcl-2 expression in colorectal carcinoma: correlation with tumour stage and patient survival. *Br J Cancer* 1995; 72:981–985.
39. Sinicrope FA, Hart J, Michelassi F, Lee JJ. Prognostic value of bcl-2 oncoprotein expression in stage II colon carcinoma. *Clin Cancer Res* 1995; 1:1103–1110.
40. Reed JC. Bcl-2: prevention of apoptosis as a mechanism of drug resistance. *Haematol Oncol Clin N America* 1995; 9(2):451–473.
41. Merritt AJ, Jones LS, Potten CS. Apoptosis in murine intestinal crypts. In: (Cotter, T.G., Martin, S.J., eds.) Techniques in Apoptosis. Portland Press, London, 1996, pp. 269–300.
42. Gavrieli Y, Sherman Y, Ben-Sasson SA. Identification of programmed cell death in situ via specific labeling of nuclear DNA fragmentation. *J Cell Biol* 1992; 119(3):493–501.
43. Hall PA, Coates PJ, Ansari B, Hopwood D. Regulation of cell number in the mammalian gastrointestinal tract: the importance of apoptosis. *J Cell Science* 1994; 107:3569–3577.
44. Potten CS, Allen TD. Ultrastructure of cell loss in intestinal mucosa. *J Ultrastruct Res* 1977; 60:272–277.
45. Han H, Iwanaga T, Uchiyama Y, Fujita T. An aggregation of macrophages in the tips of intestinal villi in guinea pigs: their possible role in the phagocytosis of effete epithelial cells. *Cell Tissue Res* 1993; 271:407–416.
46. Iwanaga T, Han H, Adachi K, Fujita T. A novel mechanism for disposing of effete epithelial cells in the small intestine of guinea pigs. *Gastroenterology* 1993; 105:1089–1097.
47. Shibahara T, Sato N, Waguri S, Iwanaga T, Nakahara A, Fukutomi H, Uchiyama Y. The fate of effete epithelial cells at the villus tips of the human small intestine. *Arch Histol Cytol* 1995; 58:205–219.
48. Potten CS. The significance of spontaneous and induced apoptosis in the gastrointestinal tract of mice. *Cancer Metastasis Rev* 1992; 11:179–195.
49. Potten CS. Effects of radiation on murine gastrointestinal cell proliferation. In: (Potten, C.S, Hendry, J.H., ed.) Radiation and Gut. Elsevier Science, Amsterdam. 1995, pp. 61–84.
50. Clarke AR, Howard LA, Harrison DJ, Winton DJ. p53, mutation frequency and apoptosis in the murine small intestine. *Oncogene* 1997; 14:2015–2018.

51. Ijiri K, Potten CS. Response of intestinal cells of differing topographical and hierarchical status to ten cytotoxic drugs and five sources of radiation. *Br J Cancer* 1983; 47:175–185.
52. Ijiri K, Potten CS. Further studies on the response of intestinal crypt cells of different hierarchical status to eighteen different cytotoxic agents. *Br J Cancer* 1987; 55:113–123.
53. Lee FD. Importance of apoptosis in the histopathology of drug related lesions in the large intestine. *J Clin Pathol* 1993; 46:118–122.
54. Lee FD. Drug-related pathological lesions of the intestinal tract. *Histopathology* 1994; 25:303–308.
55. Pritchard DM, Watson AJM, Potten CS, Jackman AL, Hickman JA. Inhibition by uridine but not thymidine of p53-dependent intestinal apoptosis initiated by 5-fluorouracil: evidence for the involvement of RNA perturbation. *Proc Natl Acad Sci USA* 1997; 94:1795–1799.
56. Bagrij T, Kralovansky J, Gyergyay F, Kiss E, Peters GJ. Influence of uridine treatment in mice on the protection of gastrointestinal toxicity caused by 5-fluorouracil. *Anticancer Res* 1993; 13:789–794.
57. Martin DS, Stoffi RL, Sawyer RC, Spiegelman S, Young CW. High dose 5-fluorouracil with delayed uridine 'rescue' in mice. *Cancer Res* 1982; 42:3964–3970.
58. Kralovansky J, Prajda N, Kerpel-Fronius S, Bagrij T, Kiss E, Peters GJ. Biochemical consequences of 5-fluorouracil gastrointestinal toxicity in rats: effects of high-dose uridine. *Cancer Chemother Pharmacol* 1993; 32:243–248.
59. Houghton JA, Houghton PJ, Wooten RS. Mechanism of induction of gastrointestinal toxicity in the mouse by 5-fluorouracil, 5-fluorouridine and 5-fluoro-2'-deoxyuridine. *Cancer Res* 1979; 39:206–2413.
60. Linke SP, Clarkin KC, Wahl GM. p53 mediates arrest over multiple cell cycles in response to gamma-irradiation. *Cancer Res* 1997; 57:1171–1179.
61. Jackman AL, Farrugia DC, Gibson W, Kimbell R, Harrap KR, Stephens TC, Azab M, Boyle FT. ZD1694 (Tomudex): a new thymidylate synthase inhibitor with activity in colorectal cancer. *Eur J Cancer* 1995; 31A:1277–1272.
62. Cunningham D, Zalcberg JR, Rath U, Olver I, Van Cutsem E, Svensson C, Seitz JF, Harper P, Kerr D, Perez-Manga G, Azab M, Seymour L, Lowery K. 'Tomudex' (ZD1694): results of a randomised trial in advanced colorectal cancer demonstrate efficacy and reduced mucositis and leucopenia. *Eur J Cancer* 1995; 31A:1945–1954.
63. Yin M, Voigt W, Panadero A, Vanhoefer U, Frank C, Pajovic S, Azizkhan J, Rutsum YM. p53 and WAF1 are induced and Rb protein is hypophosphorylated during cell growth inhibition by the thymidylate synthase inhibitor ZD1694 (Tomudex). *Mol Pharmacol* 1997; 51:630–636.
64. Matsui S, Arredondo MA, Wrzosek C, Rutsum YM. DNA damage and p53 induction do not cause ZD1694-induced cell cycle arrest in human colon carcinoma cells. *Cancer Res* 1996; 56:4715–4723.

Index

A

acquired immunodeficiency syndrome, 51
acute lymphoblastic leukemia, 37, 38, 43–48, 352–355
acute myeloid leukemia, 38, 44–48, 352–355
adenosyl-methionine decarboxylase, 20
AG2032, 288, 289
AG2034, 8–11, 281–291, 296, 305–308, 368, 376
AG2084
    cell cycle effects, 286, 287
    preclinical antitumor activity and toxicity, 285-288, 290
AG331, 377, 384
AG337, see Thymitaq
5-aminoimidazole-4-carboxamide ribonucleotide, 6, 9, 21, 27, 39, 184–186, 212, 341, 368
4-amino-4-deoxy-N10-methyl pteroic acid, 41
aminopterin, 2, 3, 14, 50, 59–61, 270, 294, 341, 349
aminopterin analogs, nonpolyglutamatable, 63–93
antifolate transport, 4, 7, 38–40, 62, 156, 157, 187, 188, 203, 206, 208, 214–216, 243, 248, 253–255, 265, 282, 284, 289, 290, 293–311, 340, 343
apoptosis, 8, 10, 11, 20, 114, 190, 289, 437–448
AZT (azidothymidine), in combination with antifolates, 373, 374, 377

B

bcl-2, 11, 426, 440–448
benzoquinazolines, 204–211
benzylacyclouridine, 103, 104
betaine-homocysteine methyltransferase, 16, 17
bifunctional C1-tetrahydrofolatesynthase, 23
bi-functional DHFR-TS, 22
BW1843U89, see GW1843

C

C1-tetrahydrofolate synthase, 23, 24
capecitabine, 106, 271
carboxypeptidase G1, 41
caspases, 430, 438, 439
caveolin, 301, 302
CB3717, 113, 114, 148–153, 168, 206–209, 229, 230, 244, 245, 247, 271, 287, 296, 304–309, 341, 384, 385, 391, 410, 413, 414
    analogs, 149–152
cell cycle
    arrest, 10, 20, 114, 189, 190, 282, 284, 288–291, 399, 416, 417, 423–428, 431, 443
    checkpoints, 9–11, 48, 49, 114, 189, 190, 288–291, 399, 416, 425, 426
cisplatin and antifolates, 370–372, 374–377
cobalamin, 18
combination chemotherapy, 9, 10, 43, 51, 119–129, 178, 179, 365–378
conjugases, see folylpolyglutamate hydrolases
coronary disease—homocysteine, 16
CPT-11 in combination with antifolates, 114, 119, 120, 127–129, 132, 374, 376, 378
cyclophosphamide, 370, 371
cystathionine-β-synthase, 19

D

DDATHF, see Lometrexol
DDMP, see Metoprine
deoxyuridine, plasma surrogate marker of thymidine, 159, 160, 390, 391
desamino-CB3717, 150–152
2-desamino-2-methylaminopterin, 22
2-desamino-2-methyl-N10-propargyl-5,8-dideazafolic acid, see ICI 198583
6-diazo-5-oxo-L-norleucine (DON), 39
5,10-dideazatetrahydrifilate, see lometrexol
dihydrofolate reductase, 1–8, 13–15, 20–23, 37–40, 43–51, 147–149, 324, 325, 343, 346, 374, 399, 400
dihydrofolate reductase inhibitors, 37–52, 59–95, 120, 122, 185, 186, 287, 294, 298, 304–309, 324, 325, 341, 368–371, 399
dihydrofolate synthetase, 3
dihydropyrimidine dehydrogenase and its inhibitors, 105, 106, 131, 372, 389, 390, 432

dimethylglycine dehydrogenase, 29
dipyridamole, 413
DNA methylation, 19
dUTP, 10, 22, 113, 114, 157, 410–417, 425
dUTPase, 113, 411–417

E

E2F, 23, 48, 49, 399, 400
edatrexate, 4, 50, 51, 183, 296, 305–309, 325, 341, 349, 350, 368, 371
endocytosis, 301, 309
10-ethyl-10-deazaaminopterin, see edatrexate
etoposide and antifolates, 370

F

fas/fas ligand, 20, 429–432, 438, 439
5-fluorodeoxyuridine, 110, 111, 115, 116, 371, 373, 399, 410, 412, 414, 427
5-fluorouracil, 5, 9, 101–132, 270, 323, 324, 326, 327, 332, 369–373, 376, 398–400, 410, 412, 423, 432, 438, 443–448
    anabolism/catabolism, 102–106
    apoptosis, 114, 115, 426, 438–448
    chronomodulation, 390
    clinical pharmacology, 116–119
    in combination, 9, 119–129, 369, 372–374, 376, 378
    predictors of response, 383–392
    prodrugs, 102–106
folate receptor vehicle and macromolecular transport, 301, 302
folate receptors, 4, 38, 39, 264, 265, 282, 284, 286, 289, 290, 294–297, 300–303, 340, 343
folate status, humans, 270
folate transport, 293–311
folic acid
    modulation of, 190, 191, 216, 219, 220, 221, 269–278, 282, 288, 289, 324, 325, 332–334
    pharmacokinetics and metabolism, 332–334
folylpolyglutamate hydrolase, 6, 30, 39, 46, 244, 342, 344, 345, 350–353
    inhibitors, 357
folylpolyglutamate synthetase, 6, 7, 10, 18, 29, 30, 39, 46, 108, 153, 184, 187, 188, 203, 210, 211, 213, 243, 248, 262–264, 282, 303, 324, 342–357, 374, 386, 388
    inhibitors, 294, 304, 356, 357
formiminotransferase–cycloideamnase, 28
10-formyl-5,8,10-triazapteroic acid, 27
5-formyl-tetrahydrofolate, see leucovorin
10-formyltetrahydrofolate dehydrogenase, 24, 25
Ftorafur, 106

G

GARFT, X-ray crystal structure, 282
gemcitabine, combination with antifolates, 377
gene amplification, 5, 45, 47–48, 110, 343, 399
γ-glutamyl hydrolase, see folylpolyglutamate hydrolase
glycinamide ribonucleotide formyltransferase (GARFT), 25–27, 39, 262, 263, 281
    inhibitors, 3, 8, 9, 11, 184–186, 189, 212, 216, 261–278, 281–291, 368
glycine cleavage system, 28
glycine N-methyltransferase, 19
GW1843, 11, 114, 122, 124, 183, 203–225, 296, 305–309, 325–342, 356, 414
    cellular uptake and efflux, 214, 215, 296, 305–309
    clinical activity, 221–224
    clinical pharmacokinetics, 222–224
    in vivo antitumor activity and toxicity, 216–221
    polyglutamation, 213, 214, 356
    TS inhibition, 212, 213

H

high capacity/low affinity, 300
homocysteine, 16–19, 270
7-hydroxy methotrexate, 41
hypoxanthine rescue, 265, 282, 284

I

ICI 198583, 150, 247, 248, 296, 305, 356
    analogs, 150–153, 247, 248, 305–309
immunotherapy, 309, 310
interferon-α and -γ, 114, 372, 402
ironotecan, see CPT11

K

Kisliuk effect, 9, 10, 287, 288

L

leucovorin, 4, 40–43, 50–52, 101, 106–111, 114–132, 160, 161, 214, 216, 250, 275, 297, 307–309, 323–334, 369, 372, 398, 399
    pharmacokinetics and metabolism, 326–329
    rescue, 40–43, 50–52, 63, 67, 158, 160, 161, 186, 187, 216, 325, 326, 369

lometrexol, 4, 7, 8, 9, 25, 30, 184, 188, 262–278, 281–284, 286, 287, 289, 290, 296, 305–308, 325, 347, 348, 356
   clinical evaluation, 272–275
   pharmacokinetics, 276
low-folate diet, 190, 191, 268, 270, 330
low pH transport route, 303, 304
LY231514, 114, 122, 124, 183–199, 263, 264, 296, 305–309, 325, 377
   clinical pharmacokinetics, 195
   clinical studies, 194–197
   in vivo antitumor activity and toxicity, 190–194
   metabolism and pharmacokinetics, 191–193
   toxicity, 190–194
LY309887, 183, 188, 189, 261–278
   clinical evaluation, 276, 277
   disposition in liver, 268, 269
   in vivo antitumor activity and toxicity, 265–268

M

MDM2, 428, 429
membrane folate-binding proteins, *see* folate receptors
methionine, 16–19
methionine adenosyl transferase, 19
methionine synthase, 16–18, 20
methionyl tRNAfmet formyltransferase, 28
methotrexate, 4–14, 18, 30, 37–52, 59–61, 147–149, 186, 187, 189, 191, 214, 216, 270, 290, 294, 296, 298, 300, 304–309, 325, 341–357, 368–374, 399, 401, 410–412, 414, 427
   analogs, non-polyglutamatable, 59–93
   and cisplatin, 370
   entereohepatic circulation, 41
   and 5-fluorouracil, 120–122, 369, 370
   high dose, 41–43, 323–325
   polyglutamation, 38, 39, 43–46, 325, 341–357
   resistance, 43–52, 345–357
   toxicity, 41–43
   transport, 38–40, 46, 47, 293–309
methylenetetrahydrofolate, 16, 17
5,10-methylenetetrahydrofolate synthetase, 25, 26
methyltetrahydrofolate, 16–18
metoprine, 60, 63
modulation of antifolate toxicity, 325, 326, 447
MOv18-guided immunotherapy 309
multitargeted antifolate (MTA), *see* LY231514

N

neural tube defects, 16
Neutrexin, *see* trimetrexate
nitrous oxide, 18
Nolatrexed dihydrochloride, *see* Thymitaq
non-polyglutamatable dihydrofolate reductase inhibitors, 59–93, 377
non-polyglutamatable thymidylate synthase inhibitors, 229–239, 243–257

O

ornithine decarboxylase, 20
oxonic acid, 106

P

p21, 425, 426 440, 446
p53, 9–11, 19, 49, 111, 126, 288, 289, 291, 404, 423–432, 439–448
PALA, 125, 372, 373, 404, 412, 423, 427
passive diffusion of folates/antifolates, 304
p-glycoprotein, 8, 47
pharmacodynamics, 383–392
piritrexim, 60, 412
platinum and antifolates, 126, 127, 131, 132, 374–376
Pneumocystis carnii pneumonia, 1, 8, 51
polyamines, 18–20
polyglutamates/polyglutamation, 3, 6, 9, 14, 16–22, 38, 39, 43–46, 123, 150, 152, 156, 158, 159, 187, 188, 208, 213, 262, 263, 290, 294, 302, 304, 325, 339–357, 368, 371
pRB, 48, 49
predictors of response to antifolates, 383–392
prostate-specific membrane antigen, 30
PT-430, 46, 47
PT523, 84–91, 183, 296, 304–309
pyrimethamine, 2, 4, 7, 48, 60

Q

quinazolines, 65–67, 148–154, 207–210, 245–248

R

raltitrexed, 1, 7, 11, 111, 114, 122, 124, 126, 154–161, 176–178, 183, 186, 187, 214, 216, 230, 243–248, 250, 251, 253–255, 271, 325, 346, 347, 356, 374–376, 384, 388, 391, 398, 401, 412, 438
   apoptosis, 438, 447, 448
   clinical activity, 167–179

clinical pharmacology, 167–179
preclinical pharmacology, 158–161
predictors of response, 388, 389
reduced-folate carrier, 4, 7, 62, 156, 157, 188, 203, 214, 243, 248, 253–255, 265, 284, 294–310, 340, 343
biodistribution, 299, 300
resistance to antifolates, 5, 43–52, 106–112, 187, 188, 299, 300, 325, 339–357, 384–386

S

S-1, 106
sarcosine dehydrogenase, 29
serine hydroxymethyltransferase, 3, 20, 21

T

taxanes and antifolates, combinations, 371, 373
thymidine kinase deficient tumors, 150–153, 158, 159, 218, 219, 233, 251, 252
thymidine phosporylase, 106, 217
thymidine rescue, 41, 126, 160, 161, 186, 187, 250, 265, 447
thymidylate synthase, 1–9, 20–22, 40, 104, 108–115, 343, 371, 383–392, 397–405, 409–417, 424
  gene expression, predictors of response, 386–392
  inhibitors, 147–161, 183–190, 203–218, 229–231, 243–257, 294, 304–309, 341, 345, 368, 371–377, 383–392, 427, 428
  regulation of expression, 397–405
  ternary complex crystal structure, 211, 212, 230, 231, 224–250, 384
thymineless death, 2, 409–417, 423–432

Thymitaq, 4, 7, 10, 114, 122, 160, 183, 229–239, 248, 250, 288, 325, 377, 384, 391
TMQ, see trimetrexate
Tomudex, see raltitrexed
topoisomerase inhibitors and antifolates, 127–129, 376, 377
topotecan, 374
translational autoregulation, 40, 111, 127–129, 401, 402
triazinate, 60
trifunctional C1-tetrahydrofolate synthase, 23
trimethoprim, 2, 4, 7, 41, 60, 287
trimetrexate, 1, 4, 7, 10, 47, 50–52, 60, 122, 183, 287, 288, 290, 368, 370, 371, 376, 378

U

UFT, 27, 106
uracil-DNA glycosylase, 113, 114, 410, 416, 417
uracil misincorporation into DNA, 10, 113–115, 409–417
uridine and 5-fluorouracil, 124, 125, 444

Z

ZD1694, see raltitrexed
ZD9331, 183, 243–257, 296, 305–309, 325, 391, 356, 414–416
ZD9331
  antitumor activity, 251–253
  clinical studies, 256, 257
  preclinical pharmacokinetics and metabolism, 255, 256
  toxicity, 255